Mammalian Heme Peroxidases

T0136399

Oxidative Stress and Disease

Series Editors:
Lester Packer, PhD
Enrique Cadenas, MD, PhD
University of Southern California School of Pharmacy
Los Angeles, California

For more information about this series, please visit: https://www.crcpress.com/Oxidative-Stress-and-Disease/book-series/CRCOXISTRDIS

Mammalian Heme Peroxidases
Diverse Roles in Health and Disease

Edited by
Clare L. Hawkins
William M. Nauseef

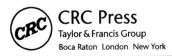

CRC Press
Taylor & Francis Group
Boca Raton London New York

CRC Press is an imprint of the
Taylor & Francis Group, an **informa** business

First edition published 2022
by CRC Press
6000 Broken Sound Parkway NW, Suite 300, Boca Raton, FL 33487-2742

and by CRC Press
2 Park Square, Milton Park, Abingdon, Oxon, OX14 4RN

Library of Congress Cataloging-in-Publication Data
Names: Hawkins, Clare, editor. | Nauseef, William M., 1950- editor.
Title: Mammalian heme peroxidases: diverse roles in health and disease / edited by Clare Hawkins, William M. Nauseef.
Description: Boca Raton: CRC Press, Taylor & Francis Group, [2021] |
Series: Oxidative stress and disease |
Includes bibliographical references and index. |
Summary: "Peroxidasins are a family of heme peroxidases that play a novel role in tissue biogenesis and matrix assembly. Mammalian heme peroxidase enzymes are critical for immune responses and disease prevention. Although highly beneficial, overproduction drives the development of pathologies, including cardiovascular, neurodegenerative, respiratory, kidney and inflammatory bowel diseases by triggering the initiation of stress-related pathways leading to cell damage and dysfunction. This book highlights the roles of mammalian heme peroxidases, as well as their involvement in immunity and disease, and potential therapeutic approaches to modulate and prevent damaging reactions"— Provided by publisher.
Identifiers: LCCN 2021014716 (print) | LCCN 2021014717 (ebook) |
ISBN 9780367820367 (hardback) | ISBN 9781032079646 (paperback) |
ISBN 9781003212287 (ebook)
Subjects: LCSH: Peroxidase.
Classification: LCC QP603.P4 M35 2021 (print) |
LCC QP603.P4 (ebook) | DDC 572/.791—dc23
LC record available at https://lccn.loc.gov/2021014716
LC ebook record available at https://lccn.loc.gov/2021014717

ISBN: 9780367820367 (hbk)
ISBN: 9781032079646 (pbk)
ISBN: 9781003212287 (ebk)

DOI: 10.1201/9781003212287

Typeset in Joanna
by codeMantra

CONTENTS

EDITORS

Clare L. Hawkins is a Professor in the Department of Biomedical Sciences, University of Copenhagen. Clare moved to Denmark in 2017, previously holding the position of Scientific Director and the Inflammation Group Leader at the Heart Research Institute, Sydney. Clare is a former Australian Research Council Future Fellow and Principal Research Fellow in Sydney Medical School, University of Sydney. She completed her PhD in Chemistry at the University of York (UK) before moving to the Heart Research Institute in Sydney, where she worked for nearly 20 years. She has authored several book chapters and more than 100 peer-reviewed journal articles in high-quality journals. Her research is focused on understanding how chemical oxidants modulate cellular function under inflammatory conditions and the role of these reactions in the pathogenesis of inflammatory diseases, including atherosclerosis.

William M. Nauseef is a Professor in the Department of Internal Medicine and the Department of Immunology and Microbiology at the University of Iowa. He also serves as the Director of the Inflammation Program at the University of Iowa. He received his MD from the SUNY Upstate Medical Center, Syracuse, New York. He is Board Certified by the American Board of Internal Medicine in Infectious Diseases. He is the author or coauthor of over 180 peer-reviewed papers, and coauthor of two books and dozens of book chapters. His research program over the past four decades has focused on elucidating the cell and molecular biology of human neutrophils within the context of innate host defense against infection.

CONTRIBUTORS

MOLLY ALLISON
College of Veterinary Medicine
Kansas State University
Manhattan, Kansas

STEPHAN BALDUS
Department for Internal Medicine III
Heart Centre Cologne
University Hospital Cologne
Cologne, Germany
and
Center for Molecular Medicine Cologne
CMMC, University of Cologne
Cologne, Germany

GAUTAM BHAVE
Division of Nephrology
Department of Medicine
Vanderbilt University Medical Center
Nashville, Tennessee
and
Department of Cell and Developmental Biology
Vanderbilt University
Nashville, Tennessee

JOSHUA D. CHANDLER
Center for CF and Airways Disease Research
Children's Healthcare of Atlanta
Atlanta, Georgia
and
Department of Pediatrics
Division of Pulmonology,
 Allergy & Immunology
Cystic Fibrosis and Sleep Medicine
Emory University
Atlanta, Georgia

JOHN W. CHEN
Department of Radiology
Institute for Innovation in Imaging
Massachusetts General Hospital
Boston, Massachusetts
and
Center for Systems Biology
Massachusetts General Hospital and Harvard
 Medical School
Boston, Massachusetts

DOMINIC J. CIAVATTA
UNC Kidney Center
UNC Chapel Hill, North Carolina
and
Department of Genetics
UNC Chapel Hill, North Carolina

CATHERINE COREMANS
Faculty of Pharmacy
Université Libre de Bruxelles
Brussels, Belgium

MICHAEL J. DAVIES
Department of Biomedical Sciences
University of Copenhagen
Copenhagen, Denmark

BRIAN J. DAY
Department of Medicine
National Jewish Health, Denver, Colorado

CÉDRIC DELPORTE
Faculty of Pharmacy
Université Libre de Bruxelles
Brussels, Belgium

NINA DICKERHOF
Department of Pathology & Biomedical
    Science
Centre for Free Radical Research
University of Otago
Christchurch, New Zealand

RONALD J. FALK
Department of Medicine
Division of Nephrology and Hypertension
UNC Chapel Hill, North Carolina
and
UNC Kidney Center
UNC Chapel Hill, North Carolina

DAVID A. FORD
Edward A. Doisy Department of Biochemistry
    and Molecular Biology
Saint Louis University School of Medicine
St. Louis, Missouri
and
Center for Cardiovascular Research
Saint Louis University School of Medicine
St. Louis, Missouri

MEGHAN E. FREE
Department of Medicine
Division of Nephrology and Hypertension
UNC Chapel Hill, North Carolina
and
UNC Kidney Center
UNC Chapel Hill, North Carolina
and
Department of Pathology and Laboratory
    Medicine
UNC Chapel Hill, North Carolina

PAUL G. FURTMÜLLER
Department of Chemistry
Institute of Biochemistry
University of Natural Resources
    and Life Sciences
Vienna, Austria

SIMON GEIßEN
Department for Internal Medicine III
Heart Centre Cologne
University Hospital Cologne
Cologne, Germany
and
Center for Molecular Medicine
    Cologne
CMMC, University of Cologne
Cologne, Germany

BRIAN V. GEISBRECHT
Department of Biochemistry & Molecular
    Biophysics
Kansas State University
Manhattan, Kansas

MIKLÓS GEISZT
Department of Physiology
Faculty of Medicine
Semmelweis University
Budapest, Hungary

MARK B. HAMPTON
Department of Pathology & Biomedical Science
Centre for Free Radical Research
University of Otago
Christchurch, New Zealand

CLARE L. HAWKINS
Department of Biomedical Sciences
University of Copenhagen
Copenhagen, Denmark

STEFAN HOFBAUER
Department of Chemistry
Institute of Biochemistry
University of Natural Resources
    and Life Sciences
Vienna, Austria

J. CHARLES JENNETTE
UNC Kidney Center
UNC Chapel Hill, North Carolina
and
Department of Pathology and Laboratory
    Medicine
UNC Chapel Hill, North Carolina

ANNA KLINKE
Agnes Wittenborg Institute for Translational
    Cardiovascular Research
Clinic for General and Interventional Cardiology/
    Angiology
Heart and Diabetes Center NRW
University Hospital of Ruhr-University
    Bochum
Bad Oeynhausen, Germany

HAJNAL A. KOVÁCS
Department of Physiology
Faculty of Medicine
Semmelweis University
Budapest, Hungary

ENRICO G. KUELLENBERG
Department of Radiology
Institute for Innovation in Imaging
Massachusetts General Hospital
Boston, Massachusetts
and
Center for Systems Biology
Massachusetts General Hospital and Harvard
    Medical School
Boston, Massachusetts

RICHARD A. MAKI
Sanford Burnham Prebys Medical Discovery
    Institute
La Jolla, California

DENNIS MEHRKENS
Department for Internal Medicine III
Heart Centre Cologne
University Hospital Cologne
Cologne, Germany
and
Center for Molecular Medicine
    Cologne
CMMC, University of Cologne
Cologne, Germany

NITIN MISHRA
Department of Biochemistry & Molecular
    Biophysics
Kansas State University
Manhattan, Kansas

MARTIN MOLLENHAUER
Department for Internal Medicine III
Cluster for Inflammation and Redox-Signaling
Heart Centre Cologne
University Hospital Cologne
Cologne, Germany

NEGIN JALALI MOTLAGH
Department of Radiology
Institute for Innovation in Imaging
Massachusetts General Hospital
Boston, Massachusetts
and
Center for Systems Biology
Massachusetts General Hospital and Harvard
    Medical School
Boston, Massachusetts

WILLIAM M. NAUSEEF
Department of Medicine
Iowa Inflammation Program
Roy J. and Lucille A. Carver College of Medicine
University of Iowa
Iowa City, Iowa

CHRISTIAN OBINGER
Department of Chemistry
Institute of Biochemistry
University of Natural Resources and Life Sciences
Vienna, Austria

DANIEL P. PIKE
Edward A. Doisy Department of Biochemistry
    and Molecular Biology
Saint Louis University School of Medicine
St. Louis, Missouri
and
Center for Cardiovascular Research
Saint Louis University School of Medicine
St. Louis, Missouri

BENJAMIN S. RAYNER
Heart Research Institute
Newtown, Australia
and
Sydney Medical School
University of Sydney
Sydney, Australia

WANDA F. REYNOLDS
Sanford Burnham Prebys Medical Discovery
    Institute
La Jolla, California

VOLKER RUDOLPH
Heart & Diabetes Center Nordrhein-Westfalen
University Hospital of Ruhr-University Bochum
Bad Oeynhausen, Germany

HEATHER L. SHEARER
Department of Pathology & Biomedical Science
Centre for Free Radical Research
University of Otago
Christchurch, New Zealand

GÁBOR SIROKMÁNY
Department of Physiology
Faculty of Medicine
Semmelweis University
Budapest, Hungary

PIERRE VAN ANTWERPEN
Faculty of Pharmacy
Université Libre de Bruxelles
Brussels, Belgium

CUIHUA WANG
Department of Radiology
Institute for Innovation in Imaging
Massachusetts General Hospital
Boston, Massachusetts
and
Center for Systems Biology
Massachusetts General Hospital and Harvard
    Medical School
Boston, Massachusetts

MARCEL ZÁMOCKÝ
Department of Chemistry
Institute of Biochemistry
University of Natural Resources and Life Sciences
Vienna, Austria
and
Institute of Molecular Biology
Slovak Academy of Sciences
Bratislava, Slovakia

KARIM ZOUAOUI BOUDJELTIA
Laboratoire de Médecine Experimentale
    (ULB 222 Unit)
ISPPC CHU de Charleroi
Montigny-Le-Tilleul, Belgium

CONTRIBUTORS

PART ONE

Introduction to Mammalian Heme Peroxidases

CHAPTER ONE

Evolution, Structure and Biochemistry of Human Peroxidases

Paul G. Furtmüller
University of Natural Resources and Life Sciences

Marcel Zámocký
University of Natural Resources and Life Sciences
Slovak Academy of Sciences

Stefan Hofbauer and Christian Obinger
University of Natural Resources and Life Sciences

CONTENTS

ABBREVIATIONS

DdPoxA:	Peroxidase A from *Dictyostelium discoideum*
$E^{\circ\prime}$:	Standard reduction potential
EPO:	Eosinophil peroxidase
HRP:	Horseradish peroxidase
LPO:	Lactoperoxidase
LspPOX:	Peroxidase from the cyanobacterium *Lyngbya* sp. PCC 8105
MPO:	Myeloperoxidase
proMPO:	Promyeloperoxidase
PXDN:	Human peroxidasin 1
RR:	Resonance Raman
TPO:	Thyroid peroxidase

HEME PEROXIDASES

Heme peroxidases use heme *b* or post-translationally modified heme as a redox cofactor to catalyse the hydrogen peroxide–mediated one- and two-electron oxidation of a myriad of molecules, including aromatic molecules (e.g. coniferyl alcohol or tyrosine), cations (e.g. Mn^{2+}), anions (e.g. ascorbate or halides) or even proteins (e.g. cytochrome *c*). During turnover, H_2O_2 is reduced to water and one-electron donors (AH_2) are oxidized to the respective radicals (·AH) (Reaction 1), whereas two-electron donors such as halides (X^-) are oxidized to the corresponding hypohalous acids (HOX) (Reaction 2). Besides

DOI: 10.1201/9781003212287-2

these *peroxidatic* reactivities, very few heme peroxidases also show a reasonable *catalatic* reactivity (Reaction 3) and use a second hydrogen peroxide molecule as two-electron donor, thereby releasing dioxygen. One additional activity catalysed by a special group of heme peroxidases is the peroxygenation reaction, i.e. the selective introduction of peroxide-derived oxygen functionalities into organic molecules (Reaction 4).

$$H_2O_2 + 2AH_2 \rightarrow H_2O + 2\ ^{\bullet}AH \qquad \text{Reaction 1}$$

$$H_2O_2 + X^- + H^+ \rightarrow H_2O + HOX \qquad \text{Reaction 2}$$

$$H_2O_2 + H_2O_2 \rightarrow 2H_2O + O_2 \qquad \text{Reaction 3}$$

$$H_2O_2 + RH \rightarrow H_2O + ROH \qquad \text{Reaction 4}$$

In the last decade, an ever-increasing number of heme peroxidase sequences were automatically assigned to related families based on typical conserved motifs. It has been demonstrated that at least four heme peroxidase superfamilies arose independently during the evolution, which each differ in overall fold, active site architecture and enzymatic activities [1]: (i) the peroxidase-catalase superfamily [2,3], (ii) the peroxidase-cyclooxygenase superfamily [4], (iii) the peroxidase-peroxygenase superfamily [5,6] and (iv) the recently described dye-decolourizing peroxidases [7]. This review focuses on Families 1 and 2 of the peroxidase-cyclooxygenase superfamily [1,4,8].

EVOLUTION AND FUNCTIONS OF PEROXIDASES FROM THE PEROXIDASE-CYCLOOXYGENASE SUPERFAMILY

The peroxidase-cyclooxygenase superfamily has Pfam accession PF03098 (IPR019791), and its members are widely distributed among all domains of life [1,4]. It counts over 22,000 representatives in various sequence databases (June 2021) and shows the highest diversity regarding domain architectures and composition. The former denomination of these proteins as the "animal heme-dependent peroxidase family" is misleading but still present in some public databases. The superfamily comprises seven families, which – in contrast to the other heme peroxidase (super)families – are mostly multidomain proteins with one heme peroxidase domain of predominantly α-helical fold with a central heme-containing core of five α-helices. Moreover, this superfamily is unique in having the prosthetic heme group posttranslationally modified [9–13]. The heme is covalently bound to the protein via one or two ester linkages formed by conserved Asp and Glu residues. In one representative (i.e. myeloperoxidase), a third heme to protein linkage is formed [14,15]. As a consequence of these modifications, the heme is electronically and structurally modified, and these peroxidases exhibit unique spectral, redox and catalytic properties [16–18]. All representatives catalyse Reactions 1 and 2, but halide oxidation seems to be the dominating physiological enzymatic activity for most studied members.

The evolution of the peroxidase-cyclooxygenase superfamily starts with bacterial peroxicins (assigned previously as Family 5) [1]. From Family 5 via Family 6 (i.e. bacterial peroxidockerins), next evolutionary steps involved the formation of solely eukaryotic Family 3 (peroxinectins), Family 2 (peroxidasins) and, finally, Family 1 (chordata peroxidases), which includes thyroid peroxidase (TPO), lactoperoxidase (LPO), eosinophil peroxidase (EPO) and myeloperoxidase (MPO). The physiological roles of Families 5 and 6 peroxidases remain unknown. Peroxinectins (Family 3) were shown to exhibit cell adhesion functions and to be involved in invertebrate immune response by production of hypohalous acids according to Reaction 2 [19]. Peroxinectins are fusion proteins of a heme peroxidase domain with an integrin-binding motif that probably co-evolved from the ancestral dockerin part of peroxidockerins (Family 6) together with the peroxidase domain. Peroxinectins are widely distributed mainly among arthropods and nematodes where they are synthesized and stored in secretory granules in an inactive form, released in response to stimuli and activated outside the cells to mediate haemocyte attachment and spreading.

It has to be mentioned that an alternative evolutionary path led from Family 5 towards Family 4, which contains bacterial and animal cyclooxygenases as well as plant alpha dioxygenases, whereas animal dual oxidases (Family 7) already segregated from peroxidockerins at the level of basal eukaryotes that are still extant [1].

Family 2 (peroxidasins) and Family 1 (chordata peroxidases) represent the youngest addition in evolution of this superfamily. For this review, we performed a phylogenetic reconstruction of

100 selected sequences from the peroxidase-cyclooxygenase superfamily with MEGA X suite [20] by using the maximum likelihood method (Figure 1.1). From this tree, it is obvious that peroxidasins diverged quite early from the common ancestor of Family 1. Whereas genes for Family 1 peroxidases were detected only among mammalian genomes, Family 2 has deep phylogenetic origins that can be followed beyond mammals back within lower vertebrates.

Peroxidasins show a broad and rather abundant distribution in various Eumetazoan phyla [8]. They were segregated in one minor clade of (yet putative) short peroxidasins and up to five distinct clades of long (multi-domain) peroxidasins with four invertebrate clades as well as one vertebrate clade that also includes two different human representatives. The domain assembly in the various invertebrate peroxidasins is variable. In the vertebrate clade, the peroxidase domain is fused N-terminally with domains of leucine-rich repeats (LRR), immunoglobulin (Ig) domains and a C-terminal von Willebrand factor type C (VWC), commonly found in extracellular matrix proteins. The physiological functions attributed to peroxidasins include antimicrobial defense as well as extracellular matrix formation and consolidation at various developmental stages [21–23]. Human peroxidasin 1 (PXDN) uses Reaction 2 to catalyse specifically the essential formation of sulfilimine bonds in collagen IV [22]. Cross-linked collagen IV scaffold is essential for epithelial tissue genesis and stabilization. Systematic analysis showed that both collagen IV cross-link formation

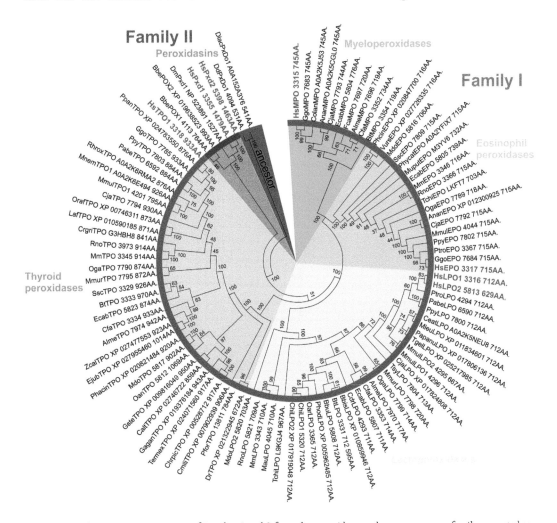

Figure 1.1 Phylogenetic reconstruction of Families 1 and 2 from the peroxidase-cyclooxygenase superfamily presented as a circle tree.

and tissue-specific peroxidasin evolution probably arose at the point of divergence between Metazoan phyla Porifera and Cnidaria. In animal tissues, PXDN is involved in structural stabilization of the extracellular matrix [23].

Family 1 comprises secreted (single domain) chordata peroxidases that have been under investigation for more than 40 years [24–26]. In the course of evolution, TPOs segregated first from the common ancestor of Family 1 (Figure 1.1). Finally, LPOs, EPOs and MPOs formed well-separated evolutionary branches. In Figure 1.1, unique sequences of Cephalochordata peroxidases are also presented that constitute phylogenetic intermediates between Family 1 and Family 2. These animal non-vertebrate peroxidases segregated very early in the evolution of Family 2 ancestors, before differentiation of peroxidasins within vertebrates and before evolution of TPOs from Family 1.

The overall phylogenetic distribution of peroxidase orthologs in the four mammalian monophyletic clades is in accordance with the general evolution and speciation of these organisms with a positive selection detected at specific amino acid sites for slight functional shifts [27]. Dimeric membrane-anchored TPO catalyses iodination of tyrosine residues in thyroglobulin and, finally, the synthesis of the thyroid hormones triiodothyronine and thyroxine [28–30]. In mammals, homodimeric MPO [24] and monomeric LPO [31] and EPO [32] have been shown to be essential parts of host defense in the innate immune system. By releasing highly reactive and oxidizing reaction products such as hypohalous acids (Reaction 2), they comprise the front-line defence against invading pathogens [24,31,32].

STRUCTURE OF THE PEROXIDASE DOMAIN OF HUMAN PEROXIDASES

The most typical sequence of the peroxidase domain that allows the correct assignment to Families 1, 2 and 3 of the peroxidase-cyclooxygenase superfamily is –X-G-**Q**-X-X-**D-H-D**-X- which includes the distal catalytic histidine that is neighboured by two aspartates, the first being involved in ester bond formation with the prosthetic group and the second in Ca^{2+} binding. The highly conserved glutamine seems to be involved in halide binding [14,33] (Figure 1.2).

Additional typical distal residues include the catalytic arginine and a conserved glutamate that is

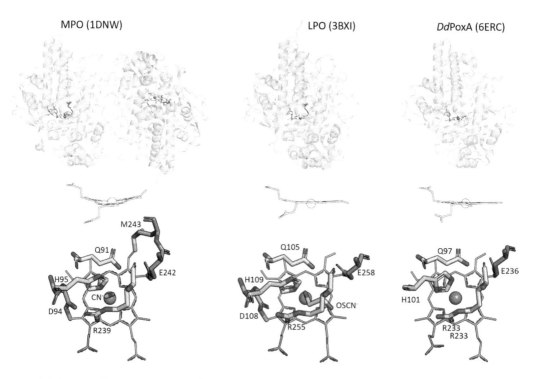

Figure 1.2 Overall and active site structures of dimeric myeloperoxidase (MPO), monomeric lactoperoxidase (LPO) and peroxidase from *Dictyostelium discoideum* (DdPoxA).

MAMMALIAN HEME PEROXIDASES: DIVERSE ROLES IN HEALTH AND DISEASE

involved in formation of the second ester bond with the heme group. The typical sequence is –X-**R**-X-X-**E**-X- [1]. The proximal ligand is a histidine hydrogen bonded to an asparagine. Figure 1.2 compares the crystal structures of human MPO [14], bovine LPO [34] and the peroxidase from *Dictyostelium discoideum* (DdPoxA), which belongs to more distantly related Family 6 [13]. In all three representatives, the fully conserved distal catalytic triad Q91-H95-R239 (MPO numbering) is at almost identical position. The mammalian enzymes MPO and LPO (as well as EPO and TPO) have two heme-to-protein ester bonds between the above-mentioned aspartate (D94) and glutamate (E242) residues and the 5- and 1-methyl groups of the heme. DdPoxA is a rare exception of a heme peroxidase with only one covalent linkage [13]. The clade of myeloperoxidases of Family 1 is unique in having a third covalent bond, i.e. a sulfonium ion linkage – between the sulfur of a methionine (M243) and the β-carbon of the 2-vinyl substituent of the post-translationally modified heme [1,4,14,15,35–37]. The typical sequence motif for the Family 1 clade of myeloperoxidases is –X-R-X-X-E-M-X-.

In addition to the heme to protein linkages, the overall fold of Family 1 and Family 2 peroxidases is stabilized by a calcium-binding site in the distal heme cavity with a typically pentagonal bipyramidal coordination [15,37]. The proximal heme iron ligand (H336) interacts with the amine side chain of a conserved asparagine (N421), whereas the carbonyl group interacts with the guanidinium group of a conserved arginine (R333). Furthermore, this arginine may form a salt bridge between its guanidinium group and the 7-propionic substituent of pyrrole ring D [15,37]. This interaction requires an anionic proximal histidine, which is facilitated by lowering its pK_a by coordination of the ferric heme iron. The pronounced imidazolate character of the proximal histidine might help to bridle the high reactivity of the redox intermediate Compound I (see below).

Note that except for MPO, LPO and DdPoxA, no crystal structures of peroxidases with posttranslationally modified heme are available. Table 1.1 summarizes all crystal structures of mammalian peroxidases so far deposited in the Protein Data Bank (September 2020) (https://www.rcsb.org/).

TABLE 1.1

Available crystal structures and PDB codes of heme peroxidases from family 1 of the peroxidase-cyclooxygenase superfamily with important ligands at the active site

PDB code	Protein	Source	Resolution (Å)	Ligand
1MYP	MPO	*Canis lupus*	3	Ca^{2+}
1MHL	MPO	*Homo sapiens*	2.25	Ca^{2+}
1DNW	MPO	*Homo sapiens*	1.9	Ca^{2+}, CN^-, SCN^-,
3F9P	MPO	*Homo sapiens*	2.9	Ca^{2+}
5MFA	proMPO	*Homo sapiens*	1.2	Ca^{2+}
2R5L	LPO	*Capra hircus*	2.4	Ca^{2+}, I^-
3BXI	LPO	*Bos taurus*	2.3	Ca^{2+}, SCN^-
3FAQ	LPO	*Bubalus bubalis*	2.7	Ca^{2+}, CN^-, I^-, SCN^-
3I6N	LPO	*Bos taurus*	2.7	Ca^{2+}, CN^-, I^-, SCN^-, isoniazid
5B72	LPO	*Bos taurus*	1.98	Ca^{2+}, I^-
5WV3	LPO	*Bos taurus*	2.07	Ca^{2+}, I^-, Br^-
6L9E	LPO	*Bos taurus*	1.7	Ca^{2+}, Zn^{2+}, SCN^-, I^-, H_2O_2
6LF7	LPO	*Capra hircus*	1.79	Ca^{2+}, SCN^-, I^-, HOOH, HOSCN
7BYZ	LPO	*Bos mutus*	1.55	Ca^{2+}, SCN^-, HOOH, HOCl
6ERC	DdPoxA	*Dictyostelium discoideum*	2.5	Ca^{2+}

MPO, myeloperoxidase; proMPO, promyeloperoxidase; LPO, lactoperoxidase; HOOH, hydrogen peroxide. For comparison DdPoxA, peroxidase A from *Dictyostelium discoideum* is shown.

Nevertheless, in human EPO, TPO, LPO, human peroxidasin 1 and bacterial *Lyngbya* sp., *Lsp*POX (Family 6), proteolytic and mass spectrometric evidence has demonstrated the presence of covalent ester bonds between the heme 1- and 5-methyl and the carboxyl groups of the respective glutamate and aspartate residues [10,11,38–41].

It is well known that covalent heme binding by ester bonds is the result of an autocatalytic posttranslational maturation process. The first evidence was the finding that in recombinant proteins, only a fraction of the protein molecules had covalently bound heme. However, a higher level of covalently bound heme was obtained when a freshly isolated protein was incubated with H_2O_2. This has been demonstrated for LPO [41,42], EPO [39], TPO [40], human peroxidasin 1 [11,43] and bacterial *Lsp*POX [10,38]. In this context, it has to be mentioned that crystallographic studies on leukocyte MPO [15], its precursor promyeloperoxidase [37] and bovine LPO [44] showed low electron density for the ester bond between the heme 1-methyl and the carboxyl groups of the respective glutamate residue, suggesting that it had high mobility and that the ester bond to this residue might have a relatively low occupancy *per se*.

The mechanism of formation of these posttranslational modifications has been postulated by Ortiz de Montellano [45–47]. It is a free-radical mechanism, which is initiated by the two-electron oxidation of the ferric heme *b* peroxidase by hydrogen peroxide to Compound I [i.e. an oxoiron(IV) porphyrin radical intermediate]. Compound I oxidizes an adjacent side-chain carboxylic acid to a carboxylate radical, concomitantly quenching the porphyrin radical to a Compound II-like state [i.e. oxoiron(IV) porphyrin] (Figure 1.3) [46].

In turn, the carboxylate radical abstracts a hydrogen atom from a methyl group, yielding a methylene radical and regenerating the carboxylic acid. Subsequently, intramolecular transfer of the unpaired electron from the methylene to the iron produces a methylene cation with concomitant reduction of the iron to the resting ferric state. Finally, the carboxylate anion traps the methyl cation to form the ester bond (Figure 1.3) [46]. Two cycles are needed for formation of two ester bonds. In eukaryotes, this posttranslational modification most probably occurs after heme insertion in the endoplasmic reticulum [37,40]. As outlined above, ester bond formation can also be promoted by addition of H_2O_2 to purified recombinant protein. However, typically only a small stoichiometric excess of H_2O_2 should be added slowly in a stepwise manner, otherwise heme bleaching occurs [10–12,38]. This indicates that ester bond formation *in vivo* is a slow process that needs (sub)micromolar concentrations of H_2O_2. The mechanism of formation of the MPO-typical M243-vinyl bond remains unclear, but it is generally assumed that it follows also an autocatalytic mechanism [46,47].

The question remains whether there is a distinct sequence of posttranslational modification and, finally, bond formation. In the case of MPO, this was investigated by expression and characterization of D94N, D94V and E242Q mutants [48–50]. The E242Q mutant has, based on its spectroscopic properties, a normal methionine-vinyl bond [48]. This indicates that E242 is not essential for formation of the methionine-vinyl bond. This is also suggested by the crystal structures of wild-type MPO and LPO that clearly show 100% formation of the sulfonium ion linkage but less occupancy of the ester bond with E242 [15,37,44].

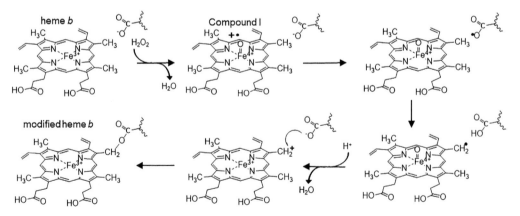

Figure 1.3 Proposed mechanism for the H_2O_2-mediated formation of ester bonds in human peroxidases [46].

It could be demonstrated that D94 is not essential for formation of either the E242-methyl link or the M243-vinyl link in MPO [49,50]. This is also supported by the fact that in DdPoxA, which lacks the respective aspartate for bond formation, the ester bond between the conserved glutamate and the heme 1-methyl is fully established. Finally, in a recent study on bacterial LspPOX (Family 6) and the mutants D109A, E238A and D109A/E238A, it was shown that both heme-to-protein ester bonds can form independently from each other [12].

In contrast to Family 1 peroxidases, no crystal structure of a Family 2 enzyme (peroxidasins) is available so far. Human peroxidasin 1 is a multi-domain peroxidase, which in – addition to the peroxidase domain with covalently bound heme – comprises LRRs, four Ig domains and a C-terminal VWC. Peroxidasin forms homotrimers involving two redox-sensitive cysteine residues and undergoes posttranslational C-terminal proteolytic cleavage [11,43,51]. A recent study on several recombinantly produced truncated peroxidasin variants [51] showed (i) that the VWC is not required for trimer formation, whereas the alpha-helical linker region located between the peroxidase domain and the VWC is crucial for trimerization and that (ii) oligomerization occurs intracellularly before C-terminal cleavage. Overall solution structures of monomeric and trimeric truncated peroxidasin variants suggest a triangular arrangement of the peroxidase domains to each other within the homotrimer as well as high flexibility of the Ig domains that interact with the peroxidase domain [51].

BIOPHYSICAL PROPERTIES OF HUMAN PEROXIDASES

Posttranslational modification of the heme group and formation of covalent links with the protein clearly increase the overall conformational and thermal stability of the enzymes. This was demonstrated for MPO [52], proMPO [52], LPO [53] and LspPOX [10,38]. MPO is unique, since it forms a third covalent sulfonium ion linkage in addition to the two ester bonds. Therefore, MPO has the highest thermal and conformational stability [52], and the prosthetic group assumes a bow-shaped structure and a pronounced out-of-plane location of the ferric high-spin heme iron (Figure 1.2) [14,15,36,37]. The two ester bonds in LPO cause a less distorted heme (Figure 1.2) [34,44].

As a consequence of these posttranslational modifications, peroxidases of Family 1 and Family 2 from the peroxidase-cyclooxygenase superfamily exhibit completely different spectral characteristics and redox properties compared with heme *b* peroxidases that also have a histidine as proximal ligand, such as the well-studied horseradish peroxidase, ascorbate peroxidase or cytochrome *c* peroxidase from the peroxidase-catalase superfamily [1,33]. In contrast to the heme *b* peroxidases, the Soret bands of mammalian peroxidases are red-shifted due to the covalent heme to protein linkages. The Soret band of ferric LPO exhibits a maximum at 412 nm, and the visible spectrum shows maxima at 500, 542, 590 and 630 nm [33,54]. The bandwidth and wavelength of the Soret band as well as the wavelength of the charge transfer band at 630 nm are characteristic of a six-coordinate high-spin aquo ferric heme [55]. This is reflected by the crystal structures of LPO (and MPO) that contain a water molecule weakly bound to the heme iron, which is at about 2.7–2.9 Å and hydrogen bonded to the N_ε of the distal histidine [14,37]. EPO [33,56], TPO [40], human peroxidasin 1 (PDXN) [11,43] and bacterial LspPOX [10,38] all exhibit spectral features very similar to those of LPO, suggesting similar heme cavity architectures, i.e. the presence of two ester bonds between the protein and the prosthetic group.

The electronic absorption maxima of ferric MPO are even more red-shifted compared with LPO and other representatives with two ester bonds. Its Soret maximum is at 430 nm, and the spectrum shows additional bands at 496, 570, 620 and 690 nm [35,57,58]. However, upon mutation of M243, the UV-vis spectrum becomes similar to LPO, confirming that the MPO-typical sulfonium ion linkage is responsible for these spectral properties [43,58–60]. In addition to the sulfonium ion linkage, its neighbouring residue E242 contributes to the distortion from the planar conformation and the lowered symmetry [61]. The electronic absorption spectrum of the D94V MPO variant shows a splitting of the Soret absorption band into two maxima, one wild-type-like and the other similar to the M243T mutant [62], suggesting that exchange of D94 not only causes loss of the ester bond but also affects to some extent the sulfonium ion linkage [48,62]. Mutational studies on bovine LPO indicate that the two ester bonds in LPO are not equivalent. Loss of the glutamate linkage shows a much stronger impact on the spectral and catalytic properties than the loss of the aspartate linkage [63].

The effect of the covalent bonds on the symmetry lowering of the heme group was demonstrated by resonance Raman (RR) spectroscopy in wild-type MPO and the variants M243T and D94V [60]. RR spectra of MPO are extremely rich, since the three linkages significantly lower the heme group symmetry [35,48,60,64]. The richness of the RR spectra of MPO is due to the activation of almost all the porphyrin skeletal frequencies induced by the distortion imposed by the simultaneous presence of protein–porphyrin covalent bonds and the charged sulfonium group [60]. Exchange of M243 reduces the complexity of the Raman spectra. Nevertheless, in both LPO and M243 variants of MPO, the RR spectra maintain some unusual features compared with other heme proteins such as a remarkable enhancement of several out-of-plane low-frequency modes arising from a protein-induced distortion mediated by the two covalent ester bonds [9,60].

In general, the spectroscopic characteristics of ferric LPO and MPO are maintained in the ferrous forms. The electronic absorption spectrum of Fe(II) MPO is rather unique, being red-shifted with respect to other heme proteins, with a Soret maximum at 472 nm and an α-band at 636 nm. Concomitantly, its vibrational spectrum is very complex [64]. Ferrous LPO has absorption maxima at 434 nm (Soret band), 561 and 593 nm [65]. This stable Fe(II) species is formed via a transient ferrous intermediate with peak maxima at 444, 561 and 593 nm. The rate of this conversion significantly increases with decreasing pH [66] and was suggested to be the result of structural changes from a relatively open, unrestricted pocket to a constrained one [67].

The low-frequency RR spectrum of a five-coordinated high-spin ferrous heme protein is characterized by the presence of a strong band due to the iron-imidazole stretching mode that is found in the 200–250 cm^{-1} region. Its frequency correlates with the bond strength between the iron and the imidazole ring, and a shift of this band correlates with a change in the hydrogen-bonding status of the proton on the proximal imidazole [68]. In both MPO and LPO, the ν(Fe-Im) stretching mode is found at fairly high frequencies (248–244 cm^{-1}) [69,70] with ν(Fe-Im) of LPO being slightly higher than ν(Fe-Im) of MPO, suggesting a substantial imidazolate character of the

proximal histidine. This fully reflects the crystal structures of both MPO and LPO which – together with molecular dynamics simulations [15] – demonstrate the interaction of an anionic proximal histidine with the amine group of the side chain of a conserved asparagine.

Besides spectral characteristics, modifications of heme have a strong impact on the redox properties of the respective heme peroxidases. Although not directly involved in the catalytic cycle, the redox behaviour of the Fe(III)/Fe(II) couple of several heme peroxidases has been analysed in a much greater detail than that of the short-living high-potential intermediates Compounds I and II [71], whose reduction potentials are more difficult to measure experimentally. Nevertheless, there is a general agreement that the molecular factors that determine $E^{\circ\prime}$[Fe(III)/Fe(II)] also influence the standard reduction potential ($E^{\circ\prime}$) of the catalytically relevant Compound I/Fe(III) and Compound I/Compound II redox couples. Indeed, the hierarchy observed for $E^{\circ\prime}$[Fe(III)/Fe(II)], namely MPO>EPO>LPO, is also reflected in $E^{\circ\prime}$[Compound I/Fe(III)] and $E^{\circ\prime}$[Compound I/Compound II] (Table 1.2) [16,17].

Typically, heme b peroxidases feature negative $E^{\circ\prime}$[Fe(III)/Fe(II)] values to stabilize the ferric state for efficient reaction with H$_2$O$_2$, e.g. in horseradish peroxidase (HRP) $E^{\circ\prime}$[Fe(III)/Fe(II)] −0.306 V [72]. Posttranslational modifications may increase the standard reduction potential significantly (Table 1.2). MPO is unique because the corresponding $E^{\circ\prime}$ value is +0.005 V (pH 7.0) in mature dimeric leukocyte MPO and +0.001 V in recombinant monomeric proMPO [73]. Variable-temperature experiments, which allow calculation of the protein and solvent-derived contributions to enthalpic ($\Delta H^{\circ\prime}_{rc}$) and entropic ($\Delta S^{\circ\prime}_{rc}$) changes during reduction of Fe(III) to Fe(II), demonstrate that the sulfonium ion linkage drastically decreases the level of enthalpic stabilization of the ferric form. The positive charge of the sulfur atom electrostatically destabilizes the ferric heme. Moreover, the electron-withdrawing effect of the sulfonium linkage reduces the basicity of the four pyrrole nitrogens, thereby decreasing the electron density at the heme iron. This effect might be enhanced by the pronounced distortion of the porphyrin ring. In MPO reduction, $\Delta H^{\circ\prime}_{rc}$ and $\Delta S^{\circ\prime}_{rc}$ almost perfectly offset each other. Entropic changes during reduction suggest that Fe(III) reduction is accompanied by limited

TABLE 1.2

Standard reduction potentials (E°′) of all relevant redox couples of myeloperoxidase (MPO) and mutants D94N, E242Q and M243V, lactoperoxidase (LPO), eosinophil peroxidase (EPO) and recombinant human peroxidasin (PXDN)

	Fe(III)/Fe(II) (mV)	Cpd I/Fe(III) (mV)	Cpd I/Cpd II (mV)	Cpd II/Fe(III) (mV)
MPO	5 [73]	1,160 [80]	1,350 [81]	970 [81]
D94N	−55 [17]	N/A	N/A	N/A
E242Q	−94 [17]	N/A	N/A	N/A
M243V	−182 [17]	N/A.	N/A	N/A
LPO	−176 [76]	1,090 [79]	1,140 [79]	1,040 [79]
EPO	−126 [76]	1,100 [80]	N/A	N/A
PXDN	−128 [43]	N/A	N/A	N/A
LspPOX	−158 [12]	N/A	N/A	N/A
E238A	−209 [12]	N/A	N/A	N/A
D109A/E238A	−212 [12]	N/A	N/A	N/A
DdPoxA	−276 [13]	N/A	N/A	N/A
HRP	−306 [78]	883 [78]	898 [78]	869 [78]

For comparison E°′ of recombinant peroxidase from wild-type *Lyngbya* sp. PCC 8106 (Family 6 of the peroxidase-cyclooxygenase superfamily) and mutants E238A and D109A/E238A, recombinant peroxidase from Dictyostelium discoideum (DdPoxA, of the peroxidase-cyclooxygenase superfamily) and horseradish peroxidase (heme b peroxidase from the peroxidase-catalase superfamily) are presented.

Cpd I, Compound I; Cpd II, Compound II; N/A, not available.

solvent reorganization, indicating that the hydrogen bond network of water molecules in the substrate channel leading to the distal heme site is quite rigid. This low mobility of the water molecules has been proposed to be crucial in fixing the position of the small anionic substrate chloride and in helping the transfer and incorporation of the oxyferryl oxygen into HOCl [73]. It is important to notice that mature dimeric leukocyte MPO and recombinant monomeric, partially unprocessed proMPO share the same redox thermodynamic features, suggesting almost identical heme cavity and substrate channel architectures. Recently, this could be confirmed by the crystal structure of promyeloperoxidase [37]. This is also reflected by very similar catalytic properties [74]. Thus, proMPO can be used in the design and testing of MPO inhibitors [75].

As outlined above, upon disruption of the sulfonium ion linkage in the M243V variant, the UV-vis and RR spectral features are considerably blue-shifted and similar to those found in LPO and EPO. In MPO M243V, the measured E°′ value (−0.182 V) [17] is significantly lower than in the wild-type protein and almost identical to LPO (Table 1.2) [76]. Redox thermodynamic studies show that protein intrinsic factors of

M243V enthalpically stabilize the oxidized form more efficiently than the recombinant wild-type proMPO form. This agrees with the effects of disruption of the sulfonium linkage, because deletion of the (positive and electron-withdrawing) bond should stabilize the ferric form of the heme both electrostatically and electronically. Furthermore, reduction of the variant M243V is entropically favoured as a consequence of a significant reduction-induced solvent reorganization within the heme cavity not observed in wild-type MPO, underlining the proposed role of the sulfonium ion linkage in fixing the positioning of the anionic halide ions [73].

The E°′ value of the MPO variant E242Q is −0.094 V [17]. Disruption of the ester bond at pyrrole ring A also induces an increase in protein-based enthalpic stabilization of the ferric form, which, however, is lower than in M243V. Since in the E242Q mutant, the sulfonium linkage is still present [61], the observed effect is not related to electrostatics. As suggested by RR studies [60,77], the decreased level of distortion of the heme in E242Q compared with wild-type MPO might enhance the interaction of the metal ion with the pyrrole nitrogens, thereby enthalpically stabilizing the Fe(III) form. Reduction of E242Q is entropically favoured suggesting that E242 (besides M243) is important in fixing the position of water molecules in the distal heme cavity and optimizing the position of the substrate. Indeed, the glutamate 242 ester bond is close to the bromide-binding site in MPO [14], and its disruption generally decreases the halogenation activity of E242Q compared with the wild-type enzyme [61].

The standard reduction potential of the Fe(III)/Fe(II) couple of the D94V mutant is -0.055 V (Table 1.2) [17]. Variable-temperature experiments show that elimination of this ester bond stabilizes the ferric form by protein intrinsic factors, which also reflects less distortion in D94V compared with the wild-type protein. Reduction of D94V is entropically unfavoured, suggesting that this ester bond plays a minor role in stabilization of the distal H-bonding network. This is in agreement with the observation that the halide-binding (and oxidation) site is close to the δ-meso bridge and thus almost opposite to D94 (Figure 1.1). The observed negative reduction entropy [17] might be related to the destabilization of the Ca^{2+}-binding site at the distal heme cavity that involves D96 in the proximity of D94 and catalytic H95 (Figure 1.2). It is reasonable to assume that disruption of the ester bond at pyrrole ring C increases the mobility of the polypeptide in this region. In any case, exchange of D94 slows the chlorination and bromination reaction (see below) [62], suggesting that this ester bond contributes to the high oxidation capacity of MPO.

Heme peroxidases with two ester bonds typically have $E^{\circ\prime}[Fe(III)/Fe(II)]$ values between -0.120 and -0.180 V, significantly more negative than MPO but more positive compared with heme b peroxidases, e.g. EPO (-0.126 V) [76], PXDN (-0.128 V) [11] and LPO (-0.176 V) [76] (Table 1.2). The reduction potential of bacterial LspPOX could only be estimated to be about -0.160 V [12]. In any case, studies on the LspPOX variants D109A, E238A and D109A/E238 demonstrate that elimination of the ester bonds decreases the $E^{\circ\prime}$ value (Table 1.2) [12], thus underscoring the impact of these posttranslational modifications on the redox properties of the heme iron. In the recently studied DdPoxA [13] that has only one (glutamate) ester linkage (Figure 1.2), the standard reduction potential of the Fe(III)/Fe(II) redox couple was determined to be -0.276 V. These studies clearly demonstrate the correlation between the nature and number of heme to

protein linkage and $E^{\circ\prime}[Fe(III)/Fe(II)]$, following the hierarchy $E^{\circ\prime}$(MPO; three linkages) $> E^{\circ\prime}$ (EPO, PXDN, LspPOX, LPO; two linkages) $> E^{\circ\prime}$ (DdPoxA: one linkage) $\sim E^{\circ\prime}$ (heme b peroxidases).

Studies on MPO, EPO, LPO and HRP clearly suggest that the hierarchy of $E^{\circ\prime}$ values of Fe(III)/Fe(II) couples reflects the hierarchy of the reduction potentials of the catalytically relevant couples Compound I/Fe(III), Compound I/Compound II and Compound II/Fe(III), respectively. The lowest $E^{\circ\prime}$ value of the redox couples Compound I/Fe(III) and Compound I/Compound II was obtained for HRP (0.883 and 0.898 V, respectively) [78]. The presence of two ester bonds significantly increases the respective $E^{\circ\prime}$ values as determined for LPO (1.090 and 1.140 V, respectively) [79]. For EPO, $E^{\circ\prime}$ [Compound I/Fe(III)] was determined to be 1.100 V [80]. As EPO exhibits structural similarities to LPO, it is reasonable to assume that the couple Compound I/Compound II has a similar $E^{\circ\prime}$ value to LPO. The highest standard reduction potentials of the couples Compound I/Fe(III) (1.160 V) [81] and Compound I/Compound II (1.350 V) [82] were obtained for MPO. As will be outlined below, these very positive reduction potentials reflect the high oxidation capacity of MPO and its extraordinary role in substrate oxidation during bacterial killing [24,26].

Generally, in MPO and LPO, the capacity to oxidize one-electron donors is higher for Compound I than for Compound II, and this is reflected by the higher redox potential for the Compound I/Compound II couple with respect to the Compound II/Fe(III) couple. In HRP, an $E^{\circ\prime}$ value of about 0.900 V was determined for both redox intermediates (Table 1.2) [78], whereas differences are seen in MPO [81] and LPO [79]. Especially in MPO, $E^{\circ\prime}$[Compound I/Compound II] is significantly more positive compared with $E^{\circ\prime}$[Compound II/Fe(III)], which is exploited in the design of reversible MPO inhibitors [75,83]. In LPO, the difference in $E^{\circ\prime}$[Compound I/Compound II] and $E^{\circ\prime}$[Compound II/Fe(III)] is less pronounced [79].

CATALYTIC PROPERTIES OF HUMAN PEROXIDASES

Peroxidases of the peroxidase-cyclooxygenase superfamily efficiently catalyse one- and two-electron oxidation reactions according to Reactions 1 and 2. Compound I [oxoiron(IV) porphyrin radical species] is the central redox intermediate formed by reaction of the ferric resting state form with hydrogen peroxide according to Reaction 5. In this reaction, the fully conserved distal histidine–arginine couple (Figure 1.2) plays a critical role in the binding, orientation and activation of H_2O_2. The histidine acts as proton acceptor from one oxygen and a donor to the other, while the arginine modulates the ionization of the histidine by decreasing its pK_a of the imidazole N_δ and polarizes the O-O bond to promote the nucleophilic attack at the heme and subsequently heterolytic cleavage [84,85]. In this reaction, the impact of posttranslational modification is negligible.

The k_{app} values of this bimolecular reaction are within $(0.3–4.6)\times 10^7$ M^{-1} s^{-1} at pH 7.0 for posttranslationally modified heme peroxidases [12,13,33,43,54,56,74,86–88] (Table 1.3), but very similar values are found for heme b peroxidases [84].

The minor role of heme modification in Compound I formation is underscored by the fact that MPO mutants lacking D94 and M243 exhibit rates of Compound I formation very similar to wild-type MPO [59]. Since in the E242Q variant the rates of Compound I formation but also Compound I reduction (Table 1.3) as well as formation of the cyanide complex are decreased, it was hypothesized that this might be related to blocking of the substrate accessibility to the heme cavity [61]. Recombinant bacterial LspPOX is an interesting model protein because it can be produced as heme b protein and subsequently posttranslationally modified by addition of H_2O_2 [12]. Upon using LspPOX, it has been demonstrated that the determined apparent rate constant for Compound I formation (and cyanide binding) significantly increases upon posttranslational modification, suggesting the necessity of structural rearrangement for optimum activity of the catalytic histidine–arginine pair during heterolytic cleavage of H_2O_2.

$$[\text{Por}\ldots\text{Fe}(\text{III})] + H_2O_2$$

$$\rightarrow [^{+\bullet}\text{Por}\ldots\text{Fe}(\text{IV})=\text{O}] + H_2O \quad \text{Reaction 5}$$

$$[^{+\bullet}\text{Por}\ldots\text{Fe}(\text{IV})=\text{O}] + X^- + H^+$$

$$\rightarrow [\text{Por}\ldots\text{Fe}(\text{III})] + \text{HOX} \quad \text{Reaction 6}$$

In contrast to Compound I formation, the heme-to-protein linkages play an important role in Compound I reduction. Family 1 peroxidases such as MPO, EPO, LPO and TPO as well as PXDN are unique in their ability to efficiently oxidize (pseudo-)halides (X^-, namely Cl^-, Br^-, I^-, SCN^-) to (pseudo-) hypohalites (HOX, namely HOCl, HOBr, HOI, HOSCN) according to Reaction 6. Standard reduction potentials for the redox couples HOX/X^-, H_2O at pH 7.0 are 1.28 V ($X^-=Cl^-$), 1.13 V (Br^-), 0.78 V (I^-) and 0.56 (SCN^-) V [16]. The reduction potential of these couples increases with decreasing pH (~0.03 V per pH unit) as two electrons and one proton are involved in the corresponding half-reaction. At pH 7.0, HOCl ($pK_a=7.53$), HOBr ($pK_a=8.8$), HOI ($pK_a=10.0$) exist predominantly in the undissociated form, whereas HOSCN ($pK_a=5.3$) is dissociated [16].

The ease of oxidation of (pseudo)halide ions is the following: $SCN^->I^->Br^->Cl^-$ [16]. Therefore, Compound I of all peroxidases, regardless whether the heme group is covalently bound or not, can oxidize iodide and thiocyanate. In representatives of the peroxidase-cyclooxygenase superfamilies studied thus far, the rates for thiocyanate oxidation are extremely high ($>9.6\times 10^6$ M^{-1} s^{-1}), with LPO, EPO and DdPoxA being $>10^8$ M^{-1} s^{-1} (Table 1.3). Similarly, oxidation of iodide is very fast ($>7.2\times 10^6$ M^{-1} s^{-1}), with EPO and DdPoxA showing the highest rates (Table 1.3). Except for MPO, elimination of the aspartate ester bond has no impact on thiocyanate or iodide oxidation [62], whereas disruption of the glutamate ester bond [61] significantly reduces the oxidation of both electron donors. By contrast, elimination of the sulfonium ion linkage increases the rates of SCN^- and I^- oxidation [59], clearly demonstrating that this MPO-typical structural feature is not essential in oxidation of two-electron donors with $E^{\circ\prime}$ [XOH/X^-, H_2O; pH 7.0] < 0.8 V. Elimination of E242 in MPO affected halide oxidation in general, most probably due to hampering proper binding and access of the electron donors [61].

In contrast to hypothiocyanite and hypoiodous acid formation, oxidation of chloride and bromide strongly depends on posttranslational modification of the prosthetic group. Only MPO Compound I is able to react with chloride at pH 7.0 at reasonable rates (Table 1.3) [85,86,88], which reflects the high reduction potential of the MPO redox couple Compound I/Fe(III) discussed above [73,80,82]. At acidic pH, Compound I reduction is accelerated significantly, which is also reflected by an increase in the steady-state chlorination activity

TABLE 1.3

Apparent second-order rate constants for Compound I formation and reduction as well as Compound II reduction by human peroxidases

Substrate	MPO	E242Q	M243V	D94N	D94V	LPO	EPO	PXDN	LspPOX	D109A	E238A	D109A/ E238A	DdPOX	HRP
References	[85,86,88,91, 93,98]	[61]	[50]	[49]	[49]	[54,97]	[56,92,99]	[43,96]	[12,38,]	[12]	[12]	[12]	[13]	[91,94,95]
							Compound I formation ($\times 10^4$ M^{-1} s^{-1})							
H$_2$O$_2$	1,800	78	2,200	1,600	870	1,100	4,300	1,800	6,000	3,200	2,520	1,020	320	1,700
						Compound I reduction by two-electron donors ($\times 10^4$ M^{-1} s^{-1})								
Chloride	2.5	0.0065	–	0.2	0.15	–	0.31	–	–	–	–	N/A	–	–
Bromide	110	5.4	13	41	15	41	1,900	560	126	54	2.1	N/A	0.0015	–
Iodide	720	64	10,000	1,800	590	1,200	9,300	1,680	4,190	1,540	2,860	N/A	10,000	0.26
Thiocyanate	960	22	10,000	1,200	490	20,000	10,000	1,830	2,450	816	1,185	N/A	10,000	N/A
						Compound I reduction by tyrosine and nitrite ($\times 10^4$ M^{-1} s^{-1})								
Tyrosine	77	0.028	N/A	42	16	11	35	2.2	62	N/A	N/A	N/A	N/A	5
Serotonin	1,700	N/A	N/A	N/A	N/A	200	N/A	48	N/A	N/A	N/A	N/A	N/A	810
Nitrite	200	N/A	N/A	N/A	N/A	2,300	N/A	19	N/A	N/A	N/A	N/A	N/A	0.45
						Compound II reduction by tyrosine and nitrite ($\times 10^4$ M^{-1} s^{-1})								
Tyrosine	1.57	0.018	N/A	0.5	1.2	1	2.7	0.043	11	N/A	N/A	N/A	N/A	1.1
Serotonin	140	N/A	N/A	N/A	N/A	30	N/A	0.77	N/A	N/A	N/A	N/A	N/A	120
Nitrite	0.055	N/A	N/A	N/A	N/A	35	0.35	0.4	N/A	N/A	N/A	N/A	N/A	0.013

Myeloperoxidase (MPO) and mutants E242Q and M243V; lactoperoxidase (LPO); eosinophil peroxidase (EPO); human peroxidasin 1 (PXDN). For comparison, kinetic data of other representatives of the peroxidase-cyclooxygenase superfamily are shown: peroxidase from *Lyngbya* sp. PCC 8106 (LspPOX) and mutants D109A, E238A, E238A and D109A/E238A; peroxidase from *Dictyostelium discoideum* (DdPOX). Finally, data from the heme *b* peroxidase horseradish peroxidase (HRP) are presented.

–, no reaction; N/A, data not available.

of MPO [89,90]. At pH 5, also EPO Compound I is able to oxidize chloride but only at poor rates [56].

The importance of the MPO-typical sulfonium ion linkage in Compound I reduction mediated by chloride is seen in various M243 mutants that lost the chlorination activity almost completely [58,59]. This is also underscored by the LPO-like $E^{o\prime}$ values of the redox couple Fe(III)/Fe(II) of the respective M243 mutants [17]. As already outlined above, exchange of E242 also decreased the chlorination activity dramatically, whereas exchange of D94 by asparagine has almost no impact on chloride oxidation, since the sulfonium ion linkage in these mutants is (partially) intact [59].

Efficient oxidation of bromide by Compound I ($>10^6$ M^{-1} s^{-1}) is seen in several heme peroxidases with two ester linkages following the hierarchy EPO>PXDN>LspPOX>MPO at pH 7 (Table 1.3). These peroxidases have $E^{o\prime}$ values of the redox couple Fe(III)/Fe(II) >−0.160 V, and the hierarchy in $E^{o\prime}$ values reflects the apparent rate constants for Compound I reduction at pH 7.0 (compare Tables 1.2 and 1.3). The standard reduction potential of $E^{o\prime}$[Compound I/Fe(III)] of EPO is 1.10 V. LPO, with $E^{o\prime}$ [Fe(III)/Fe(II)=−0.176 V [79] and $E^{o\prime}$[Compound I/Fe(III)]=1.090 V [79], shows barely detectable activity with bromide at neutral pH, suggesting that besides thermodynamics, also structural features must contribute to the poor bromide oxidation capacity of LPO. The heme peroxidase from *Dictyostelium discoideum* with $E^{o\prime}$ [Fe(III)/Fe(II)=−0.276 V [13] and only one ester linkage is unable to oxidize bromide.

The importance of heme modification in the capacity to oxidize bromide was also demonstrated with bacterial LspPOX [12,38]. In the reconstituted heme *b* form of the wild-type enzyme, Compound I reacts slowly with bromide, whereas upon incubation with H_2O_2 and establishment of the two ester bonds, the rate of Compound I reduction was increased by a factor of 6,300. This suggests that posttranslational modification − besides increasing the reduction potential of the redox couple Compound I/Fe(III) − also optimizes the heme cavity architecture for access, binding and oxidation of bromide.

Although for Family 1 and 2 enzymes, the halogenation cycle (i.e. Reactions 5 and 6) seems to be related to the physiological function, these heme peroxidases can also follow the peroxidase cycle that includes Reactions 5, 7 and 8. In the peroxidase cycle, Compound I is reduced

by two one-electron donors (AH$_2$; e.g. tyrosine, serotonin, ascorbate, urate, nitrite, etc.) via Compound II [oxoiron(IV)species] to the ferric resting state, thereby releasing the corresponding radicals ($^{\bullet}$AH) [9,16,33,74,85,91–99].

$$\left[^{+\bullet}Por\ldots Fe(IV)=O \right]+AH_2$$

$$\rightarrow \left[Por\ldots Fe(IV)-OH \right]+ {}^{\bullet}AH \qquad \text{Reaction 7}$$

$$\left[Por\ldots Fe(IV)-OH \right]+AH_2$$

$$\rightarrow \left[Por\ldots Fe(III) \right]+ {}^{\bullet}AH+H_2O \qquad \text{Reaction 8}$$

Typically, significant differences in rates of Reaction 7 are observed between heme *b* peroxidases and posttranslationally modified enzymes but also within the latter group [91–99]. For example, MPO Compound I is a significantly better one-electron oxidant compared with LPO Compound I. By contrast, the determined rates of Compound II reduction (Reaction 8) are similar [91], which is also reflected by the fact that the standard reduction potentials of the redox couple Compound II/Fe(III) enzyme for MPO and LPO are similar, with MPO (0.970 V) being even 0.070 V lower than LPO (1.040 V) (Table 1.2) [79,81]. Regarding Compound II reduction mediated by tyrosine [$E^{o\prime}$ (tyrosyl radical/tyrosine)=0.94 V at pH 7], both LPO and MPO show rate constants that are similar to that of the heme *b* enzyme HRP (Table 1.3) [93,95]. Regarding Compound I reduction by tyrosine, significant differences are observed, with MPO Compound I being an extremely strong oxidant of one-electron donors, which is reflected by the very positive reduction potential of the Compound I/Compound II couple (Table 1.2). Compound I of MPO is able to oxidize substrates with a reduction potential ca. 1.2 V and even higher [83,91]. This again underscores the role of the sulfonium ion linkage in further increasing the electron deficiency of the porphyrin π-cation radical of Compound I. In Compound II, the porphyrin radical is quenched, but the heme iron is still in its low-spin form, which favours a more in-plane position compared with its native high-spin state. This could partially explain the large difference of $E^{o\prime}$ of the Fe(III)/Fe(II) couple between MPO and LPO despite the similar $E^{o\prime}$ values for the Compound II/Fe(III) couple. The binding and oxidation site for the (aromatic) substrates should be identical in Compound I and II, namely a hydrophobic region at the entrance to the distal cavity almost centred above the pyrrole ring D 8-methyl group [83,100–102].

The marked difference in $E^{\circ\prime}$ value of the MPO Compound I/Compound II and Compound II/Fe(III) couple is unique among heme peroxidases and is exploited in the design of reversible inhibitors of MPO [75,83,100–102]. These inhibitors of typically very positive reduction potential compete with the substrate chloride and are efficiently oxidized by MPO Compound I. Thereby, Compound II is formed, which is unable to oxidize both chloride and these inhibitors. As a consequence, MPO is trapped in the Compound II state and the chlorination activity of MPO is dampened.

CONCLUSION

Heme peroxidases from the peroxidase-cyclooxygenase superfamily are widely distributed among all domains of life and show diversity in domain architectures and composition. It comprises seven families with five human peroxidases (MPO, EPO, LPO, TPO and peroxidasin 1) belonging to Families 1 and 2. These heme enzymes are unique in having the prosthetic heme group posttranslationally modified by a peroxide-driven autocatalytic radical mechanism. Typically, they have two or three covalent heme–protein bonds which structurally rearrange and electronically modify the prosthetic heme group. This may lead to heme distortion, lowering of its symmetry and promotion of out-of-plane location of the iron ion as well as optimization of the binding of small anionic substrates such as halides. As a consequence, these oxidoreductases show peculiar spectral features and typically high reduction potentials of the redox couples Fe(III)/Fe(II), Compound I/Fe(III) and Compound I/Compound II. The capacity to oxidize two- and one-electron donors by the catalytically relevant redox intermediate Compound I is higher than in heme b enzymes. There is only one clade of Family I enzymes, i.e. MPOs, that have in addition to two ester linkages an electron-withdrawing sulfonium ion linkage. Its prosthetic group is strongly distorted and the relevant $E^{\circ\prime}$ values are very positive, enabling MPO to play a prominent role in innate immunity of neutrophils by producing antimicrobial hypochlorous acids. Monomeric EPO and homotrimeric multidomain PXDN efficiently oxidize bromide to hypobromous acid used for either unspecific microbial defence (EPO) or specific sulfilimine bond formation in collagen IV (PXDN). Thiocyanate is the main substrate for LPO in host defence, whereas membrane-anchored TPO uses hypoiodous acid in specific thyroid hormone biosynthesis.

ACKNOWLEDGEMENTS

This work was supported by the Austrian Science Fund FWF [Doctoral Program BioToP – Biomolecular Technology of Proteins (W1224)] and with project P 31707-B32.

REFERENCES

1. Zámocký, M., Hofbauer, S., Schaffner, I. et al. 2015. Independent evolution of four heme peroxidase superfamilies. *Arch. Biochem. Biophys.* 574:108–119.
2. Welinder, K.G. 1992. Superfamily of plant, fungal and bacterial peroxidases. *Curr. Opin. Struct. Biol.* 2:388–393.
3. Zámocký, M., Gasselhuber, B., Furtmüller, P.G. et al. 2014. Turning points in the evolution of peroxidase–catalase superfamily: Molecular phylogeny of hybrid heme peroxidases. *Cell. Mol. Life Sci* 71:4681–4696.
4. Zámocký, M., Jakopitsch, C., Furtmüller, P.G. et al. 2008. The peroxidase-cyclooxygenase superfamily: Reconstructed evolution of critical enzymes of the innate immune system. *Proteins* 71:589–605.
5. Piontek, K., Strittmatter, E., Ullrich, R. 2013. Structural basis of substrate conversion in a new aromatic peroxygenase. *J. Biol. Chem.* 288:34767–34776.
6. Hofrichter, M., Ullrich, R. 2014. Oxidations catalyzed by fungal peroxygenases. *Curr. Opinion Chem. Biol.* 19:116–125.
7. Singh, R., Eltis, L.D. 2015. The multihued palette of dye-decolorizing peroxidases. *Arch. Biochem. Biophys.* 574:56–65.
8. Soudi, M., Zámocký, M., Jakopitsch, C. et al. 2012. Molecular evolution, structure, and function of peroxidasins. *Chem. Biodivers.* 9:1776–1793.
9. Zederbauer, M., Furtmüller, P.G., Brogioni, S. et al. 2007. Heme to protein linkages in mammalian peroxidases: Impact on spectroscopic, redox and catalytic properties. *Nat. Prod. Rep.* 24:571–584.

10. Auer, M., Gruber, C., Bellei, M. et al. 2013. A stable bacterial peroxidase with novel halogenating activity and an autocatalytically linked heme prosthetic group. *J. Biol. Chem.* 288:27181–27199.

11. Soudi, M., Paumann-Page, M., Delporte, C. et al. 2015. Multidomain human peroxidasin 1 is a highly glycosylated and stable homotrimeric high spin ferric peroxidase. *J. Biol. Chem.* 290:10876–10890.

12. Nicolussi, A., Auer, M. Weissensteiner, J. et al. 2017. Posttranslational modification of heme *b* in a bacterial peroxidase: The role of heme to protein ester bonds in ligand binding and catalysis. *Biochemistry* 56:4525–4538.

13. Nicolussi, A., Dunn, J.D., Mlynek, G. et al. 2018. Secreted heme peroxidase from *Dictyostelium discoideum*: Insights into catalysis, structure, and biological role. *J. Biol. Chem.* 293:1330–1345.

14. Fiedler, T.J., Davey, C.A., Fenna, R.E. 2000. X-ray Crystal structure and characterization of halide-binding sites of human myeloperoxidase at 1.8 Å resolution. *J. Biol. Chem.* 275:11964–11971.

15. Carpena, X., Vidossich, P., Schroettner, K. et al. 2009. Essential role of proximal histidine-asparagine interaction in mammalian peroxidases. *J. Biol. Chem.* 284:25929–25937.

16. Arnhold, J., Monzani, E., Furtmüller, P.G. et al. 2006. Kinetics and thermodynamics of halide and nitrite oxidation by mammalian heme peroxidases. *Eur. J. Inorg. Chem.* 19:3801–3811.

17. Battistuzzi, G., Stampler, J., Bellei, M. et al. 2011. Influence of the covalent heme-protein bonds on the redox thermodynamics of human myeloperoxidase. *Biochemistry* 50:7987–7994.

18. Nicolussi, A., Auer, M., Sevcnikar, B. 2018. Posttranslational modification of heme in peroxidases – Impact on structure and catalysis. *Arch. Biochem. Biophys.* 643:14–23.

19. Vizzini, A., Parrinello, D., Sanfratello, M.A. et al. 2013. *Ciona intestinalis* peroxinectin is a novel component of the peroxidase-cyclooxygenase gene superfamily upregulated by LPS. *Dev. Comput. Immunol.* 41:59–67.

20. Kumar, S., Stecher, G., Li, M. et al. 2018. MEGA X: Molecular Evolutionary Genetics Analysis across computing platforms. *Mol. Biol. Evol.* 35:1547–1549.

21. Nelson, R.E., Fessler, L.I., Takagi, Y. et al. 1994. Peroxidasin: A novel enzyme-matrix protein of *drosophila* development. *EMBO J.* 13:3438–3447.

22. Bhave, G., Cummings, C.F., Vanacore, R.M. et al. 2012. Peroxidasin forms sulfilimine chemical bonds using hypohalous acids in tissue genesis. *Nat. Chem. Biol.* 8:784–790.

23. Fidler, A.L., Vanacorea, R.M., Chetyrkinaet, S.V. et al. 2014. A unique covalent bond in basement membrane is a primordial innovation for tissue evolution. *Proc. Natl. Acad. Sci. USA* 111:331–336.

24. Klebanoff, S.J. 2005. Myeloperoxidase: Friend and Foe. *J. Leukoc. Biol.* 77:598–625.

25. Obinger, C. 2006. Chemistry and biology of human peroxidases. *Arch. Biochem. Biophys* 445:197–198.

26. Davies, M.J. Hawkins C.L., Pattison, D.I. et al. 2008. Mammalian heme peroxidases: From molecular mechanisms to health implications. *Antioxid. Redox Signal.* 10:1199–1234.

27. Loughran, N.B., O'Connor, B., Ó'Fágáin, C. et al. 2008. The phylogeny of the mammalian heme peroxidases and the evolution of their diverse functions. *BMC Evol. Biology* 8:101.

28. Ruf, J., Carayon, P. 2006. Structural and functional aspects of thyroid peroxidase. *Arch. Biochem. Biophys.* 445:269–277.

29. Kessler, J., Obinger, C., Eales, G. 2008. Factors influencing the study of peroxidase-generated iodine species and implications for thyroglobulin synthesis. *Thyroid* 18:769–774.

30. Mondal, S., Raja, K., Schweizer, U. et al. 2016. Chemistry and biology in the biosynthesis and action of thyroid hormones. *Angew. Chem. Int. Ed.* 55:7606–7630.

31. Ihalin, R., Loimaranta, V., Tenovuo, J. 2006. Origin, structure, and biological activities of peroxidases in human saliva. *Arch. Biochem. Biophys.* 445:261–268.

32. Malik, A., Batra, J.K. 2012. Antimicrobial activity of human eosinophil granule proteins: Involvement in host defence against pathogens. *Crit. Rev. Microbiol.* 38:168–181.

33. Furtmüller, P.G., Zederbauer, M., Jantschko, W. et al. 2006. Active site structure and catalytic mechanisms of human peroxidases. *Arch. Biochem. Biophys.* 445:199–213.

34. Singh, A.K., Singh, N., Sharma, S., et al. 2008. Crystal structure of lactoperoxidase at 2.4 Å resolution. *J. Mol. Biol.* 376:1060–1075.

35. Kooter, I.M., Koehler, B.P., Moguilevsky, N., et al. 1999. The Met243 sulfonium ion linkage is responsible for the anomalous magnetic circular dichroism and optical spectral properties of myeloperoxidase. *J. Biol. Inorg. Chem.* 4:684–691.

36. Fenna, R., Zeng, J., Davey, C. 1995. Structure of the green heme in myeloperoxidase. *Arch. Biophys. Biochem.* 316:653–656.

37. Grishkovskaya, I., Paumann-Page, M., Tscheliessnig, R. et al. 2017. Structure of human promyeloperoxidase (proMPO) and the role of the propeptide in processing and maturation. *J. Biol. Chem.* 292:8244–8261.

38. Auer, M., Nicolussi, A., Schütz, G. et al. 2014. How covalent heme to protein bonds influence the formation and reactivity of redox intermediates of a bacterial peroxidase. *J. Biol. Chem.* 289:31480–31491.

39. Oxvig, C., Thomsen, A.R., Overgaard, M.T. et al. 1999. Biochemical evidence for heme linkage through esters with Asp-93 and Glu-241 in human eosinophil peroxidase. The ester with Asp-93 is only partially formed in vivo. *J. Biol. Chem.* 274:16953–16958.

40. Fayadat, L., Niccoli-Sire, P., Lanet, J. et al. 1999. Role of heme in intracellular trafficking of thyroperoxidase and involvement of H_2O_2 generated at the apical surface of thyroid cells in autocatalytic covalent heme binding. *J. Biol. Chem.* 274:10533–10538.

41. DePillis, G.D., Ozaki, S., Kuo, J.M. et al. 1997. Autocatalytic processing of heme by lactoperoxidase produces the native protein-bound prosthetic group. *J. Biol. Chem.* 272:8857–8860.

42. Colas, C., Kuo, J.M., Ortiz de Montellano, P.R. 2002. Asp-225 and Glu-375 in autocatalytic attachment of the prosthetic heme group of lactoperoxidase. *J. Biol. Chem.* 277:7191–7200.

43. Paumann-Page, M., Katz, R.-S., Bellei, M. et al. 2017. Pre-steady-state kinetics reveal the substrate specificity and mechanism of halide oxidation of truncated human peroxidasin 1. *J. Biol. Chem.* 292:4583–4592.

44. Singh, P.K., Sirohi, H.V., Iqbal, N. et al. 2017. Structure of bovine lactoperoxidase with a partially linked heme moiety at 1.98 Å resolution. *Biochim. Biophys. Acta Proteins Proteom.* 1865:329–335.

45. Colas, C., Ortiz de Montellano, P.R. 2003. Autocatalytic radical reactions in physiological prosthetic heme modification. *Chem. Rev.* 103:2305–2332.

46. Ortiz de Montellano, P.R. 2016. Self-processing of peroxidases. in: E. Raven, B. Dunford (Eds.), *Heme Peroxidases*, 3–30. Royal Society of Chemistry, Cambridge, UK.

47. Colas, C., Ortiz de Montellano, P.R. 2004. Horseradish peroxidase mutants that autocatalytically modify their prosthetic heme group: Insights into mammalian peroxidase heme-protein covalent bonds. *J. Biol. Chem.* 279:24131–24140.

48. Kooter, I.M., Moguilevsky, N., Bollen, A. et al. 1999. Characterization of the Asp94 and Glu242 mutants in myeloperoxidase, the residues linking the heme group via ester bonds. *Eur. J. Biochem.* 264:211–217.

49. Zederbauer, M., Furtmüller, P.G., Bellei, M. et al. 2007. Disruption of the aspartate to heme ester linkage in human myeloperoxidase: Impact on ligand binding, redox chemistry, and interconversion of redox intermediates. *J. Biol. Chem.* 282:17041–17052.

50. Zederbauer, M., Furtmüller, P.G., Ganster, B. et al. 2007. The vinyl-sulfonium bond in human myeloperoxidase: Impact on Compound I formation and reduction by halides and thiocyanate. *Biochem. Biophys. Res. Commun.* 356:450–456.

51. Paumann-Page, M., Tscheliessnig, R., Sevcnikar, B. et al. 2020. Monomeric and homotrimeric solution structures of truncated human peroxidasin 1 variants. *Biochim. Biophys. Acta Proteins Proteom.* 1868:140249.

52. Banerjee, S., Stampler, J., Furtmüller, P.G. et al. 2011. Conformational and thermal stability of mature dimeric human myeloperoxidase and a recombinant monomeric form from CHO cells. *Biochim. Biophys. Acta Proteins Proteom.* 1814:375–387.

53. Banerjee, S., Furtmüller, P.G., Obinger, C. 2011. Bovine lactoperoxidase - a versatile one- and two-electron catalyst of high structural and thermal stability. *Biotechnol. J.* 6:231–243.

54. Furtmüller, P.G., Jantschko, W., Regelsberger, G. et al. 2002. Reaction of lactoperoxidase compound I with halides and thiocyanate. *Biochemistry* 41:11895–11900.

55. Smulevich, G., Neri, F., Willemsen, O. et al. 1995. Effect of the His175-Glu mutation on the heme pocket architecture of cytochrome *c* peroxidase. *Biochemistry* 34:13485–13490.

56. Furtmüller, P.G., Burner, U., Regelsberger, G. et al. 2000. Spectral and kinetic studies on the formation of eosinophil peroxidase compound I and its reaction with halides and thiocyanate. *Biochemistry* 39:15578–15584.

57. Wever, R., Plat, H. 1981. Spectral properties of myeloperoxidase and its ligand complexes. *Biochim. Biophys. Acta Proteins Proteom.* 661:235–239.

58. Kooter, I.M., Moguilevsky, N., Bollen, A. et al. 1999. The sulfonium ion linkage in myeloperoxidase. Direct spectroscopic detection by isotopic labeling and effect of mutation. *J. Biol. Chem.* 274:26794–26802.

59. Zederbauer, M., Furtmüller, P.G., Ganster, B. et al. 2007. The vinyl-sulfonium bond in human myeloperoxidase: Impact on compound I formation and reduction by halides and thiocyanate. *Biochem. Biophys. Res. Commun.* 356:450–456.

60. Brogioni, S., Feis, A., Marzocchi, M.P. et al. 2006. Resonance Raman assignment of myeloperoxidase and the selected mutants Asp94Val and Met243Thr. Effect of the heme distortion. *J. Raman Spectrosc.* 37:263–276.

61. Zederbauer, M., Jantschko, W., Neugschwandtner, K. et al. 2005. Role of the covalent glutamic acid 242-heme linkage in the formation and reactivity of redox intermediates of human myeloperoxidase. *Biochemistry* 44:6482–6491.

62. Zederbauer, M., Furtmüller, P.G., Bellei, M. et al. 2007. Disruption of the aspartate to heme ester linkage in human myeloperoxidase: Impact on ligand binding, redox chemistry, and interconversion of redox intermediates. *J. Biol. Chem.* 282:17041–17052.

63. Suriano, G., Watanabe, S., Ghibaudi, E. et al. 2001. Glu375Gln and Asp225Val mutants: About the nature of the covalent linkages between heme group and apo-protein in bovine lactoperoxidase. *Bioorg. Med. Chem. Lett.* 11:2827–2831.

64. Floris, R., Mogulevsky, N., Puppels, G. et al. 1995. Heme-protein interaction in myeloperoxidase: Modification of spectroscopic properties and catalytic activity by single residue mutation. *J. Am. Chem. Soc.* 117:3907–3912.

65. Jantschko, W., Furtmüller, P.G., Zederbauer, M. et al. 2005. Reaction of ferrous lactoperoxidase with hydrogen peroxide and dioxygen: An anaerobic stopped-flow study. *Arch. Biochem. Biophys.* 434:51–59.

66. Ohlsson, P.I. 1984. Lactoperoxidase, a dithionite ion dismutase. *Eur. J. Biochem.* 142:233–238.

67. Abu-Soud, H.M., Hazen, S.L. 2001. Interrogation of heme pocket environment of mammalian peroxidases with diatomic ligands. *Biochemistry* 40:10747–10755.

68. Smulevich, G., Feis, A., Howes, B.D. 2005. Fifteen years of Raman spectroscopy of engineered heme containing peroxidases: What have we learned. *Acc. Chem. Res.* 38:433–440.

69. Kitagawa, T., Hashimoto, S., Teraoka, J., et al. 1983. Distinct heme-substrate interactions of lactoperoxidase probed by resonance Raman spectroscopy: Difference between animal and plant peroxidases. *Biochemistry* 22:2788–2792.

70. Kitagawa, K., Nagai, K., Tsubaki, M. 1979. Assignment of the Fe-epsilon (His F8) stretching band in the resonance Raman spectra of deoxy myoglobin. *FEBS Lett.* 104:376–378.

71. Battistuzzi, G., Bellei, M., Bortolotti, C.A., et al. 2010. Redox properties of heme peroxidases. *Arch. Biochem. Biophys.* 500:21–36.

72. Battistuzzi, G., Borsari, M., Ranieri, J. et al. 2001. Redox thermodynamic of the Fe^{3+}/Fe^{2+} couple in horseradish peroxidase and its cyanide complex. *J. Am. Chem. Soc.* 124:26–27.

73. Battistuzzi, G., Bellei, M., Zederbauer, M., et al. 2006. Redox thermodynamics of the Fe(III)/Fe(II) couple of human myeloperoxidase in its high-spin and low-spin forms. *Biochemistry* 45:12750–12755.

74. Furtmüller, P.G., Jantschko, W., Regelsberger, G. et al. 2001. A transient kinetic study on the reactivity of recombinant unprocessed monomeric myeloperoxidase. *FEBS Lett.* 503:147–150.

75. Malle, E., Furtmüller, P.G., Sattler, W. et al. 2007. Myeloperoxidase: A target for new drug development? *Br. J. Pharmacol.* 152:838–854.

76. Battistuzzi, G., Bellei, M., Vlasits, J. et al. 2010. Redox thermodynamics of lactoperoxidase and eosinophil peroxidase. *Arch. Biochem. Biophys.* 494:72–77.

77. Brogioni, S., Stampler, J., Furtmüller, P.G. et al. 2008. The role of the sulfonium linkage in the stabilization of the ferrous form of myeloperoxidase: A comparison with lactoperoxidase. *Biochim. Biophys. Acta Proteins Proteom.* 1784:843–849.

78. Farhangrazi, Z.S. Fossett, M.E. Powers, L.S. et al. 1995. Variable-temperature spectro-electrochemical study of horseradish peroxidase. *Biochemistry* 34:2866–2871.

79. Furtmüller, P.G., Arnhold, J., Jantschko, W. et al. 2005. Standard reduction potentials of all couples of the peroxidase cycle of lactoperoxidase. *J. Inorg. Biochem.* 99:1220–1229.

80. Arnhold, J., Furtmüller, P.G., Regelsberger, G. et al. 2001. Redox properties of the couple Compound I/native enzyme of myeloperoxidase and eosinophil peroxidase. *Eur. J. Biochem.* 268:5142–5148.

81. Furtmüller, P.G., Arnhold, J., Jantschko, W. et al. 2003. Redox properties of the couples Compound I/Compound II and Compound II/native enzyme of human myeloperoxidase. *Biochem. Biophys. Res. Commun.* 301:551–557.

82. Arnhold, J., Furtmüller, P.G., Obinger, C. 2003. Redox properties of myeloperoxidase. *Redox Rep.* 8:179–186.

83. Jantschko, W., Furtmüller, P.G., Zederbauer, M. et al. 2005. Exploitation of the unusual thermodynamic properties of human myeloperoxidase in inhibitor design. *Biochem. Pharmacol.* 69:1149–1157.

84. Poulos, T.L., Kraut, J. 1980. The stereochemistry of peroxidase catalysis. *J. Biol. Chem.* 255:8199–8205.

85. Marquez, L.A., Huang, J.T., Dunford, H.B. 1994. Spectral and kinetic studies on the formation of myeloperoxidase compounds I and II: Roles of hydrogen peroxide and superoxide. *Biochemistry* 33:1447–1454.

86. Furtmüller, P.G., Burner, U., Obinger, C. 1998. Reaction of myeloperoxidase compound I with chloride, bromide, iodide, and thiocyanate. *Biochemistry* 37:17923–17930.

87. Furtmüller, P.G., Burner, U., Regelsberger, G. et al. 2000. Spectral and kinetic studies on the formation of eosinophil peroxidase Compound I and its reaction with halides and thiocyanate. *Biochemistry* 39:15578–15584.

88. Furtmüller, P.G., Obinger, C., Hsuanyu, Y. et al. 2000. Mechanism of reaction of myeloperoxidase with hydrogen peroxide and chloride ion. *Eur. J. Biochem.* 267:5858–5864.

89. Lee, H.C., Booth, K.S., Caughey, W.S. et al. 1991. Interaction of halides with the cyanide complex of myeloperoxidase: A model for substrate binding to Compound I. *Biochim. Biophys. Acta* 1076:317–320.

90. Ramos, D.R., García, M.V., Canle, M.V. et al. 2007. Myeloperoxidase-catalyzed taurine chlorination: Initial versus equilibrium rate. *Arch. Biochem. Biophys.* 466:221–233.

91. Jantschko, W., Furtmüller, P.G., Allegra, M. et al. 2002. Redox intermediates of plant and mammalian peroxidases: A comparative transient-kinetic study of their reactivity toward indole derivatives. *Arch. Biochem. Biophys.* 398:12–22.

92. Furtmüller, P.G., Jantschko, W., Regelsberger, G. et al. 2001. Spectral and kinetic studies on eosinophil peroxidase compounds I and II and their reaction with ascorbate and tyrosine. *Biochim. Biophys. Acta* 1548:121–128.

93. Marquez, L.A., Dunford, H.B. 1995. Kinetics of oxidation of tyrosine and dityrosine by myeloperoxidase Compounds I and II. Implications for lipoprotein peroxidation. *Studies J. Biol. Chem.* 270:30434–30440.

94. Roman, R., Dunford, H.B. 1972. pH dependence of the oxidation of iodide by compound I of horseradish peroxidase. *Biochemistry* 11:2017–2079.

95. Ralston, I., Dunford, H.B. 1978. Horseradish peroxidase. XXXII. pH dependence of the oxidation of L-(-)-tyrosine by compound I. *Can. J. Biochem.* 56:1115–1119.

96. Sevcnikar, B., Paumann-Page, M., Hofbauer, S. et al. 2020. Reaction of human peroxidasin 1 compound 1 and compound II with one-electron donors. *Arch. Biochem. Biophys.* 681:108267.

97. Brück, T.B., Felding, R.J., Symons, M.C.R. et al. 2001. Mechanism of nitrite-stimulated catalysis of lactoperoxidase. *Eur. J. Biochem.* 268:3214–3222.

98. Burner, U., Furtmüller, P.G., Kettle, A.J. et al. 2000. Mechanism of reaction of myeloperoxidase with nitrite. *J. Biol. Chem.* 275:20597–20601.

99. Van Dalen, C., Winterbourne, C.C., Kettle, A.J. 2006. Mechanism of nitrite oxidation by eosinophil peroxidase: Implications for oxidant production and nitration by eosinophils. *Biochem. J.* 394:707–713.

100. Soubhye, J., Prevost, J.M., Van Antwerpen, P. et al. 2010. Structure-based design, synthesis, and pharmacological evaluation of 3-(aminoalkyl)-5-fluoroindoles as myeloperoxidase inhibitors. *J. Med. Chem.* 53:8747–8759.

101. Aldib, I., Soubhye, J., Zouaoui Boudjeltia, K. et al. 2012. Evaluation of new scaffolds of myeloperoxidase inhibitors by rational design combined with high-throughput virtual screening. *J. Med. Chem.* 55:7208–7218.

102. Soubhye, J., Aldiba, I., Elfving, B. et al. 2013. Design, synthesis, and structure-activity relationship studies of novel 3-alkylindole derivatives as selective and highly potent myeloperoxidase inhibitors. *J. Med. Chem.* 56: 3944–3958.

CHAPTER TWO

Biosynthesis of Mammalian Heme Proteins, Peroxidases, and NADPH Oxidases

William M. Nauseef
University of Iowa

CONTENTS

ABBREVIATIONS

CCP:	Complement control protein
CGD:	Chronic granulomatous disease
CLN:	Calnexin
CRT:	Calreticulin
DUOX:	Dual oxidase
EGF:	Epidermal growth factor
EPO:	Eosinophil peroxidase
ER:	Endoplasmic reticulum
Eros:	essential for reactive oxygen species
FAD:	Flavin adenine dinucleotide
FRD:	Ferric reductases
HEK:	Human embryonal kidney
LPO:	Lactoperoxidase
MPO:	Myeloperoxidase
NADPH:	Nicotinamide adenine dinucleotide phosphate
NEM:	N-ethylmaleimide
NOX:	NADPH oxidase
PRR:	Proline-rich region
SH3:	src homology 3
TPO:	Thyroid peroxidase

DOI: 10.1201/9781003212287-3

INTRODUCTION

Many physiologic processes depend on a collaboration between members of two important protein families, namely heme peroxidases and NADPH oxidases (NOX proteins). The fundamental biochemistry whereby a peroxidase utilizes H_2O_2 generated by a NOX enzyme to modify a substrate figures widely throughout biology. A few examples demonstrate the extent of this biochemical principle in biology. Cross-linking of extracellular matrix with dityrosine bond formation catalyzed by ovoperoxidase in the presence of H_2O_2 from the dual oxidase Udx1 protects the fertilized sea urchin egg from polyspermy [1,2]. A DUOX enzyme in *Rhodnius prolixus*, a vector for Chagas disease, provides the H_2O_2 in ovarian follicle epithelium to support peroxidase-dependent tyrosine cross-linking to harden the insect eggshell [3]. The reaction of myeloperoxidase (MPO) with H_2O_2 from NOX2 oxidizes chloride to create the potent microbicide HOCl and promotes optimal oxygen-dependent antimicrobial activity in human neutrophils [4]. In the presence of H_2O_2 derived from DUOX2, thyroid peroxidase (TPO) oxidizes iodide and produces thyroid hormone, and the absence or dysfunction of either TPO or DUOX2 results in thyroid hormone deficiency and clinical hypothyroidism (reviewed in Ref. [5]). Hypothiocyanate produced in airways by lactoperoxidase (LPO) and DUOX-generated H_2O_2 contributes to the antimicrobial activity in the respiratory tract [reviewed in Refs. [6,7]. Although there are other examples of physiology and pathology that result from the joint activities of peroxidases and NADPH oxidases, these few illustrate the remarkably diverse biology dependent on these enzymes.

This review summarizes features of the biosynthesis of specific members of these two protein families. Where possible, features shared by peroxidases and NOX proteins are highlighted, as are those areas where understanding of specific steps is lacking.

PEROXIDASES

Members of the Chordata peroxidase subfamily [8], MPO, eosinophil peroxidase (EPO), LPO, and TPO, participate in many physiologic processes. Initially purified from the pyometra of experimentally infected dogs and named by its discoverer Kjell Agner verdoperoxidase because of its intense green color [9], MPO has been extensively studied, with advances in elucidating its structure, biochemistry, and activities in physiologic and pathologic settings (reviewed in Refs. [4,10,11]). Similarly, its biosynthesis has been examined in considerable detail using both cultured cells producing endogenous MPO and heterologous systems expressing wild-type or mutant MPO (reviewed in Ref. [12]). Biosynthesis of the two related peroxidase family members that like MPO are soluble enzymes, EPO and LPO, has been studied less extensively than has MPO but likely shares many features.

Myeloperoxidase

MPO constitutes ~2%–5% of the dry weight of human neutrophils [9,13], where MPO reaches millimolar concentrations in the azurophilic granules along with serine proteases and other enzymes that contribute to antimicrobial defense [14]. The $MPO/H_2O_2/Cl^-$ system generates the potent microbicide HOCl (reviewed in Ref. [11]), and X-ray crystal structure has demonstrated direct binding of halides, including chloride, bromide, iodide, and the pseudohalide thiocyanate, to the enzyme active site ([15,16] and reviewed in Ref. [17]). Under normal circumstances, MPO biosynthesis occurs only during the promyelocytic stage of myeloid differentiation in the bone marrow [18–22] and terminates as more mature myeloid cells arise [23]. Mature MPO is a glycosylated homodimer, with each monomer composed of a heavy (59-kDa) and a light (13.5-kDa) subunit, and the dimer linked together by a single disulfide bond between C319 in the heavy subunit of each monomer. A single heme prosthetic group in each half of MPO has three covalent bonds to the peptide backbone (D280, E408, M409[1]). The two ester bonds are conserved in EPO, LPO, and TPO, but the sulfonium linkage at M409 is unique to MPO and is responsible for its signature spectral properties and chlorinating potential [15,24–26]. In the endoplasmic reticulum (ER), nascent apoproMPO, the heme-free precursor of mature MPO, undergoes N-linked glycosylation at six sites, one in the propeptide (N139) and five in what will be

---

[1] Numbering of amino acid residues uses that of human MPO and includes the 41 amino acid presumed signal peptide plus the 125 amino acid propeptide.

the heavy subunit of the mature enzyme, to generate a 90-kDa product (Figure 2.1).

Removal of oligosaccharides side chains by treatment with glycosidases reduces binding to ceruloplasmin, chlorinating activity, and staphylocidal action [27,28]. Perhaps more clinically relevant is the contribution of glycosylation to the immunogenicity of human MPO in the context of vasculitic disorders secondary to anti-neutrophil cytoplasmic autoantibodies (ANCA, reviewed in Ref. [29]). Carbohydrate analysis of tryptic digests of recombinant MPO demonstrates heterogeneity among the glycans recovered. A detailed analysis of human MPO isolated from healthy subjects highlights features that are relatively uncommon for extracellular glycoproteins, including phosphorylated high-mannose forms and truncated small glycans [30]. The authors propose that atypical oligosaccharides on MPO, released into the circulation from neutrophils, may contribute to the promotion of ANCA-related disease. Several studies support the notion that the glycosylation of MPO in the pathogenesis of ANCA vasculitis [31], a topic reviewed in Free et al. (see Chapter 16 in this book).

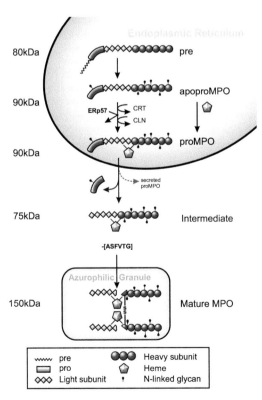

Figure 2.1 Schematic summary of myeloperoxidase biosynthesis.

In the context of biosynthesis, glycosylation serves an important service in the stability and productive folding of MPO precursors during their long half-life in the ER [32–34]. ApoproMPO associates transiently with several ER molecular chaperones, including ERp57, calreticulin, and calnexin, presumably in part via interactions with oligosaccharide side chains on apoproMPO, and inhibition of N-linked glycosylation by tunicamycin prevents these associations [35–37]. Missense mutations in MPO result in prolonged interactions between molecular chaperones and MPO precursors and their retention in the ER, thus suggesting a role of the chaperones in quality control in MPO synthesis [38–42]. Of note, whereas ERp57, calreticulin, and calnexin associate with apoproMPO, only calnexin interacts also with proMPO. Furthermore, calnexin retains in the ER MPO mutants that fail to incorporate heme, a finding that suggests a role for calnexin in heme incorporation into apoproMPO [36].

In studies of MPO biosynthesis employing in vitro culture systems, incorporation of heme into apoproMPO to produce the enzymatically active proMPO is the rate-limiting step and a prerequisite for the transport of precursors out of the ER en route to production of mature MPO [43–45]. Analysis of the crystal structure of proMPO demonstrates the presence of features nearly identical to those in mature MPO [46], indicating that the process of heme incorporation is effectively completed within the ER. As in mature MPO, three covalent bonds link the heme group to the peptide backbone in proMPO. The autocatalytic oxidation that promotes ester bond formation requires a source of H_2O_2 ([47,48] and reviewed in Ref. [26]), which may be ER oxidoreductase Ero1 (reviewed in Ref. [49]) or, as discussed later, NOX4 [50].

ProMPO exits the ER destined for one of two fates. Approximately 10% of the proMPO produced in a variety of experimental settings, including human bone marrow cultured in vitro [51], stable cell lines of myeloid precursors [37,52–56], or in heterologously transfected cell lines [57–59], is secreted constitutively. Although the specific activities of intracellular and secreted proMPO are identical [60] and the same as that of mature MPO [46], the two species of proMPO differ with respect to their glycosylation. In contrast to the carbohydrate side chains on intracellular proMPO, which retain their high mannose structure [56,61,62], secreted proMPO has some

N-linked oligosaccharides that are modified during passage through the Golgi and are complex [55], the functional significance of which is not defined at this time.

The 116 amino acid propeptide of proMPO contributes to structural stability within the ER but does not serve to direct the precursor to its final destination in the neutrophil azurophilic granule. Chimeric proteins with the propeptide at the N-terminus are not redirected to different cellular compartments [54,55,63], and the propeptide alone does not function as an intramolecular chaperone [54]. Instead, the propeptide serves a critical role in the eventual homodimerization of MPO precursors [46].

ProMPO possesses seven disulfide bonds, one more than is present in mature MPO. The additional bond links C158 in the propeptide with C319 in the eventual heavy subunit [46]. Rearrangement of disulfide bonds results in formation of C319-C319 linkage and creation of a dimer, leaving C158 unpaired. A subtilisin-like proprotein convertase cleaves the propeptide from proMPO to generate a short-lived 75-kDa intermediate species that is enzymatically active (vide infra). The identity of the convertase responsible for proprotein cleavage remains unknown, and its characterization as a subtilisin-like enzyme rests on studies using the inhibitor CMK-RVKR and site-directed mutagenesis of a presumed convertase target motif in proMPO.

Using single-letter abbreviations for the amino acids, the motif recognized by proprotein convertases is $(K/R) -X_n-(K/R)$, where X is any amino acid (although rarely C) and $n = 0, 2, 4,$ or 6 residues [64–66]. The propeptide in proMPO contains a sequence consistent with the motif, ^{128}RKLRSLWR^{136}, where n could be 0, 2, or 6. Addition of CMK-RVKR to cultured transfectants expressing wild-type MPO blocks biosynthesis at the proMPO stage, as does site-directed mutagenesis of residues in the putative cleavage site [59]. The presumed convertase cleavage site is exposed in the crystal structure of proMPO [46], thus rendering it accessible to proteolytic attack.

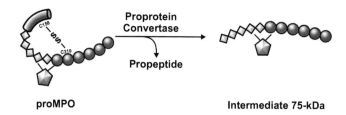

Figure 2.2 Propeptide cleavage from proMPO.

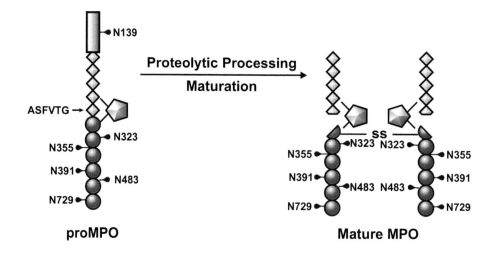

Figure 2.3 Steps in conversion of proMPO to mature MPO.

Just as the specific convertase responsible for propeptide cleavage remains unidentified, the subcellular compartment where processing occurs is unknown. Proteolytic removal of the propeptide occurs after proMPO exits the ER, since brefeldin A, an agent that disrupts ER-Golgi transport [67–69], blocks processing of proMPO [43]. Seminal studies by Akin and Kinkade demonstrate the presence of a 74-kDa MPO-related protein generated by processing of proMPO in granules at neutral pH [53,70]. Inhibition of cysteine protease activity with N-acetyl-leucyl-leucyl-methionine, N-acetyl-leucyl-leucyl-norleucine, or E64 blocks processing of the 75-kDa intermediate to mature MPO [59]. Presumably, an endopeptidase with cysteine protease action mediates excision of the hexapeptide ASFVTG from the 75-kDa species to yield the mature MPO protomer with heavy and light subunits. Of note, the ASFVTG peptide is on the surface of the crystal structure of proMPO [46] and thus accessible for excision.

Taken together, available evidence suggests that three processing events – namely removal of the propeptide, dimerization, and excision of ASFVTG (illustrated in Figure 2.3) – occur in a post-ER compartment that is enriched in preparations of granules from human promyelocytes [53,70,71]. Whether removal of ASFVTG precedes or follows dimerization is unknown.

BIOSYNTHESIS OF RELATED PEROXIDASES

As closely related members of the Chordata peroxidase protein subfamily, MPO, EPO, LPO, and TPO share features in the heme-binding pocket, including two ester linkages between the heme and the protein, and additional conserved motifs essential to the structure and function of the mammalian peroxidases (reviewed in detail in Ref. [8]). However, the individual peroxidases differ in their structural organization, subcellular location, and tissue distribution (Table 2.1).

Eosinophil Peroxidase

EPO shares the most sequence homology with MPO and has N-linked oligosaccharides on two of its four potential glycosylation sites, both homologous with two sites in MPO (N355, N391) [72]. The propeptide of EPO has 67% identity with the MPO propeptide and includes a proconvertase cleavage site motif sequence, EKLQPQRS, where n in the motif equals 4. Biosynthetic radiolabeling studies using human bone marrow cells [73] or transfected K562 cells [74] demonstrate the presence of an ~80-kDa precursor that undergoes proteolytic processing to yield mature EPO, a heterodimer with heavy (55-kDa) and light (15-kDa) chains [73,75–78].

Esterification of the heme linkages is incomplete in EPO purified from eosinophils of individuals with eosinophilia, with fewer than one-third of molecules having links to the D232 in the light chain (the homologue of D260 in MPO) [79]. In contrast, linkage at E380 in the heavy subunit (homologue of E408 in MPO) is always present. Of note, addition of exogenous H_2O_2 drives formation of the ester linkage to the light chain, consistent with the autocatalytic reaction described as the general mechanism for heme group incorporation into mammalian peroxidases [47]. However, approximately threefold more H_2O_2 is required to complete ester linkage formation in EPO compared with that for LPO [79], suggesting that the process is less efficient in EPO than in LPO. The structural and functional implications of the different efficiency of esterification by added H_2O_2 or of the infrequency of ester linkage to the light subunit of endogenous EPO have not been elucidated.

The overall pattern of disulfide bonds in EPO mirrors that in MPO. EPO possesses intramolecular disulfide bonds in both the light (1) and heavy (5) subunits but, as in MPO, none is between the light and heavy subunits. Two unpaired cysteine

TABLE 2.1

Features of mammalian peroxidases

Peroxidase	Organization	State	Location	Tissue/cell
MPO	Homodimer	Soluble	Granule	Neutrophil/monocyte
EPO	Monomer	Soluble	Granule	Eosinophil
LPO	Monomer	Soluble	Secreted	Airway surface liquid, milk, tears, saliva, vaginal secretions
TPO	Homodimer	Transmembrane	Plasma membrane	thyrocytes

residues in EPO, C131 and C291 are equivalent to C158 and C319 in MPO, the cysteines with critical roles in proMPO stability and dimerization [46]. Further study needs to determine if an intramolecular bond between C131 in the propeptide of proEPO and C291 in the heavy subunit contributes to proEPO proteolytic maturation in the same way as the C158–C319 disulfide does in proMPO.

Lactoperoxidase

Present in secretions, including airway surface liquid, milk, tears, saliva, and vaginal fluids, LPO contributes to the natural antimicrobial activity in these bodily fluids (reviewed in Refs. [80,81]). Recent interest has highlighted the synergy between LPO and the H_2O_2-generating NOX protein family member DUOX as an important physiologic feature of airway host defense [6,7]. Studies of LPO structure frequently utilize enzyme isolated from milk because of the high concentrations, ~30 mg/L in bovine milk, and ease of purification. Observations from structural and functional studies using recombinant LPO expressed in CHO cells [82] or Sf9 insect cells [83] parallel those made on enzyme purified from natural sources. However, the lack of in vitro culture systems to express LPO has limited study of its biosynthesis. Splice variants for LPO have been identified in cultured primary airway epithelial cells [84], and recombinant LPO expressed in CHO cells recapitulates the 4 N-linked sites seen in native LPO but lacks the expected O-glycosylation present in the naturally occurring enzyme [82].

The distal heme-binding site in LPO preferentially binds SCN^- as opposed to Cl^- (as in MPO) and supports the generation of $OSCN^-$ by LPO in the presence of H_2O_2 [85], a property that contributes to the observed antimicrobial action of LPO in the respiratory tract. LPO contains a site for high-affinity binding of calcium, and removal of calcium from purified LPO results in its precipitation and loss of activity [86]. The calcium-binding site is conserved among the peroxidases [8] and resides near the distal histidine in the heme-binding pocket [87]. Site-directed mutagenesis of the site in LPO (or MPO) markedly decreases secretion of the recombinant protein from Sf9 cells [87], suggesting that the integrity of the calcium-binding site may be critical for proper folding of the precursor and productive biosynthesis of LPO.

Thyroid Peroxidase

Expressed in the apical membrane of thyrocytes and the only member of the peroxidase protein family that is a transmembrane protein, TPO has two additional features not seen in the other members of the mammalian peroxidases, namely a complement control protein (CCP)-like motif and an epidermal growth factor (EGF)-like domain in its C-terminus [88]. In the presence of H_2O_2 generated by DUOX2, TPO catalyzes the iodination of thyroglobulin (reviewed in Ref. [89]), and its dysfunction or absence results in hypothyroidism [90,91]. In addition, TPO can serve as an antigenic target for autoantibody production in the development of autoimmune thyroid disease (reviewed in Ref. [30]), and several structural features have been suggested to drive its antigenicity [92].

Heme incorporation and N-linked glycosylation of proTPO occur in the ER, and heme acquisition is a prerequisite for its exit from the ER and targeting to the plasma membrane [93]. Glycosylation of proTPO supports its interactions with several ER molecular chaperones, including calreticulin, calnexin, ERp57, and BiP [94–96]. After proTPO exits the ER, O-glycosylation and propeptide cleavage occur [97]. The role of the propeptide in the biosynthesis or integrity of TPO is unclear, as studies using CHO transfectants have yielded conflicting results. One study found that propeptide deletion mutants are not enzymatically active or properly delivered to the plasma membrane [97], whereas another group reported that propeptide deletion mutants behave just as the holoprotein does with respect to activity and targeting [98]. The basis for these conflicting findings is unknown, as are the roles of propeptide in the production, targeting, or activity of TPO.

Structural data regarding TPO are limited to those from analysis of crystals of baculovirus-expressed recombinant TPO [99] and enzyme purified from patients with Graves' disease [100]. Mature TPO exists as a homodimer in thyrocyte plasma membrane, with a single disulfide at C296 binding the monomers [92,101]. Of note, C296 is equivalent to C319 in MPO, echoing a recurrent feature in the structure of members of this peroxidase family.

NOX PROTEINS

NADPH oxidases (NOX) are heme-containing integral membrane proteins that operate as electron transferases in a wide variety of living organisms, shuttling electrons from cytoplasmic NADPH, via flavin adenine dinucleotide (FAD), sequentially across two heme groups to molecular oxygen to generate superoxide anion (reviewed in Refs. [102–104]). Homologues of ferric reductases (FRD) [105], NOX proteins possess 6 or 7 transmembrane helices and a cytosolic carboxy terminus with domains that bind FAD and NADPH [106], factors essential for enzyme activity.

The two heme groups in NOX2 are stacked, with one closer to the cytoplasmic side of the membrane and the other closer to the extracytoplasmic surface, and inequivalent, with $E_{m7}=-225$ and $-265\,mV$ [107]. Although the structure of the heme-binding transmembrane regions of NOX proteins has not been elucidated, Magnani et al. have solved the crystal structure of the transmembrane helical domain of NOX5 from the cyanobacterium *Cylindrospermum stagnale* [108] (csNOX5), which has 40% sequence identity to human NOX5 [109]. The red shift in spectroscopy of the reduced csNOX5 suggests the presence of hexacoordination of the hemes; H313-H385 and H299-H372 in helices 3 and 5 support the outer and inner heme groups, respectively. Of note, the pairs of histidines identified in csNOX5 are conserved in human NOX2 (H115-H222 and H101-H209). Indirect evidence based on the effect of mutagenesis of these histidines on the production of functional NOX2 in cultured human promyelocytic cells implicated these specific histidines as the sites of heme coordination [110]. It is likely, but not demonstrated, that the same organization of hemes applies to all members of the NOX protein family.

Despite similarities in structure and shared purpose in electron transfer for FRD and NOX proteins, the homologues have distinct activities. For example, NOX2 and FRE1, the ferric reductase of *Saccharomyces cerevisiae* [111], are structural homologues, share similar spectral properties, and have low redox potentials but deliver electrons to different targets, oxygen in the case of NOX2 and Fe^{+3} for FRE1. FRE1 has the capacity to reduce oxygen, albeit inefficiently (20–100 pmol min^{-1} (mg wet weight)$^{-1}$ [112]), but NOX2 lacks detectable ferric reductase activity [113]. Detailed description of structural features that distinguish members of the FRD superfamily and the evolution of the FRD domain within the context of NOX proteins has been reviewed recently [109].

NOX proteins transport electrons from cytoplasmic NADPH across membranes (plasma, phagosomal, or endosomal) to molecular oxygen to generate superoxide anion as the immediate product (reviewed in Ref. [114]):

$$NADPH + 2O_2 \rightarrow NADP^+ + 2O_2^-$$

Depending on the cellular context, superoxide anion can be consumed to produce other oxidants, including H_2O_2, HOCl, or peroxynitrite.

NOX2

The recognition that chronic granulomatous disease (CGD), a rare clinical disorder with significant morbidity and mortality (reviewed in Ref. [115]), reflects the inability of neutrophils to generate oxidants to fuel killing of ingested microbes catalyzed the discovery and characterization of NOX2 (the history reviewed in Ref. [116]). In addition to the strong biomedical incentive to understand the biochemical basis of the inherited defect, the robust activity of the enzyme complex plus the ease with which large numbers of functional neutrophils can be isolated from human blood facilitated work by investigators to elucidate features of the phagocyte oxidase. Studies over the past two decades have identified NOX2 expression in non-phagocytes and have expanded to include its role in cell signaling in addition to supporting microbicidal action [117].

Encoded by CYBB, NOX2 (aka gp91^{phox}) is a glycosylated integral membrane protein produced in the ER. Studies of its biosynthesis using the cultured human promyelocytic cell line PLB-985 [118] demonstrate a 55-kDa primary translation product that undergoes co-translational N-linked glycosylation and association with p22^{phox} to produce the heterodimer gp65-p22^{phox} [110,119–121]. It is important to appreciate that unlike human NOX2, the murine protein is not glycosylated and remains a 55-kDa protein in association with p22^{phox} [122,123]. Maturation of the carbohydrate side chains of gp65 to generate the gp91^{phox} found in mature human neutrophils occurs after exit from the ER and during transit through the Golgi. Although glycosylation is not required for heterodimer formation or catalytic activity [121], successful advance from ER to Golgi requires two interrelated modifications in the ER that are essential for the activity of NOX2. First, heterodimer formation stabilizes the individual subunits and is prerequisite for NOX2 maturation and targeting. Most patients with CGD due to mutations in either *CYBB* or *CYBA*, the gene encoding p22^{phox}, lack both gp91^{phox} and p22^{phox}; free gp65 and p22^{phox} do not exit the ER [115,124–126]. Second, nascent gp65 must acquire heme. When PLB-985 cells are cultured in the presence of the heme synthesis inhibitor succinyl acetone, heterodimers fail to form, and the unassociated subunits are degraded [121]. If and how heme acquisition promotes heterodimer formation remain unknown.

Recently published work has described a novel protein that plays an essential role in the biosynthesis of NOX2. Thomas et al. have reported that Eros (essential for reactive oxygen species), an ortholog of a protein required for the expression of components of the photosynthetic photosystem I complex in plants, contributes to the stability of the gp91^{phox}-p22^{phox} heterodimer in the ER [127]. In mice that lack Eros expression, the gp91^{phox}-p22^{phox} heterodimer protein is reduced despite no change in mRNA, thus suggesting that Eros regulates in some way gp91^{phox}-p22^{phox} heterodimer degradation. Flag-tagged Eros coprecipitates with gp91^{phox} in the ER of HEK293 transfectants, thereby functioning as a molecular chaperone. Underscoring the biological and clinical relevance of Eros in NOX2 biosynthesis, two laboratories have independently identified patients with mutations in CYBC1, the gene encoding Eros, who have the clinical phenotype of CGD [128,129]. Whether biosynthesis of other members of the NOX protein family similarly depend on the presence of Eros in ER is currently unknown.

Other NOX Protein Family Members

Like NOX2, mature and functional forms of NOX1, NOX3, and NOX4 exist as heterodimers associated with p22^{phox}. NOX1, NOX2, and NOX3 similarly share a dependence on cytoplasmic subunits for maximal agonist-dependent activity, although the specific factors for NOX2 differ from those for NOX1 and NOX3 (reviewed in Ref. [130]).

For NOX proteins 1–4, the association of p22^{phox} with heme-containing NOX precursors occurs in the ER and serves at least two purposes. First, heterodimer formation provides stability to nascent NOX proteins in the ER and permits subsequent trafficking out of ER and successful targeting to its subcellular destination. Second, once finally in the targeted membranes, p22^{phox} provides a docking site for assembly of cytoplasmic subunits by virtue of interactions between its proline-rich region (PRR) and src-homology 3 (SH3) domains of p47^{phox} (for NOX2) or NOXO1 (for NOX1 and NOX3). Evidence for these two features rests on a variety of experimental approaches, including site-directed mutagenesis, transfections with specific mutants in PRR of p22^{phox}, and use of siRNA [131–134].

NOX1

NOX1 directly interacts with p22^{phox}, and mutations in histidines necessary for heme acquisition block its targeting and activity [132,135]. Furthermore, CRISPR/cas9-mediated suppression of endogenous p22^{phox} in transfectants expressing NOX1 eliminates NOX1 activity [136], demonstrating that the requirement for NOX1-p22^{phox} heterodimer is not an artifact of using heterologous expression systems. The latter point is an important one, since plasma membrane expression of terminally tagged NOX1 occurs in CHO transfectants independent of p22^{phox} [137]. The affinity of p22^{phox} for NOX1 appears to be less than that for NOX2, but co-expression of p22^{phox} results in maturation of N-linked oligosaccharides in NOX1. Unglycosylated mutants of NOX1 target to plasma membrane and support depressed superoxide production, demonstrating that glycosylation is not required for either property of the heterodimer [137,138].

NOX3

Expressed exclusively in spiral ganglions and the vestibular and cochlear epithelia [139], NOX3 serves a very specialized role in otoconial development [140,141]. Consequently, NOX3 biosynthesis has been the subject of relatively few studies. Transfected in human embryonic kidney cells (HEK-293) in the presence of required cytoplasmic subunits, NOX3 associates with p22^{phox} in the ER, localizes to the plasma membrane, and is functional [142]. Furthermore, siRNA targeting of p22^{phox} or co-expression of p22^{phox} with mutations in PRR blocks the oxidase activity of NOX3-expressing transfectants [132,143]. NOX3 is constitutively active, but only at very low levels, and its activity is greatly amplified by co-expression of cytosolic cofactors NOXO1 and NOXA1 [144], thus demonstrating the essential role of p22^{phox} association for productive delivery to target membranes and to support assembly of the soluble components at the cytoplasmic face of the membrane.

NOX4

The structural organization of NOX4 resembles that of NOX1, 2, and 3 in that association with p22^{phox} is required [50,135,145,146], and heme incorporation in the ER is a prerequisite for formation of a functional heterodimer [147]. However, in contrast to the other NOX proteins, NOX4 is constitutively active [148] and does not depend on cytoplasmic subunits for activity [149,150]. NOX4 possesses many of the structural features conserved across the NOX protein family and supports electron transfer from NADPH to FAD and then sequentially across the two heme groups coordinated within transmembrane helices. Because heme supports only single electron transfers, NOX4 must generate a superoxide anion as the initial product of oxygen reduction. However, H_2O_2 is the product of NOX4 activity typically recovered [150], a consequence perhaps of the action of one of the extracytoplasmic loops providing superoxide dismutase-like activity and thereby promoting dismutation of the superoxide anion to H_2O_2.

Expressed in plasma membranes, NOX4 has been detected also in mitochondria [151], nucleus [152], cytoskeleton [153], and ER [50], although such widespread expression should be interpreted cautiously, as the fidelity of antibodies against NOX4 has been a challenge in the field [154]. In the ER along with ERO1, the NOX4-p22^{phox} complex could provide H_2O_2 to create the oxidative environment necessary to support the folding of nascent proteins during their biosynthesis [155].

Several proteins co-localize with NOX4, including Poldip2 [156] and PDI [157], but do not participate in NOX4 biosynthesis. In contrast, experimental data indicate that the ER molecular chaperone calnexin interacts with NOX4 in the ER of a transfected cell system as well as in settings that assess the interactions of endogenous NOX4 [158]. As mentioned in the section on MPO biosynthesis, calnexin, but not calreticulin or ERp57, associates with proMPO, suggesting that calnexin

may facilitate heme acquisition for heme proteins synthesized in ER [36]. Calnexin does not associate with NOX1, NOX2, or NOX5 under the experimental conditions used, which suggests that it may be a feature of NOX4 biosynthesis that is not shared by related NOX protein family members. In support of the notion that NOX4 biosynthesis has unique features, the Y121H mutant of p22^{phox} [159] associates productively with NOX4 but not with NOX2 or NOX1 [131]. Detailed structural analysis of NOX4-p22^{phox} interactions identified specific amino acid requirements for heterodimer stability [131,134].

NOX5

NOX5 on the plasma membrane generates the superoxide anion extracellularly, and tagged constructs of NOX5 form tetramers at the plasma membrane of transfectants [160]. Unlike NOX1, 2, 3 and 4, NOX5 expression and activity are independent of p22^{phox} and cytoplasmic subunits [161,162]. Calmodulin-regulated changes in cytoplasmic free calcium modulate NOX5 activity via the four unique EF-hand motifs at its N-terminus [139,163]. Of note, NOX5 is absent from rodents [150,164], thus eliminating use of many typical experimental approaches. However, rabbit NOX5 has been cloned and sequenced, and rabbits are characterized as a suitable animal model for the further study of NOX5 [165].

Despite NOX5 expression in many tissues and implications for its important physiological activity, particularly in the cardiovascular system [166–168], little is known about its biosynthesis. Mature NOX5 is not glycosylated and is detected in ER-like structures in transfected cell systems [169] or cultured tumor cell lines [169–173]. Hsp90, the cytoplasmic heat shock protein that functions as a molecular chaperone in a variety of cellular settings [174], and several supporting chaperones coprecipitate with the C-terminal region of NOX5 and thereby modulate NOX5 oligomerization and oxidant production [175,176]. Of note, expression of grp94, an Hsp90 protein family member that resides in ER [177], does not contribute to NOX5 expression or activity [175]. Whether grp94 operates as a bona fide molecular chaperone during NOX5 biosynthesis or as a cytoplasmic factor that stabilizes NOX5 folding and function is not known currently.

DUOX

The dual oxidases DUOX1 and DUOX2 (83% similar in sequence [178]) possess two cytosolic EF-hand motifs that mediate calcium-dependent regulation of their activity. They differ from the other members of the NADPH oxidase family in several important ways. Not only do the DUOX proteins lack an association with $p22^{phox}$ or functional dependence on cytosolic subunits, but they also possess an additional (a seventh) transmembrane helix and an associated long N-terminal extracellular domain with limited sequence homology with mammalian peroxidases (*vide infra*).

Productive expression of DUOX proteins requires the presence of the corresponding maturation factor, i.e., DUOXA1 for DUOX1, DUOXA2 for DUOX2 [179]. In the absence of maturation factors, the corresponding DUOX remains in the ER and undergoes proteolytic degradation. Heterodimerization of DUOX-DUOXA stabilizes the complex during its maturation along the biosynthetic pathway and productively contributes to oxidant production [180,181]. The maturation factors associate with nascent DUOXes in the ER and are required for successful transport into the Golgi [179]. However, unlike *bona fide* molecular chaperones, which interact transiently with their targets and are not retained with the mature product [182], DUOXA proteins form a covalent complex with the corresponding DUOX protein at the target plasma membrane [180,183]. Heterodimer formation between DUOX and DUOXA in stable transfectants requires heme acquisition by DUOX [180], a finding that mirrors studies of other NOX protein family members. Furthermore, heterodimer formation influences the oxidants detected by DUOX activation, whether superoxide anion or H_2O_2 [181].

Whereas NOX proteins 1–5 possess six transmembrane domains, the DUOX proteins have a seventh that is N-terminal to the motifs homologous with the other NOX protein family members. The extracellular N-terminal segment of DUOX2 (amino acids 1–599) includes cysteine residues (C^{124}, C^{351}, C^{370}, C^{568}, and C^{582}), which are required for the structural and functional integrity of DUOX2-DUOXA2. Mutations of any of the four cysteines in the peroxidase homology domain (C^{351}, C^{370}, C^{568}, and C^{582}) cause ER retention of the precursor [184,185].

Two interesting features of the N-terminal extracellular region of DUOX merit comment. The region, which encompasses the initial 599 amino acids of the protein, has ~25% amino acid sequence homology with MPO and related peroxidases, and the presence of limited sequence homology prompted its designation as *peroxidase homology domain* (PHD) or *peroxidase-like domain*. However, many of the residues that are conserved across the peroxidase family, integral to peroxidase structure, and critical for peroxidase activity in animal peroxidases, are replaced. For example, using MPO for comparison, the histidine residues that support proximal and distal bonds with the heme group, H^{502} and H^{261}, are replaced with serine residues in human DUOX protein (Table 2.2).

Residues that form covalent linkages with the heme group in MPO, namely D^{260}, E^{408}, and M^{409} in human MPO, are not conserved in the human DUOX proteins. When expressed in a baculovirus system, the human DUOX1 peroxidase homology domain ($DUOX1_{1-593}$) lacks a heme spectrum, has no peroxidase activity, and binds exogenously added heme only weakly [186]. In contrast to human DUOX proteins, the proximal heme, catalytic arginine, and one of the two distal ester linkage sites critical for MPO and related peroxidases are conserved in *C. elegans* DUOX (Table 2.2). *C. elegans* DUOX1 exhibits weak peroxidase activity, ~0.4% of that of LPO [186], and forms two covalent bonds

TABLE 2.2
Sequence homologies of residues essential for peroxidase activity

Functional role	Human MPO	Human DUOX	*C. elegans* DUOX
Distal heme	Histidine 261	Serine	Tyrosine
Proximal heme	Histidine 502	Serine	Histidine
Catalytic arginine	Arginine 405	Arginine	Arginine
Ester linkage	Aspartate 260	Leucine	Alanine
Ester linkage	Glutamate 408	Arginine	Glutamate

Residues identical to those in MPO are in **red** font.

with heme [186]. Based on these data comparing the features of peroxidase homology domains purified from a baculovirus expression system, the peroxidase activity essential for the cross-linking of extracellular matrix in *C. elegans* [187] is not conserved in human DUOX1. Of note, the physiology of thyroid hormone synthesis demonstrates that DUOX2 lacks peroxidase activity. If DUOX2 possessed intrinsic peroxidase activity, it could support thyroid hormone production in the absence of TPO. However, the absence of functional TPO results in hypothyroidism [188].

The second noteworthy structural features of DUOX relate to extracellular cysteine residues and their relationship to biosynthesis and protein stability (Figure 2.4).

Six cysteine residues, including five in the peroxidase homology domain and C^{1162} on an extracellular loop, make essential contributions to interactions between DUOX and DUOXA. Individual replacement of C^{351}, C^{370}, C^{568}, or C^{582} compromises proper targeting of DUOX1 to the plasma membrane [184,185,189], despite each mutant maintaining the same specific enzymatic activity as that of wild-type DUOX1 [189]. Studies using recombinant human $DUOX1_{1-593}$ expressed in baculovirus suggest that C^{364} is critical for homodimerization of $DUOX1_{1-593}$, which is a prerequisite for heterodimer formation with DUOXA1 in the ER [189]. Furthermore, intramolecular disulfide bonding between C^{124} in the peroxidase homology domain and C^{1162} on an extracellular loop supports the subsequent formation of intermolecular bridges with DUOXA [183]. Such shuffling of intramolecular disulfide bonds to create intermolecular linkages critical to structural stability is reminiscent of the importance of C^{319} in the transformation of proMPO

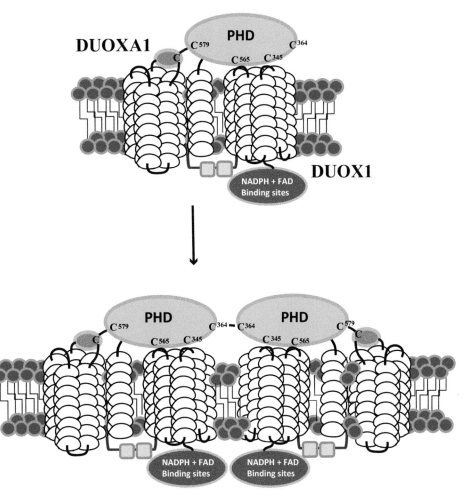

Figure 2.4 Schematic of associations between DUOX1 and DUOXA1.

to the mature dimeric form, discussed earlier. Cryo-electron microscopy (cryo-EM) studies of full-length murine DUOX1-DUOXA1 complexes demonstrate the presence of a dimer-of-dimer configuration both in the absence and presence of added NADPH [190] (see Figure 2.4).

The peroxidase homology domain of two DUOX1s directly interacts, forming a homodimer reminiscent of the organization of dimeric MPO (*vide supra*). The report of the elegant cryo-EM studies lacks mention of the disulfide bonds highlighted in work on recombinant human DUOX1-human DUOXA1 [189], leaving unsettled if and how intra- or intermolecular disulfides contribute to the structure of native DUOX-DUOXA complexes. Nonetheless, compelling data from several independent labs highlight events essential for proper DUOX-DUOXA formation, maturation, and targeting that occur in the oxidizing environment of the ER. In the context of a discussion of disulfide bonding in DUOX, it is interesting that the coprecipitation of DUOX and TPO from the membranes of thyrocytes is disrupted after treatment with the reducing agent N-ethylmaleimide (NEM) [191]. Of course, NEM could indirectly affect the DUOX-TPO interaction, but it is possible that a C-C interaction between TPO and the peroxidase homology domain of DUOX mediates formation of a complex that supports thyroid hormone synthesis [191].

CONCLUSIONS

Understanding the steps in the biosynthesis of mammalian peroxidases and NOX proteins has advanced, particularly with respect to MPO, TPO, NOX2, and DUOX. However, insights into how the precursors of these proteins acquire heme are lacking. Presumably, heme synthesized in the mitochondria reaches the apoforms of the precursors in the ER, perhaps involving heme transporters [192–194] or via direct docking of mitochondria with ER at specific contact structures (reviewed in Ref. [195]). Such structures have been implicated in heme transport between intracellular compartments in yeast [196] and may have homologues in mammalian systems.

If such transport mechanisms support heme delivery to the peroxidase and NOX protein precursors in the ER, what regulates the association between mitochondria and ER in human myeloid precursors? What specific transporters shuttle heme from mitochondria to ER? Do molecular chaperones in ER promote heme incorporation, as suggested for calnexin during biosynthesis of MPO or NOX4? Elucidation of how peroxidases and NOX proteins acquire heme may pave the way to understanding the principles that apply to other hemoproteins synthesized in the ER.

ACKNOWLEDGMENTS

Thanks to Professor Ulla Knaus for her thoughtful and constructive input on the original version of this manuscript. Work in the Nauseef lab is supported by National Institute of Health grants AI132335 and AI116546, Veterans Affairs Merit Review award BX000513, and use of facilities at the Iowa City Department of Veterans Affairs Medical Center, Iowa City, IA.

REFERENCES

1. E. Turner, C.E. Somers, B.M. Shapiro, 1985, The relationship between a novel NAD(P)H oxidase activity of ovoperoxidase and the CN$^-$-resistant respiratory burst that follows fertilization of sea urchin eggs, J. Biol. Chem. 260: 13163–13171.

2. J.L. Wong, R. Créton, G.M. Wessel, 2004, The oxidative burst at fertilization is dependent upon activation of the dual oxidase Udx1, *Dev. Cell* 7: 801–814.

3. F.A. Dias, A.C. Gandara, F.G. Queiroz-Barros, et al., 2013, Ovarian dual oxidase (Duox) activity is essential for insect eggshell hardening and waterproofing, J. Biol. Chem. 288: 35058–35067.

4. W.M. Nauseef, 2014, Myeloperoxidase in human neutrophil host defence, *Cell. Microbiol.* 16: 1146–1155.

5. X. De Deken, F. Miot, 2019, DUOX Defects and their roles in congenital hypothyroidism, *Methods Mol. Biol.* 1982: 667–693.

6. C. Wijkstrom-Frei, S. El-Chemaly, R. Ali-Rachedi, et al., 2003, Lactoperoxidase and human airway host defense, *Am. J. Respir. Cell Mol. Biol.* 29: 206–212.

7. D. Sarr, E. Tóth, A. Gingerich, B. Rada, 2018, Antimicrobial actions of dual oxidases and lactoperoxidase, J. Microbiol. 56: 373–386.

8. M. Zamocky, C. Jakopitsch, P.G. Furtmüller, C. Dunand, C. Obinger, 2008, The peroxidase-cyclooxygenase superfamily: Reconstructed evolution of critical enzymes of the innate immune system, *Prot. Struct. Funct. Gene.* 72: 589–605.

9. K. Agner, 1941, Verdoperoxidase: A ferment isolated from leukocytes, *Acta Physiol. Scand.* 2: 1–62.

10. L.V. Forbes, A.J. Kettle, 2018, Myeloperoxidase: Unleashing the Power of Hydrogen Peroxide, in: M.C.M. Vissers, M.B. Hampton, A.J. Kettle (Eds.), *Hydrogen Peroxide Metabolism in Health and Disease*, CRC Press, Boca Raton, pp. 281–304.

11. S.J. Klebanoff, A.J. Kettle, H. Rosen, C.C. Winterbourn, W.M. Nauseef, 2013, Myeloperoxidase: A front-line defender against phagocytosed microorganisms, *J. Leuk. Biol.* 93: 185–198.

12. W.M. Nauseef, 2018, Biosynthesis of human myeloperoxidase, *Arch. Biochem. Biophys.* 642: 1–9.

13. J. Schultz, K. Kaminker, 1962, Myeloperoxidase of the leucocyte of normal human blood, *Arch. Biochem. Biophys.* 96: 465–467.

14. W.M. Nauseef, 2007, How human neutrophils kill and degrade microbes: An integrated view, *Immunol. Rev.* 219: 88–102.

15. T.J. Fiedler, C.A. Davey, R.E. Fenna, 2000, X-ray crystal structure and characterization of halide-binding sites of human myeloperoxidase at 1.8 Å resolution, *J. Biol. Chem.* 275: 11964–11971.

16. J. Dekker, M. De Boer, D. Roos, 2001, Gene-scan method for the recognition of carriers and patients with p47 phox -deficient autosomal recessive chronic granulomatous disease, *Exp. Hematol.* 29: 1319–1325.

17. M.J. Davies, C.L. Hawkins, D.I. Pattison, M.D. Rees, 2008, Mammalian heme peroxidases: From molecular mechanisms to health implications, *Antioxid. Redox Signal.* 10: 1199–1234.

18. J.D. Zhu, 1999, Myeloid cell-lineage and premylocytic-stage-specific- expression of the mouse myeloperoxidase gene is controlled at initiation as well as elongation levels of transcription, *Cell Res.* 9: 107–134.

19. G.E. Austin, W.G. Zhao, W. Zhang, et al., 1995, Identification and characterization of the human myeloperoxidase promoter, *Leukemia* 9: 848–857.

20. G.E. Austin, W.G. Zhao, A. Adjiri, J.P. Lu, 1996, Control of myeloperoxidase gene expression in developing myeloid cells, *Leuk. Res.* 20: 817–820.

21. G.E. Austin, W.C. Chan, W. Zhao, M. Racine, 1994, Myeloperoxidase gene expression in normal granulopoiesis and acute leukemias, *Leuk. Lymphoma* 15: 209–226.

22. M. Lübbert, C.W. Miller, H.P. Koeffler, 1991, Changes of DNA methylation and chromatin structure in the human myeloperoxidase gene during myeloid differentiation, *Blood* 78: 345–356.

23. K.M. Lin, G.E. Austin, 2002, Functional activity of three distinct myeloperoxidase (MPO) promoters in human myeloid cells, *Leukemia* 16: 1143–1153.

24. M. Blair-Johnson, T. Fiedler, R. Fenna, 2001, Human myeloperoxidase: Structure of a cyanide complex and its interaction with bromide and thiocyanate substrates at 1.9 Å resolution, *Biochemistry* 40: 13990–13997.

25. X. Carpena, P. Vidossich, K. Schroettner, et al., 2009, Essential role of proximal histidine-asparagine interaction in mammalian peroxidases, *J. Biol. Chem.* 284: 25929–25937.

26. P.R. Ortiz de Montellano, 2016, Self-processing of Peroxidases, in: E. Raven, B. Duford (Eds.), *Heme Peroxidases*, Royal Society of Chemistry, Cambridge, UK, pp. 3–30.

27. J. Wang, J.N. Li, Z. Cui, M.H. Zhao, 2018, Deglycosylation influences the oxidation activity and antigenicity of myeloperoxidase, *Nephrology*, 23: 46–52.

28. P. Van Antwerpen, M.C. Slomianny, K.Z. Boudjeltia, et al., 2010, Glycosylation pattern of mature dimeric leukocyte and recombinant monomeric myeloperoxidase. Glycosylation is required for optimal enzymatic activity, *J. Biol. Chem.* 285: 16351–16359.

29. D. Nakazawa, S. Masuda, U. Tomaru, A. Ishizu, 2019, Pathogenesis and therapeutic interventions for ANCA-associated vasculitis, *Nat. Revi. Rheumatol.*, 15: 91–101.

30. K.R. Reiding, V. Franc, M.G. Huitema, et al., 2019, Neutrophil myeloperoxidase harbors distinct site-specific peculiarities in its glycosylation, *J. Biol. Chem.* 294: 20233–20245.

31. O.M. Lardinois, L.J. Deterding, J.J. Hess, et al., 2019, Immunoglobulins G from patients with ANCA-associated vasculitis are atypically glycosylated in both the Fc and Fab regions and the relation to disease activity, *PLoS One* 14: e0213215.

32. W.M. Nauseef, I. Olsson, K. Strömberg-Arnljots, 1988, Biosynthesis and processing of myeloperoxidase – A marker for myeloid differentiation, *Eur. J. Haematol.* 40: 97–110.

33. W.M. Nauseef, 1998, Insights into myeloperoxidase biosynthesis from its inherited deficiency, *J. Mol. Med.* 76: 661–668.

34. U. Gullberg, N. Bengtsson, E. Bülow, et al., 1999, Processing and targeting of granule proteins in human neutrophils, *J. Immunol. Meth.* 232: 201–210.

35. W.M. Nauseef, S.J. McCormick, R.A. Clark, 1995, Calreticulin functions as a molecular chaperone in the biosynthesis of myeloperoxidase, J. Biol. Chem. 270: 4741–4747.

36. W.M. Nauseef, S.J. McCormick, M. Goedken, 1998, Coordinated participation of calreticulin and calnexin in the biosynthesis of myeloperoxidase, J. Biol. Chem. 273: 7107–7111.

37. W.M. Nauseef, 1986, Myeloperoxidase biosynthesis by a human promyelocytic leukemia cell line: Insight into myeloperoxidase deficiency, Blood 67: 865–872.

38. W.M. Nauseef, S. Brigham, M. Cogley, 1994, Hereditary myeloperoxidase deficiency due to a missense mutation of arginine 569 to tryptophan, J. Biol. Chem. 269: 1212–1216.

39. F.R. DeLeo, M. Goedken, S.J. McCormick, W.M. Nauseef, 1998, A novel form of hereditary myeloperoxidase deficiency linked to endoplasmic reticulum/proteasome degradation, J. Clin. Invest. 101: 2900–2909.

40. W.M. Nauseef, S. McCormick, M. Goedken, 2000, Impact of missense mutations on biosynthesis of myeloperoxidase, Redox Rep. 5: 197–206.

41. M. Romano, P. Dri, L. Dadalt, P. Patriarca, F.E. Baralle, 1997, Biochemical and molecular characterization of hereditary myeloperoxidase deficiency, Blood 90: 4126–4134.

42. W. Nauseef, 2004, Lessons from MPO deficiency about functionally important structural features, Jpn. J. Infect. Dis. 57: S4–S5.

43. W.M. Nauseef, S. McCormick, H. Yi, 1992, Roles of heme insertion and the mannose-6-phosphate receptor in processing of the human myeloid lysosomal enzyme, myeloperoxidase, Blood 80: 2622–2633.

44. V.L. Castañeda, R.T. Parmley, I.B. Pinnix, et al., 1992, Ultrastructural, immunochemical, and cytochemical study of myeloperoxidase in myeloid leukemia HL-60 cells following treatment with succinylacetone, an inhibitor of heme biosynthesis, Exp. Hematol. 20: 916–924.

45. I.B. Pinnix, G.S. Guzman, H.L. Bonkovsky, S.R. Zaki, J.M. Kinkade, Jr., 1994, The post-translational processing of myeloperoxidase is regulated by the availability of heme, Arch. Biochem. Biophys. 312: 447–458.

46. I. Grishkovskaya, M. Paumann-Page, R. Tscheliessnig, et al., 2017, Structure of human promyeloperoxidase (proMPO) and the role of the propeptide in processing and maturation, J. Biol. Chem. 292: 8244–8261.

47. G.D. DePillis, S. Ozaki, J.M. Kuo, D.A. Maltby, P.R. Ortiz de Montellano, 1997, Autocatalytic processing of heme by lactoperoxidase produces the native protein-bound prosthetic group, J. Biol. Chem. 272: 8857–8860.

48. C. Colas, P.R. Ortiz de Montellano, 2002, Asp-225 and Glu-375 in autocatalytic attachment of the prosthetic heme group of lactoperoxidase, J. Biol. Chem. 277: 7191–7200.

49. E.D. Yoboue, R. Sitia, T. Simmen, 2018, Redox crosstalk at endoplasmic reticulum (ER) membrane contact sites (MCS) uses toxic waste to deliver messages, Cell Death Dis. 9: 331.

50. K. Chen, M.T. Kirber, H. Xiao, Y. Yang, J.F. Keaney, Jr., 2008, Regulation of ROS signal transduction by NADPH oxidase 4 localization, J. Cell Biol. 181: 1129–1139.

51. I. Olsson, A.M. Persson, K. Strömberg, 1984, Biosynthesis, transport, and processing of myeloperoxidase in the human leukemia promyelocytic cell line HL-60 and normal marrow cells, Biochem. J. 223: 911–920.

52. M. Yamada, S.J. Hur, H. Toda, 1990, Isolation and characterization of extracellular myeloperoxidase precursor in HL-60 cell cultures, Biochem. Biophys. Res. Commun. 166: 852–859.

53. D.T. Akin, J.M. Kinkade, Jr., 1986, Processing of a newly identified intermediate of human myeloperoxidase in isolated granules occurs at neutral pH, J. Biol. Chem. 261: 8370–8375.

54. E. Bülow, W.M. Nauseef, M. Goedken, et al., 2002, Sorting for storage in myeloid cells of nonmyeloid proteins and chimeras with the propeptide of myeloperoxidase precursor, J. Leukoc. Biol. 71: 279–288.

55. E. Andersson, L. Hellman, U. Gullberg, I. Olsson, 1998, The role of the propeptide for processing and sorting of human myeloperoxidase, J. Biol. Chem. 273: 4747–4753.

56. W.M. Nauseef, 1987, Posttranslational processing of a human myeloid lysosomal protein, myeloperoxidase, Blood 70: 1143–1150.

57. N. Moguilevsky, L. Garcia-Quintana, A. Jacquet, et al., 1991, Structural and biological properties of human recombinant myeloperoxidase produced by Chinese hamster ovary cell lines, Eur. J. Biochem. 197: 605–614.

58. M. Goedken, S. McCormick, K.G. Leidal, et al., 2007, Impact of two novel mutations on the structure and function of human myeloperoxidase, J. Biol. Chem. 282: 27994–28003.

59. S. McCormick, A. Nelson, W.M. Nauseef, 2012, Proconvertase proteolytic processing of an enzymatically active myeloperoxidase precursor, Arch. Biochem. Biophys. 527: 31–36.

60. P.G. Furtmuller, W. Jantschko, G. Regelsberger, et al., 2001, A transient kinetic study on the reactivity of recombinant unprocessed monomeric myeloperoxidase, FEBS Lett. 503: 147–150.

61. K. Strömberg, A.M. Persson, I. Olsson, 1986, The processing and intracellular transport of myeloperoxidase, Eur. J. Cell Biol. 39: 424–431.

62. A. Hasilik, R. Pohlmann, R.L. Olsen, K. Von Figura, 1984, Myeloperoxidase is synthesized as larger phosphorylated precursor, EMBO J. 3: 2671–2676.

63. U. Bening, R. Castino, N. Harth, C. Isidoro, A. Hasilik, 1998, Lysosomal segregation of a mannose-rich glycoprotein imparted by the prosequence of myeloperoxidase, J. Cell. Biochem. 71: 158–168.

64. M. Rholam, C. Fahy, 2009, Processing of peptide and hormone precursors at the dibasic cleavage sites, Cell. Mol. Life Sci. 66: 2075–2091.

65. N.G. Seidah, G. Mayer, A. Zaid, et al., 2008, The activation and physiological functions of the proprotein convertases, Int. J. Biochem. Cell Biol. 40: 1111–1125.

66. P. Duckert, S. Brunak, N. Blom, 2004, Prediction of proprotein convertase cleavage sites, Protein Eng. Des. Sel. 17: 107–112.

67. T. Fujiwara, K. Oka, S. Yokota, A. Takatsuki, Y. Ikehara, 1988, Brefeldin A causes dissembly of the Golgi complex and accumulation of secretory proteins in the endoplasmic reticulum, J. Biol. Chem. 263: 18545–18552.

68. J. Lippincott-Schwartz, L.C. Yuan, J.S. Bonifacino, R.D. Klausner, 1989, Rapid redistribution of Golgi proteins into the ER in cells treated with brefeldin A: Evidence for membrane recycling from Golgi to ER, Cell 56: 801–813.

69. R.W. Dams, G. Russ, J.W. Yewell, 1989, Brefeldin A redistributes resident and itinerant Golgi proteins to the endoplasmic reticulum, J. Cell Biol. 109: 61–72.

70. D.T. Akin, J.M. Kinkade, Jr., 1987, Evidence for the involvement of an acidic compartment in the processing of myeloperoxidase in human promyelocytic leukemia HL-60 cells, Arch. Biochem. Biophys. 255: 428–436.

71. K.L. Taylor, G.S. Guzman, C.A. Burgess, J.M. Kinkade, Jr., 1990, Assembly of dimeric myeloperoxidase during posttranslational maturation in human leukemic HL-60 cells, Biochemistry 29: 1533–1539.

72. A.R. Thomsen, L. Sottrup-Jensen, G.J. Gleich, C. Oxvig, 2000, The status of half-cystine residues and locations of N-glycosylated asparagine residues in human eosinophil peroxidase, Arch. Biochem. Biophys. 379: 147–152.

73. I. Olsson, A.M. Persson, K. Stromberg, et al., 1985, Purification of eosinophil peroxidase and studies of biosynthesis and processing in human marrow cells, Blood 66: 1143–1148.

74. M. Romano, F.E. Baralle, P. Patriarca, 2000, Expression and characterization of recombinant human eosinophil peroxidase. Impact of the R286H substitution on the biosynthesis and activity of the enzyme, Eur. J. Biochem. 267: 3704–3711.

75. M.G. Carlson, C.G. Peterson, P. Venge, 1985, Human eosinophil peroxidase: Purification and characterization, J. Immunol. 134: 1875–1879.

76. R.L. Olsen, C. Little, 1983, Purification and some properties of myeloperoxidase and eosinophil peroxidase from human blood, Biochem. J. 209: 781–787.

77. R. Wever, H. Plat, M.N. Hamers, 1981, Human eosinophil peroxidase: A novel isolation procedure, spectral properties and chlorinating activity, FEBS Lett. 123: 327–331.

78. R.M. Ten, L.R. Pease, D.J. McKean, M.P. Bell, G.J. Gleich, 1989, Molecular cloning of the human eosinophil peroxidase. Evidence for the existence of a peroxidase multigene family, J. Exp. Med. 169: 1757–1769.

79. C. Oxvig, A.R. Thomsen, M.T. Overgaard, et al., 1999, Biochemical evidence for heme linkage through esters with Asp-93 and Glu-241 in human eosinophil peroxidase, J. Biol. Chem. 274: 16953–16958.

80. K.D. Kussendrager, A.C. van Hooijdonk, 2000, Lactoperoxidase: Physico-chemical properties, occurrence, mechanism of action and applications, Br. J. Nutr. 84 Suppl 1: S19–S25.

81. R. Ihalin, V. Loimaranta, J. Tenovuo, 2005, Origin, structure, and biological activities of peroxidases in human saliva, Arch. Biochem. Biophys. 445: 261–268.

82. S. Watanabe, F. Varsalona, Y.C. Yoo, et al., 1998, Recombinant bovine lactoperoxidase as a tool to study the heme environment in mammalian peroxidases, *FEBS Lett.* 441: 476–479.

83. K. Shin, H. Hayasawa, B. Lönnerdal, 2000, PCR cloning and baculovirus expression of human lactoperoxidase and myeloperoxidase, *Biochem. Biophys. Res. Commun.* 271: 831–836.

84. M.A. Fragoso, A. Torbati, N. Fregien, G.E. Conner, 2009, Molecular heterogeneity and alternative splicing of human lactoperoxidase, *Arch. Biochem. Biophys.* 482: 52–57.

85. I.A. Sheikh, A.K. Singh, N. Singh, et al., 2009, Structural evidence of substrate specificity in mammalian peroxidases. Structure of the thiocyanate complex with lactoperoxidase and its interactions at 2.4 Å resolution, *J. Biol. Chem.* 284: 14849–14856.

86. K.S. Booth, S. Kimura, H.C. Lee, M. Ikeda-Saito, W.S. Caughey, 1989, Bovine myeloperoxidase and lactoperoxidase each contain a high affinity binding site for calcium, *Biochem. Biophys. Res. Commun.* 160: 897–902.

87. K. Shin, H. Hayasawa, B. Lönnerdal, 2001, Mutations affecting the calcium-binding site of myeloperoxidase and lactoperoxidase, *Biochem. Biophys. Res. Commun.* 281: 1024–1029.

88. M. Godlewska, M. Góra, A.M. Buckle, et al., 2014, A redundant role of human thyroid peroxidase propeptide for cellular, enzymatic, and immunological activity, *Thyroid* 24: 371–382.

89. J. Ruf, P. Carayon, 2006, Structural and functional aspects of thyroid peroxidase, *Arch. Biochem. Biophys.* 445: 269–277.

90. F.S. Belforte, M.B. Miras, M.C. Olcese, et al., 2012, Congenital goitrous hypothyroidism: Mutation analysis in the thyroid peroxidase gene, *Clin. Endocrinol. (Oxf.)* 76: 568–576.

91. C. Ris-Stalpers, H. Bikker, 2010, Genetics and phenomics of hypothyroidism and goiter due to TPO mutations, *Mol. Cell. Endocrinol.* 322: 38–43.

92. S.N. Le, B.T. Porebski, J. McCoey, et al., 2015, Modelling of thyroid peroxidase reveals insights into its enzyme function and autoantigenicity, *PLoS One* 10: e0142615.

93. L. Fayadat, P. Niccoli-Sire, J. Lanet, J.L. Franc, 1999, Role of heme in intracellular trafficking of thyroperoxidase and involvement of H_2O_2 generated at the apical surface of thyroid cells in autocatalytic covalent heme binding, *J. Biol. Chem.* 274: 10533–10538.

94. V. Le Fourn, S. Siffroi-Fernandez, M. Ferrand, J.L. Franc, 2006, Competition between calnexin and BiP in the endoplasmic reticulum can lead to the folding or degradation of human thyroperoxidase, *Biochemistry* 45: 7380–7388.

95. L. Fayadat, S. Siffroi-Fernandez, J. Lanet, J.L. Franc, 2000, Calnexin and calreticulin binding to human thyroperoxidase is required for its first folding step(s) but is not sufficient to promote efficient cell surface expression, *Endocrinology* 141: 959–966.

96. L. Fayadat, P. Niccoli-Sire, J. Lanet, J.L. Franc, 1998, Human thyroperoxidase is largely retained and rapidly degraded in the endoplasmic reticulum. Its N-glycans are required for folding and intracellular trafficking, *Endocrinology* 139: 4277–4285.

97. V. Le Fourn, M. Ferrand, J.L. Franc, 2005, Endoproteolytic cleavage of human thyroperoxidase: Role of the propeptide in the protein folding process, *J. Biol. Chem.* 280: 4568–4577.

98. M. Godlewska, M. Gora, A.M. Buckle, et al., 2014, A redundant role of human thyroid peroxidase propeptide for cellular, enzymatic, and immunological activity, *Thyroid* 24: 371–382.

99. E. Hendry, G. Taylor, K. Ziemnicka, et al., 1999, Recombinant human thyroid peroxidase expressed in insect cells is soluble at high concentrations and forms diffracting crystals, *J. Endocrinol.* 160: R13–R15.

100. A. Gardas, M.K. Sohi, B.J. Sutton, A.M. McGregor, J.P. Banga, 1997, Purification and crystallisation of the autoantigen thyroid peroxidase from human Graves' thyroid tissue, *Biochem. Biophys. Res. Commun.* 234: 366–370.

101. J.R. Baker, P. Arscott, J. Johnson, 1994, An analysis of the structure and antigenicity of different forms of human thyroid peroxidase, *Thyroid* 4: 173–178.

102. J.D. Lambeth, A.S. Neish, 2014, NOX Enzymes and new thinking on reactive oxygen: A double-edged sword revisited, *Annu. Rev. Pathol.* 9: 119–145.

103. H. Buvelot, V. Jaquet, K.H. Krause, 2019, Mammalian NADPH Oxidases, *Methods Mol. Biol.* 1982: 17–36.

104. F. Magnani, A. Mattevi, 2019, Structure and mechanisms of ROS generation by NADPH oxidases, *Curr. Opin. Struct. Biol.* 59: 91–97.

105. K.P. Shatwell, A. Dancis, A.R. Cross, R.D. Klausner, A.W. Segal, 1996, The FRE1 ferric reductase of Saccharomyces cerevisiae is a cytochrome b similar to that of NADPH oxidase, *J. Biol. Chem.* 271: 14240–14244.

106. A.A. Finegold, K.P. Shatwell, A.W. Segal, R.D. Klausner, A. Dancis, 1996, Intramembrane bis-heme motif for transmembrane electron transport conserved in a yeast iron reductase and the human NADPH oxidase, *J. Biol. Chem.* 271: 31021–31024.

107. A.R. Cross, J. Rae, J.T. Curnutte, 1995, Cytochrome b-245 of the neutrophil superoxide-generating system contains two nonidentical hemes. Potentiometric studies of a mutant form of gp91phox, *J. Biol. Chem.* 270: 17075–17077.

108. F. Magnani, S. Nenci, E. Millana Fananas, et al., 2017, Crystal structures and atomic model of NADPH oxidase, *Proc. Natl. Acad. Sci. U. S. A.* 114: 6764–6769.

109. X. Zhang, K.H. Krause, I. Xenarios, T. Soldati, B. Boeckmann, 2013, Evolution of the ferric reductase domain (FRD) superfamily: Modularity, functional diversification, and signature motifs, *PLoS One* 8: e58126.

110. K.J. Biberstine-Kinkade, F.R. DeLeo, R.I. Epstein, et al., 2001, Heme-ligating histidines in flavocytochrome b 558, *J. Biol. Chem.* 276: 31105–31112.

111. A. Dancis, D.G. Roman, G.J. Anderson, A.G. Hinnebusch, R.D. Klausner, 1992, Ferric reductase of Saccharomyces cerevisiae: Molecular characterization, role in iron uptake, and transcriptional control by iron, *Proc. Natl. Acad. Sci. U. S. A.* 89: 3869–3873.

112. E. Lesuisse, M. Casteras-Simon, P. Labbe, 1996, Evidence for the Saccharomyces cerevisiae ferrireductase system being a multicomponent electron transport chain, *J. Biol. Chem.* 271: 13578–13583.

113. F.R. DeLeo, O. Olakanmi, G.T. Rasmussen, et al., 1999, Despite structural similarities between gp91 phox and FRE1, flavocytochrome b 558 does not mediate iron uptake by myeloid cells, *J. Lab. Clin. Med.* 134: 275–282.

114. W.M. Nauseef, 2008, Biological roles for the NOX family NADPH oxidases, *J. Biol. Chem.* 283: 16961–16965.

115. D. Roos, 2019, Chronic Granulomatous disease, *Methods Mol. Biol.* 1982: 531–542.

116. W.M. Nauseef, R.A. Clark, 2019, Intersecting stories of the phagocyte NADPH oxidase and chronic granulomatous disease, in: U.G. Knaus, T.L. Leto (Eds.), *Methods Mol. Biol.* 1982: 3–16.

117. W.M. Nauseef, 2019, The phagocyte NOX2 NADPH oxidase in microbial killing and cell signaling, *Curr. Opin. Immunol.* 60: 130–140.

118. K.A. Tucker, M.B. Lilly, L. Heck, T.A. Rado, 1987, Characterization of a new human diploid myeloid leukemia cell line (PLB-985) with granulocytic and monocytic differentiating capacity, *Blood* 70: 372–378.

119. L. Yu, M.C. Dinauer, 1997, Biosynthesis of the phagocyte NADPH oxidase cytochrome b 558, *J. Biol. Chem.* 272: 27288–27294.

120. L. Yu, F.R. DeLeo, K.J. Biberstine-Kinkade, et al., 1999, Biosynthesis of flavocytochrome b558, *J. Biol. Chem.* 274: 4364–4369.

121. F.R. DeLeo, J.B. Burritt, L. Yu, et al., 2000, Processing and maturation of flavocytochrome b 558 include incorporation of heme as a prerequisite for heterodimer assembly, *J. Biol. Chem.* 275: 13986–13993.

122. J.D. Pollock, D.A. Williams, M.A.C. Gifford, et al., 1995, Mouse model of X-linked chronic granulomatous disease, an inherited defect in phagocyte superoxide production, *Nat. Genet.* 9: 202–209.

123. H. Björgvinsdóttir, L. Zhen, M.C. Dinauer, 1996, Cloning of murine gp91 phox cDNA and functional expression in a human X-linked chronic granulomatous disease cell line, *Blood* 87: 2005–2010.

124. P.G. Heyworth, A.R. Cross, J.T. Curnutte, 2003, Chronic granulomatous disease, *Curr. Opin. Immunol.* 15: 578–584.

125. D. Roos, D.B. Kuhns, A. Maddalena, et al., 2010, Hematologically important mutations: The autosomal recessive forms of chronic granulomatous disease (second update), *Blood Cells Mol. Dis.* 44: 291–299.

126. D. Roos, M. de Boer, 2014, Molecular diagnosis of chronic granulomatous disease, *Clin. Exp. Immunol.* 175: 139–149.

127. D.C. Thomas, S. Clare, J.M. Sowerby, et al., 2017, Eros is a novel transmembrane protein that controls the phagocyte respiratory burst and is essential for innate immunity, *J. Exp. Med.* 214: 1111–1128.

128. G.A. Arnadottir, G.L. Norddahl, S. Gudmunds dottir, et al., 2018, A homozygous loss-of-function mutation leading to CYBC1 deficiency causes chronic granulomatous disease, *Nat. Commun.* 9: 4447.

129. D.C. Thomas, L.M. Charbonnier, A. Schejtman, et al., 2018, EROS mutations: Decreased NADPH oxidase function and chronic granulomatous disease, J. Allergy Clin. Immunol. 143: 782–785.

130. H. Sumimoto, R. Minakami, K. Miyano, 2019, Soluble regulatory proteins for activation of NOX Family NADPH oxidases, Methods Mol. Biol. 1982: 121–137.

131. K. von Löhneysen, D. Noack, A.J. Jesaitis, M.C. Dinauer, U.G. Knaus, 2008, Mutational analysis reveals distinct features of the Nox4-p22 phox complex, J. Biol. Chem. 283: 35273–35282.

132. T. Kawahara, D. Ritsick, G. Cheng, J.D. Lambeth, 2005, Point mutations in the proline-rich region of p22 phox are dominant inhibitors of NOX1- and NOX2-dependent reactive oxygen generation, J. Biol. Chem. 280: 31859–31869.

133. Y. Zhu, C. Marchal, A.J. Casbon, et al., 2006, Deletion mutagenesis of p22 phox subunit of flavocytochrome b558: Identification of regions critical for gp91 phox maturation and NADPH oxidase activity, J. Biol. Chem. 281: 30336–30346.

134. K. von Lohneysen, D. Noack, M.R. Wood, J.S. Friedman, U.G. Knaus, 2010, Structural insights into NOX4 and NOX2: Motifs involved in function and cellular localization, Mol. Cell. Biol. 30: 961–975.

135. R.K. Ambasta, P. Kumar, K.K. Griendling, et al., 2004, Direct interaction of the novel NOX proteins with p22phox is required for the formation of a functionally active NADPH oxidase, J. Biol. Chem. 279: 45935–45941.

136. K.K. Prior, M.S. Leisegang, I. Josipovic, et al., 2016, CRISPR/Cas9-mediated knockout of p22phox leads to loss of Nox1 and Nox4, but not NOX5 activity, Redox Biol. 9: 287–295.

137. K. Miyano, H. Sumimoto, 2014, N-Linked glycosylation of the superoxide-producing NADPH oxidase Nox1, Biochem. Biophys. Res. Commun. 443: 1060–1065.

138. M. Matsumoto, M. Katsuyama, K. Iwata, et al., 2014, Characterization of N-glycosylation sites on the extracellular domain of NOX1/NADPH oxidase, Free Radic. Biol. Med. 68: 196–204.

139. B. Banfi, B. Malgrange, J. Knisz, et al., 2004, NOX3, a superoxide-generating NADPH oxidase of the inner ear, J. Biol. Chem. 279: 46065–46072.

140. R.A. Bergstrom, Y. You, L.C. Erway, M.F. Lyon, J.C. Schimenti, 1998, Deletion mapping of the head tilt (het) gene in mice: A vestibular mutation causing specific absence of otoliths, Genetics 150: 815–822.

141. R. Paffenholz, R.A. Bergstrom, F. Pasutto, et al., 2004, Vestibular defects in head-tilt mice result from mutations in NOX3, encoding an NADPH oxidase, Genes Dev. 18: 486–491.

142. Y. Nakano, B. Banfi, A.J. Jesaitis, et al., 2007, Critical roles for p22 phox in the structural maturation and subcellular targeting of NOX3, Biochem. J. 403: 97–108.

143. T. Ueyama, M. Geiszt, T.L. Leto, 2006, Involvement of Rac1 in activation of multicomponent NOX1- and NOX3-based NADPH oxidases, Mol. Cell Biol. 26: 2160–2174.

144. N. Ueno, R. Takeya, K. Miyano, H. Kikuchi, H. Sumimoto, 2005, The NADPH oxidase NOX3 constitutively produces superoxide in a p22 phox -dependent manner: Its regulation by oxidase organizers and activators, J. Biol. Chem. 280: 23328–23339.

145. M. Zana, Z. Peterfi, H.A. Kovacs, et al., 2018, Interaction between p22(phox) and Nox4 in the endoplasmic reticulum suggests a unique mechanism of NADPH oxidase complex formation, Free Radic. Biol. Med. 116: 41–49.

146. Y. Nisimoto, B.A. Diebold, D. Constentino-Gomes, J.D. Lambeth, 2014, NOX4: A hydrogen peroxide-generating oxygen sensor, Biochemistry 53: 5111–5120.

147. S. O'Neill, M. Mathis, L. Kovačič, et al., 2018, Quantitative interaction analysis permits molecular insights into functional NOX4 NADPH oxidase heterodimer assembly, J. Biol. Chem. 293: 8750–8760.

148. K. von Löhneysen, D. Noack, P. Hayes, J.S. Friedman, U.G. Knaus, 2012, Constitutive NADPH oxidase 4 activity resides in the composition of the B-loop and the penultimate C terminus, J. Biol. Chem. 287: 8737–8745.

149. L. Serrander, L. Cartier, K. Bedard, et al., 2007, NOX4 activity is determined by mRNA levels and reveals a unique pattern of ROS generation, Biochem. J. 406: 105–114.

150. K.D. Martyn, L.M. Frederick, K. von Loehneysen, M.C. Dinauer, U.G. Knaus, 2006, Functional analysis of NOX4 reveals unique characteristics compared to other NADPH oxidases, Cell. Signal. 18: 69–82.

151. K. Block, Y. Gorin, H.E. Abboud, 2009, Subcellular localization of Nox4 and regulation in diabetes, Proc. Natl. Acad. Sci. USA 106: 14385–14390.

152. J. Kuroda, K. Nakagawa, T. Yamasaki, et al., 2005, The superoxide-producing NAD(P)H oxidase NOX4 in the nucleus of human vascular endothelial cells, *Genes Cells* 10: 1139–1151.

153. L.L. Hilenski, R.E. Clempus, M.T. Quinn, J.D. Lambeth, K.K. Griendling, 2004, Distinct subcellular localizations of Nox1 and Nox4 in vascular smooth muscle cells, *Arterioscler. Thromb. Vasc. Biol.* 24: 677–683.

154. B.A. Diebold, S.G. Wilder, X. De Deken, et al., 2019, Guidelines for the detection of NADPH oxidases by immunoblot and RT-qPCR, *Methods Mol. Biol.* 1982: 191–229.

155. C. Giulivi, K. Davies, 2001, Mechanism of the formation and proteolytic release of H2O2-induced dityrosine and tyrosine oxidation products in hemoglobin and red blood cells, *J. Biol. Chem.* 276: 24129–24136.

156. A. Lyle, N. Deshpande, Y. Taniyama, et al., 2009, Poldip2, a novel regulator of nox4 and cytoskeletal integrity in vascular smooth muscle cells, *Circ. Res.* 105: 249–259.

157. M. Janiszewski, L.R. Lopes, A.O. Carmo, et al., 2005, Regulation of NAD(P)H oxidase by associated protein disulfide isomerase in vascular smooth muscle cells, *J. Biol. Chem.* 280: 40813–40819.

158. K.K. Prior, I. Wittig, M.S. Leisegang, et al., 2016, The endoplasmic reticulum chaperone calnexin is a NADPH oxidase NOX4 interacting protein, *J. Biol. Chem.* 291: 7045–7059.

159. Y. Nakano, C.M. Longo-Guess, D.E. Bergstrom, et al., 2008, Mutation of the cyba gene encoding p22phox causes vestibular and immune defects in mice, *J. Clin. Invest.* 118: 1176–1185.

160. T. Kawahara, H.M. Jackson, S.M.E. Smith, P.D. Simpson, J.D. Lambeth, 2011, Nox5 forms a functional oligomer mediated by self-association of its dehydrogenase domain, *Biochemistry* 50: 2013–2025.

161. G. Cheng, Z. Cao, X. Xu, E. Van Meir, J. Lambeth, 2001, Homologs of gp91 phox: Cloning and tissue expression of Nox3, Nox4, and Nox5, *Gene* 269: 131–140.

162. B. Bánfi, G. Molnár, A. Maturana, et al., 2001, A Ca^{2+}-activated NADPH oxidase in testis, spleen, and lymph nodes, *J. Biol. Chem.* 276: 37594–37601.

163. B. Bánfi, F. Tirone, I. Durussel, et al., 2004, Mechanism of Ca^{2+} activation of the NADPH oxidase 5 (NOX5), *J. Biol. Chem.* 279: 18583–18591.

164. T. Kawahara, M.T. Quinn, J.D. Lambeth, 2007, Molecular evolution of the reactive oxygen-generating NADPH oxidase (Nox/Duox) family of enzymes, *BMC Evol. Biol.* 7: 109.

165. F. Chen, C. Yin, C. Dimitropoulou, D.J. Fulton, 2016, Cloning, characteristics, and functional analysis of rabbit NADPH oxidase 5, *Front. Physiol.* 7: 284.

166. D.J.R. Fulton, 2019, The molecular regulation and functional roles of NOX5, *Methods Mol. Biol.* 1982: 353–375.

167. R.M. Touyz, A. Anagnostopoulou, F. Rios, A.C. Montezano, L.L. Camargo, 2019, NOX5: Molecular biology and pathophysiology, *Exp. Physiol.* 104: 605–616.

168. H.K. Li, I. Rombach, R. Zambellas, et al., 2019, Oral versus intravenous antibiotics for bone and joint infection, *N. Engl. J. Med.* 380: 425–436.

169. D. Jagnandan, J.E. Church, B. Banfi, et al., 2007, Novel mechanism of activation of NADPH oxidase 5(NOX5): Calcium-sensitization via phosphorylation, *J. Biol. Chem.* 282: 6494–6507.

170. L. Serrander, V. Jaquet, K. Bedard, et al., 2007, NOX5 is expressed at the plasma membrane and generates superoxide in response to protein kinase C activation, *Biochimie* 89: 1159–1167.

171. R.S. BelAiba, T. Djordjevic, A. Petry, et al., 2007, NOX5 variants are functionally active in endothelial cells, *Free Radic. Biol. Med.* 42: 446–459.

172. T. Kawahara, J.D. Lambeth, 2008, Phosphatidylinositol (4,5)-bisphosphate modulates Nox5 localization via an N-terminal polybasic region, *Mol. Biol. Cell* 19: 4020–4031.

173. S.S. Brar, Z. Corbin, T.P. Kennedy, et al., 2003, NOX5 NAD(P)H oxidase regulates growth and apoptosis in DU 145 prostate cancer cells, *Am. J. Physiol. Cell Physiol.* 285: C353–C369.

174. F.H. Schopf, M.M. Biebl, J. Buchner, 2017, The HSP90 chaperone machinery, *Nat. Rev. Mol. Cell Biol.* 18: 345–360.

175. F. Chen, D. Pandey, A. Chadli, et al., 2011, Hsp90 regulates NADPH oxidase activity and is necessary for superoxide but not hydrogen peroxide production, *Antioxid. Redox Signal.* 14: 2107–2119.

176. F. Chen, S. Haigh, Y. Yu, et al., 2015, Nox5 stability and superoxide production is regulated by C-terminal binding of Hsp90 and CO-chaperones, *Free Radic. Biol. Med.* 89: 793–805.

177. M. Marzec, D. Eletto, Y. Argon, 2012, GRP94: An HSP90-like protein specialized for protein

folding and quality control in the endoplasmic reticulum, *Biochim. Biophys. Acta* 1823: 774–787.

178. J. Cohn, G. Sessa, G.B. Martin, 2001, Innate immunity in plants, *Curr. Opin. Immunol.* 13: 55–62.

179. H. Grasberger, S. Refetoff, 2006, Identification of the maturation factor for dual oxidase, *J. Biol. Chem.* 281: 18269–18272.

180. S. Luxen, D. Noack, M. Frausto, et al., 2009, Heterodimerization controls localization of duox-duoxA NADPH oxidases in airway cells, *J. Cell Sci.* 122: 1238–1247.

181. S. Morand, T. Ueyama, S. Tsujibe, et al., 2009, Duox maturation factors form cell surface complexes with Duox affecting the specificity of reactive oxygen species generation, *FASEB J.* 23: 1205–1218.

182. V. Dahiya, J. Buchner, 2019, Functional principles and regulation of molecular chaperones, *Adv. Protein Chem. Struct. Biol.* 114: 1–60.

183. A. Carré, R.A. Louzada, R.S. Fortunato, et al., 2015, When an intramolecular disulfide bridge governs the interaction of DUOX2 with its partner DUOXA2, *Antioxid. Redox Signal.* 23: 724–733.

184. S. Morand, D. Agnandji, M.S. Noel-Hudson, et al., 2004, Targeting of the dual oxidase 2 N-terminal region to the plasma membrane, *J. Biol. Chem.* 279: 30244–30251.

185. R.S. Fortunato, E.C.L. de Souza, R.A. Hassani, et al., 2010, Functional consequences of dual oxidase-thyroperoxidase interaction at the plasma membrane, *J. Clin. Endocrinol. Metab.* 95: 5403–5411.

186. J.L. Meitzler, P.R. Ortiz de Montellano, 2009, *Caenorhabditis elegans* and human dual oxidase 1 (DUOX1) "peroxidase" domains. Insights into heme binding and catalytic activity, *J. Biol. Chem.* 284: 18634–18643.

187. W.A. Edens, L. Sharling, G. Cheng, et al., 2001, Tyrosine cross-linking of extracellular matrix is catalyzed by Duox, a multidomain oxidase/peroxidase with homology to the phagocyte oxidase subunit gp91 phox, *J. Cell Biol.* 154: 879–891.

188. S.M. Park, V.K.K. Chatterjee, 2005, Genetics of congenital hypothyroidism, *J. Med. Genet.* 42: 379–389.

189. J.L. Meitzler, S. Hinde, B. Banfi, W.M. Nauseef, P.R. Ortiz de Montellano, 2013, Conserved cysteine residues provide a protein-protein interaction surface in dual oxidase (DUOX) proteins, *J. Biol. Chem.* 288: 7147–7157.

190. J. Sun, 2020, Structures of mouse DUOX1-DUOXA1 provide mechanistic insights into enzyme activation and regulation, *Nat. Struct. Mol. Biol.* 27: 1086–1093.

191. Y. Song, J. ruf, P. Lothaire, et al., 2010, Association of duoxes with thyroid peroxidase and its regulation in thyrocytes, *J. Clin. Endocrinol. Metab.* 95: 375–382.

192. S. Severance, I. Hamza, 2009, Trafficking of heme and porphyrins in metazoa, *Chem. Rev.* 109: 4596–4616.

193. A. Rajagopal, A.U. Rao, J. Amigo, et al., 2008, Haem homeostasis is regulated by the conserved and concerted functions of HRG-1 proteins, *Nature* 453: 127–131.

194. T. Korolnek, J. Zhang, S. Beardsley, G.L. Scheffer, I. Hamza, 2014, Control of metazoan heme homeostasis by a conserved multidrug resistance protein, *Cell Metab* 19: 1008–1019.

195. H. Wu, P. Carvalho, G.K. Voeltz, 2018, Here, there, and everywhere: The importance of ER membrane contact sites, *Science* 361: eaan5835.

196. O. Martinez-Guzman, M.M. Willoughby, A. Saini, et al., 2020, Mitochondrial-nuclear heme trafficking in budding yeast is regulated by GTPases that control mitochondrial dynamics and ER contact sites, *J. Cell Sci.* 133: jcs237917.

CHAPTER THREE

Peroxidasin: Structure and Function

Gábor Sirokmány, Hajnal A. Kovács, and Miklós Geiszt
Semmelweis University

CONTENTS

THE DISCOVERY OF PXDN

PXDN was first purified from the conditioned media of *Drosophila* Kc cells [1]. Electrophoretic analysis under reducing and nonreducing conditions showed a molecular weight of 170 kD and suggested the formation of trimers through disulfide bridges. The existence of trimers was also confirmed by electron microscopy [1]. Analysis of PXDN's domain architecture showed a unique composition of protein modules, which are characteristic for extracellular matrix (ECM) proteins, and a peroxidase domain displaying close homology to other members of the peroxidase-cyclooxygenase superfamily [1,2]. The *Drosophila* PXDN consists of 1,512 amino acids and contains the sequence of six leucine-rich repeats (LRRs), followed by four immunoglobulin (Ig) domains (Figure 3.1). The peroxidase domain of PXDN is located after the Ig domains, followed by an amphipathic alpha-helix and a short von Willebrand factor C domain (vWFC). The purified protein exhibited peroxidase activity, which

was tested by o-dianisidine oxidation, dityrosine formation, and protein iodination. The expression of PXDN was studied by *in situ* hybridization, and the mRNA was found to be localized mainly in hemocytes during embryogenesis [1].

The human gene encoding PXDN was initially cloned from a colon cancer cell line as a p53-responsive gene product, but its function was not studied further [3]. The PXDN gene was also identified as melanoma-associated gene (MG50) from melanoma samples, but the possible peroxidase function of the encoded protein was not assessed [4]. Cheng et al. described the mammalian PXDN as vascular peroxidase 1 (VPO1), because they found high PXDN expression in vascular cells [5]. Although the specific expression pattern of other peroxidases warrants the tissue-based nomenclature conventionally used, the expression of mammalian PXDN is so widespread that the VPO1 name is no longer accurate. The size and domain architecture of mammalian PXDN is highly similar to its *Drosophila* counterpart, suggesting a conserved function (Figure 3.1).

DOI: 10.1201/9781003212287-4

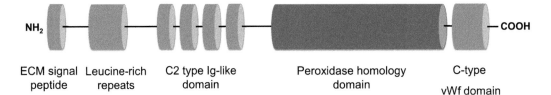

Figure 3.1 Domain structure of human peroxidasin (PXDN).

STRUCTURAL FEATURES OF HUMAN PXDN

The human PXDN protein contains 1,479 amino acids with a calculated molecular weight of 165 kD. The protein contains an N-terminal signal peptide followed by the LRR domain. LRRs are short sequence repeats found in a wide variety of proteins, and they frequently mediate protein–protein interactions. Next to the LRR domain, there are four Ig domains. Ig domains are present in hundreds of proteins with diverse functions. The Ig domains can be categorized into four types: variable (V set), constant (C1 and C2 sets), and intermediate (I set). The Ig domains of PXDN are classified as I set, members of which are frequently recognized in cell adhesion proteins and cell surface receptors [6]. The properties of the peroxidase domain will be discussed later. The C-terminal vWFC domain is a cysteine-rich, highly conserved protein module, which is present in many secreted, extracellular proteins, including thrombospondins and Von Willebrand factor. Proteins with vWFC domains are frequently found in multi-protein complexes.

Two groups, including ours, showed that the human PXDN functions in homotrimers formed through disulfide bridges [7,8]. Both heterologously and endogenously expressed PXDNs were described to form homotrimers. Site-directed mutagenesis of cysteines highlighted the importance of Cys736 and Cys1315 in trimer formation [8]. In support of the importance of the C-terminus in the process, a PXDN construct truncated at amino acid position 1,288 did not form homotrimers [7]. Trimer formation might be required for optimal cross-linking, as the C736S, C1315S double-mutant PXDN showed reduced activity [8].

Similar to other members of the peroxidase-cyclooxygenase superfamily, PXDN is also N-glycosylated: seven glycosylation sites have been experimentally verified in the peroxidase domain, and three additional glycosylation sites were identified in the second Ig domain, in

the region between the peroxidase and vWFC domains and in the vWFC domain [7].

THE PEROXIDASE ACTIVITY OF PXDN

Each PXDN monomer has an active peroxidase domain with a covalently bound heme group [7]. The catalytic domain is homologous to other mammalian peroxidases (MPO, EPO, TPO, LPO), but is most similar to LPO. In the distal heme cavity of the peroxidase domain, His827 and Arg977 are essential for the cleavage of hydrogen peroxide, and Gln823 is necessary for the binding of halides [2]. PXDN can catalyze reactions through the halogenation cycle and the peroxidase cycle as well. In both cycles compound I is the intermediate [9,10]. The first discovered physiological function of PXDN is the cross-linking of collagen IV molecules in the basement membrane [11]. The cross-link is a sulfilimine covalent bond between Met93 and hydroxylysine(Hyl)211 of two adjacent NC1 domains at the C-terminal end of collagen IV [12], and it is formed through the halogenation cycle via hypobromous acid (Figure 3.2).

A convenient method for detecting the cross-linking reaction is the Western blot analysis of NC1 domains after collagenase I digestion, using collagen IV isoform-specific antibodies [8,13] (Figure 3.3).

The halogenation cycle starts with the oxidation of the resting enzyme by hydrogen peroxide to produce compound I (oxoiron(IV) with porphyrin π-cation radical). After this step compound I can undergo a direct reaction with two-electron donors, such as bromide or pseudohalide (SCN^-) to form hypobromous acid or hypothiocyanite, but chloride is not a substrate of the enzyme [9]. It is possible that during this reaction, other domains of PXDN (e.g., LRR- and Ig domains) help to position the production of hypohalous acid close to the site of sulfilimine bond formation. It is essential to produce this potentially harmful oxidizing agent close to its physiological substrate so as

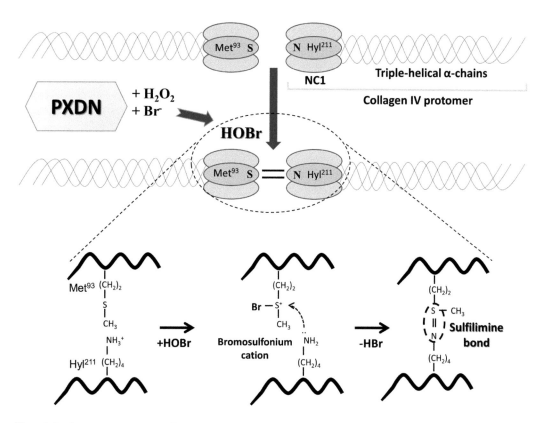

Figure 3.2 Schematic representation of collagen IV cross-linking by PXDN. PXDN catalyzes sulfinimine bond formation between Met93 and Hyl211 residues of adjacent NC1 domains through the formation of HOBr. HOBr reacts with Met93 to form a halosulfonium intermediate, which reacts with Hyl211 of the opposing protomer's NC1 domain to form the sulfilimine bond.

not to damage other off-target molecules [14,15]. The PXDN pre-steady-state kinetics and substrate specificity were analyzed with the help of a highly active truncated variant, which consists of four Ig and the peroxidase domains. This study revealed that compound I can be reduced by bromide $(5.6 \times 10^6 \ \mathrm{M^{-1}s^{-1}})$, iodide $(1.68 \times 10^7 \ \mathrm{M^{-1}s^{-1}})$, and thiocyanate $(1.83 \times 10^7 \ \mathrm{M^{-1}s^{-1}})$ but not by chloride, even when applied at physiological concentrations (more than 100 mM) [9]. Based on *in vitro* experiments with PFHR9 cells, PXDN prefers using bromide in the enzymatic cross-linking of collagen IV [11]. The bromide preference of PXDN was also proven *in vivo* in *Drosophila*, which resulted in the discovery of the first known function of bromine in live organisms [16]. The normal plasma bromide concentration is 10–100 μM in humans, enough to support the sulfilimine bond formation based on the experiments with *Drosophila*. During sulfilimine bond formation, the halide is oxidized to hypohalous acid, which then reacts with Met93 to form a halosulfonium

intermediate that either reacts with water to form a methionine sulfoxide (a "dead end" in cross-linking) or reacts with the ε-NH_2 of Hyl211 to form the sulfilimine bond (Figure 3.2).

The selectivity for bromide occurs because PXDN cannot form HOCl, instead it forms HOBr. HOBr reacts with Met93 to form a bromosulfonium intermediate, which has a low energetic barrier to sulfiliminie bond formation. Other halides such as fluoride are inert to sulfilimine bond formation; meanwhile, iodide and thiocyanate can inhibit the reaction *in vitro*, probably because of the competition with bromide for the active site and because their corresponding hypohalous acids do not react significantly with Met residues [11,16,17]. The plasma iodide level is 0.2–0.4 μM, which means it is not high enough to compete with bromide *in vivo*, but thiocyanate may interfere *in vivo* with the cross-linking, as its level normally varies between 10 and 50 μM and can be even higher (70–300 μM) in smokers [18]. As was mentioned before, PXDN can also participate

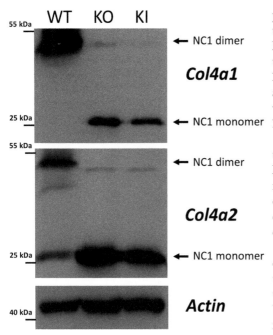

Figure 3.3 Analysis of collagen IV NC1 dimers and monomers by Western blot. Tissues from the fingers of wild-type (WT) and PXDN-deficient knock-out (KO) animals were collagenase digested in hypotonic lysis buffer and processed for Col4a1 and Col4a2 Western blots. Before collagenase I digestion, small aliquots were taken for actin Western blot.

in the peroxidase cycle. In this reaction, the first step is also compound I formation by hydrogen peroxide, which is then reduced in two steps via compound II into the ferric resting state of the enzyme by two one-electron donors. The common redox intermediate in both cycles is compound I. Clearly, the halogenation cycle seems to be directly involved in sulfilimine bond catalysis, but peroxidase substrates can alter the bromination activity of PXDN by promoting compound I to become compound II to follow the peroxidase cycle instead of the halogenation cycle. This shift to the peroxidase cycle was observed in cell culture experiments, where the presence of urate decreased the formation of collagen IV cross-links (the dimerization was inhibited to a maximum of 35% with an IC_{50} of 20 μM) [14]. Based on kinetic measurements, endogenous molecules, such as serotonin and nitrite, can be moderate peroxidase substrates for PXDN, and other molecules such as urate or tyrosine are poor substrates for the peroxidase cycle at physiological pH [10].

Another important question related to the cross-linking reaction is the source of hydrogen

peroxide. The oxidant source and PXDN both have to be placed close to the NC1 domains of collagen IV to localize the reaction to the expected targets. Our group investigated the role of NOX/DUOX enzymes in sulfilimine bond formation as possible hydrogen peroxide sources, but we found normal cross-linking activity in the NOX/DUOX knock-out models that we studied [13]. We also found that under *in vitro* conditions, sulfilimine bond formation is normal at low oxygen concentrations. The flavoprotein inhibitor diphenylene iodonium or expression of targeted catalase constructs to the cytosol or the mitochondrial matrix did not affect the cross-linking activity of PXDN [13].

A further intriguing question is whether PXDN catalyzes the bromination of proteins *in vivo* in addition to that in sulfilimine bond formation. The renal tubule basement membranes, Bowman's capsule basement membranes, and glomerular basement membranes of mouse and normal human kidneys are enriched in bromine, and the accumulation of bromide is PXDN-dependent [19]. The COL4A2 NC1 domains isolated from these kidneys contain brominated Tyr residues (Tyr 1485 in mouse, Tyr 1490 in human), which are essentially absent from the kidney of the PXDN KO mouse [19]. In vitro experiments with PFHR9 cells also show that the ECM of these cells contains 3-Br-Tyr residues produced by PXDN [20]. These residues were also present in significant amounts in the intracellular extract, which can indicate that PXDN might be active intracellularly too [20].

PROTEIN INTERACTIONS OF PXDN

The ability of PXDN to catalyze the formation of NC1 cross-links is unique among members of the peroxidase-cyclooxygenase superfamily. Although eosinophil peroxidase (EPO) produces HOBr, its cross-linking effectiveness lags far behind PXDN [21]. This observation indicates the importance of other structural elements in collagen IV cross-linking. In an overlay test system, where different truncated variants of PXDN were expressed in HEK293T cells, a mutant PXDN construct lacking seven N-terminal amino acids in the first Ig domain failed to cross-link collagen IV [21]. This result highlights the importance of this region in PXDN's function.

Although the critical role of PXDN in basement membrane formation is now proven, we know little about the protein interactions of PXDN within this complex environment. This is an important issue because proper positioning of HOBr formation is probably crucial for the generation of oxidative modification in a spatiotemporally confined manner. Considering the function of PXDN, binding to collagen IV would be plausible; however, Ero-Tolliver et al. found no evidence for a strong interaction between the two proteins [21]. Furthermore, the degradation of the collagen IV network by collagenase treatment did not solubilize PXDN from the ECM produced by PFHR9 cells [21]. Based on their well-recognized role in mediating protein–protein interactions, it is reasonable to believe that the N-terminal LRR and Ig motifs are important in positioning PXDN in the ECM. Sevcnikar et al. recently reported the binding of PXDN to laminin, a key component of basement membranes [22]. Although the exact mechanism of this interaction remains to be clarified, it might be crucial in positioning PXDN for the cross-linking reaction. The vWF C-type domain, which is located at the C-terminal part of the protein, is also a candidate for mediating protein–protein interactions. This domain, however, might not be present in the secreted protein, because PXDN contains a proprotein-convertase (furin) cleavage site at Arg1336, and PXDN is cleaved at this location during its post-translational processing [23]. Thus, the vWF C-type domain is probably not an integral part of extracellularly localized PXDN, although it is possible that a fraction of the full-length protein also becomes secreted.

FUNCTIONAL ASPECTS: ROLE OF PXDN IN THE ORGANIZATION OF BASEMENT MEMBRANES

As yet, the only known intentional molecular target of the HOBr produced by PXDN is the C-terminal, non-collagenous NC1 domain of collagen IV α-chains [11]. Three of these α-chains form a collagen IV protomer, and these protomers are cross-linked through the NC1 parts by the HOBr-catalyzed sulfilimine cross-links. A very intriguing and fundamental question is how this very precisely characterized biochemical function relates to the phenotypic changes observed in the development, morphology, and physiology of PXDN mutant animals? Simply put, what could be the biological role of the sulfilimine cross-link in collagen IV?

Type IV collagen is mainly known as a major component of a unique form of the ECM, the basement membrane. We can observe this complex, three-dimensional sheet of extracellular proteins underlying the basolateral side of epithelial cells in all epithelial tissues [24] (Figure 3.4).

Basement membrane is present under the endothelial cells of blood vessels and under the epithelium of the gastrointestinal, urogenital, and respiratory tract [24]. Importantly we can find collagen IV in other locations as well. All striated – skeletal and heart – muscle cells are surrounded by a collagen-IV-containing ECM sheet. Smooth muscle cells found in different tissues also synthesize significant amounts of collagen IV [25]. Neuromuscular synapses contain collagen IV in the synaptic cleft [26]. There is also a connective tissue envelope rich in collagen IV around each fat cell in the adipose tissue. Accordingly, PXDN shows a ubiquitous expression pattern, and it is especially highly expressed in smooth-muscle-containing organs, such as the urinary bladder, uterus, aorta. PXDN is also strongly expressed in the heart and in adipose tissue (for human expression data, we refer to The Broad Institute's www.gtexportal.org/home/ database).

The long, triple-helical collagen IV protomers are held together in an intricate network structure by several different types of interactions [27]. The N-terminal 7S part of the protomer is rich in cysteines and lysines or hydroxy-lysine residues. Four protomers form tetramers through disulfide bonds and lysine cross-links between the N-terminal 7S domains. The long, collagenous part of the protomers contains several short interruptions of the Gly-Xaa-Yaa triple repeats. These interruptions also serve as binding sites for other molecules and receptors and interchain cross-linking of the protomers [27,28]. Interestingly, different α-chain isoforms contain different numbers of these interruptions, making them more or less suitable for cross-linking in the collagenous domain. These lateral interactions between long protomers are reinforced by the cross-linking activity of lysyl-oxidase and lysyl-oxidase-like enzymes secreted into the ECM [28]. Finally, the C-terminal NC1 trimers of neighboring protomers are covalently cross-linked by the unique sulfilimine bond, forming NC1 hexamers.

As we can see, several structural elements are responsible for the mechanical complexity and strength of the collagen IV network. Therefore,

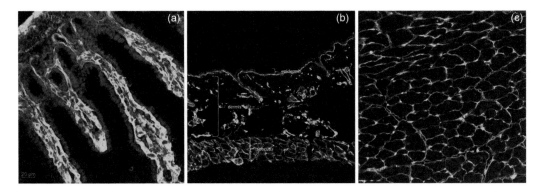

Figure 3.4 Immunofluorescent labeling of collagen IV in different tissues: (a) mouse frozen small intestine section, (b) mouse skin sagittal paraffin section, and (c) mouse skeletal muscle paraffin section. The green color in a–c indicates collagen IV staining, and the red color in c indicates nuclear staining.

it must be stressed that the sulfilimine covalent cross-link is by far not the only stabilizing force of the collagen IV network. Importantly, it was shown by electron microscopy that there are no obvious ultrastructural morphological changes in the glomerular basal membrane (GBM) in the kidneys of PXDN-deficient mice [29]. This observation indicates that this essential basal membrane structure is not destroyed by the lack of the sulfilimine bond [29]. However, it is also important to note that the adult GBM is very rich in the α4 collagen IV isoform, which is much better suited for numerous lateral interactions between the triple-helical domains than other, more ubiquitous isoforms, such as the α1 and α2 chains [27]. This composition can also contribute to the mechanical integrity of the GBM, even in the absence of the sulfilimine cross-links between the NC1 domains.

What has been described above about the supramolecular structure of collagen IV also suggests that the sulfilimine cross-link might have a biological function not necessarily related solely to the mechanical resistance or tensile strength of the collagen network. Instead, it might also contribute to the growth factor binding activity of basal membranes. Several morphogens and growth factors are bound, embedded, and gradually released from the ECM and basement membranes. The TGFβ superfamily of morphogens are often present in large preproprotein forms in the ECM, embedded into the matrix through various protein–protein interactions. The biologically active ligands are released through a series of proteolytic steps [30]. A member of this superfamily, bone morphogenetic protein 4 (Bmp4), was shown to directly interact with collagen IV [31].

Morphogen gradients in the developing embryos are important determinants of tissue and organogenesis. Therefore, any influence of collagen IV sulfilimine cross-links on morphogen gradients could provide a lucid explanation for the several developmental defects observed in PXDN mutant animal models discussed later.

Proteolytic enzymes, such as matrix metalloproteases (MMPs), continuously cleave matrix components, releasing numerous biologically active peptides and protein fragments from matrix proteins. Among them, some collagen IV NC1 isoforms released from collagen protomers (arrestin, canstatin, and tumstatin) were reported to have antiangiogenic and antitumor activity, and they were also described to regulate branching morphogenesis of exocrine glands [32,33]. These released NC1 domains can exert their effects by binding to integrin receptors on cell surfaces [34]. It is reasonable to assume that the lack or presence of sulfilimine cross-linking between the NC1 domains released by MMPs can impact their receptor binding and biological activity. This could provide an additional mechanism for how the sulfilimine cross-link might influence the biological function of collagen IV.

PXDN FUNCTIONS: EXAMPLES FROM DIFFERENT SPECIES

A seminal approach to study the significance and biological role of a biochemical modification such as the collagen IV sulfilimine cross-link is the analysis of the evolutionary appearance of the molecular substituents involved in the reaction. Thereby, it might be possible to identify environmental challenges and important tissue and organ evolutionary steps where the particular biochemical reaction played a fundamental role. A detailed and meticulous study analyzed the evolutionary occurrence of the sulfilimine cross-link and PXDN expression in 31 species across 11 major phyla [35]. To determine PXDN expression, available genomic data were analyzed, or next-generation RNA sequencing was used for de novo transcriptome assembly. For the detection of NC1 dimers and the presence of the sulfilimine bond, NC1 dimer extracts were prepared following collagenase I digestion of tissue samples (NC1 domains – in contrast to the collagenous domains – are resistant to collagenase I digestion). Coomassie staining and anti-collagen IV NC1 immunoblotting were used to detect the NC1 dimers, and high-resolution Orbitrap mass spectrometry was applied with Fourier transform-based analysis to identify the presence of cross-linked amino acids in tryptic digests of NC1 dimer extracts. It was found that cross-links and PXDN expression are both conserved throughout Eumetazoa – an animal clade that displays defining features such as an embryonic development that goes through a gastrula stage, the presence of true tissues organized into germ layers, and the emergence of nerve cells. This biochemical feature of the collagen IV network appeared over 500 million years ago at the divergence of Porifera and Cnidaria. In some of the non-eumetazoan Porifera and Placozoa species, there are already peroxidase domain-containing sequences, but these encode much shorter proteins than the multidomain PXDN. Furthermore, in the collagen IV NC1 sequences of these species, the conserved Met and Lys residues are absent. Among the eight Cnidarian species tested in the study, there was only one (Hydra magnipapillata) not expressing PXDN and not containing the conserved amino acid residues. The fragile, highly flexible nature of Hydra is based on its mesoglea, a gelatinous, largely acellular layer between endo- and ectoderm. Later in triploblastic Bilateralia, the development of the mesoderm and multicellular muscle tissues along with the more complex tissue organization probably required the occurrence of the additional sulfilimine bond in the collagen IV structure [35].

Next, we discuss a few examples of the developmental and functional defects observed in the absence of functional PXDN. In the extensively used nematode model, Caenorhabditis elegans (C. elegans), ethyl-methanesulfonic acid (EMS)-based mutagenesis was used to generate mutants to screen for defects in the elongation phase, the last major stage of C. elegans embryonic morphogenesis. Seven lethal mutations were mapped to the pxn-2 gene in this screen [36]. To rescue these mutants by transfection of peroxidasin transgenes, the intact peroxidase activity of the transgenes was indispensable. Time-lapse video analysis revealed that epidermal elongation and epidermal–muscle interactions are severely disturbed between the twofold and threefold stages of development resulting in larval arrest and muscle detachment. Weaker pxn-2 mutations also sensitized the embryos for loss-of-function mutations of other basement membrane components such as the laminin αA (lam-3) [36].

PXN-2 was found also to be involved in selective axon guidance choices, but was not essential for axon outgrowth during development. In partial loss-of-function pxn-2 adult animals, the axon regrowth after laser axotomy was significantly enhanced, indicating that pxn-2 might inhibit adult axon regrowth after injury. Remarkably, there is also another peroxidasin-like protein, pxn-1, expressed in C. elegans [36]. Mutation of this gene did not result in obvious developmental defects or structural changes of basal membranes. Interestingly, the pxn-1, pxn-2 double mutants showed reduced phenotype, while pxn-1 overexpression in pxn-2 mutants aggravated the phenotype, indicating antagonistic functions of the two proteins [36]. In human and many other mammalian species, there is also a peroxidasin-like (PXDNL) gene, but it is absent in some often used rodent experimental models such as mice and rats [37]. Importantly, in all primate PXDNL sequences, some catalytically critical amino acids are replaced, eliminating its peroxidase activity.

Peroxidasin protein was first characterized after successful purification from the supernatant of immortalized Drosophila melanogaster cells of hemocyte origin [1]. It had been proposed that Drosophila PXDN was important in both host defense and tissue remodeling during development. It was rightly assumed that "secreted peroxidasin has a role in the consolidation of ECM" [1]. In a later study, describing PXDN as the enzyme that catalyzes the sulfilimine cross-linking, a severely hypomorphic Drosophila Pxn allele was analyzed [11]. Larvae homozygous for this mutant allele survived until the third instar larval stage. Using a GFP-labeled collagen IV transgene (Drosophila

Viking), it was shown that the collagen networks were severely distorted and torn within the basement membrane of midgut visceral muscles [11].

The highly translucent tissues of the developing embryo of the zebrafish (*Danio rerio*) make these animals convenient models for time-lapse video analysis of tissue morphogenesis. Injection of morpholino oligomers into developing embryos successfully inhibited PXDN translation and resulted in a decrease or disappearance of the collagen IV NC1 dimers. Twenty-four hours post-fertilization there were severe developmental defects, such as cardiac edema, decreased eye size, and gross trunk patterning effects [35].

It is interesting to note that in both the *Drosophila* and zebrafish studies, inhibition of PXDN function resulted not only in a decrease in cross-linked NC1 dimers but also in a general decrease in the total amount of collagen IV detected by anti-NC1 collagen IV antibodies [11,35]. This implies that the cross-link has an impact also on the stability or turnover of collagen IV protomers.

In mouse PXDN mutants reported so far, the most apparent phenotype is disturbed ocular development [38,39]. The newborn animals are blind, and there are clear anatomical and histological findings of severe anterior segment dysgenesis (ASD). Beyond this, there is also a pigmentation problem, whereby naturally black mouse strains (C57BL/6) develop white belly spots. Also, the PXDN mutant animals are usually smaller and display increased perinatal lethality.

Normal development of the mammalian eye requires a precise biomechanical organization of developing structures and fine-tuned signaling by morphogens and growth factors. Interestingly, TGFβ isoforms (especially TGFβ2) and bone morphogenetic proteins (BMPs) are indispensable for eye development and differentiation [40]. TGFβ2 mutations lead to a severe ASD phenotype, just as does the PXDN mutation in mice [41]. In human patients with PXDN mutations, the eye phenotype (ASD) is also an obligate sign [42,43]. Probably the high precision that is required for proper development and function of the eye is a significant reason why the eye phenotype is the most prominent and penetrant abnormality in mammalian PXDN mutant models. However, one can assume that based on the ubiquitous expression of PXDN and the presence of the sulfilimine cross-link in most tissues, PXDN mutations lead to severe, albeit less pronounced, differences in many other tissues as well.

CONCLUSION

As discussed above, PXDN combines an active peroxidase domain with protein modules capable of enabling protein–protein interactions in the extracellular space. With its already discovered collagen IV cross-linking function in the basement membrane, this unique structure placed PXDN in the center of interest. We can assume that sulfilimine bond formation is not the only function of this protein. To resolve if there are also other biochemical modifications catalyzed by PXDN, novel, innovative experimental approaches will be required. Future studies on the exact biological function of the "sulfilimine knot" and PXDN will pave the way for a more profound understanding of matrix biology. This knowledge will advance several fields, such as clinical diagnostics and therapeutics or *in vitro* tissue engineering techniques.

REFERENCES

1. R.E. Nelson, L.I. Fessler, Y. Takagi, et al., 1994, Peroxidasin: A novel enzyme-matrix protein of Drosophila development, *EMBO J.* 13: 3438–3447.

2. M. Zamocky, C. Jakopitsch, P.G. Furtmüller, C. Dunand, C. Obinger, 2008, The peroxidase-cyclooxygenase superfamily: Reconstructed evolution of critical enzymes of the innate immune system, *Proteins* 72: 589–605.

3. N. Horikoshi, J. Cong, N. Kley, T. Shenk, 1999, Isolation of differentially expressed cDNAs from p53-dependent apoptotic cells: Activation of the human homologue of the Drosophila peroxidasin gene, *Biochem. Biophys. Res. Commun.* 261: 864–869.

4. M.S. Mitchell, J. Kan-Mitchell, B. Minev, C. Edman, R.J. Deans, 2000, A novel melanoma gene (MG50) encoding the interleukin 1 receptor antagonist and six epitopes recognized by human cytolytic T lymphocytes, *Cancer Res.* 60: 6448–6456.

5. G. Cheng, J.C. Salerno, Z. Cao, P.J. Pagano, J.D. Lambeth, 2008, Identification and characterization of VPO1, a new animal heme-containing peroxidase, *Free Radic. Biol. Med.* 45: 1682–1694.

6. Y. Harpaz, C. Chothia, 1994, Many of the immunoglobulin superfamily domains in cell adhesion molecules and surface receptors belong to a new structural set which is close to that containing variable domains, *J. Mol. Biol.* 238: 528–539.

7. M. Soudi, M. Paumann-Page, C. Delporte, et al., 2015, Multidomain human peroxidasin 1 is a highly glycosylated and stable homotrimeric high spin ferric peroxidase, *J. Biol. Chem.* 290: 10876–10890.

8. E. Lázár, Z. Péterfi, G. Sirokmány, et al., 2015, Structure-function analysis of peroxidasin provides insight into the mechanism of collagen IV crosslinking, *Free Radic. Biol. Med.* 83: 273–282.

9. M. Paumann-Page, R.S. Katz, M. Bellei, et al., 2017, Pre-steady-state kinetics reveal the substrate specificity and mechanism of halide oxidation of truncated human Peroxidasin 1, *J. Biol. Chem.* 292: 4583–4592.

10. B. Sevcnikar, M. Paumann-Page, S. Hofbauer, et al., 2020, Reaction of human peroxidasin 1 compound I and compound II with one-electron donors, *Arch. Biochem. Biophys.* 681: 108267.

11. G. Bhave, C.F. Cummings, R.M. Vanacore, et al., 2012, Peroxidasin forms sulfilimine chemical bonds using hypohalous acids in tissue genesis, *Nat. Chem. Biol.* 8: 784–790.

12. R. Vanacore, A.J. Ham, M. Voehler, et al., 2009, A sulfilimine bond identified in collagen IV, *Science* 325: 1230–1234.

13. G. Sirokmány, H.A. Kovács, E. Lázár, et al., 2018, Peroxidasin-mediated crosslinking of collagen IV is independent of NADPH oxidases, *Redox Biol.* 16: 314–321.

14. B. Bathish, R. Turner, M. Paumann-Page, A.J. Kettle, C.C. Winterbourn, 2018, Characterisation of peroxidasin activity in isolated extracellular matrix and direct detection of hypobromous acid formation, *Arch. Biochem. Biophys.* 646: 120–127.

15. D.I. Pattison, M.J. Davies, 2004, Kinetic analysis of the reactions of hypobromous acid with protein components: Implications for cellular damage and use of 3-bromotyrosine as a marker of oxidative stress, *Biochemistry* 43: 4799–4809.

16. A.S. McCall, C.F. Cummings, G. Bhave, et al., 2014, Bromine is an essential trace element for assembly of collagen IV scaffolds in tissue development and architecture, *Cell* 157: 1380–1392.

17. O. Skaff, D.I. Pattison, M.J. Davies, 2009, Hypothiocyanous acid reactivity with low-molecular-mass and protein thiols: Absolute rate constants and assessment of biological relevance, *Biochem. J.* 422: 111–117.

18. C.J. Vesey, Y. Saloojee, P.V. Cole, M.A. Russell, 1982, Blood carboxyhaemoglobin, plasma thiocyanate, and cigarette consumption: Implications for epidemiological studies in smokers, *Br. Med. J. (Clin. Res. Ed.)* 284: 1516–1518.

19. C. He, W. Song, T.A. Weston, et al., 2020, Peroxidasin-mediated bromine enrichment of basement membranes, *Proc. Natl. Acad. Sci. U.S.A.* 117: 15827–15836.

20. B. Bathish, M. Paumann-Page, L.N. Paton, A.J. Kettle, C.C. Winterbourn, 2020, Peroxidasin mediates bromination of tyrosine residues in the extracellular matrix, *J. Biol. Chem.* 295: 12697–12705.

21. I.A. Ero-Tolliver, B.G. Hudson, G. Bhave, 2015, The ancient immunoglobulin domains of peroxidasin are required to form sulfilimine cross-links in collagen IV, *J. Biol. Chem.* 290: 21741–21748.

22. B. Sevcnikar, I. Schaffner, C.Y. Chuang, et al., 2020, The leucine-rich repeat domain of human peroxidasin 1 promotes binding to laminin in basement membranes, *Arch. Biochem. Biophys.* 689: 108443.

23. S. Colon, G. Bhave, 2016, Proprotein convertase processing enhances peroxidasin activity to reinforce collagen IV, *J. Biol. Chem.* 291: 24009–24016.

24. V.S. LeBleu, B. Macdonald, R. Kalluri, 2007, Structure and function of basement membranes, *Exp. Biol. Med. (Maywood)* 232: 1121–1129.

25. D.B. Borza, O. Bondar, Y. Ninomiya, et al., 2001, The NC1 domain of collagen IV encodes a novel network composed of the alpha 1, alpha 2, alpha 5, and alpha 6 chains in smooth muscle basement membranes, *J. Biol. Chem.* 276: 28532–28540.

26. J.R. Sanes, 1982, Laminin, fibronectin, and collagen in synaptic and extrasynaptic portions of muscle fiber basement membrane, *J. Cell. Biol.* 93: 442–451.

27. J. Khoshnoodi, V. Pedchenko, B.G. Hudson, 2008, Mammalian collagen IV, *Microsc. Res. Tech.* 71: 357–370.

28. C. Añazco, A.J. López-Jiménez, M. Rafi, et al., 2016, Lysyl Oxidase-like-2 cross-links collagen iv of glomerular basement membrane, *J. Biol. Chem.* 291: 25999–26012.

29. G. Bhave, S. Colon, N. Ferrell, 2017, The sulfilimine cross-link of collagen IV contributes to kidney tubular basement membrane stiffness, *Am. J. Physiol. Renal Physiol.* 313: F596–F602.

30. V.M. Paralkar, S. Vukicevic, A.H. Reddi, 1991, Transforming growth factor beta type 1 binds to collagen IV of basement membrane matrix: Implications for development, *Dev. Biol.* 143: 303–308.

31. X. Wang, R.E. Harris, L.J. Bayston, H.L. Ashe, 2008, Type IV collagens regulate BMP signalling in Drosophila, *Nature* 455: 72–77.

32. T.M. Mundel, R. Kalluri, 2007, Type IV collagen-derived angiogenesis inhibitors, *Microvasc. Res.* 74: 85–89.

33. I.T. Rebustini, C. Myers, K.S. Lassiter, et al., 2009, MT2-MMP-dependent release of collagen IV NC1 domains regulates submandibular gland branching morphogenesis, *Dev. Cell* 17: 482–493.

34. Y. Wu, G. Ge, 2019, Complexity of type IV collagens: From network assembly to function, *Biol. Chem.* 400: 565–574.

35. A.L. Fidler, R.M. Vanacore, S.V. Chetyrkin, et al., 2014, A unique covalent bond in basement membrane is a primordial innovation for tissue evolution, *Proc. Natl. Acad. Sci. U.S.A.* 111: 331–336.

36. J.R. Gotenstein, R.E. Swale, T. Fukuda, et al., 2010, The C. elegans peroxidasin PXN-2 is essential for embryonic morphogenesis and inhibits adult axon regeneration, *Development* 137: 3603–3613.

37. Z. Péterfi, Z.E. Tóth, H.A. Kovács, et al., 2014, Peroxidasin-like protein: A novel peroxidase homologue in the human heart, *Cardiovasc. Res.* 101: 393–399.

38. X. Yan, S. Sabrautzki, M. Horsch, et al., 2014, Peroxidasin is essential for eye development in the mouse, *Hum. Mol. Genet.* 23: 5597–5614.

39. H.K. Kim, K.A. Ham, S.W. Lee, et al., 2019, Biallelic deletion of Pxdn in Mice leads to anophthalmia and severe eye malformation, *Int. J. Mol. Sci.* 20: 6144.

40. S. Saika, 2006, TGFbeta pathobiology in the eye, *Lab. Invest.* 86: 106–115.

41. J.C. Sowden, 2007, Molecular and developmental mechanisms of anterior segment dysgenesis, *Eye (Lond)* 21: 1310–1318.

42. K. Khan, A. Rudkin, D.A. Parry, et al., 2011, Homozygous mutations in PXDN cause congenital cataract, corneal opacity, and developmental glaucoma, *Am. J. Hum. Genet.* 89: 464–473.

43. A. Choi, R. Lao, P. Ling-Fung Tang, et al., 2015, Novel mutations in PXDN cause microphthalmia and anterior segment dysgenesis, *Eur. J. Hum. Genet.* 23: 337–341.

PART TWO

Reactivity of Peroxidase Oxidants

Reactivity of Peroxidase-Derived Oxidants with Proteins, Glycoproteins and Proteoglycans

Michael J. Davies
University of Copenhagen

CONTENTS

ABBREVIATIONS

ApoA1:	Apolipoprotein A1
3ClTyr:	3-chlorotyrosine
CRP:	C-reactive protein
3,5diClTyr:	3,5-dichlorotyrosine
di-Tyr:	o-o'-di-tyrosine
ECM:	Extracellular matrix
EPO:	Eosinophil peroxidase
GAPDH:	Glyceraldehyde-3-phosphate dehydrogenase
HDL:	High-density lipoproteins
H_2O_2:	Hydrogen peroxide
HOBr:	Hypobromous acid
HOCl:	Hypochlorous acid
HOI:	Hypoiodous acid
HOSCN:	Hypothiocyanous acid
HOSeCN:	Hyposelenocyanous acid
LDL:	Low-density lipoproteins
LPO:	Lactoperoxidase
MAPK:	Mitogen-activated protein kinase
MMP:	Matrix metalloproteinase

DOI: 10.1201/9781003212287-6

INTRODUCTION

Mammalian heme peroxidases are a family of enzymes that play a key role in the destruction, by the innate immune system, of bacteria, yeasts, fungi, parasites and other invading pathogens [1–3]. The major mammalian heme peroxidases are myeloperoxidase (MPO), eosinophil peroxidase (EPO), lactoperoxidase (LPO), thyroid peroxidase (TPO) and peroxidasin (PXDN, also previously known as vascular peroxidase, VPO) [2,4]. Each of these species catalyzes the reaction of hydrogen peroxide (H_2O_2) with one or more members of the halide/pseudo-halide anion family (chloride, Cl^-; bromide, Br^-; iodide, I^-; thiocyanate, SCN^-; selenocyanate, $SeCN^-$) via a catalytic cycle often termed the "halogenation cycle" (Figure 4.1) [2,5]. In some cases, the selectivity of the peroxidase for a particular anion is high (e.g. TPO primarily oxidizes I^- [6,7]), but in most cases, these enzymes oxidize multiple

species, with the extent of formation of particular oxidized products dependent on the anion concentration (i.e. they act as competitive substrates) [8].

SOURCES AND OUTLINE OF BIOLOGICAL FUNCTIONS OF HEME PEROXIDASES

Heme peroxidases are synthesized and released by a number of different cell types to carry out specific biological functions. MPO is released into the phagolysosome compartment and to a more limited extent extracellularly, by activated neutrophils (in which it is a very abundant protein accounting for ~ 5% by dry mass), monocytes and some tissue macrophages [9,10]. The function of the oxidants generated by this enzyme is believed to be primarily pathogen killing, with genetic deficiencies in this enzyme associated with chronic and persistent infections and particularly with the fungus *Candida albicans* [3,9–11].

EPO is released extracellularly by activated eosinophils to kill (predominantly) parasites as a result of enzyme attachment to the target [12,13]. LPO is excreted into a number of biological fluids including breast milk, tears, vaginal fluid, saliva, airway lung fluid and other mucosal excretions, where it acts as an antimicrobial defense system [1,14,15]. TPO, as its name indicates, is specifically found in the thyroid where it employs I^- to iodinate thyroglobulin to yield thyroxine (T_4) or

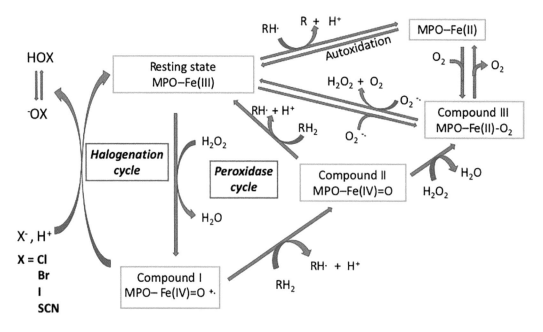

Figure 4.1 Catalytic cycles of heme peroxidases.

triiodothyronine (T_3) [7,16]. The final member of the family PXDN is found in the vessel wall of arteries and associated with the extracellular matrix (ECM), where it plays a key role in tissue synthesis and development via cross-linking of type IV collagen chains, to form a complex three-dimensional ECM structural network [17–21]. Disruption of the PXDN system is embryonically lethal in *Drosophila* and *C. elegans* [19].

CATALYTIC CYCLES OF HEME PEROXIDASE ENZYMES

The peroxidase catalytic cycle of heme peroxidases involves the initial two-electron oxidation of the resting state Fe^{3+} (ferric) form of the enzyme by H_2O_2 to a species, which is formally a Fe^{5+} species, but which is better described as an Fe^{4+}-oxo species and a porphyrin radical cation (Figure 4.1) [22]. This species is, for historical reasons, commonly called Compound I. This oxidation is fast (e.g. k 1.4×10^7 $M^{-1}s^{-1}$ for MPO) and limited to H_2O_2 (i.e. does not occur rapidly with other peroxides) by the constrained nature of the access channel to the iron protoporphyrin IX prosthetic group [22]. The Compound I species then has two major pathways that result in reduction back to the resting Fe^{3+} form – either direct two-electron reduction at the expense of an oxidizable halide/pseudohalide species or two sequential one-electron reduction reactions [2].

The first process – direct two-electron reduction of Compound I – results in the formation of the corresponding hypohalous acids (hypochlorous acid, HOCl, from Cl^-; hypobromous acid, HOBr, from Br^-; hypoiodous acid, HOI, from I^-; hypothiocyanous acid, HOSCN, from SCN^-; and hyposelenocyanous acid, HOSeCN, from $SeCN^-$) (Figure 4.1) (reviewed in Ref. [2]). Each of these hypohalous acids exists as an equilibrium with its conjugate anion, ^-OX (X=Cl, Br, I, SCN, SeCN)

at physiological pH values, though the pK_a value varies with these species, such that some are predominantly ionized at pH 7.4 (HOSCN, HOSeCN), some are nearly equal mixtures (HOCl) and some are predominantly neutral (HOBr) (Table 4.1) (reviewed in Ref. [2]). These hypohalous acids also vary markedly in their oxidizing power as indicated by their two electron reduction potentials (Table 4.1) (reviewed in Refs. [2,8,23]).

The second pathway involves two sequential one-electron oxidations of electron-rich substrates (Figure 4.1) (reviewed in Refs. [2,22,24]). The first step results in restitution of the porphyrin radical cation, leaving an Fe^{4+}-oxo species – commonly called Compound II. The latter can then induce a second one-electron oxidation, with reformation of the Fe^{3+} resting state. As both of these steps are one-electron reactions, the species that are oxidized are converted to radicals (or less commonly, converted from a radical to a non-radical species [2]). These reactions occur with a wide variety of electron-rich species such as inorganic anions (such as NO_2^-, which is oxidized to $NO_2^\bullet$ [25,26]) and aromatic compounds (e.g. phenols, indoles, urate, flavonoids, dye molecules and related species [22,27]). Further reduction of the resting state Fe^{3+} form has also been characterized for species such as MPO, to yield Fe^{2+} forms including Fe^{2+}-O_2 and deoxy-Fe^{2+}complexes [28]; the formation and reactions of these species have been reviewed elsewhere [23].

SUBSTRATE SPECIFICITIES OF HEME PEROXIDASES

There are major differences in the specificity of the heme peroxidase family for different halide and pseudohalide anions. MPO primarily generates HOCl and HOSCN at neutral pH values (7–7.4) with normal plasma ion concentrations (100–140 mM Cl^-, 20–100 µM Br^-, < 1 µM I^- and

TABLE 4.1
Physical chemical properties of hypohalous acids

Parameter	HOCl	HOBr	HOSCN
Standard two-electron reduction potential (E°) for reaction couple HOX/X^- (V)	1.28	1.13	0.56
pK_a	7.59	8.7	4.85

E° values from Ref. [8] at pH 7.0 and 25°C. pK_a values from Refs. [68,208,209]. The pK_a for HOSCN reported is lower than an earlier value (5.3) reported in Ref. [112].

20–100 μM SCN⁻) [2,29]; HOBr is formed only at low concentrations, but this is pH-dependent [30]. The rate constants for reaction of these halide/pseudohalide ions with Compound I of MPO have been determined (Table 4.2) [8], and it is clear from these data that the predominance of HOCl as a product is driven by the concentration of the parent halide, rather than a high rate constant for oxidation of this anion. Indeed, the rate constants for oxidation increase down the order $Cl^- < Br^- < I^- < SCN^-$ (i.e. the rate constants follow the ease of oxidation of these anions) [2,5,8,31]. This allows manipulation of the oxidants formed by MPO, via alteration of the anion concentrations (see below). The relatively modest rate of oxidation of Cl^- by Compound I arises from the high two-electron reduction potential of this anion, and this can only be achieved at significant rates by the distorted heme structure of MPO [32,33]. The heme distortion arises from the cross-linking of the iron protoporphyrin IX group, via a sulfonium group and ester linkages, to the surrounding protein [33,34]. The absence of this heme distortion and bonding results in very low levels of Cl^- oxidation by the other members of the heme peroxidase family [33,34].

EPO primarily oxidizes Br^- and SCN^- to yield HOBr and HOSCN [13,35], whereas LPO shows considerable selectivity for SCN^- [1]. TPO produces predominantly HOI, though it can also oxidize SCN^- [7,24], whereas PXDN preferentially generates HOBr, though it can also oxidize SCN^-, I^- and other electron-rich species, but not Cl^- (although initial reports suggested that it did) [18,19,36,37].

These preferences are, however, sensitive to the anion concentrations [31] and local pH values (e.g. [30]). Thus, high concentrations of SCN^- are known, for example, to perturb the generation of HOCl by MPO [31,38,39] and iodinating species by TPO such that, in the latter case, hypothyroidism can result [40].

TARGETS OF HYPOHALOUS ACIDS

Although formation of HOCl, HOBr, HOSCN and HOI are critical for tissue development, metabolism and immunity, inappropriate formation of these reactive species can cause host tissue damage [3,41]. The generation of these species is therefore usually subject to specific control and localization. However, there is now abundant evidence that collateral damage arising from the formation of these species is a common and widespread event. Thus, evidence has been presented for neutrophil proteins being a major target for damage by HOCl generated during phagocytosis of pathogens [11,42], with this likely to be a major contributing factor to the short lifetime of activated neutrophils at sites of infection and inflammation. Similarly, inappropriate activation of leukocytes (e.g. in the absence of a pathogen: "sterile inflammation") and chronic low-grade inflammation are associated with extensive heme-peroxidase-mediated damage [43,44]. This is particularly the case with MPO and EPO as these generate the most damaging hypohalous acids, HOCl and HOBr (see below). The evidence for major host tissue damage by the less reactive species (HOSCN,

TABLE 4.2

Selected apparent second-order rate constants for the formation and subsequent reactions of Compound I of MPO

Reaction	Rate constant ($M^{-1} s^{-1}$)	Conditions	Reference
Native enzyme + H_2O_2 → Compound I	1.4×10^7	pH 7, 15°C	[210]
	1.8×10^7	pH 6.5, 25°C	[211]
Compound I + Cl^- → Native enzyme + HOCl	2.5×10^4	pH 7, 15°C	[210]
Compound I + Br^- → Native enzyme + HOBr	1.1×10^6	pH 7, 15°C	[210]
Compound I + I^- → Native enzyme + HOI	7.2×10^6	pH 7, 15°C	[210]
Compound I + SCN^- → Native enzyme + HOSCN	9.6×10^6	pH 7, 15°C	[210]
Compound I + RH → Compound II + $R^•$	Tyr 7.7×10^5	pH 7, 25°C	[212]
	Trp 4.5×10^5	pH 7, 25°C	[212]
	NO_2^- 2.0×10^6	pH 7, 15°C	[213]
Compound I + $O_2^{•-}$ → Compound II + O_2	5×10^6	pH 7.4, 37°C	[87]
Compound I + H_2O_2 → Compound II + $O_2^{•-}$	8.1×10^4	pH 7.1, 25°C	[211]

HOI, HOSeCN) is less compelling; these species are however both cytostatic and cytotoxic to many bacteria [45–49].

As with the initial formation of hypohalous acids from the corresponding anions, the *abundance* of different biological targets is a major driving force in determining which host cell, tissue and biological fluid species are modified by the oxidants generated by heme peroxidases [50,51]. The preponderance of proteins in nearly all biological situations results in these being major targets (cf. data for plasma presented in Figure 4.2), with this being exacerbated by the (proportional and absolute) high rate constants for reaction of most hypohalous acids with some protein side chains (see below) [50,52]. The absolute reactivity across the hypohalous acid series, for those species with significant kinetic data available, decreases along the series: HOCl~HOBr>HOSCN [50,53]. Less data are available for HOI and HOSeCN; unpublished data suggests that these sit between HOBr and HOSCN (Ignasiak et al., unpublished data; Seitner et al., unpublished data). A number of secondary reactive species (e.g. chloramines, RNHCl) are also formed from these hypohalous acids; these also vary markedly in terms of their reactivity [50,53–55], but these also appear to predominantly target proteins and peptides.

The reactivity and associated selectivity of each of the hypohalous acids, and reactive species derived from them, are discussed in greater detail below, together with information on the products formed from these reactions.

REACTIVITY AND SELECTIVITY

Kinetic data have been determined for reaction of HOCl with free or protected amino acids and models of these, in an attempt to understand the reactivity of side chains on peptides and proteins (and also versus other targets). Most of the available data are at neutral pH (7–7.4) [50,52,53], though some analyses of the pH dependence of these reactions have also been published [52,56,57]. HOCl is more reactive than its corresponding anion $^-$OCl, and therefore (in the absence of other factors) the rate of reaction decreases at higher pH values [52,56,57]. At low pH values, analysis is complicated by the formation of free Cl_2 from acidified solutions of HOCl [58]. This is however only significant under markedly acidic conditions. The presence of ionizable groups on the side chain can perturb this overall picture, with this being particularly significant for those species with pK_a values near neutral – this is important for the thiol group of Cys and the imidazole side chain

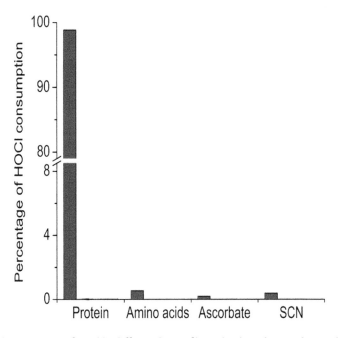

Figure 4.2 Calculated consumption of HOCl by different classes of biomolecules in human plasma. These are calculated for 10 μM HOCl, and are expressed as the percentage of the total, with this showing little variation over a large range of HOCl concentrations. (Data from Ref. [51].)

of His. In the former case, the ionized (thiolate) form is more reactive than the neutral species, and for the imidazole ring, protonation at acidic pH values decreases the reactivity [52,56,57]. Thus, for both species, due to the opposing pH dependence of the HOCl/$^-$OCl pair, a bell-shaped curve is obtained and a complex pH dependence; this is further complicated by the fact that the pK_a values of both Cys and His are markedly dependent on the protein environment and neighboring groups.

Figure 4.3 illustrates the wide variation in rate constants for reaction of HOCl with amino acid side chains and how these compare with reaction with other biological targets. The data for the protein side chains vary by ten orders of magnitude between the most reactive (cysteine, Cys and its selenium analogue, selenocysteine, Sec) and the least reactive (aliphatic side chains such as Ala, Val, Leu, and Ile) [50,52,53,59–61]. Data for the

aliphatic side chains are not included in this plot as they are too slow to measure. It should be noted that there are significant caveats on these data – these have been obtained for the free amino acids, protected species or model compounds and may not always reflect the situation within proteins where other factors can have a significant modulating effect (e.g. as a result of steric or electronic interactions, the effect of neighboring groups and conformation). The example of cystine (the disulfide formed from Cys) illustrates the latter well [61]: the values obtained for reaction with HOCl vary by four orders of magnitude (between 10^4 and 10^8 M^{-1}s^{-1}) as a result of two factors – stabilization of the reaction intermediate by remote lone pairs of electrons (e.g. carboxylate anions, neutral amines) and stabilization by lone pairs of electrons on the neighboring sulfur in the disulfide, with the latter only being a significant factor when the disulfide is

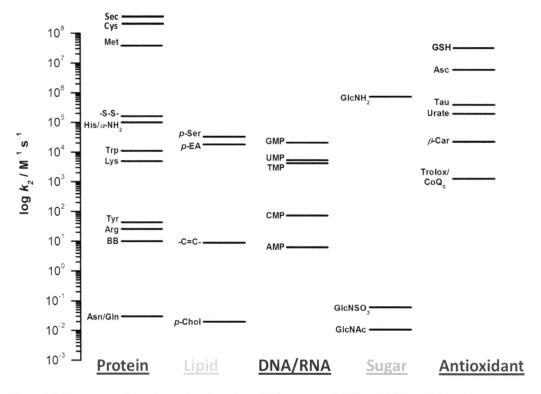

Figure 4.3 Rate constants (vertical axis, plotted on a log scale) for reaction of HOCl with different biological components as indicated on the horizontal axis. (Data from Refs. [50,52,53,59–61].) Abbreviations used: Sec, selenocysteine; Cys, cysteine; Met, methionine; -S-S-, cystine (disulfide bond); His, histidine; α-NH$_2$, α-amino group; Trp, tryptophan; Lys, lysine; Tyr, tyrosine; Arg, arginine; BB, backbone amide; Asn, asparagine; Gln, glutamine; p-Ser, phosphorylserine; p-EA, phosphorylethanolamine; -C=C-, double bond; p-Chol, phosphorylcholine; GMP, guanosine monophosphate; UMP, uridine monophosphate; TMP, thymidine monophosphate; CMP, cytidine monophosphate; AMP, adenosine monophosphate; GlcNH$_2$, glucosamine; GlcNSO$_3$, N-sulfated glucosamine; GlcNAc, N-acetylated glucosamine; GSH, glutathione; Asc, ascorbic acid; Tau, taurine; Urate, uric acid; β-Car, β-carotene; Trolox, (+)6-hydroxy-2,5,7,8-tetramethylchromane-2-carboxylic acid: a water-soluble analogue of α-tocopherol; CoQ0, ubiquinol-0.

in a conformation that allows good orbital overlap [61]. Thus, the approximate order of reactivity of the amino acid side chains is: Cys>Met>cystine> His>α-amino>Trp>Lys>Tyr~Arg>Gln~Asn [50,52,53,59–61]. The amide groups of the protein backbone are also a target for HOCl, although the rate constant is low and environment-dependent [50,52]. This implies that HOCl gives rise to very limited backbone fragmentation of proteins, and this conclusion is supported by experimental data, with the detection of low-molecular-mass bands on sodium dodecyl sulfate-polyacrylamide gel elec-trophoresis (SDS-PAGE) gels only detected at high molar excesses of HOCl compared to the protein [62] (see also below).

These data indicate that HOCl can damage a wide variety of sites on proteins, though there is a degree of selectivity between sites, with the sul-fur- (and rare selenium-) containing amino acids being the most reactive. With low levels of HOCl, these species will therefore be the major sites that are modified, and this effect is enhanced by sec-ondary reactions (see below). The high reactivity of the sulfur-containing species is mitigated, to some extent, by the (typically) lower levels of these side chains compared with others. Thus, the major plasma protein human serum albumin (HSA) contains only a single Cys and Trp residue, compared with 6 Met, 17 cystine, 16 His, 59 Lys and 18 Tyr. Thus, it would be expected that there would be proportionally greater damage at cys-tine, His and Lys, due to their abundance, than might be expected purely on the basis of the rate constant values [51].

The selectivity of HOBr has some similarities to that for HOCl. However, the rate constants reported for Cys and Met are lower than for HOCl, by approximately ten-fold, and that for Tyr increased by ~ 5,000-fold. Some of the other amino acid side chains also react with somewhat higher (30–100 times greater) rate constants than for HOCl [63]. HOBr, therefore, also shows limited selectivity in terms of the amino acid side chains that are subject to damage [63]. How PDXN, which utilizes HOBr to generate essential cross-links in Type IV col-lagen at specific Met residues (see above), achieves selectivity of modification (if this is indeed the case) remains to be established, but there is some data to indicate that this arises (at least in part) by specific localization of the enzyme to the sites of cross-link formation. This may occur via interac-tions, possibly mediated by the immunoglobulin [64] or leucine-rich repeats [65] present in the protein sequence, with other ECM species such as laminins [65]. Evidence has also been presented for MPO binding to specific ECM proteins, though probably via different mechanisms [66].

In contrast to HOCl and HOBr, HOSCN is a weak oxidant and displays a marked selectivity for the thiol group of Cys residues (and particularly those that are ionized, i.e. present as the thiolate anion, RS$^-$) [67]. These reactions are considerably slower than with HOCl (by a factor of 10^2–10^4 [67,68]), and therefore HOSCN is likely to be much less damaging overall than equal concentrations of HOCl or HOBr, and as discussed below, the dam-age induced by HOSCN is predominantly reversible, rather than irreversible (e.g. [69,70]). HOSCN also reacts with the selenium-containing amino acids, selenocysteine (Sec) and selenomethionine, with reaction with the former being more rapid than with Cys [71]. This pattern of reactivity mirrors the two-electron reduction potentials of these species (Table 4.1). The related species HOSeCN appears to be somewhat more reactive than HOSCN, but the kinetics and specificity of this species remain to be determined. Initial experiments suggest that this species can induce damage at Cys, Trp and Tyr resi-dues (Seitner, unpublished data).

The kinetics of reaction of HOI and its selectiv-ity are less well established. It is known that HOI iodinates proteins readily (cf. the function of TPO in generating thyroid hormones), and there is evidence for rapid oxidation of sulfur-containing amino acids, His and Trp residues (Ignasiak et al., unpublished data) This species would therefore be expected to modify multiple sites on proteins, if formed in high yields. However, the very low plasma concentration of I$^-$ limits this, and high yields are only likely to be formed in the thyroid, where I$^-$ is concentrated (by the sodium/iodine symporter of thyroid cells) to 20–50-fold higher levels than are present in plasma (see above) [72]. Whether "collateral damage" (i.e. oxidation at other residues apart from Tyr) occurs at other sites on thyroglobulin is unclear and, if not, how TPO (or other factors) prevents this. This may be via specific enzyme–target protein interactions [7].

Reaction of HOCl and HOBr (and possibly also the other hypohalous acids) with nitrogen cen-ters (e.g. the amine groups present on the Lys side chain, the guanidine group of Arg, the imidazole ring of His, the N-terminus of proteins/peptides/ amino acids and to a lesser extent amide groups on Gln, Asn and polypeptide backbones) can give rise to semi-stable chloramine/bromamine and chloramide/bromamide species [i.e. species with weak N-X bonds, RNHCl or R'NCl-C(O)R" in the case of chlorination] [73]. Similar species can be formed on other biological targets including nucleobases, nucleosides and nucleotides and the amine head groups of phospholipids [74–79]. These species retain some of the oxidizing capacity of the parent hypohalous acids, but are less powerful oxidants and react more slowly [50,55,80,81]. The difference in reactivity is however markedly structure-dependent with some species showing considerable reactivity (e.g. His chloramines [55,82,83]), whereas others (e.g. taurine chloramine [81]) are only weakly reactive. The further reactions of these species are discussed in the "Products" section below. Di-halogenation can also occur (e.g. to give $RNCl_2$) [84]. The latter are also modest oxidants and undergo similar reactions to the monochlorinated species. However, as the formation of dichloramines requires two equivalents of hypohalous acid, they are likely to be low-yield species in most biological situations where the target concentration is large. Formation of these species is however a significant process in circumstances where the oxidant is in excess (e.g. during water disinfection in swimming pools or waste treatment plants, where high levels of oxidant may be used relative to low levels of organic contaminants) [85,86] or possibly in the neutrophil phagolysosome [87].

PRODUCTS FORMED ON MODIFICATION OF AMINO ACID SIDE CHAINS

Sulfur-Containing Side Chains: Cys, Met and Cystine

HOCl reacts with the thiol group of Cys to give an initial, short-lived, sulfenyl chloride (RS-Cl) (Figure 4.4). This undergoes rapid reaction with other nucleophiles (as Cl^- is a good leaving group) with this resulting in the formation of a sulfenic acid with H_2O, disulfides, when the attacking species is another thiol, and sulfenamides (RSNR'), when the attacking species is an amine (e.g. on Lys or the N-terminus) (Figure 4.4). Both sulfenic acids and sulfenamides undergo rapid secondary reactions involving further oxidation or hydrolysis, with these yielding sulfinic (RSO_2H) and sulfonic acids (RSO_3H) [88,89] and sulfinamides

(RS(O)NR') and sulfonamides ($RS(O)_2NR'$) [90–92], respectively (Figure 4.4). Sulfenic and sulfinic acids can be reduced enzymatically within cells, but sulfonic acid formation is irreversible [93,94].

Sulfenyl chlorides decompose to give thiyl radicals (RS) when heated, or in the presence of reducing metal ions [95]. The reactions with other thiols and amines can occur with both low molecular mass species, as well as these groups on the same or other proteins, with this being an important source of intra- and intermolecular cross-links. HOBr reacts similarly to yield highly reactive sulfenyl bromides (RS-Br), and HOSCN yields less reactive sulfenyl thiocyanates (RS-SCN) [96,97]. The lower reactivity of the latter results in a greater selectivity, with only good nucleophiles (e.g. thiolate anions) undergoing significant reaction; disulfides are therefore major products [97], though sulfenic acids, and hence high oxy acids, can also be formed [69,98].

As described above, cystine and other disulfides are oxidized by HOCl and HOBr at very variable rates [61,99]. The initial intermediate is believed to be an adduct ($RS^+(X)SR'$, X=Cl, Br) that is rapidly hydrolyzed to a thiosulfinate (RS(O) SR') [61,99]. The latter are weak oxidants and can undergo nucleophilic attack by water (hydrolysis) or further oxidation to yield sulfinic and sulfonic acids or reaction with thiols to yield a new mixed disulfide (Figure 4.4) [99]. Each of these processes results in cleavage of the disulfide bond, which may have important consequences for protein structure and function, given the key role that disulfides play in stabilizing and maintaining protein structure. Reaction with HOSCN and HOSeCN is slow or not detected, and whether reaction occurs with HOI is unclear.

The major product formed from Met side chains by HOCl and HOBr is methionine sulfoxide, probably via an initial halogen adduct and subsequent very rapid hydrolysis [100]. HOI probably reacts in a similar manner, whereas HOSCN and HOSeCN do not appear to react significantly with this amino acid [67], though reaction occurs with selenomethionine and HOSCN to yield the selenoxide [71]. Met sulfoxide can be oxidized further to the sulfone, though this is a slower reaction and hence is typically only seen with large molar excess of oxidant [50,101]. HOCl also generates dehydromethionine, a cyclic azasulfonium salt, when Met is present at the N-terminus of peptides and proteins [102,103].

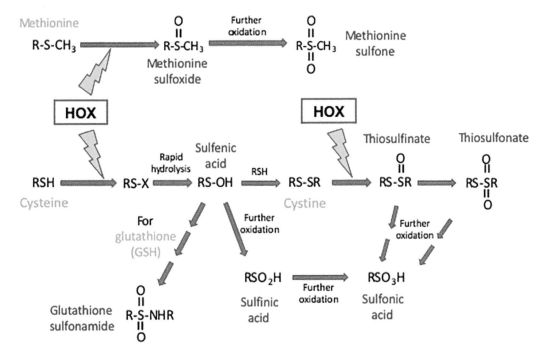

Figure 4.4 Selected products of oxidation of sulfur amino acids by HOX. Parent amino acids are indicated in green text. It should be noted that not all known products are illustrated.

This species is reported to be specific for HOCl and has been used as a biomarker for MPO activity, for example, in the bronchoalveolar fluid from children with cystic fibrosis [104], where it is detected (together with methionine sulfoxide) at the N-terminus of the S100A8 monomer of calprotectin. It should however be noted that HOBr may react similarly, and hence this may not be solely a HOCl biomarker [102].

Amines and Amides (Lys, N-Terminus, Gln, Asn)

The products detected from amines arise primarily from the initial halamines and halamides formed from these groups, particularly by HOCl and HOBr [105,106]. The halamines and halamides undergo two major types of behavior (Figure 4.5). They undergo redox reactions similar to those of the parent hypohalous acids (but at slower rates), with this resulting in, for example, oxidation of Cys and Met and chlorine transfer to other amine/amide/aromatic groups both on the same protein, or on other proteins or targets (e.g. [54,55,82,83]). These reactions result in additional damage to the target residues and regeneration of the amine/amide function [55,106]. Due to this regeneration, the occurrence and significance of these types of

reactions – particularly in complex systems – can be difficult to discern and quantify, but it is likely that these are significant processes due to the high abundance of amine residues and particularly Lys residues on some proteins.

The second process is cleavage of the N-X bond (Figure 4.5). Thermolysis can give two radical species, whereas one-electron reduction of the N-X bond (e.g. by metal ions such as Fe^{2+} and Cu^+ or by $O_2^{\bullet-}$) can give either a nitrogen-centered radical ($RNH^\bullet$ or $RN^\bullet C(O)R'$) and a halide anion or the alternative pairing of a nitrogen anion and a halide radical; the former pairing appears to predominate [62,107,108]. Heterolytic cleavage is also a major process with this resulting in elimination of, for example, HCl, with the proton being lost from a neighboring carbon, and formation of an imine (Figure 4.5) [106,109]. The latter undergo rapid hydrolysis to form carbonyl compounds and free ammonium ions [109,110]. In the case of Lys residues, this gives rise to protein-bound 2-aminoadipic acid semialdehyde (2-aminoadipate-6-semialdehyde, 2-ammonio-6-oxohexanoate) [110]. This is likely to be a major contributor to the (relatively modest) yield of carbonyl groups detected on hypohalous-acid-treated proteins [62,107]. Decomposition of protein

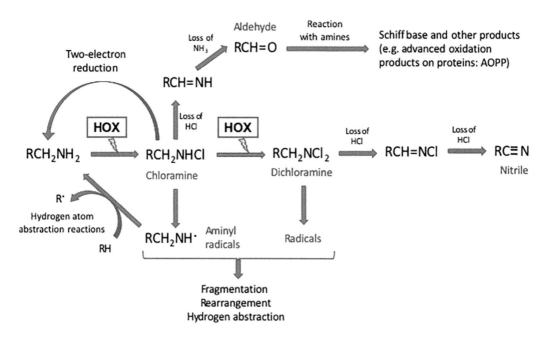

Figure 4.5 Overview of chloramine and dichloramine decomposition pathways.

dichloramines by two successive reactions results in modest yields of nitriles (R-CN) [110,111]. These reactions are summarized in Figure 4.5.

The products formed from RN-SCN species generated by HOSCN [112] are less well characterized. These intermediates appear to be short-lived at physiological pH values; these have been detected on poly-Lys, but evidence for their presence on proteins is lacking [113]. These species have been reported to decompose to regenerate the parent amine [112].

Guanidine (Amidine, Arg Side Chains)

The guanidine group of Arg can be converted to N-chlorinated species by HOCl [114,115], albeit at relatively slow rates when compared with amine groups [52]. The resulting chlorinated species have been suggested to be of pathophysiological significance as they can function (at least in simplified systems) as inhibitors of endothelial nitric oxide synthase (eNOS) activity, thereby depressing production of the key signaling molecule, nitric oxide (NO$^{\bullet}$) [115,116]. Whether sufficient Arg-derived N-chloro species can be formed in vivo to induce such effects is unclear. As the concentration of free Arg in plasma is modest (low micomolar) compared with other targets such as other protein side chains, formation of N-chloro species is unlikely to be a major

pathway. Direct modification of eNOS, at the heme center, or the tetrahydrobiopterin/flavin/calmodulin cofactors, may be more significant factors [117,118].

Imidazole Groups (His)

Ring-derived (endo cyclic) halamines are formed from the imidazole group of His by both HOCl and HOBr [82,83]. These species show considerable reactivity and have been reported to be key species in chlorine transfer reactions (e.g. to Lys and Tyr residues) within and between proteins [55,82,83]. These transfer reactions result in the regeneration of the parent imidazole. These halamines have also been postulated to undergo hydrolysis reactions to give multiple products including 2-oxo-His [100]. This species can undergo further reactions resulting in ring opening to give eventually Asp residues [119]. Chlorine transfer can also occur to other biological molecules, including the exocyclic amine groups of DNA nucleobases [120]; this type of reaction may be of particular significance with regard to damage transfer from histone proteins to bound DNA. The imidazole ring of His has also been reported to be modified by a LPO/H_2O_2/SCN$^-$ system, with these reactions yielding thiocyanatosulfonamide (R-SO$_2$NH-SCN) and thiocyanatimine (ring RNH-SCN) species, which retain some of the oxidizing capacity of HOSCN [112]. These reactions were only examined in isolated systems (i.e. in the absence of other potential targets), so the physiological relevance of these reactions is unclear, and other studies have indicated that His residues on proteins are not targets for reagent HOSCN [113].

Indole Groups (Trp)

Trp residues are modest targets for HOCl [27,52, 121,122], HOBr [63], HOI and probably HOSeCN, but only a minor target for HOSCN at neutral pH [113] (the latter is more favorable at pH < 3 due to the formation of thiocyanogen, $(SCN)_2$, in place of HOSCN [123]). In each case, hydroxylated species appear to be formed (e.g. 2-hydroxytryptophan, 2-OH Trp, oxindolyalanine) and, at least in some case, further deoxygenated and ring-opened products such as N-formylkynurenine and its hydrolysis product, kynurenine. These may arise, at least in part, from initial halogen adducts at the indole nitrogen or as a result of chlorine transfer from other residues [88,113,123–125]. These reactions may be of biological significance as modification of the Trp residues of the apolipoprotein A1 (apoA1) protein present in high-density lipoproteins (HDL), by HOCl, to yield 2-OHTrp derivatives, appears to be associated with a reduced capacity of apoA1 to bind lipids and cholesterol and thereby induce cholesterol efflux from lipid-laden macrophages in the context of lipid accumulation in the artery wall during the development of atherosclerosis [126,127]. Modification of apoA1 to yield 2-OHTrp occurs at a specific residue, Trp72, with this modification being present on ~ 20% of the apoA1 extracted from human atherosclerotic lesions [127]. Why this specific alteration occurs in such high yields is unclear at present, but may be due to neighboring group effects (see below). Trp modification on apoA1 has also been reported with HOSCN, with similar effects on cholesterol efflux capacity [128]. Evidence for modulation by neighboring amino acids has been demonstrated in systems where a Trp residue is flanked by Gly or Ala residues, with the presence of these species resulting in the formation of cyclized products on exposure to HOCl [126]. Limited data have also been presented for indole chlorination by HOCl, with chlorotryptophan reported to be formed on ECM proteins isolated from renal tissue in models of experimental diabetes [129]. Other mass spectrometric studies have, however, not detected chlorotryptophans on ECM proteins (e.g. fibronectin and laminins) treated with either reagent HOCl or $MPO/H_2O_2/Cl^-$ [130,131].

Aromatic Side Chains (Tyr)

Although Tyr is a relatively poor target for HOCl and a more significant target for HOBr and HOI, extensive studies have been carried out on these reactions, as the resulting products are (at least for the protein-bound species) stable carbon–halogen species that are used extensively as biomarkers of heme-peroxidase-mediated reactions in vivo (e.g. [132–135]). Thus, reaction of reagent HOCl or $MPO/H_2O_2/Cl^-$ with peptide or protein Tyr residues yields the stable chlorinated products 3ClTyr and 3,5-dichlorotyrosine (3,5diClTyr) [136–139]. The latter is a secondary product that is only formed at significant levels at very high levels of oxidant exposure. These species can be formed either by direct reaction of HOCl or via intermediate chloramines [139]. This chlorination process appears to be specific for HOCl or $MPO/H_2O_2/Cl^-$ in mammals, but other pathways can give rise to chlorination in non-mammalian systems (e.g. via chloroperoxidase enzymes in fungi [140,141]). Reaction of HOCl and $MPO/H_2O_2/Cl^-$ with protein Tyr residues also results in the formation of the dimer species, o-o'-dityrosine (di-Tyr) [142–144]. The mechanism of formation of this species by HOCl is unclear, as this product is believed to arise solely via radical–radical dimerization of Tyr phenoxyl radicals [144]. This species when formed intermolecularly contributes to protein aggregation [145]. For the enzymatic system, the generation of this species can be readily rationalized, as Compound I of MPO can induce (Cl^- independent) one-electron, radical-transfer reactions, with this resulting in the formation of protein radicals on both MPO and other proteins [146]; similar processes occur with LPO [146] and other heme proteins [147–150]. The radicals formed in these cases are likely to be localized at Trp and Tyr residues due to the low one-electron reduction potentials of these residues [151]. It is likely that di-Trp and mixed Tyr-Trp cross-links are also formed, as these are alternative products of Tyr and Trp radicals (see, e.g. [152–154]). It is important to note that the situation with the free amino acid is different from that for peptide/protein Tyr. In this case, reaction at the free amine group is kinetically more rapid with this resulting in chloramine formation, and hence a (deaminated) carbonyl species, rather than chlorination of the aromatic ring to yield 3ClTyr [136].

HOBr induces similar reactions, but more rapidly (ca. 5,000-fold) [63], to yield 3-bromoTyr (3BrTyr) and the corresponding 3,5diBrTyr species with peptide/protein Tyr, and aldehydes from the free amino acid [155]. These brominated products have been used extensively as biomarkers of HOBr and EPO-mediated reactions [30,156]. However, direct oxidation of Br$^-$ by HOCl to yield HOBr is rapid [157], and hence the detection of 3BrTyr may not always reflect EPO-mediated reactions. These oxidant systems also yield di-Tyr via similar pathways to those indicated above [155]. Modification of Tyr by the TPO enzymatic system, to yield 3-iodoTyr and subsequent multiply iodinated species, also appears to be rapid and efficient, but the kinetics of these reactions are unknown [7]. The LPO/H$_2$O$_2$/SCN$^-$ system has also been reported to modify Tyr [158], though this may occur via (SCN)$_2$ or via Compound I single-electron transfer reactions (as above), as such modifications have not been detected with reagent HOSCN [69].

PRODUCTS FORMED FROM SUGAR RESIDUES

The sugar residues present on glycoproteins and proteoglycans are also known targets of HOCl and HOBr, though little evidence is available for significant reaction with the other hypohalous acids [159–164]. The most reactive targets are amino sugars containing free or substituted amines. The free amine species are more reactive than N-sulfated or amide species; other sugar residues are essentially unreactive [162]. As might be expected from the discussion above, reaction with both HOCl and HOBr generates chloramines (and derivatives) at these residues [162]. Dichlorinated species can also be generated [159]. These species are reactive and undergo subsequent reactions as indicated above for protein chloramines (i.e. redox reactions with Cys/Met, chlorine atom transfer, radical formation and loss of HX to yield an imine, which subsequently undergoes hydrolysis; cf. Figure 4.5) [159,160,162]. In the case of sugar polymers (glycosaminoglycans, GAGs), these reactions result in fragmentation of the sugar backbone, with this occurring specifically at the amino sugars [159–161]. Thus, fragmentation occurs at regular disaccharide intervals in hyaluronan, with distinct ladders detected on gels [160]. Similar reactions occur with HOBr

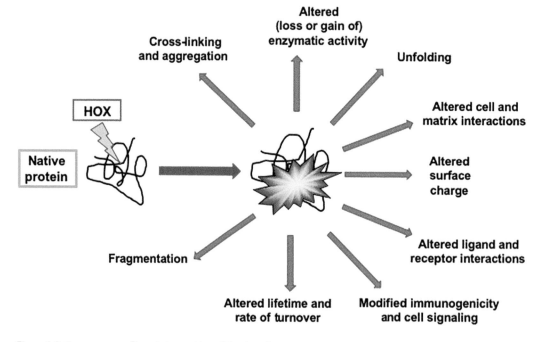

Figure 4.6 Consequences of hypohalous acid modification of proteins.

[165]. For GAGs containing sulfated or amidated sugars, the lower reactivity of these species results is preferential reaction at the protein core in at least some proteoglycans (e.g. perlecan) [166]. These reactions are of potential importance in hypohalous acid-mediated degradation of tissue ECM [165,167].

CONSEQUENCES OF THE REACTION OF HYPOHALOUS ACIDS WITH PROTEINS

The reaction of hypohalous acids with protein side chains can modulate the structure and function of proteins. This can occur via a number of different mechanisms, summarized in Figure 4.6, including both gross changes, such as formation of intra- or intermolecular cross-links and fragmentation reactions (though, as noted above, these are rather limited) and more subtle effects.

Cross-Linking and Aggregation

Heme peroxidase-induced protein cross-linking and aggregation can arise from the formation of covalent linkages involving disulfides by all members of the hypohalous acid family, as well as via direct enzyme reactions [62,107]. Noncovalent aggregates have also been reported [168]. Disulfide formation is typically a reversible event, though there may be situations where the disulfide is inaccessible to biological reductants. Although it is commonly assumed that disulfides are the only readily reduced protein cross-links, it should be noted that other cross-links formed by hypohalous acids, such as sulfenamides, can also be reduced, albeit less rapidly [169]. The formation of disulfides has been *associated* with the inactivation of some intracellular enzymes (reviewed in Ref. [170]), but whether this is causal, or even a major process, is not always clear, as direct oxidation of (active site) Cys residues (see below) and other perturbations may also be significant. Reaction of calprotectin, a protective and highly abundant protein (up to 60% of the cytosolic content) present in, and released by, activated neutrophils with HOCl (and other MPO-derived oxidants) results in disulfide bond formation between Cys residues on the S100A8 and S100A9 monomers [91,104,171]. The presence of these cross-links increases the susceptibility of calprotectin to proteolysis by neutrophil proteases and results in a loss of the iron, zinc and manganese-binding capacity of this protein and its antibacterial and antifungal function [104]. This cross-linked species has been detected both in the saliva of healthy adults and in bronchoalveolar lavage fluid from people with respiratory diseases [171].

HOCl and HOBr, and to a lesser extent other hypohalous acids, can induce irreversible cross-links; these have been associated with tissue damage during the development of chronic inflammatory pathologies (reviewed in Ref. [2]), but causality is often not established. A number of these cross-links involve the most reactive amino acid targets Cys and Met. Thus, intra- and intermolecular sulfinamide (RS(O)-NR′) and sulfonamide [RS(O_2)-NR′] linkages can be formed between Cys and Lys (or Arg); these have been implicated in HOCl-induced low-density lipoprotein (LDL) aggregation [90], and sulfinamides have been reported between S100A8 and S100A9 of calprotectin [91,104,171,172]. Related intra- and intermolecular sulfilimine (RS=NR′) links involving Met and Lys residues have been reported to be induced by both HOCl [173] and HOBr and bromamines [173] and during the cross-linking of the NC1 domains of collagen IV during ECM assembly by peroxidasin [18,19]. These links may therefore be beneficial or detrimental depending on the context.

Heme peroxidase-induced protein cross-linking has also been observed via aromatic amino acid side chains and particularly Tyr (see above). Di-Tyr cross-links have been observed on exposure of reconstituted human blood to HOCl with cross-linked material detected containing α-, β- and γ-fibrinogen chains, apoA1 and complement C3 [174,175] as well as both HDL and LDL [145,176,177]. However, di-Tyr does not account for all the irreversible HOCl-induced cross-links [178], with evidence available for aggregation involving Trp residues in HOCl-treated ceruloplasmin [179]. Similarly, decomposition of Lys-derived chloramines has been shown to give rise to cross-links involving Schiff bases, via carbonyl formation and reaction with a second amine group [109,175].

In many cases, both reversible and irreversible cross-links are likely to be formed. This is exemplified by studies on phosphatase and tensin homologue (PTEN), where exposure to HOCl results in a loss of phosphatase activity that correlates with the formation of aggregates. However, this was only partially reversed on addition of reducing agents to remove disulfide bonds, suggesting that multiple processes are involved [180].

Non-covalent aggregate formation has also been reported [168] possibly as a result of unfolding or ionic interactions. Unfolding is a known consequence of many oxidative reactions as the inclusion of either oxygen atoms (e.g. on conversion of Met to the sulfoxide, Trp to 2OHTrp, N-formylkynurenine or kynurenine, His to 2-oxoHis) or halogenation (e.g. Tyr to 3ClTyr) can increase the polarity and hence hydrophilicity of a side chain (reviewed in Refs. [2,29]). In addition, incorporation of sterically bulky substituents (e.g. chlorine and bromine) can result in additional steric interactions and alterations to side chain interactions and packing [142,168,181].

Fragmentation

Reaction of HOCl and HOBr with backbone amide groups (peptide bonds) is relatively slow (see above) and results in the formation of N-halamides, which can play a role in backbone fragmentation via multiple mechanisms (reviewed in Ref. [100]). Backbone halamides can decompose (see above) to yield nitrogen-centered radicals, which undergo rearrangement reactions to cause backbone fragmentation [62,107,114]. Protein fragmentation has also been reported to occur via chloramines formed from Lys side-chain chloramines, with decomposition of these species to radicals and subsequent hydrogen atom abstraction from the α-carbon site on the backbone [62,107,114]. Similar processes occur with HOBr and bromamines [155]. These α-carbon radicals are well-established intermediates in O_2-dependent backbone scission reactions involving peroxyl and alkoxyl radicals [182]. Backbone cleavage is typically only observed with high molar excesses of oxidant, but the extent has been suggested to be dependent on the amino acid composition of the protein and particularly the number of reactive amino acid side chains, which can act as competitive targets for the oxidant [100]. Thus, fragmentation of ribonuclease A occurs much more readily than with serum albumin, consistent with the greater number of HOCl/HOBr-reactive side chains in albumin [62].

Other Modifications to Protein Structure

Modifications induced by hypohalous acids also alter side chain charge, which can modify interactions within a protein or between proteins. Thus, chlorination of Tyr decreases the pK_a of Tyr residues to 8.3 [183] such that at physiological pH values this residue becomes partially ionized, oxidation of Cys residues generates negatively charged oxy acids and conversion of neutral- or positively charged His residues yields negatively charged ring-opened species such as Asp [100]. Reaction with hypohalous acids can also alter protein surface charge, as reaction with (positively charged) Lys, Arg and His residues can result in the loss of charge and formation of neutral (e.g. carbonyl, nitrile) or acidic groups [100]. Such alterations underlie the marked changes in electrophoretic mobility seen for LDL treated with increasing doses of HOCl [109,184].

Exposure of C-reactive protein (CRP), a major acute phase protein, to HOCl, induces protein unfolding and greater hydrophobicity, together with the formation of aggregates; these species contain new ligand-binding sites and have an enhanced capacity to activate platelets and promote thrombosis [185]. This process may be of particular significance at sites of chronic inflammation [185]. Each of these types of modification can alter the overall protein structure, with implications for function and activity. Some of these effects may be remote from an enzyme-active site, but still impinge on a catalytic center and therefore induce overall biological effects.

Direct modification of active site residues is also well established – and this is particularly prevalent for the many enzymes reliant on Cys or His for their activity. Thus, exposure to HOCl has been linked with inactivation of a number of Cys-dependent, intracellular enzymes, including GAPDH (glyceraldehyde-3-phosphate dehydrogenase), creatine kinase, the sarco/endoplasmic reticulum Ca^{2+}-ATPase (SERCA), which contributes to the control of intracellular Ca^{2+} levels, protein tyrosine phosphatases (PTPs) and kinases and a number of proteolytic enzymes including caspases and cathepsins B and L (reviewed in Refs. [2,186]). Proteins with Cys residues that are present predominantly in their ionized form (i.e. have a low pK_a) appear to be particularly susceptible to inactivation, with a loss of activity occurring in parallel with loss of this residue [81]. Alterations to the activity of some redox-sensitive transcription factors, such as nuclear factor κB (NFκB) and nuclear factor erythroid 2-related factor 2 (Nrf2), and mitogen-activated protein kinase (MAPK) signaling, have also been associated with thiol oxidation, with these changes perturbing cell function and intra- and intermolecular cell signaling [2,186].

Oxidation of Met has also been associated with enzyme inactivation, with a well-established example being α1-antitrypsin, with the active site Met residue being susceptible to HOCl-induced oxidation [187]. Similar inactivation reactions have been reported for cathepsin G [188] and lysozyme [142], but not soybean trypsin inhibitor activity [142]. In other cases, oxidation of Met residues may protect critical residues from damage [189].

Modifications to proteins can also modulate the rate of protein turnover, with low extents of alteration typically increasing the rate of protein turnover, as a result of recognition of damage and subsequent catabolism by proteasomes or lysosomes, but extensive changes can result in a decreased rate of turnover (below basal rate), and this has been associated with extensive cross-linking (e.g. [190]). Modification of proteolysis recognition sites may also play a role.

Although protein modification is often associated with *adverse* effects on protein structure and function, examples are known where alteration results in a *gain* of function [191–193]. In particular, it is known that hypohalous acid treatment can activate the "cysteine switch" of the matrix metalloproteinase (MMP) family of enzymes, with HOCl shown to convert pro-MMP-7 to active MMP-7 [192,193]. This can result in a marked *increase* in enzyme activity and enhanced ECM degradation. Inactivation of enzyme inhibitors (e.g. tissue inhibitors of matrix metalloproteinases, TIMPs; trypsin inhibitor) results in an enhancement of overall enzyme activity [193,194]. These increases in activity can be deleterious (e.g. as a result of increased ECM degradation) or positive if they result in an activation of stress response or protective pathways.

Protein alterations can influence immunity by increasing the immunogenicity of proteins [195] and promote the activation and degranulation of neutrophils and other leukocytes [196]; such modulation may be either positive or negative with regard to tissue inflammation, damage and disease.

The formation of specific epitopes on, for example, HSA and apo-transferrin, has been reported to modulate both the innate and adaptive immune systems [196]. HOCl exposure of these proteins results in the binding of the modified proteins to endocytic receptors on antigen-presenting dendritic cells and macrophages [195]. This increased immunogenicity may indicate a pathway through which the immune system can detect pathogens that have escaped detection by pattern recognition receptors [195]. HSA exposure to HOCl can also alter immune cell function directly, with HOCl-modified HSA reported to trigger activation and degranulation of neutrophils [196] and to induce macrophage differentiation into dendritic-like cells [197]. These pathways may act as a trigger and regulator of the inflammatory response.

Modifications to the major ECM proteins fibronectin and laminin, by HOCl and MPO/H_2O_2/halide ion systems, and the biological consequences of these reactions, have been studied in detail [66,130,131,198,199]. These studies were based on the high abundance of these proteins in the artery wall, data indicating a very high level of modification to ECM materials [200,201] and the known association of heme peroxidases, with ECM materials (both via electrostatic interactions in the case of MPO [66] and via potential domain interactions in the case of PXDN [64,65]). Furthermore, studies on human atherosclerotic lesions have provided evidence for the colocalization of these ECM proteins with epitopes recognized by an antibody raised against HOCl-induced damage [66,199]. Data obtained using LC-MS peptide mass mapping indicates that damage occurs in a dose-dependent manner, at a considerable number of different types of residue (Met, Cys, Trp, Tyr, His) and sites along the protein sequences, though at relatively modest levels [130,131]. It should be noted that not all residues of any particular type suffer modification (i.e. that damage is partially selective) with some residues suffering no significant modification [130,131]. This may be due to steric or electronic shielding, inclusion in buried domains or a high level of exposure on the protein surface. In the case of the MPO enzymatic system, this may also arise from binding to specific ECM components [66,202–204], with differences in the pattern and extent of damage observed with different MPO to ECM ratios [205] and also on comparison of reagent HOCl with the enzymatic system [205]. Of particular note is the observation that a considerable number of the modifications occur within functionally important domains (e.g. those associated with cell binding and interaction with other ECM materials [130,131,205]).

The potential functional effects of this broad spectrum of damage have been explored, with these changes shown to result in the activation of specific genes in naïve cells (i.e. cells that have not been directly exposed to the oxidant, only the modified ECM generated by oxidant treatment) [199,206]. Whether this is protective or deleterious is not clear, with both protective and potentially damaging proteins (e.g. MMPs) being upregulated [199,206]. Furthermore, HOCl-modified ECM has been shown to decrease cell adhesion and proliferation with multiple cell types [199,206,207], but in the case of human coronary artery smooth muscle cells, an initial decrease in adhesion was followed by *enhanced* proliferation and a change in cell phenotype (from contractile and quiescent, to proliferative and synthetic) [206]. This phenotypic change mirrors that seen in the development of human atherosclerotic lesions.

CONCLUSIONS

Overall, these data indicate that different members of the hypohalous acid family have vastly different reactivities, different specificities and induce different extents of damage with this being oxidant-dependent. A wide range of products are formed from multiple residues in some cases (HOCl and HOBr) and a very limited number in others (HOSCN). Some of these species can act as specific biomarkers of modification. Studies on the biological effects of the oxidants indicate that highly reactive oxidants such as HOCl and HOBr induce biological effects via the formation of *low levels of multiple different modifications spread across a wide range of sites*, rather than a high level of modification at a single or small number of sites. In contrast, highly specific oxidants, such as HOSCN, may induce biological effects via *high levels of modification at a single site*. While considerable data has been garnered over the last few decades on the chemistry and biological effects of these materials, a significant number of important questions remain unanswered.

ACKNOWLEDGMENTS

The author is grateful to his many colleagues and research team members who have contributed to the studies reviewed here, and the Novo Nordisk Foundation (Grants: NNF13OC0004294 and NNF19OC0058493) and the Independent Research Fund Denmark (Danmarks Frie Forskningsfond; Grant: DFF-7014-00047) for financial support.

REFERENCES

1. B.J. Day, 2019, The science of licking your wounds: Function of oxidants in the innate immune system, *Biochem. Pharmacol.* 163: 451–457.
2. M.J. Davies, C.L. Hawkins, 2020, The role of myeloperoxidase (MPO) in biomolecule modification, chronic inflammation and disease, *Antioxid. Redox Signal.* 32: 957–981.
3. D. Roos, C.C. Winterbourn, 2002, Immunology. Lethal weapons, *Science* 296: 669–671.
4. M. Zamocky, S. Hofbauer, I. Schaffner, et al., 2015, Independent evolution of four heme peroxidase superfamilies, *Arch. Biochem. Biophys.* 574: 108–119.
5. M.J. Davies, C.L. Hawkins, D.I. Pattison, M.D. Rees, 2008, Mammalian heme peroxidases: From molecular mechanisms to health implications, *Antioxid. Redox Signal.* 10: 1199–1234.
6. J.T. Neary, M. Soodak, F. Maloof, 1984, Iodination by thyroid peroxidase, *Methods Enzymol.* 107: 445–475.
7. M. Morrison, G.R. Schonbaum, 1976, Peroxidase-catalyzed halogenation, *Annu. Rev. Biochem.* 45: 861–888.
8. J. Arnhold, E. Monzani, P.G. Furtmuller, et al., 2006, Kinetics and thermodynamics of halide and nitrite oxidation by mammalian heme peroxidases, *Eur. J. Inorg. Chem.* 2006: 3801–3811.
9. J. Arnhold, J. Flemmig, 2010, Human myeloperoxidase in innate and acquired immunity, *Arch. Biochem. Biophys.* 500: 92–106.
10. S.J. Klebanoff, A.J. Kettle, H. Rosen, C.C. Winterbourn, W.M. Nauseef, 2013, Myeloperoxidase: A front-line defender against phagocytosed microorganisms, *J. Leukocyte Biol.* 93: 185–198.
11. J.N. Green, A.J. Kettle, C.C. Winterbourn, 2014, Protein chlorination in neutrophil phagosomes and correlation with bacterial killing, *Free Radic. Biol. Med.* 77: 49–56.

12. E.C. Jong, W.R. Henderson, S.J. Klebanoff, 1980, Bactericidal activity of eosinophil peroxidase, *J. Immunol.* 124: 1378–1382.

13. J. Wang, A. Slungaard, 2006, Role of eosinophil peroxidase in host defense and disease pathology, *Arch. Biochem. Biophys.* 445: 256–260.

14. C. Gerson, J. Sabater, M. Scuri, et al., 2000, The lactoperoxidase system functions in bacterial clearance of airways, *Am. J. Respir. Cell. Mol. Biol.* 22: 665–671.

15. G.E. Conner, M. Salathe, R. Forteza, 2002, Lactoperoxidase and hydrogen peroxide metabolism in the airway, *Am. J. Respir. Crit. Care Med.* 166: S57–61.

16. J.L. Michot, J. Osty, J. Nunez, 1980, Regulatory effects of iodide and thiocyanate on tyrosine oxidation catalyzed by thyroid peroxidase, *Eur. J. Biochem.* 107: 297–301.

17. M. Soudi, M. Zamocky, C. Jakopitsch, P.G. Furtmuller, C. Obinger, 2012, Molecular evolution, structure, and function of peroxidasins, *Chem. Biodivers.* 9: 1776–1793.

18. G. Bhave, C.F. Cummings, R.M. Vanacore, et al., 2012, Peroxidasin forms sulfilimine chemical bonds using hypohalous acids in tissue genesis, *Nat. Chem. Biol.* 8: 784–790.

19. A.S. McCall, C.F. Cummings, G. Bhave, et al., 2014, Bromine is an essential trace element for assembly of collagen IV scaffolds in tissue development and architecture, *Cell* 157: 1380–1392.

20. G. Cheng, J.C. Salerno, Z. Cao, P.J. Pagano, J.D. Lambeth, 2008, Identification and characterization of VPO1, a new animal heme-containing peroxidase, *Free Radic. Biol. Med.* 45: 1682–1694.

21. Z. Peterfi, M. Geiszt, 2014, Peroxidasins: Novel players in tissue genesis, *Trends Biochem. Sci.* 39: 305–307.

22. H.B. Dunford, 1982, Peroxidases, *Adv. Inorg. Biochem.*: 41–68.

23. J. Arnhold, P.G. Furtmuller, C. Obinger, 2003, Redox properties of myeloperoxidase, *Redox Rep.* 8: 179–186.

24. P.J. O'Brien, 2000, Peroxidases, *Chem. Biol. Interact.* 129: 113–139.

25. C.J. van Dalen, C.C. Winterbourn, R. Senthilmohan, A.J. Kettle, 2000, Nitrite as a substrate and inhibitor of myeloperoxidase. Implications for nitration and hypochlorous acid production at sites of inflammation, *J. Biol. Chem.* 275: 11638–11644.

26. A. van der Vliet, J.P. Eiserich, B. Halliwell, C.E. Cross, 1997, Formation of reactive nitrogen species during peroxidase-catalyzed oxidation of nitrite. A potential additional mechanism of nitric oxide-dependent toxicity, *J. Biol. Chem.* 272: 7617–7625.

27. A.J. Kettle, L.P. Candaeis, 2000, Oxidation of tryptophan by redox intermediates of myeloperoxidase and inhibition of hypochlorous acid production, *Redox Rep.* 5: 179–184.

28. A.J. Kettle, R.F. Anderson, M.B. Hampton, C.C. Winterbourn, 2007, Reactions of superoxide with myeloperoxidase, *Biochemistry* 46: 4888–4897.

29. C.L. Hawkins, 2020, Hypochlorous acid-mediated modification of proteins and its consequences, *Essays Biochem.* 64: 75–86.

30. R. Senthilmohan, A.J. Kettle, 2006, Bromination and chlorination reactions of myeloperoxidase at physiological concentrations of bromide and chloride, *Arch. Biochem. Biophys.* 445: 235–244.

31. C.J. van Dalen, M.W. Whitehouse, C.C. Winterbourn, A.J. Kettle, 1997, Thiocyanate and chloride as competing substrates for myeloperoxidase, *Biochem. J.* 327: 487–492.

32. P.G. Furtmuller, J. Arnhold, W. Jantschko, H. Pichler, C. Obinger, 2003, Redox properties of the couples compound I/compound II and compound II/native enzyme of human myeloperoxidase, *Biochem. Biophys. Res. Commun.* 301: 551–557.

33. A. Nicolussi, M. Auer, B. Sevcnikar, et al., 2018, Posttranslational modification of heme in peroxidases - Impact on structure and catalysis, *Arch. Biochem. Biophys.* 643: 14–23.

34. P.G. Furtmuller, M. Zederbauer, W. Jantschko, et al., 2006, Active site structure and catalytic mechanisms of human peroxidases, *Arch. Biochem. Biophys.* 445: 199–213.

35. C.J. van Dalen, A.J. Kettle, 2001, Substrates and products of eosinophil peroxidase, *Biochem. J.* 358: 233–239.

36. M. Paumann-Page, R.S. Katz, M. Bellei, et al., 2017, Pre-steady-state kinetics reveal the substrate specificity and mechanism of halide oxidation of truncated human peroxidasin 1, *J. Biol. Chem.* 292: 4583–4592.

37. B. Sevcnikar, M. Paumann-Page, S. Hofbauer, et al., 2020, Reaction of human peroxidasin 1 compound I and compound II with one-electron donors, *Arch. Biochem. Biophys.* 681: 108267.

38. J. Talib, D.I. Pattison, J.A. Harmer, D.S. Celermajer, M.J. Davies, 2012, High plasma thiocyanate levels modulate protein damage induced by myeloperoxidase and perturb measurement of 3-chlorotyrosine, *Free Radic. Biol. Med.* 53: 20–29.

39. P.E. Morgan, D.I. Pattison, J. Talib, et al., 2011, High plasma thiocyanate levels in smokers are a key determinant of thiol oxidation induced by myeloperoxidase, *Free Radic. Biol. Med.* 51: 1815–1822.

40. B. Contempre, G.M. de Escobar, J.F. Denef, J.E. Dumont, M.C. Many, 2004, Thiocyanate induces cell necrosis and fibrosis in selenium- and iodine-deficient rat thyroids: A potential experimental model for myxedematous endemic cretinism in central Africa, *Endocrinology* 145: 994–1002.

41. J.M. Pullar, M.C. Vissers, C.C. Winterbourn, 2000, Living with a killer: The effects of hypochlorous acid on mammalian cells, *IUBMB Life* 50: 259–266.

42. A.L. Chapman, M.B. Hampton, R. Senthilmohan, C.C. Winterbourn, A.J. Kettle, 2002, Chlorination of bacterial and neutrophil proteins during phagocytosis and killing of *Staphylococcus aureus*, *J. Biol. Chem.* 277: 9757–9762.

43. Y. Doring, M. Drechsler, O. Soehnlein, C. Weber, 2015, Neutrophils in atherosclerosis: From mice to man, *Arterioscler. Thromb. Vasc. Biol.* 35: 288–295.

44. A. Strzepa, K.A. Pritchard, B.N. Dittel, 2017, Myeloperoxidase: A new player in autoimmunity, *Cell. Immunol.* 317: 1–8.

45. J.D. Chandler, B.J. Day, 2012, Thiocyanate: A potentially useful therapeutic agent with host defense and antioxidant properties, *Biochem. Pharmacol.* 84: 1381–1387.

46. J.D. Chandler, B.J. Day, 2015, Biochemical mechanisms and therapeutic potential of pseudohalide thiocyanate in human health, *Free Radic. Res.* 49: 695–710.

47. J.D. Chandler, E. Min, J. Huang, et al., 2015, Antiinflammatory and antimicrobial effects of thiocyanate in a cystic fibrosis mouse model, *Am. J. Respir. Cell. Mol. Biol.* 53: 193–205.

48. B.J. Day, P.E. Bratcher, J.D. Chandler, et al., 2020, The thiocyanate analog selenocyanate is a more potent antimicrobial pro-drug that also is selectively detoxified by the host, *Free Radic. Biol. Med.* 146: 324–332.

49. T.J. Barrett, C.L. Hawkins, 2012, Hypothiocyanous acid: Benign or deadly? *Chem. Res. Toxicol.* 25: 263–273.

50. D.I. Pattison, M.J. Davies, 2006, Reactions of myeloperoxidase-derived oxidants with biological substrates: Gaining insight into human inflammatory diseases, *Curr. Med. Chem.* 13: 3271–3290.

51. D.I. Pattison, C.L. Hawkins, M.J. Davies, 2009, What are the plasma targets of the oxidant hypochlorous acid? A kinetic modeling approach, *Chem. Res. Toxicol.* 22: 807–817.

52. D.I. Pattison, M.J. Davies, 2001, Absolute rate constants for the reaction of hypochlorous acid with protein side chains and peptide bonds, *Chem. Res. Toxicol.* 14: 1453–1464.

53. D.I. Pattison, M.J. Davies, C.L. Hawkins, 2012, Reactions and reactivity of myeloperoxidase-derived oxidants: Differential biological effects of hypochlorous and hypothiocyanous acids, *Free Radic. Res.* 46: 975–995.

54. A.V. Peskin, R.G. Midwinter, D.T. Harwood, C.C. Winterbourn, 2004, Chlorine transfer between glycine, taurine, and histamine: Reaction rates and impact on cellular reactivity, *Free Radic. Biol. Med.* 37: 1622–1630.

55. A.V. Peskin, C.C. Winterbourn, 2003, Histamine chloramine reactivity with thiol compounds, ascorbate, and methionine and with intracellular glutathione, *Free Radic. Biol. Med.* 35: 1252–1260.

56. X.L. Armesto, L. Canle, J.A. Santaballa, 1993, α-Amino acids chlorination in aqueous media, *Tetrahedron* 49: 275–284.

57. X.L. Armesto, C.L. Moises, I. Fernandez, et al., 2001, Intracellular oxidation of dipeptides. Very fast halogenation of the amino-terminal residue, *J. Chem. Soc.* 2: 608–612.

58. S.L. Hazen, F.F. Hsu, K. Duffin, J.W. Heinecke, 1996, Molecular chlorine generated by the myeloperoxidase-hydrogen peroxide-chloride system of phagocytes converts low density lipoprotein cholesterol into a family of chlorinated sterols, *J. Biol. Chem.* 271: 23080–23088.

59. C. Storkey, M.J. Davies, D.I. Pattison, 2014, Reevaluation of the rate constants for the reaction of hypochlorous acid (HOCl) with cysteine, methionine, and peptide derivatives using a new competition kinetic approach, *Free Radic. Biol. Med.* 73: 60–66.

60. L. Carroll, K. Gardiner, M. Ignasiak, et al., 2020, Interaction kinetics of selenium-containing compounds with oxidants, *Free Radic. Biol. Med.* 155: 58–68

61. M. Karimi, M.T. Ignasiak, B. Chan, et al., 2016, Reactivity of disulfide bonds is markedly affected

by structure and environment: Implications for protein modification and stability, *Sci. Rep.* 6: 38572.

62. C.L. Hawkins, M.J. Davies, 1998, Hypochlorite-induced damage to proteins: Formation of nitrogen-centred radicals from lysine residues and their role in protein fragmentation, *Biochem. J.* 332: 617–625.

63. D.I. Pattison, M.J. Davies, 2004, A kinetic analysis of the reactions of hypobromous acid with protein components: Implications for cellular damage and the use of 3-bromotyrosine as a marker of oxidative stress, *Biochemistry* 43: 4799–4809.

64. I.A. Ero-Tolliver, B.G. Hudson, G. Bhave, 2015, The ancient immunoglobulin domains of peroxidasin are required to form sulfilimine cross-links in collagen IV, *J. Biol. Chem.* 290: 21741–21748.

65. B. Sevcnikar, I. Schaffner, C.Y. Chuang, et al., 2020, The leucine-rich repeat domain of human peroxidasin 1 promotes binding to laminin in basement membranes, *Arch. Biochem. Biophys.* 689: 108443.

66. H. Cai, C.Y. Chuang, C.L. Hawkins, M.J. Davies, 2020, Binding of myeloperoxidase to the extracellular matrix of smooth muscle cells and subsequent matrix modification, *Sci. Rep.* 10: 666.

67. O. Skaff, D.I. Pattison, M.J. Davies, 2009, Hypothiocyanous acid reactivity with low-molecular-mass and protein thiols: Absolute rate constants and assessment of biological relevance, *Biochem. J.* 422: 111–117.

68. P. Nagy, G.N. Jameson, C.C. Winterbourn, 2009, Kinetics and mechanisms of the reaction of hypothiocyanous acid with 5-thio-2-nitrobenzoic acid and reduced glutathione, *Chem. Res. Toxicol.* 22: 1833–1840.

69. T.J. Barrett, D.I. Pattison, S.E. Leonard, et al., 2012, Inactivation of thiol-dependent enzymes by hypothiocyanous acid: Role of sulfenyl thiocyanate and sulfenic acid intermediates, *Free Radic. Biol. Med.* 52: 1075–1085.

70. J.D. Chandler, D.P. Nichols, J.A. Nick, R.J. Hondal, B.J. Day, 2013, Selective metabolism of hypothiocyanous acid by mammalian thioredoxin reductase promotes lung innate immunity and antioxidant defense, *J. Biol. Chem.* 288: 18421–18428.

71. O. Skaff, D.I. Pattison, P.E. Morgan, et al., 2012, Selenium-containing amino acids are major targets for myeloperoxidase-derived hypothiocyanous acid: Determination of absolute rate constants and implications for biological damage, *Biochem. J.* 441: 305–316.

72. H.R. Chung, 2014, Iodine and thyroid function, *Ann. Pediatr. Endocrinol. Metab.* 19: 8–12.

73. S.T. Test, M.B. Lampert, P.J. Ossanna, J.G. Thoene, S.J. Weiss, 1984, Generation of nitrogen-chlorine oxidants by human phagocytes, *J. Clin. Invest.* 74: 1341–1349.

74. Y. Kawai, H. Kiyokawa, Y. Kimura, et al., 2006, Hypochlorous acid-derived modification of phospholipids: Characterization of aminophospholipids as regulatory molecules for lipid peroxidation, *Biochemistry* 45: 14201–14211.

75. J. Flemmig, H. Spalteholz, K. Schubert, S. Meier, J. Arnhold, 2009, Modification of phosphatidylserine by hypochlorous acid, *Chem. Phys. Lipids* 161: 44–50.

76. C.L. Hawkins, M.J. Davies, 2001, Hypochlorite-induced damage to nucleosides: Formation of chloramines and nitrogen-centered radicals, *Chem. Res. Toxicol.* 14: 1071–1081.

77. C.L. Hawkins, M.J. Davies, 2002, Hypochlorite-induced damage to DNA, RNA and polynucleosides: Formation of chloramines and nitrogen-centered radicals, *Chem. Res. Toxicol.* 15: 83–92.

78. S. Ohnishi, M. Murata, S. Kawanishi, 2002, DNA damage induced by hypochlorite and hypobromite with reference to inflammation-associated carcinogenesis, *Cancer Lett.* 178: 37–42.

79. W.A. Prutz, 1998, Interactions of hypochlorous acid with pyrimidine nucleotides, and secondary reactions of chlorinated pyrimidines with GSH, NADH, and other substrates, *Arch. Biochem. Biophys.* 349: 183–191.

80. A.V. Peskin, C.C. Winterbourn, 2001, Kinetics of the reactions of hypochlorous acid and amino acid chloramines with thiols, methionine, and ascorbate, *Free Radic. Biol. Med.* 30: 572–579.

81. A.V. Peskin, C.C. Winterbourn, 2006, Taurine chloramine is more selective than hypochlorous acid at targeting critical cysteines and inactivating creatine kinase and glyceraldehyde-3-phosphate dehydrogenase, *Free Radic. Biol. Med.* 40: 45–53.

82. D.I. Pattison, M.J. Davies, 2006, Evidence for rapid inter-and intra-molecular chlorine transfer reactions of histamine and carnosine chloramines: Implications for the prevention of hypochlorous acid mediated damage, *Biochemistry* 45: 8152–8162.

83. D.I. Pattison, M.J. Davies, 2005, Kinetic analysis of the role of histidine chloramines in hypochlorous acid mediated protein oxidation, Biochemistry 44: 7378–7387.

84. E.L. Thomas, M.M. Jefferson, J.J. Bennett, D.B. Learn, 1987, Mutagenic activity of chloramines, Mutat. Res. 188: 35–43.

85. M.M. Donnermair, E.R. Blatchley, 3rd, 2003, Disinfection efficacy of organic chloramines, Water Res. 37: 1557–1570.

86. D. Liviac, E.D. Wagner, W.A. Mitch, M.J. Altonji, M.J. Plewa, 2010, Genotoxicity of water concentrates from recreational pools after various disinfection methods, Environ. Sci. Technol. 44: 3527–3532.

87. C.C. Winterbourn, M.B. Hampton, J.H. Livesey, A.J. Kettle, 2006, Modeling the reactions of superoxide and myeloperoxidase in the neutrophil phagosome: Implications for microbial killing, J. Biol. Chem. 281: 39860–39869.

88. R. Drozdz, J.W. Naskalski, J. Sznajd, 1988, Oxidation of amino acids and peptides in reaction with myeloperoxidase, chloride and hydrogen peroxide, Biochim. Biophys. Acta 957: 47–52.

89. W.E. Pereira, Y. Hoyano, R.E. Summons, V.A. Bacon, A.M. Duffield, 1973, Chlorination studies. II. The reaction of aqueous hypochlorous acid with α-amino acids and dipeptides, Biochim. Biophys. Acta. 313: 170–180.

90. X. Fu, D.M. Mueller, J.W. Heinecke, 2002, Generation of intramolecular and intermolecular sulfenamides, sulfinamides, and sulfonamides by hypochlorous acid: A potential pathway for oxidative cross-linking of low-density lipoprotein by myeloperoxidase, Biochemistry 41: 1293–1301.

91. M.J. Raftery, Z. Yang, S.M. Valenzuela, C.L. Geczy, 2001, Novel intra- and inter-molecular sulfinamide bonds in S100A8 produced by hypochlorite oxidation, J. Biol. Chem. 276: 33393–33401.

92. D.T. Harwood, A.J. Kettle, C.C. Winterbourn, 2006, Production of glutathione sulfonamide and dehydroglutathione from GSH by myeloperoxidase-derived oxidants and detection using a novel LC-MS/MS method, Biochem. J. 399: 161–168.

93. N.O. Devarie-Baez, E.I. Silva Lopez, C.M. Furdui, 2016, Biological chemistry and functionality of protein sulfenic acids and related thiol modifications, Free Radic. Res. 50: 172–194.

94. V. Gupta, K.S. Carroll, 2014, Sulfenic acid chemistry, detection and cellular lifetime, Biochim. Biophys. Acta 1840: 847–875.

95. M.J. Davies, C.L. Hawkins, 2000, Hypochlorite-induced oxidation of thiols: Formation of thiyl radicals and the role of sulfenyl chlorides as intermediates, Free Radic. Res. 33: 719–729.

96. E.L. Thomas, T.M. Aune, 1978, Lactoperoxidase, peroxide, thiocyanate antimicrobial system: Correlation of sulfhydryl oxidation with antimicrobial action, Infect. Immun. 20: 456–463.

97. M.T. Ashby, H. Aneetha, 2004, Reactive sulfur species: Aqueous chemistry of sulfenyl thiocyanates, J. Am. Chem. Soc. 126: 10216–10217.

98. D.T. Love, T.J. Barrett, M.Y. White, et al., 2016, Cellular targets of the myeloperoxidase-derived oxidant hypothiocyanous acid (HOSCN) and its role in the inhibition of glycolysis in macrophages, Free Radic. Biol. Med. 94: 88–98.

99. M. Karimi, B. Crossett, S.J. Cordwell, D.I. Pattison, M.J. Davies, 2020, Characterization of disulfide (cystine) oxidation by HOCl in a model peptide: Evidence for oxygen addition, disulfide bond cleavage and adduct formation with thiols, Free Radic. Biol. Med. 154: 62–74.

100. C.L. Hawkins, D.I. Pattison, M.J. Davies, 2003, Hypochlorite-induced oxidation of amino acids, peptides and proteins, Amino Acids 25: 259–274.

101. D.I. Pattison, C.L. Hawkins, M.J. Davies, 2007, Hypochlorous acid-mediated protein oxidation: How important are chloramine transfer reactions and protein tertiary structure? Biochemistry 46: 9853–9864.

102. A.V. Peskin, R. Turner, G.J. Maghzal, C.C. Winterbourn, A.J. Kettle, 2009, Oxidation of methionine to dehydromethionine by reactive halogen species generated by neutrophils, Biochemistry 48: 10175–10182.

103. J.L. Beal, S.B. Foster, M.T. Ashby, 2009, Hypochlorous acid reacts with the N-terminal methionines of proteins to give dehydromethionine, a potential biomarker for neutrophil-induced oxidative stress, Biochemistry 48: 11142–11148.

104. N.J. Magon, R. Turner, R.B. Gearry, et al., 2015, Oxidation of calprotectin by hypochlorous acid prevents chelation of essential metal ions and allows bacterial growth: Relevance to infections in cystic fibrosis, Free Radic. Biol. Med. 86: 133–144.

105. E.L. Thomas, P.M. Bozeman, M.M. Jefferson, C.C. King, 1995, Oxidation of bromide by the human leukocyte enzymes myeloperoxidase and eosinophil peroxidase. Formation of bromamines, J. Biol. Chem. 270: 2906–2913.

106. E.L. Thomas, M.B. Grisham, M.M. Jefferson, 1986, Preparation and characterization of chloramines, *Methods Enzymol.* 132: 569–585.

107. C.L. Hawkins, M.J. Davies, 1998, Hypochlorite-induced oxidation of plasma proteins: Formation of nitrogen-centred radicals and their role in protein fragmentation, *Curr. Topics Biophys.* 22 (Suppl. B): 89–98.

108. D.I. Pattison, R.J. O'Reilly, O. Skaff, et al., 2011, One-electron reduction of N-chlorinated and N-brominated species is a source of radicals and bromine atom formation, *Chem. Res. Toxicol.* 24: 371–382.

109. L.J. Hazell, J.J. van den Berg, R. Stocker, 1994, Oxidation of low-density lipoprotein by hypochlorite causes aggregation that is mediated by modification of lysine residues rather than lipid oxidation, *Biochem. J.* 302: 421–428.

110. H. Lin, B.S. Levison, J.A. Buffa, et al., 2017, Myeloperoxidase-mediated protein lysine oxidation generates 2-aminoadipic acid and lysine nitrile in vivo, *Free Radic. Biol. Med.* 104: 20–31.

111. J.D. Sivey, S.C. Howell, D.J. Bean, et al., 2013, Role of lysine during protein modification by HOCl and HOBr: Halogen-transfer agent or sacrificial antioxidant? *Biochemistry* 52: 1260–1271.

112. E.L. Thomas, 1981, Lactoperoxidase-catalyzed oxidation of thiocyanate: Equilibria between oxidized forms of thiocyanate, *Biochemistry* 20: 3273–3280.

113. C.L. Hawkins, D.I. Pattison, N.R. Stanley, M.J. Davies, 2008, Tryptophan residues are targets in hypothiocyanous acid-mediated protein oxidation, *Biochem. J.* 414: 271–280.

114. C.L. Hawkins, M.J. Davies, 1998, Reaction of HOCl with amino acids and peptides: EPR evidence for rapid rearrangement and fragmentation reactions of nitrogen-centered radicals, *J. Chem. Soc. Perkin Trans.* 2: 1937–1945.

115. C. Zhang, C. Reiter, J.P. Eiserich, et al., 2001, L-arginine chlorination products inhibit endothelial nitric oxide production, *J. Biol. Chem.* 276: 27159–27165.

116. C. Zhang, R. Patel, J.P. Eiserich, et al., 2001, Endothelial dysfunction is induced by proinflammatory oxidant hypochlorous acid, *Am. J. Physiol. Heart Circ. Physiol.* 281: H1469–1475.

117. J. Xu, Z. Xie, R. Reece, D. Pimental, M.H. Zou, 2006, Uncoupling of endothelial nitric oxidase synthase by hypochlorous acid: Role of NAD(P)H oxidase-derived superoxide and peroxynitrite, *Arterioscler. Thromb. Vasc. Biol.* 26: 2688–2695.

118. J. Talib, J. Kwan, A. Suryo Rahmanto, P.K. Witting, M.J. Davies, 2014, The smoking-associated oxidant hypothiocyanous acid induces endothelial nitric oxide synthase dysfunction, *Biochem. J.* 457: 89–97.

119. H. Ihara, Y. Kakihana, A. Yamakage, et al., 2019, 2-Oxo-histidine-containing dipeptides are functional oxidation products, *J. Biol. Chem.* 294: 1279–1289.

120. N.R. Stanley, D.I. Pattison, C.L. Hawkins, 2010, Ability of hypochlorous acid and N-chloramines to chlorinate DNA and its constituents, *Chem. Res. Toxicol.* 23: 1293–1302.

121. A. Jerlich, M. Hammel, F. Nigon, M.J. Chapman, R.J. Schaur, 2000, Kinetics of tryptophan oxidation in plasma lipoproteins by myeloperoxidase-generated HOCl, *Eur. J. Biochem.* 267: 4137–4143.

122. A.J. Szuchman-Sapir, D.I. Pattison, N.A. Ellis, et al., 2008, Hypochlorous acid oxidizes methionine and tryptophan residues in myoglobin, *Free Radic. Biol. Med.* 45: 789–798.

123. V. Bonifay, T.J. Barrett, D.I. Pattison, et al., 2014, Tryptophan oxidation in proteins exposed to thiocyanate-derived oxidants, *Arch. Biochem. Biophys.* 564: 1–11.

124. X. Fu, Y. Wang, J. Kao, et al., 2006, Specific sequence motifs direct the oxygenation and chlorination of tryptophan by myeloperoxidase, *Biochemistry* 45: 3961–3971.

125. A. Aspee, E.A. Lissi, 2002, Chemiluminescence associated with amino acid oxidation mediated by hypochlorous acid, *Luminescence* 17: 158–164.

126. D.Q. Peng, G. Brubaker, Z. Wu, et al., 2008, Apolipoprotein A-I tryptophan substitution leads to resistance to myeloperoxidase-mediated loss of function, *Arterioscler. Thromb. Vasc. Biol.* 28: 2063–2070.

127. Y. Huang, J.A. DiDonato, B.S. Levison, et al., 2014, An abundant dysfunctional apolipoprotein A1 in human atheroma, *Nat. Med.* 20: 193–203.

128. K.A. Hadfield, D.I. Pattison, B.E. Brown, et al., 2013, Myeloperoxidase-derived oxidants modify apolipoprotein A-I and generate dysfunctional high-density lipoproteins: Comparison of hypothiocyanous acid (HOSCN) with hypochlorous acid (HOCl), *Biochem. J.* 449: 531–542.

129. K.L. Brown, C. Darris, K.L. Rose, et al., 2015, Hypohalous acids contribute to renal extracellular matrix damage in experimental diabetes, *Diabetes* 64: 2242–2253.

130. T. Nybo, H. Cai, C.Y. Chuang, et al., 2018, Chlorination and oxidation of human plasma fibronectin by myeloperoxidase-derived oxidants, and its consequences for smooth muscle cell function, *Redox Biol.* 19: 388–400.

131. T. Nybo, S. Dieterich, L.F. Gamon, et al., 2019, Chlorination and oxidation of the extracellular matrix protein laminin and basement membrane extracts by hypochlorous acid and myeloperoxidase, *Redox Biol.* 20: 496–513.

132. D.T. Harwood, B.A. Darlow, F.C. Cheah, et al., 2011, Biomarkers of neutrophil-mediated glutathione and protein oxidation in tracheal aspirates from preterm infants: Association with bacterial infection, *Pediatr. Res.* 69: 28–33.

133. C.C. Winterbourn, A.J. Kettle, 2000, Biomarkers of myeloperoxidase-derived hypochlorous acid, *Free Radic. Biol. Med.* 29: 403–409.

134. S.L. Hazen, J.R. Crowley, D.M. Mueller, J.W. Heinecke, 1997, Mass spectrometric quantification of 3-chlorotyrosine in human tissues with attomole sensitivity: A sensitive and specific marker for myeloperoxidase-catalysed chlorination at sites of inflammation, *Free Radic. Biol. Med.* 23: 909–916.

135. S.L. Hazen, J.W. Heinecke, 1997, 3-Chlorotyrosine, a specific marker of myeloperoxidase-catalysed oxidation, is markedly elevated in low density lipoprotein isolated from human atherosclerotic intima, *J. Clin. Invest.* 99: 2075–2081.

136. S. Fu, H. Wang, M.J. Davies, R.T. Dean, 2000, Reaction of hypochlorous acid with tyrosine and peptidyl-tyrosyl residues gives dichlorinated and aldehydic products in addition to 3-chlorotyrosine, *J. Biol. Chem.* 275: 10851–10858.

137. N.M. Domigan, T.S. Charlton, M.W. Duncan, C.C. Winterbourn, A.J. Kettle, 1995, Chlorination of tyrosyl residues in peptides by myeloperoxidase and human neutrophils, *J. Biol. Chem.* 270: 16542–16548.

138. H. Buss, R. Senthilmohan, B.A. Darlow, et al., 2003, 3-Chlorotyrosine as a marker of protein damage by myeloperoxidase in traceal aspirates from preterm infants: Association with adverse respiratory outcome, *Pediatr. Res.* 53: 455–462.

139. A.J. Kettle, 1999, Detection of 3-chlorotyrosine in proteins exposed to neutrophil oxidants, *Methods Enzymol.* 300: 111–120.

140. K.H. van Pee, 2012, Biosynthesis of halogenated alkaloids, *Alkaloids Chem. Biol.* 71: 167–210.

141. K.H. van Pee, 2012, Enzymatic chlorination and bromination, *Methods Enzymol.* 516: 237–257.

142. C.L. Hawkins, M.J. Davies, 2005, Inactivation of protease inhibitors and lysozyme by hypochlorous acid: Role of side-chain oxidation and protein unfolding in loss of biological function, *Chem. Res. Toxicol.* 18: 1600–1610.

143. J.W. Heinecke, W. Li, H.L. Daehnke, J.A. Goldstein, 1993, Dityrosine, a specific marker of oxidation, is synthesized by the myeloperoxidase-hydrogen peroxide system of human neutrophils and macrophages, *J. Biol. Chem.* 268: 4069–4077.

144. J.S. Jacob, D.P. Cistola, F.F. Hsu, et al., 1996, Human phagocytes employ the myeloperoxidase-hydrogen peroxide system to synthesize dityrosine, trityrosine, pulcherosine, and isodityrosine by a tyrosyl radical-dependent pathway, *J. Biol. Chem.* 271: 19950–19956.

145. J.W. Heinecke, W. Li, G.A. Francis, J.A. Goldstein, 1993, Tyrosyl radical generated by myeloperoxidase catalyzes the oxidative cross-linking of proteins, *J. Clin. Invest.* 91: 2866–2872.

146. O.M. Lardinois, P.R. Ortiz de Montellano, 2000, EPR spin-trapping of a myeloperoxidase protein radical, *Biochem. Biophys. Res. Commun.* 270: 199–202.

147. H. Ostdal, H.J. Andersen, M.J. Davies, 1999, Formation of long-lived radicals on proteins by radical transfer from heme enzymes-a common process? *Arch. Biochem. Biophys.* 362: 105–112.

148. H. Ostdal, M.J. Bjerrum, J.A. Pedersen, H.J. Andersen, 2000, Lactoperoxidase-induced protein oxidation in milk, *J. Agric. Food Chem.* 48: 3939–3944.

149. H. Ostdal, M.J. Davies, H.J. Andersen, 2002, Reaction between protein radicals and other biomolecules, *Free Radic. Biol. Med.* 33: 201–209.

150. H. Ostdal, L.H. Skibsted, H.J. Andersen, 1997, Formation of long-lived protein radicals in the reaction between H_2O_2 activated metmyoglobin and other proteins, *Free Radic. Biol. Med.* 23: 754–761.

151. J. Butler, E.J. Land, W.A. Prutz, A.J. Swallow, 1982, Charge transfer between tryptophan and tyrosine in proteins, *Biochim. Biophys. Acta* 705: 150–162.

152. P. Hagglund, M. Mariotti, M.J. Davies, 2018, Identification and characterization of protein cross-links induced by oxidative reactions, *Expert Rev. Proteomics* 18: 665–681.

153. F. Leinisch, M. Mariotti, M. Rykaer, et al., 2017, Peroxyl radical- and photo-oxidation of glucose 6-phosphate dehydrogenase generates cross-links and functional changes via oxidation of tyrosine and tryptophan residues, *Free Radic. Biol. Med.* 112: 240–252.

154. M. Mariotti, F. Leinisch, D.J. Leeming, et al., 2018, Mass-spectrometry-based identification of cross-links in proteins exposed to photo-oxidation and peroxyl radicals using ^{18}O labeling and optimized tandem mass spectrometry fragmentation, *J. Proteome Res.* 17: 2017–2027.

155. C.L. Hawkins, M.J. Davies, 2005, The role of reactive N-bromo species and radical intermediates in hypobromous acid-induced protein oxidation, *Free Radic. Biol. Med.* 39: 900–912.

156. W. Wu, Y. Chen, A. d'Avignon, S.L. Hazen, 1999, 3-Bromotyrosine and 3,5-dibromotyrosine are major products of protein oxidation by eosinophil peroxidase: Potential markers for eosinophil- dependent tissue injury in vivo, *Biochemistry* 38: 3538–3548.

157. K. Kumar, D.W. Margerum, 1987, Kinetics and mechanism of general acid-assisted oxidation of bromide by hypochlorite and hypochlorous acid, *Inorg. Chem.* 26: 2706–2711.

158. T.M. Aune, E.L. Thomas, M. Morrison, 1977, Lactoperoxidase-catalyzed incorporation of thiocyanate ion into a protein substrate, *Biochemistry* 16: 4611–4615.

159. M.D. Rees, M.J. Davies, 2006, Heparan sulfate degradation via reductive homolysis of its N-Chloro derivatives, *J. Am. Chem. Soc.* 128: 3085–3097.

160. M.D. Rees, C.L. Hawkins, M.J. Davies, 2003, Hypochlorite-mediated fragmentation of hyaluronan, chondritin sulfates, and related N-acetyl glycosamines, *J. Am. Chem. Soc.* 125: 13719–13733.

161. M.D. Rees, C.L. Hawkins, M.J. Davies, 2004, Hypochlorite and superoxide radicals can act synergistically to induce fragmentation of hyaluronan and chondritin sulfates, *Biochem. J.* 381: 175–184.

162. M.D. Rees, D.I. Pattison, M.J. Davies, 2005, Oxidation of heparan sulphate by hypochlorite: Role of N-chloro derivatives and dichloramine-dependent fragmentation, *Biochem. J.* 391: 125–134.

163. A. Akeel, S. Sibanda, S.W. Martin, A.W. Paterson, B.J. Parsons, 2013, Chlorination and oxidation of heparin and hyaluronan by hypochlorous acid and hypochlorite anions: Effect of sulfate groups on reaction pathways and kinetics, *Free Radic. Biol. Med.* 56: 72–88.

164. B.J. Parsons, S. Sibanda, D.J. Heyes, A.W. Paterson, 2013, Reaction of superoxide radicals with glycosaminoglycan chloramides: A kinetic study, *Free Radic. Biol. Med.* 61: 111–118.

165. M.D. Rees, T.N. McNiven, M.J. Davies, 2007, Degradation of extracellular matrix and its components by hypobromous acid, *Biochem. J.* 401: 587–596.

166. M.D. Rees, J.M. Whitelock, E. Malle, et al., 2010, Myeloperoxidase-derived oxidants selectively disrupt the protein core of the heparan sulfate proteoglycan perlecan, *Matrix Biol.* 29: 63–73.

167. M.D. Rees, E.C. Kennett, J.M. Whitelock, M.J. Davies, 2008, Oxidative damage to extracellular matrix and its role in human pathologies, *Free Radic. Biol. Med.* 44: 1973–2001.

168. A.L. Chapman, C.C. Winterbourn, S.O. Brennan, T.W. Jordan, A.J. Kettle, 2003, Characterization of non-covalent oligomers of proteins treated with hypochlorous acid, *Biochem. J.* 375: 33–40.

169. J.W. Lee, S. Soonsanga, J.D. Helmann, 2007, A complex thiolate switch regulates the Bacillus subtilis organic peroxide sensor OhrR, *Proc. Natl. Acad. Sci. USA* 104: 8743–8748.

170. B.S. Rayner, D.T. Love, C.L. Hawkins, 2014, Comparative reactivity of myeloperoxidase-derived oxidants with mammalian cells, *Free Radic. Biol. Med.* 71: 240–255.

171. T.S. Hoskin, J.M. Crowther, J. Cheung, et al., 2019, Oxidative cross-linking of calprotectin occurs in vivo, altering its structure and susceptibility to proteolysis, *Redox Biol.* 24: 101202.

172. L.H. Gomes, M.J. Raftery, W.X. Yan, et al., 2013, S100A8 and S100A9-oxidant scavengers in inflammation, *Free Radic. Biol. Med.* 58: 170–186.

173. G.E. Ronsein, C.C. Winterbourn, P. Di Mascio, A.J. Kettle, 2014, Cross-linking methionine and amine residues with reactive halogen species, *Free Radic. Biol. Med.* 70: 278–287.

174. G. Colombo, M. Clerici, D. Giustarini, et al., 2015, A central role for intermolecular dityrosine cross-linking of fibrinogen in high molecular weight advanced oxidation protein product (AOPP) formation, *Biochim. Biophys. Acta* 1850: 1–12.

175. G. Colombo, M. Clerici, A. Altomare, et al., 2017, Thiol oxidation and di-tyrosine formation

in human plasma proteins induced by inflammatory concentrations of hypochlorous acid, J. Proteomics 152: 22–32.

176. O. Ziouzenkova, L. Asatryan, M. Akmal, et al., 1999, Oxidative cross-linking of ApoB100 and hemoglobin results in low density lipoprotein modification in blood. Relevance to atherogenesis caused by hemodialysis, J. Biol. Chem. 274: 18916–18924.

177. C. Delporte, K.Z. Boudjeltia, C. Noyon, et al., 2014, Impact of myeloperoxidase-LDL interactions on enzyme activity and subsequent posttranslational oxidative modifications of apoB-100, J. Lipid Res. 55: 747–757.

178. A.M. O'Connell, S.P. Gieseg, K.K. Stanley, 1994, Hypochlorite oxidation causes cross-linking of Lp(a), Biochim. Biophys. Acta 1225: 180–186.

179. Vlasova II, A.V. Sokolov, V.A. Kostevich, E.V. Mikhalchik, V.B. Vasilyev, 2019, Myeloperoxidase-induced oxidation of albumin and ceruloplasmin: Role of tyrosines, Biochemistry (Mosc) 84: 652–662.

180. I. Verrastro, K. Tveen-Jensen, C.M. Spickett, A.R. Pitt, 2018, The effect of HOCl-induced modifications on phosphatase and tensin homologue (PTEN) structure and function, Free Radic. Res. 52: 232–247.

181. C.L. Hawkins, M.J. Davies, 2005, The role of aromatic amino acid oxidation, protein unfolding, and aggregation in the hypobromous acid-induced inactivation of trypsin inhibitor and lysozyme, Chem. Res. Toxicol. 18: 1669–1677.

182. M.J. Davies, 2016, Protein oxidation and peroxidation, Biochem. J. 473: 805–825.

183. Y. Yu, X. Lv, J. Li, et al., 2015, Defining the role of tyrosine and rational tuning of oxidase activity by genetic incorporation of unnatural tyrosine analogs, J. Am. Chem. Soc. 137: 4594–4597.

184. L.J. Hazell, R. Stocker, 1993, Oxidation of low-density lipoprotein with hypochlorite causes transformation of the lipoprotein into a high-uptake form for macrophages, Biochem. J. 290: 165–172.

185. M. Boncler, B. Kehrel, R. Szewczyk, et al., 2018, Oxidation of C-reactive protein by hypochlorous acid leads to the formation of potent platelet activator, Int. J. Biol. Macromol. 107: 2701–2714.

186. B.S. Rayner, D.T. Love, C.L. Hawkins, 2014, Comparative reactivity of myeloperoxidase-derived oxidants with mammalian cells, Free Radic. Biol. Med. 71: 240–255.

187. R.A. Clark, P.J. Stone, A. El Hag, J.D. Calore, C. Franzblau, 1981, Myeloperoxidase-catalyzed inactivation of α1-protease inhibitor by human neutrophils, J. Biol. Chem. 256: 3348–3353.

188. B. Shao, A. Belaaouaj, C.L. Verlinde, X. Fu, J.W. Heinecke, 2005, Methionine sulfoxide and proteolytic cleavage contribute to the inactivation of cathepsin G by hypochlorous acid: An oxidative mechanism for regulation of serine proteinases by myeloperoxidase, J. Biol. Chem. 280: 29311–29321.

189. B. Shao, M.N. Oda, C. Bergt, et al., 2006, Myeloperoxidase impairs ABCA1-dependent cholesterol efflux through methionine oxidation and site-specific tyrosine chlorination of apolipoprotein A-I, J. Biol. Chem. 281: 9001–9004.

190. R.A. Dunlop, R.T. Dean, K.J. Rodgers, 2008, The impact of specific oxidized amino acids on protein turnover in J774 cells, Biochem. J. 410: 131–140.

191. M. Cederlund, A. Deronic, J. Pallon, O.E. Sorensen, B. Akerstrom, 2015, A1M/alpha1-microglobulin is proteolytically activated by myeloperoxidase, binds its heme group and inhibits low density lipoprotein oxidation, Front Physiol. 6: 11.

192. X. Fu, S.Y. Kassim, W.C. Parks, J.W. Heinecke, 2001, Hypochlorous acid oxygenates the cysteine switch domain of pro- matrilysin (MMP-7). A mechanism for matrix metalloproteinase activation and atherosclerotic plaque rupture by myeloperoxidase, J. Biol. Chem. 276: 41279–41287.

193. X. Fu, W.C. Parks, J.W. Heinecke, 2008, Activation and silencing of matrix metalloproteinases, Semin. Cell Dev. Biol. 19: 2–13.

194. Y. Wang, H. Rosen, D.K. Madtes, et al., 2007, Myeloperoxidase inactivates TIMP-1 by oxidizing its N-terminal cysteine residue: An oxidative mechanism for regulating proteolysis during inflammation, J. Biol. Chem. 282: 31826–31834.

195. R. Biedron, M.K. Konopinski, J. Marcinkiewicz, S. Jozefowski, 2015, Oxidation by neutrophils-derived HOCl increases immunogenicity of proteins by converting them into ligands of several endocytic receptors involved in antigen uptake by dendritic cells and macrophages, PLoS One 10: e0123293.

196. I.V. Gorudko, D.V. Grigorieva, E.V. Shamova, et al., 2014, Hypohalous acid-modified human serum albumin induces neutrophil NADPH oxidase activation, degranulation, and shape change, Free Radic. Biol. Med. 68: 326–334.

197. S. Garibaldi, C. Barisione, B. Marengo, et al., 2017, Advanced oxidation protein products-modified albumin induces differentiation of RAW264.7 macrophages into dendritic-like cells which is modulated by cell surface thiols, *Toxins (Basel)* 9: 27.

198. H. Cai, C.Y. Chuang, S. Vanichkitrungruang, C.L. Hawkins, M.J. Davies, 2019, Hypochlorous acid-modified extracellular matrix contributes to the behavioral switching of human coronary artery smooth muscle cells, *Free Radic. Biol. Med.* 134: 516–526.

199. S. Vanichkitrungruang, C.Y. Chuang, C.L. Hawkins, et al., 2019, Oxidation of human plasma fibronectin by inflammatory oxidants perturbs endothelial cell function, *Free Radic. Biol. Med.* 136: 118–134.

200. A.A. Woods, M.J. Davies, 2003, Fragmentation of extracellular matrix by hypochlorous acid, *Biochem. J.* 376: 219–227.

201. A.A. Woods, S.M. Linton, M.J. Davies, 2003, Detection of HOCl-mediated protein oxidation products in the extracellular matrix of human atherosclerotic plaques, *Biochem. J.* 370: 729–735.

202. M.D. Rees, L. Dang, T. Thai, et al., 2012, Targeted subendothelial matrix oxidation by myeloperoxidase triggers myosin II-dependent de-adhesion and alters signaling in endothelial cells, *Free Radic. Biol. Med.* 53: 2344–2356.

203. S. Baldus, J.P. Eiserich, M.L. Brennan, et al., 2002, Spatial mapping of pulmonary and vascular nitrotyrosine reveals the pivotal role of myeloperoxidase as a catalyst for tyrosine nitration in inflammatory diseases, *Free Radic. Biol. Med.* 33: 1010–1019.

204. S. Baldus, J.P. Eiserich, A. Mani, et al., 2001, Endothelial transcytosis of myeloperoxidase confers specificity to vascular ECM proteins as targets of tyrosine nitration, *J. Clin. Invest.* 108: 1759–1770.

205. S. Vanichkitrungruang, C.Y. Chuang, C.L. Hawkins, M.J. Davies, 2020, Myeloperoxidase-derived damage to human plasma fibronectin: Modulation by protein binding and thiocyanate ions (SCN⁻), *Redox Biol.* 36: 101641.

206. H. Cai, C.Y. Chuang, S. Vanichkitrungruang, C.L. Hawkins, M.J. Davies, 2019, Hypochlorous acid-modified extracellular matrix contributes to the behavioural switching of human coronary artery smooth muscle cells, *Free Radic. Biol. Med.* 134: 516–526.

207. M.C.M. Vissers, C. Thomas, 1997, Hypochlorous acid disrupts the adhesive properties of subendothelial matrix, *Free Radic. Biol. Med.* 23: 401–411.

208. J.C. Morris, 1966, The acid ionization constant of HOCl from 5°C to 35°C, *J. Phys. Chem.* 70: 3798–3805.

209. W.A. Prutz, R. Kissner, W.H. Koppenol, H. Ruegger, 2000, On the irreversible destruction of reduced nicotinamide nucleotides by hypohalous acids, *Arch. Biochem. Biophys.* 380: 181–191.

210. P.G. Furtmuller, U. Burner, C. Obinger, 1998, Reaction of myeloperoxidase compound I with chloride, bromide, iodide, and thiocyanate, *Biochemistry* 37: 17923–17930.

211. L.A. Marquez, J.T. Huang, H.B. Dunford, 1994, Spectral and kinetic studies on the formation of myeloperoxidase compounds I and II: Roles of hydrogen peroxide and superoxide, *Biochemistry* 33: 1447–1454.

212. W. Jantschko, P.G. Furtmuller, M. Allegra, et al., 2002, Redox intermediates of plant and mammalian peroxidases: A comparative transient-kinetic study of their reactivity toward indole derivatives, *Arch. Biochem. Biophys.* 398: 12–22.

213. U. Burner, P.G. Furtmuller, A.J. Kettle, W.H. Koppenol, C. Obinger, 2000, Mechanism of reaction of myeloperoxidase with nitrite, *J. Biol. Chem.* 275: 20597–20601.

CHAPTER FIVE

Reactivity of Hypochlorous Acid (HOCl) with Nucleic Acids, RNA and DNA

Clare L. Hawkins
University of Copenhagen

CONTENTS

ABBREVIATIONS

5ClC:	5-chloro-cytidine
5ClUra:	5-chloro-uracil
5CldC:	5-chloro-2′-deoxycytidine
5CldU:	5-chloro-2′-deoxyuridine
8ClA:	8-chloro-adenosine
8ClG:	8-chloro-guanosine
8CldA:	8-chloro-2′-deoxyadenosine
8CldG:	8-chloro-2′-deoxyguanosine
DNA:	Deoxyribonucleic acid
HCAEC:	Human coronary artery endothelial cells
H_2O_2:	Hydrogen peroxide
HOBr:	Hypobromous acid
HOCl:	Hypochlorous acid
hTDG:	Human thymine DNA glycosylase
LPS:	Lipopolysaccharide
MeCP:	Methyl-CpG-binding protein
MPO:	Myeloperoxidase
MRM:	Multiple reaction monitoring
RNA:	Ribonucleic acid
SSB:	Single-stranded DNA binding protein
UDG:	Uracil DNA glycosylase

INTRODUCTION

The production of oxidants by neutrophils (and other phagocytes) is a major defensive pathway in innate immunity to facilitate

DOI: 10.1201/9781003212287-7

the destruction of bacteria and other invading pathogens [1]. Myeloperoxidase (MPO) plays a key role in this process by catalyzing the conversion of hydrogen peroxide to hypochlorous acid (HOCl), which is a potent bactericidal agent [2,3]. However, in addition to promoting the destruction of pathogens, HOCl also reacts readily with host tissue, particularly under chronic inflammatory conditions, causing modification and damage to a wide range of biological molecules (reviewed in Ref. [4]). Nucleic acids are important targets for HOCl, as evidenced by the detection of a range of different stable chlorinated nucleobase products both in model in vitro cellular systems [5–8] and in vivo in humans [8–11].

Damage to nucleic acids resulting from the overproduction of HOCl under chronic inflammatory conditions has been implicated in the development of a number of human diseases, including atherosclerosis [10], diabetes [11] and various types of cancers [12–14]. Indeed, it has been estimated, on the basis of epidemiological data, that more than 20% of all cancers are caused by chronic inflammation, which can be attributed in some cases to chronic infection [15]. Although the underlying cellular mechanisms responsible for this association are complex [16], the modification of nucleic acids by neutrophil-derived oxidants, particularly HOCl, is nonetheless believed to play an important role in carcinogenesis [12,14]. For example, chlorinated nucleobases cause base mis-pairing and mutagenesis (e.g. [14,17,18]) and have also been implicated in the perturbation of epigenetic signaling [19,20]. Whether the chlorination of nucleic acids also plays a role in the development of other human diseases remains to be established. However, recent studies support a potential pathological role for some chlorinated nucleobase products [21–24].

This chapter will provide an overview of the reactivity of HOCl with isolated nucleosides, RNA and DNA, including a description of the products formed, the kinetics of the reactions and the detection methods used for quantification of stable chlorinated products. The chapter will also describe the structural and functional consequences of nucleic acid modification by HOCl, including the biological effects and therapeutic applications of chlorinated nucleobases.

FORMATION OF CHLORINATED PRODUCTS

Reactive Intermediates – N-Chloramines and Nitrogen-Centered Radicals

The reaction of HOCl with RNA, DNA and the related nucleobases, nucleosides and nucleotides results in the formation of both unstable and stable chlorinated products. The initial reaction involves the interaction of HOCl with the heterocyclic and exocyclic nitrogen atoms of the nucleobases. This results in the generation of a nitrogen–chlorine bond and formation of the N-chloramine (RR′N-Cl; Figure 5.1) [25–30]. The rate of these reactions is dependent on the nucleobase structure, particularly the location of the nitrogen atom. The second-order rate constants for these reactions can be classified into two groups, with k_2 for heterocyclic nitrogen atoms typically ca. 10^3–10^4 $M^{-1}s^{-1}$, while the reaction with exocyclic nitrogen atoms, such as found in cytidine, is much slower ($k_2 < 100$ $M^{-1}s^{-1}$) (Table 5.1).

The stability of the nucleobase N-chloramines is dependent on the site of reaction and the structure of the nucleobase [29]. Thus, the N-chloramines formed on the exocyclic amine groups are more stable than the corresponding ring-derived species formed on the heterocyclic amine groups [29]. For example, with pyrimidine nucleobases, the N-chloramines formed on uridine and thymidine decompose more rapidly than those formed on cytidine, which contains an exocyclic amine group [29]. For the purine nucleobases, multiple species are formed, with more complex chloramine decay curves observed, consistent with the formation of both ring-derived and exocyclic N-chloro-species [29]. In experiments with RNA and DNA, the formation of chloramines accounts for ca. 50%–65% of the added HOCl, with biphasic decomposition kinetics observed, consistent with the formation of both heterocyclic and exocyclic chloramines [30]. In experiments with isolated RNA and DNA, the chloramines decompose over a period of 2 h at 37°C [30], suggesting that the lifetime of these species in vivo will be limited. However, immunological staining is consistent with the presence of N4,5 di-halogenated 2′deoxycytidine species (halogenation of the ring N atoms) in the

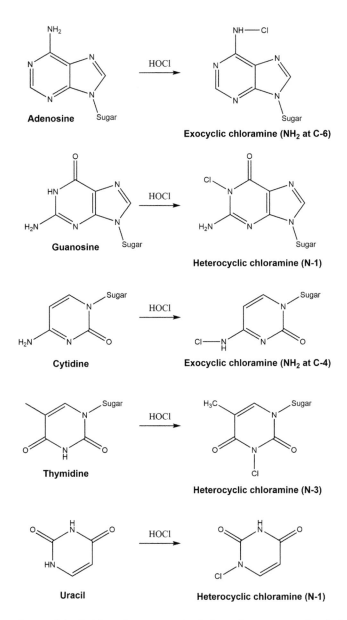

Figure 5.1 Structures of some of the N-chloramines proposed to be formed on exposure of nucleobases and nucleosides to HOCl.

lung and liver tissue of mice exposed to lipopolysaccharide (LPS), suggesting that these species can be observed in vivo [31].

Nucleobase-derived chloramines decompose by several pathways, which are summarized in Figure 5.2. The heterocyclic chloramines readily undergo intra- and intermolecular chlorine transfer reactions (Figure 5.2). There is evidence for the occurrence of chlorine transfer from the heterocyclic, ring-derived N-chloro species to form more stable exocyclic N-chloro species [29]. These transfer reactions and the interconversion of N-chloramines are of potential importance in the reaction of RNA and DNA with HOCl [30]. Nucleobase-derived chloramines can also decompose by transferring chlorine to other substrates,

TABLE 5.1
TABLE 5.1
Second-order rate constants for the reactions of HOCl with nucleobases

Substrate	pH	k_2 (M^{-1}s^{-1})	Product	Reference
Uracil	5	0.28	5-chlorouracil	[27]
	7	5.1		
	9	5.0		
Uridine monophosphate	6.9	5.5×10^3	Heterocyclic chloramine (N-3)	[32]
Guanosine monophosphate	6.9	2.1×10^4	Heterocyclic chloramine (N-1)	[56]
		2.4	Exocyclic chloramine (NH$_2$ at C-2)	
Thymidine monophosphate	6.9	4.3×10^3	Heterocyclic chloramine (N-3)	[56]
Adenosine monophosphate	6.9	6.4	Exocyclic chloramine (NH$_2$ at C-6)	[56]
Cytidine monophosphate	6.9	83	Exocyclic chloramine (NH$_2$ at C-4)	[32]
		66		[56]
Poly(C)	6.9	308	Exocyclic chloramines (NH$_2$ at C-4)	[32]
Poly(U)	6.9	1.3×10^3	Heterocyclic chloramine (N-3)	[32]
DNA	6.9	~10	Mixed chloramines	[56]

including thiol and thioether moieties [32,33]. This results in the formation of S-chloro species, which react further to form disulfides and sulfoxides, respectively [32,33]. In addition, nucleobase chloramines may transfer chlorine to aromatic functional groups, such as phenols, to form stable chlorinated products, analogous to reactions reported for related heterocyclic amino acid-derived N-chloro species [34].

In addition to decomposition via chlorine transfer, the N-Cl bonds of nucleobase chloramines can undergo homolysis to form nitrogen-centered radicals (Figure 5.2) [29,30,35]. This type of decomposition reaction can occur thermally or

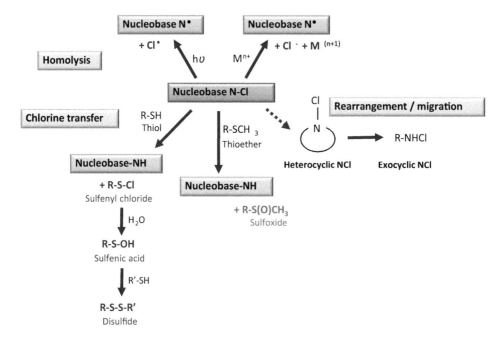

Figure 5.2 Scheme showing the proposed decomposition and interconversion pathways of nucleobase-derived N-chloramines.

be initiated by UV light or transition metal ions (e.g. Cu^+, Fe^{2+}, Ti^{3+}). Radicals can be formed on both exocyclic and heterocyclic nitrogen atoms and can undergo rapid rearrangement reactions to form secondary carbon-centered radicals. These secondary radicals can promote the formation of cross-linked species and the transfer of damage to other substrates [29,30,36].

Stable Products – Chlorinated Nucleobases

The reaction of HOCl with nucleobases, nucleosides, nucleotides, RNA and DNA results in the formation of a number of stable chlorinated products, including 8-chloro-(2′-deoxy)-adenosine, 8Cl(d)A [6,37–39], 8-chloro-(2′-deoxy)-guanosine, 8Cl(d)G [6,11,39], 5-chloro-(2′-deoxy)-cytidine, 5Cl(d)C [6,8,25,39,40] and 5-chlorouracil, 5ClUra [9,10,25,27,41] (Figure 5.3). These products can also be formed on exposure of DNA to low-molecular-mass chloramines, for example, those formed following exposure of Nα-acetyl-histidine to HOCl [5]. HOCl can react with free nucleosides and DNA to form other oxidized products, including aminoimidazolone nucleoside and 2,5-diimino-4-[(2-deoxy-β-D-erythro-pentofuranosyl)amino]-2H, 5H-imidazole from 2′-deoxyguanosine [42] and the pyrimidine oxidation products thymine

glycol, 5-hydroxycytosine, 5-hydroxyhydantoin and 5-hydroxyuracil [43]. These products are formed as a result of hydroxylation or ring-opening reactions but are also observed on exposure of DNA and related nucleic acids to other oxidants.

As the formation of chlorinated nucleobases is specific for MPO-derived chlorinated oxidants in mammalian systems, this has led to their use as biomarkers for HOCl-induced damage under pathological conditions (e.g. [8–11,41]). However, the relatively low abundance of these products can pose a challenge for their reliable detection and quantification (reviewed in Ref. [44]). Thus, even in experiments with isolated DNA, the formation of stable chlorinated products accounts for <10% of the HOCl consumed [5,37,39,45]. This may reflect the propensity of the chlorinated products to undergo further HOCl-mediated oxidation reactions [38], which is an additional limitation on the utilization of these materials as biomarkers in vivo [44]. Similarly, there is likely to be some degradation of these materials during the sample processing required before quantification. For example, experiments with oligonucleotides containing 5ClC show a 20% loss of this chlorinated product as a result of hydrolysis, with the recovery of only trace amounts of the deamination product, 5ClUra [46].

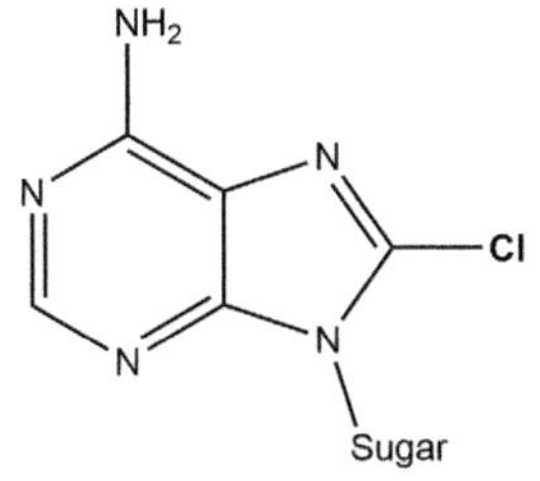

8-chloro-(2'-deoxy)-adenosine
8Cl(d)A

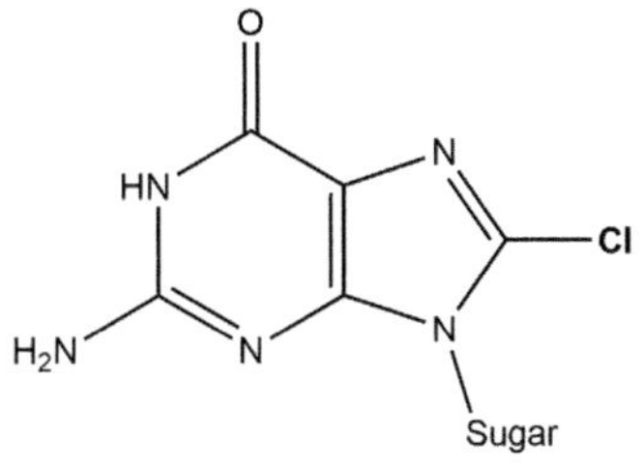

8-chloro-(2'-deoxy)-guanosine
8Cl(d)G

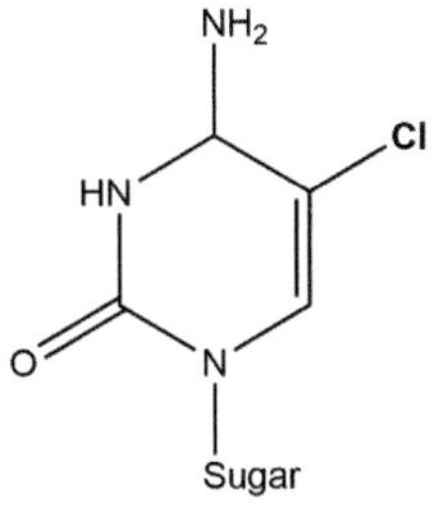

5-chloro-(2'-deoxy)-cytidine
5Cl(d)C

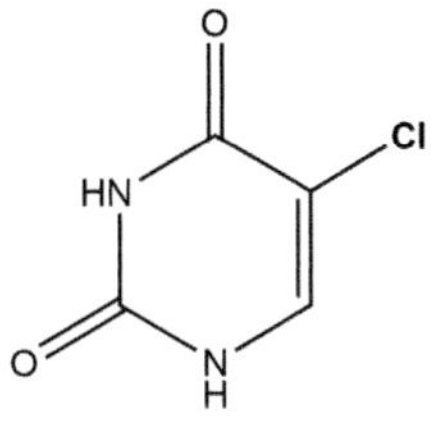

5-chloro-uracil
5ClUra

Figure 5.3 Structures of stable chlorinated nucleobases and nucleosides. The sugar is either ribose or 2-deoxyribose.

It is also important to note that there is a substrate-dependent difference in the pattern of nucleobase chlorination observed on reaction of HOCl with free nucleosides compared with RNA or DNA. Thus, 8CldG is the only product detected on reaction of HOCl with an equimolar mixture of 2′-deoxyadenosine, 2′-deoxyguanosine, 2′-deoxycytidine and 2′-deoxythymidine, whereas 5CldC is the major product formed with DNA [5]. This may further influence the relative abundance and distribution of chlorinated nucleobase products found in cells and tissues. This is highlighted in experiments with different cell types exposed to varying concentrations of HOCl, where 5ClC and 5CldC are the only products detected on RNA and DNA at sublethal oxidant concentrations [5,6,8], with evidence for the chlorination of both guanosine and cytidine in the cytoplasmic nucleotide pools. Interestingly, the extent of 5CldC formation in duplex DNA exposed to HOCl was greater at CpG dinucleotides (where cytosine is followed by guanine) compared with non-CpG sites [47], suggesting that the DNA sequence is also important in defining the chlorination pattern. This has important implications for the perturbation of epigenetic signaling (see below). It is also possible that the ability of MPO to bind to RNA or DNA could influence the selectivity and nature of products formed. This could be particularly relevant in relation to the release of extracellular traps by neutrophils and other immune cells, where enzymatically active MPO (and other granule proteins) is bound to a DNA backbone [48,49].

The mechanism by which chlorinated nucleobases are formed in vivo is generally postulated to involve reactions mediated by HOCl and/or chloramines [5,39]. Whether these reactions occur primarily within intact cells or in the extracellular environment, for example, after necrotic cell death, is not well defined. Several studies have demonstrated nucleic acid chlorination on exposure of cells to an extracellular source of HOCl at pathophysiological oxidant concentrations (e.g. [5,6,8]). It is less clear whether the internalization of MPO by cells can lead to intracellular production of HOCl and subsequent modification of DNA. There is evidence for DNA strand cleavage in human lung epithelial cells under conditions where MPO has been internalized by the cells and is present in both the nucleus and cytoplasm [50]. However, whether this strand cleavage reflects reactions mediated by HOCl or other cellular oxidants formed as a result of the activation of pro-inflammatory signaling cascades has not been established [50]. This is significant in light of other studies showing the ability of MPO to modulate cellular function independently of its catalytic activity [51].

In addition to nucleic acid modification by HOCl and chloramines, evidence has also been presented for a role of molecular chlorine, particularly at low pH, which could be relevant at inflammatory sites [40]. The presence of tertiary amines, including nicotine and trimethylamine, can enhance the chlorination of nucleobases on free nucleosides, RNA and DNA at physiological amine concentrations [10,39,52]. This is postulated to involve formation of reactive quarternary chlorammonium ions (R_3N^+-Cl) (Reaction 1), which then chlorinate heterocyclic and exocyclic nucleobase amines to form N-chloramines (Reaction 2) and subsequently transfer chlorine to form stable chlorinated products [39]. Alternatively, the quarternary chlorammonium ions could undergo hemolysis, forming tertiary amine cation radicals and chlorine radicals (Reaction 3), which react directly with the nucleobase [39].

$$HOCl + R_3N \rightarrow R_3N^+\text{-}Cl + HO^- \qquad (1)$$

$$R_3N^+\text{-}Cl + R_2'NH \rightarrow R_3N^+\text{-}H + R_2'N\text{-}Cl \qquad (2)$$

$$R_3N^+\text{-}Cl \rightarrow R_3N^{\bullet+} + Cl^\bullet \qquad (3)$$

The catalytic effects of nicotine on nucleobase chlorination were seen with HOCl, MPO/H_2O_2/Cl$^-$ and activated neutrophils, at μM amine concentrations [10,39], suggesting that these reactions may be relevant to the development of smoking-related inflammatory pathologies. In addition, it has been reported that elevated levels of 5ClC are formed on exposure of isolated DNA to peroxynitrite, in a chloride-dependent manner [45]. Whether this reaction has any relevance in vivo remains to be established.

Mass spectrometry is commonly used to detect and quantify chlorinated nucleobase products. LC-MS has been used extensively to detect and quantify the formation of 8Cl(d)A, 8Cl(d)G and 5Cl(d)C in complex biological matrices, including cells, biological fluids and tissues (e.g. [5,6,8,22–24]), whereas GC-MS has been more commonly utilized for the detection and quantification of 5ClUra (e.g. [9,10,41]). As discussed above, the low abundance of chlorinated nucleobases poses a significant challenge for detection of chlorinated nucleobases. Badouard et al. developed sensitive tandem LC-MS methodology, which allowed the quantification of all the chlorinated ribose and deoxyribose nucleobases at a limit of detection ranging from 2 to 25 fmol [6]. This high sensitivity was facilitated by using multiple reaction monitoring (MRM) that incorporated a transition corresponding to loss of a (2-deoxy)ribose moiety containing the ^{37}Cl isotope, enabling accurate determination of the chlorinated nucleobases with a level of detection of about 0.1 lesion per 10^6 nucleosides from 50 µg DNA [6]. Using this method, it was possible to quantify the presence of 8CldA and 5CldC in isolated human leukocytes [6]. More recently, Noyon et al. developed a triple quadrupole MS analysis method, which had a markedly improved sensitivity (~25-fold) for 5Cl(d)C and 8Cl(d)G but was not suitable for quantification of 8Cl(d)A [8]. Nonetheless, using this technique, it was possible to detect and quantify 5ClC (1.0 ± 0.2 nM) in the plasma from healthy individuals [8]. In some cases, immunological detection of chlorinated nucleobases is also possible (e.g. [11]), though in general, the antibodies are not commercially available, which has limited the wider application of this approach for the analysis of samples from inflammatory models and pathological conditions.

STRUCTURAL CONSEQUENCES OF NUCLEOBASE CHLORINATION

Exposure of DNA to HOCl results in alterations to structure, resulting from either dissociation of the double helix [32,53,54] or strand cleavage [30,55]. In each case, these effects appear to involve the formation of N-chlorinated nucleobase products, which cause disruption to the hydrogen-bonding interactions between the nucleobases [32,53]. Indeed, it has been suggested that the base pairing of double-stranded DNA serves to prevent, or certainly slow, the reaction of HOCl with the heterocyclic and exocyclic amines of the nucleobase on the basis that the chlorination of denatured DNA occurs more rapidly [32,56]. The formation of nucleobase chloramines can also promote fragmentation of the DNA backbone, as shown with plasmid DNA [30]. This strand cleavage is attributed to the formation of intermediate nucleobase nitrogen-centered radicals, which undergo further reaction to result in hydrogen atom abstraction from the sugar-phosphate backbone [30]. These reactions occur most readily with the unstable heterocyclic thymidine and uridine N-chloramines, but can also be promoted by chloramines formed on other substrates, including amino acids and proteins, which may be important in cellular systems [36].

There is evidence to support the formation of covalent DNA–protein cross-links, which is also associated with N-chloramine formation [36,57]. For example, the HOCl-induced covalent attachment of histidine and lysine to DNA occurs in a chloramine-dependent manner and is postulated to involve the formation and subsequent reactions of nitrogen-centered radicals [36]. It has been shown that lysine-derived, nitrogen-centered, radicals can rapidly add to the C5–C6 double bond of thymidine to generate C6-yl and C5-yl radical adducts and protein-base dimers (Figure 5.4) [36]. Long-lived intermediates such as N-chloramines have also been implicated in

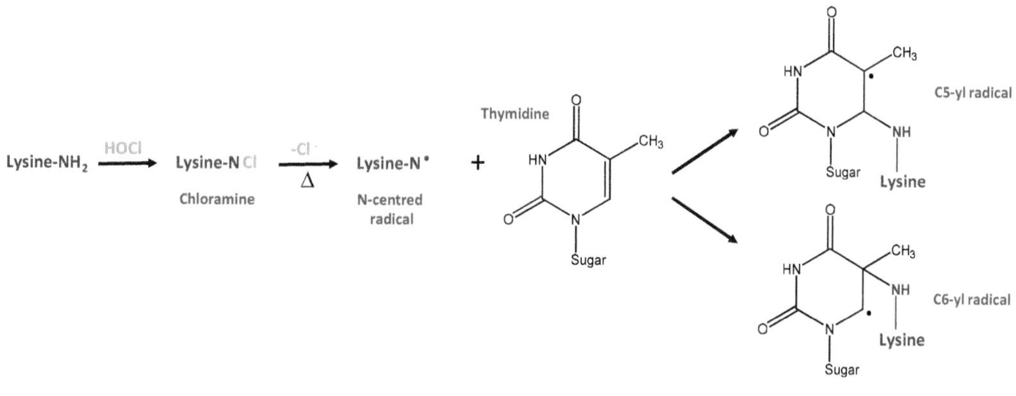

Figure 5.4 Proposed mechanism for the formation of C5-yl and C6-yl radicals on pyrimidine nucleobases (shown here for thymidine) on reaction with radicals derived from lysine-derived chloramines.

HOCl-mediated cross-linking of single-stranded DNA-binding protein (SSB) to single-stranded oligonucleotides [57]. DNA–protein cross-links have been detected on exposure of *Escherichia coli* to HOCl, suggesting that these reactions have potential significance *in vivo* [55,57]. The DNA–protein cross-links may contribute to cytotoxicity [57] or alternatively serve as an intrinsic probe for HOCl and/or other chlorinating oxidants [55]. Thus, the extent of DNA–protein complexation following exposure of bacteria to lethal concentrations of HOCl was found to be more extensive than nucleobase chlorination, as determined by quantification of 5ClUra [55].

FUNCTIONAL CONSEQUENCES OF NUCLEOBASE CHLORINATION

There is increasing evidence to support a range of downstream effects following the cellular uptake of different chlorinated nucleosides. It has been demonstrated that cells in culture can take up and phosphorylate chlorinated nucleosides, which results in their accumulation in the cellular nucleotide pool. This can lead to mutagenesis, altered function and cytotoxicity resulting from the incorporation of the chlorinated nucleobases into RNA and DNA, and/or disruption to metabolic and signaling pathways. This has important implications for both the development of certain cancers and inflammatory pathologies and the use of these compounds in a therapeutic context, as will be discussed below.

Mutagenesis

It is well established that chlorinated nucleobases are mutagenic and cause base mispairing in a manner that is dependent on the nucleoside structure. Early studies in relation to the biological effects of chlorinated nucleobases were performed with 5CldC and 5ClUra, as there was interest in the utilization of these compounds therapeutically, as a means to sensitize DNA in malignant tissue to the effects of ionizing radiation (reviewed in Ref. [58]). 5CldC is a substrate for deoxycytidine kinase, which promotes its conversion to 5Cl-dCMP and subsequent incorporation into genomic DNA [59]. Exposure of cells to 5CldC also results in the formation of 5CldU via the action of cytidine deaminases [59,60]. Similarly, the addition of 5ClUra to cells results in the formation of 5CldU from the activity

of thymidine phosphorylase, which can then be incorporated into DNA by DNA polymerases [58,61]. This incorporation of 5CldU results in mutagenesis, as this chlorinated nucleoside is a thymidine analog mutagen, which causes mispairing with guanine to cause G•C → A•T and A•T → G•C transitions [62] and sister chromatid exchanges [58,61]. On the basis of the pH dependency observed on examination of the extent of guanine mispairing in studies with synthetic oligonucleotides containing 5ClUra, it has been suggested that the presence of the electron-withdrawing chlorine substituent at the C5 position promotes the formation of an ionized base pair [63]. Interestingly, it was also demonstrated that 5ClUra was more efficiently repaired by human glycosylases when paired with guanine compared with adenine [63].

5CldC is also mutagenic by causing C → T transitions at frequencies ranging from 3% to 9%, which is dependent on the nature of the DNA polymerase [18]. In this case, the presence of 5CldC increases the probability of mispairing with adenine, owing to a specific steric interaction between 5CldC and the incoming dATP, which occurs in the active site of the polymerase [18]. This miscoding as thymidine is a mutation that is prevalent in tissues experiencing inflammatory stress and also in the genomes of some inflammation-associated cancers [18].

Less is known about the potential mutagenicity of the chlorinated purine nucleobases. However, a recent study to assess the miscoding properties of 8CldG demonstrated that this chlorinated nucleobase could also form mismatches and incorrectly base-pair in DNA duplexes [64]. The miscoding specificities were dependent on the nature of the DNA polymerase, with evidence supporting one-base deletions, as well as mispairing of 8CldC with dGMP, dAMP and dTMP, in addition to the pairing with dCMP [64]. More recently, it has been shown that 8CldG facilitates misincorporation of guanine during DNA replication [17]. In this study, the efficiency for the insertion of guanine found to be only 15-fold less than that of cytosine, suggesting that the presence of 8CldG lesions in DNA could promote a G → C transversion mutation [17].

Replication, Transcription and Translation

In addition to promoting mutagenesis, the presence of chlorinated nucleobases within DNA can affect the rate of DNA replication [58]. The incorporation of 5CldU is reported to compromise the ability of mammalian cells to proceed through DNA synthesis. Thus, the presence of 5CldU within the genomic DNA can cause cells to become delayed in S-phase, resulting in the accumulation of cells in the G2+M phase [58]. This is postulated to reflect damage during S-phase, such as DNA strand breaks, which are repaired during the G2 phase [65]. Similarly, the presence of 5CldU within the DNA of HeLa cells induced senescence by halting cell division [66,67]. This was attributed to an alteration in the nuclear matrix structure, following a change in the expression of nuclear matrix proteins [66,67]. However, these effects were not apparent in macrophage-like cells exposed to 5CldC, where there was no significant alteration in the growth or proliferation of the cells, although there was some evidence for DNA fragmentation and uracil misincorporation [22].

The presence of chlorinated nucleobases in RNA also has functional consequences. It has been shown that the incorporation of 5ClC into the RNA of endothelial or epithelial prostatic cells leads to a decrease in the activity of enzymes involved in replication, transcription and translation and a significant reduction in the translation yield [24]. The long-term consequences of 5ClC incorporation into RNA on downstream parameters such as protein synthesis have yet to be examined. However, the consequences of 5ClC formation are important to consider, given the evidence for selective chlorination of cellular RNA rather than DNA on exposure of *Escherichia coli* to an MPO/H_2O_2/Cl$^-$ system [40].

Gene Silencing and Epigenetic Regulation

In addition to its intrinsic mutagenic properties, 5ClC has also been implicated in the perturbation of epigenetic signaling via its ability to alter the affinity of sequence-specific DNA-binding proteins (reviewed in Ref. [19]). Thus, 5ClC within DNA can mimic the presence of 5-methylcytosine and, as such, can inadvertently enhance the binding of methyl-CpG-binding proteins, including methyl-CpG-binding protein 2 (MeCP2), to direct enzymatic DNA methylation [68]. This is postulated to influence the recruitment of histone-modifying enzymes that promote a cascade of reactions leading to chromatin condensation and gene silencing of tumour suppressor genes [20,68]. Similar mimicry of 5ClC for 5-methylcytosine is also observed with the maintenance methyl transferase, DNMT1, which is essential for the heritable transfer of cytosine methylation patterns to progeny cells (Figure 5.5) [69]. This is particularly significant in light of the demonstration of preferential chlorination of cytosine in CpG dinucleotides [47], as methylation of cytosine occurs predominantly in islands of concentrated CpG sequences located in promoter regions [19]. This misrecognition of 5ClC as 5-methylcytosine and subsequent hypermethylation of CpG sites has been shown to lead to heritable aberrant gene silencing *in vivo* [70]. This is particularly significant given the role of aberrant silencing of tumour suppressor genes in the development of many human cancers [19].

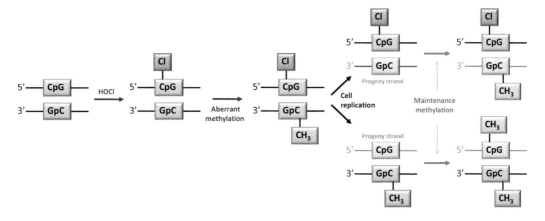

Figure 5.5 The proposed mechanism for altered maintenance methylation due to the presence of 5-chlorocytosine (5ClC) on DNA (adapted from Ref. [69]). The presence of 5ClC within a CpG site on DNA (shown in red) can be misrecognized as 5-methycytosine by methyl-binding proteins and the maintenance methyl transferase DNMT1 resulting in undesired methylation (shown in blue). This can be heritably transmitted to the progeny cell DNA (shown in gold) on cell replication resulting in the establishment of aberrant methylation patterns (shown in green).

Other Perturbations to Cellular Function

Given the role of MPO and HOCl formation in the development of numerous inflammatory pathologies, there has been some interest in examining whether the exposure of cells to chlorinated nucleosides has functional effects in addition to promoting mutation and influencing DNA replication. Recent studies have shown that a range of nonmalignant, mammalian cell types, including macrophages, endothelial cells and epithelial prostatic cells, can take up and incorporate chlorinated nucleosides into their RNA and DNA [21–24]. The incorporation of chlorinated nucleosides is dependent on the nucleotide, cell type and incubation time. With macrophages, chlorinated ribose nucleosides were incorporated into the cellular RNA within 4 h of exposure, whether present individually or as part of an equimolar mixture, with 5ClC achieving the highest concentration [22]. Similar results have been reported with other cell types, including endothelial and epithelial cells, where incorporation of 5ClC was favored over 8ClG; insertion of 8ClA was not assessed [24]. There seems to be more variation in the extent of chlorinated deoxyribose nucleoside incorporation into DNA. Thus, only 5CldC was incorporated into the cellular DNA of macrophages to a significant extent [22], and this nucleoside was favored over 8CldG in EA.hy926 endothelial cells and epithelial prostatic cells [24]. However, in human coronary artery endothelial cells (HCAEC), 8CldG was found to incorporate to the greatest extent, though evidence was also obtained for the presence of 5CldC and 8CldA [71].

These differences in the extent of incorporation could be related to cellular uptake, turnover, repair or differing affinities of the individual kinases (cytidine, adenosine and guanosine) for the chlorinated nucleosides. There are few detailed mechanistic and kinetic studies examining the cellular uptake of chlorinated nucleosides. However, with non-chlorinated nucleosides, a facilitated diffusion mechanism results in the rapid transfer across the plasma membrane [72] at a rate dependent on both the extracellular and intracellular nucleoside or nucleotide concentrations [73]. The cellular repair of chlorinated RNA and DNA lesions is also likely to play a key role in determining the extent of incorporation observed. There is some evidence for the removal of chlorinated nucleosides from RNA and DNA on further incubation of cells in the absence of an external source of nucleoside

[22,23]. With 5Cl(d)C, this is at least partially explained by deamination to form 5Cl(d)U rather than clearance, by reactions mediated by cytidine deaminase or dCMP deaminase [74].

Although there is evidence for the incorporation of significant amounts of 5Cl(d)C, 8Cl(d)A and 8Cl(d)G into cellular RNA and DNA, in most cases, this does not appear to be associated with a rapid loss of cell viability when assessed by metabolic activity assays [22,23]. An exception to this behavior is 8ClA, which decreases the metabolic activity of macrophages and HCAEC and induces apoptotic cell death [21,23] analogous to the behavior reported for various malignant cell types (e.g. [75–77]). The altered cellular metabolism and apoptotic cell death seen in malignant [75–77] and nonmalignant cell types on exposure to 8ClA [21,23] are associated with an accumulation of 8Cl-ATP. With malignant cells, this has led to the use of 8ClA therapeutically, which will be described later in the chapter.

With macrophages, 8ClA did not have a significant effect on mitochondrial respiration or glycolysis but instead altered the mRNA expression of a range of antioxidant and DNA damage repair genes [21]. This suggests that the capacity of the cells to cope with oxidative stress and repair DNA damage would likely be compromised on exposure to 8ClA, which may be relevant in inflammatory pathologies such as atherosclerosis. 8ClA also altered the expression of antioxidant genes in HCAEC, which in this case was associated with activation of the unfolded protein response and sustained endoplasmic reticulum stress, culminating in the elevation of cytosolic calcium and cell death by apoptosis [23].

Similarly, there is evidence for the differential activation of stress-related, pro-inflammatory signaling pathways in macrophages exposed to other chlorinated nucleosides. A significant increase in the expression of interleukin 1β (IL-1β) was observed, particularly in experiments with 5ClC, which was associated with the nuclear translocation of the NF-κB subunit p65 [22]. Interestingly, 5ClC treatment did not alter the expression of other NF-κB-related cytokines or chemokines, and no nuclear translocation of p65 was seen with 8ClG, which induced a more sustained elevation in the expression of IL-1β, suggesting that multiple pathways may be involved in these cellular effects [22].

Overall, these studies provide new insight into the pathways by which the excessive production of HOCl during chronic inflammation could contribute to disease development, though questions remain as to whether chlorinated nucleosides are formed in sufficient yield in vivo to induce these cellular effects. The concentrations used in in vitro studies are often based on the concentrations of chlorinated nucleosides formed in cells exposed to pathophysiological amounts of HOCl, owing to the difficulty in quantifying the molar amounts of these materials at inflammatory sites or diseased tissue. However, with 8ClA, the reported cellular effects with macrophages [21] and HCAEC [23] are seen at concentrations of nucleoside comparable to the plasma levels achieved therapeutically on supplementation with 8ClA in animal models [78] and clinical trials with the related analogue 8Cl-cAMP [79].

REMOVAL AND REPAIR OF CHLORINATED RNA AND DNA DAMAGE

There is limited information about the nature and efficacy of repair pathways for different chlorinated RNA and DNA lesions. It has been postulated that 5CldC contributes to mutagenesis and increases the probability that inflamed tissues will progress to malignancy, on the basis of a lack of a specific repair pathway for this chlorinated lesion [18]. On the other hand, the repair pathway resulting in the excision of 5CldU has been implicated as playing a causal role in the cytotoxicity associated with this chlorinated nucleoside [80]. The incorporation of chlorinated nucleosides into DNA could also be influenced by the activity of other defensive enzymes designed to prevent spontaneous mutations. For example, the human mutT homologue (hMTH1) could prevent misincorporation of 8CldG into DNA by degrading 8Cl-dGTP to form 8Cl-dGMP [81]. This type of reaction could play a role in determining the specificity or pattern of chlorinated nucleoside incorporation reported previously in studies with 5CldC and 8CldG [22,24]. It is also important to note that HOCl, N-chloramines and activated neutrophils can inhibit DNA repair enzymes and prevent nucleotide excision repair, which is also relevant to consider, particularly in inflammatory pathologies [14,82].

Damage to DNA nucleobases can be repaired by excision of the damaged base, a process initiated by damage-specific DNA glycosylases, which catalyze the cleavage of the N-glycosidic bond of the base sugar to result in the removal of the nucleobase and formation of an abasic or apurinic/

apyrimidinic (AP) site in the DNA, which becomes a substrate for other enzymes [83]. Human thymine DNA glycosylase (hTDG) removes thymine and uracil from DNA when these bases are mismatched with guanine. However, hTDG can also remove 5-halogenated uracils, including 5ClUra, particularly from CpG sites [84]. While this enzyme is active in removing 5ClUra from DNA when matched with guanine, any chlorinated base paired with adenine will likely persist in the DNA, given the inability of hTDG to repair this lesion [84]. Moreover, removal of 5ClUra by this base excision repair pathway can create a repetitive cycle of chlorinated nucleoside misincorporation and excision, which increases the number of abasic sites and DNA strand breaks, promoting sister chromatid exchange [84]. It is possible that other DNA repair enzymes may behave in a similar manner, including human methyl-CpG-binding domain 4 (hMBD4), which can also excise 5ClUra from DNA when paired with guanine [85].

Interestingly, other studies demonstrated that the cytotoxicity associated with 5CldU is an indirect result of uracil DNA glycosylase (UDG) activity, as the 5CldU was not excised from the DNA in this case [80]. Instead, the accumulation of 5CldU resulted in the inhibition of thymidylate synthase, which promoted the incorporation of uracil into the DNA by depleting dTMP from the cellular nucleotide pool. This led to the formation of DNA abasic sites and fragmentation via the excision of uracil by UDG [80]. This could also be a potential pathway to cytotoxicity on exposure of cells to 5CldC, as there is evidence for the presence of increased amounts of uracil in the DNA of macrophages exposed to this chlorinated nucleoside [22].

The pathways responsible for the removal of chlorinated lesions from RNA are poorly understood. It is postulated either that there is an active proofing process that targets the chlorinated nucleobase specifically or, perhaps more likely, that the RNA is actively or passively degraded [86]. Thus, there is some evidence for the premature degradation of mRNA following the incorporation of the chlorinated nucleotide 5Cl-UTP, into β-globin pre-mRNA. This is attributed to inhibition of the active spliceosome and splicing to the mRNA [87]. There is also evidence for premature termination of transcription in cells exposed to 8ClA. This is believed to be due to destabilization of the RNA, as 8ClA adopts a syn- rather than anti-conformation [77], which could also be relevant for 8ClG. Lastly, the incorporation of 5ClC is reported to influence RNA synthesis and translation [24].

THE ROLE OF CHLORINATED NUCLEOSIDES IN HEALTH AND DISEASE

Therapeutic Use of Chlorinated Nucleosides

There has been considerable interest in the use of some chlorinated nucleosides in a therapeutic context to treat different malignancies. Originally, the effects of the chlorinated nucleosides were believed to be specifically RNA- or DNA-directed and applicable mainly to rapidly dividing cells. Therefore, chlorinated pyrimidine nucleosides, including 5CldC, 5CldU and 5ClUra, have been used as sensitizers to improve the efficacy of tumour destruction by radiation therapy [58–60]. However, although these compounds are effective radiosensitizers, they are also highly cytotoxic and mutagenic, as outlined above, which has disfavored their clinical use.

In contrast, the RNA-directed actions of 8ClA and its ability to more selectively kill malignant cell types, including chronic lymphocytic leukemia lymphocytes [75], breast cancer [76], myeloma [77] and mantle cell lymphoma cells [88], have led to clinical trials to test the efficacy of this chlorinated nucleoside as a chemotherapeutic drug. 8ClA displays potent cytotoxic and growth inhibitory properties, following its phosphorylation by various enzymes, including adenosine kinase, to result in the cellular accumulation of 8Cl-ATP [77,89,90]. In the malignant cell types examined, this results in the depletion of ATP, which can trigger cell death by apoptosis, though 8ClA can also induce apoptotic cell death by inhibiting the transcription of antiapoptotic proteins [75–77]. 8ClA has cytotoxic efficacy in malignant cells at a concentration of $10\,\mu M$ (e.g. [88–91]), which has been shown to be a therapeutically achievable plasma concentration based on intervention studies [78] and clinical trials with 8-Cl-cAMP [79]. However, recent studies indicate that this concentration of 8ClA can also influence the function and behavior of nonmalignant cells, including macrophages [21] and endothelial cells [23], which may be relevant in light of the clinical interest in this nucleoside.

Chlorinated Nucleosides as Biomarkers of Disease

The presence of chlorinated nucleosides in models of chronic inflammation, human inflammatory fluids and diseased tissues suggests that nucleic acids are targets for MPO-derived oxidants in vivo, particularly under pathological conditions. There is evidence for increased concentrations of 5ClUra in human atherosclerotic lesions compared with healthy tissue [10] and the inflammatory exudates of humans [9] and LPS-treated rats [41]. Similarly, infection of Rag2$^{-/-}$ mice with *Helicobacter hepaticus* to mimic human inflammatory bowel disease results in an increase in the levels of 5ClC and 5CldC in colonic RNA and DNA, respectively [92]. There are also elevated amounts of 5CldC in human colonic tissue samples from patients with Crohn's disease and ulcerative colitis [93]. The development of more sensitive LC-MS-based methodologies has revealed that 5ClC is present in the plasma of healthy donors [8] and at 5–6-fold higher concentrations in the plasma of elderly patients under hemodialysis, where MPO is also elevated [24]. There is evidence for the presence of 8CldG in the liver tissue and urine of LPS-treated rats and the urine of human diabetic patients [11]. Moreover, it has been suggested that 8CldG could be a potential biomarker of early inflammation, as antibody staining consistent with the presence of this chlorinated nucleoside was seen in liver tissue from hepatocellular carcinoma patients but not from human cirrhosis patients [11].

CONCLUDING REMARKS

There is accumulating evidence for the presence of RNA and DNA damage products resulting from reactions of HOCl with these nucleic acids and related materials in a number of inflammatory pathologies. While there is little doubt as to the mutagenic capacity of chlorinated nucleobases when present in DNA and strong links with tumorigenesis, whether the formation of these compounds plays a biological role in the development of other human diseases has yet to be firmly established. However, the results from recent in vitro studies with nonmalignant cell types do lend some support to additional pathogenic properties of chlorinated nucleosides, with the caveat as to whether sufficient concentrations of these species are present at inflammatory sites to elicit such reactions. In addition, more work needs to be done to gain a better understanding of the cellular consequences of RNA chlorination, which may be more prevalent and manifest alternative cellular effects in vivo.

REFERENCES

1. S.J. Klebanoff, 1999, Oxygen metabolites from phagocytes, in: J.I. Gallin, R. Snyderman (Eds.), *Inflammation: Basic Principles and Clinical Correlates*, Lippincott Williams & Wilkins, Philadelphia, pp. 721–768.

2. M.B. Hampton, A.J. Kettle, C.C. Winterbourn, 1998, Inside the neutrophil phagosome: oxidants, myeloperoxidase, and bacterial killing, *Blood* 92: 3007–3017.

3. S.J. Klebanoff, 2005, Myeloperoxidase: friend and foe, *J. Leukocyte Biol.* 77: 598–625.

4. M.J. Davies, C.L. Hawkins, 2020, The role of myeloperoxidase in biomolecule modification, chronic inflammation, and disease, *Antioxid. Redox Signal.* 32: 957–981.

5. N.R. Stanley, D.I. Pattison, C.L. Hawkins, 2010, Ability of hypochlorous acid and N-chloramines to chlorinate DNA and its constituents, *Chem. Res. Toxicol.* 23: 1293–1302.

6. C. Badouard, M. Masuda, H. Nishino, et al., 2005, Detection of chlorinated DNA and RNA nucleosides by HPLC coupled to tandem mass spectrometry as potential biomarkers of inflammation, *J. Chromatogr. B* 827: 26–31.

7. J.P. Spencer, M. Whiteman, A. Jenner, B. Halliwell, 2000, Nitrite-induced deamination and hypochlorite-induced oxidation of DNA in intact human respiratory tract epithelial cells, *Free Radic. Biol. Med.* 28: 1039–1050.

8. C. Noyon, C. Delporte, D. Dufour, et al., 2016, Validation of a sensitive LC/MSMS method for chloronucleoside analysis in biological matrixes and its applications, *Talanta* 154: 322–328.

9. J.P. Henderson, J. Byun, J. Takeshita, J.W. Heinecke, 2003, Phagocytes produce 5-chlorouracil and 5-bromouracil, two mutagenic products of myeloperoxidase, in human inflammatory tissue, *J. Biol. Chem.* 278: 23522–23528.

10. J. Takeshita, J. Byun, T.Q. Nhan, et al., 2006, Myeloperoxidase generates 5-chlorouracil in human atherosclerotic tissue. A potential pathway for somatic mutagenesis by macrophages, *J. Biol. Chem.* 281: 3096–3104.

11. T. Asahi, H. Kondo, M. Masuda, et al., 2010, Chemical and immunochemical detection of 8-halogenated deoxyguanosines at early stage inflammation, *J. Biol. Chem.* 285: 9282–9291.

12. P. Lonkar, P.C. Dedon, 2011, Reactive species and DNA damage in chronic inflammation: reconciling chemical mechanisms and biological fates, *Int. J. Cancer* 128: 1999–2009.

13. S.A. Weitzman, L.I. Gordon, 1990, Inflammation and cancer: role of phagocyte-generated oxidants in carcinogenesis, *Blood* 76: 655–663.

14. A.M. Knaapen, N. Gungor, R.P. Schins, P.J. Borm, F.J. Van Schooten, 2006, Neutrophils and respiratory tract DNA damage and mutagenesis: a review, *Mutagenesis* 21: 225–236.

15. V. Bouvard, R. Baan, K. Straif, et al., 2009, A review of human carcinogens – Part B: biological agents, *Lancet Oncol.* 10: 321–322.

16. J.K. Kundu, Y.J. Surh, 2012, Emerging avenues linking inflammation and cancer, *Free Radic. Biol. Med.* 52: 2013–2037.

17. Y. Kou, M.C. Koag, S. Lee, 2019, Promutagenicity of 8-chloroguanine, a major inflammation-induced halogenated DNA lesion, *Molecules* 24: 3507.

18. B.I. Fedeles, B.D. Freudenthal, E. Yau, et al., 2015, Intrinsic mutagenic properties of 5-chlorocytosine: a mechanistic connection between chronic inflammation and cancer, *Proc. Natl. Acad. Sci. U.S.A.* 112: E4571–4580.

19. V. Valinluck, L.C. Sowers, 2007, Inflammation-mediated cytosine damage: a mechanistic link between inflammtion and the epigenetic alterations in human cancers, *Cancer Res.* 67: 5583–5586.

20. V. Valinluck, W. Wu, P.F. Liu, J.W. Neidigh, L.C. Sowers, 2006, Impact of cytosine 5-halogens on the interaction of DNA with restriction endonucleases and methyltransferase, *Chem. Res. Toxicol.* 19: 556–562.

21. J.L. Macer-Wright, I. Sileikaite, B.S. Rayner, C.L. Hawkins, 2020, 8-chloroadenosine alters the metabolic profile and downregulates antioxidant and DNA damage repair pathways in macrophages, *Chem. Res. Toxicol.* 33: 402–413.

22. J.L. Macer-Wright, N.R. Stanley, N. Portman, et al., 2019, A role for chlorinated nucleosides in the perturbation of macrophage function and promotion of inflammation, *Chem. Res. Toxicol.* 32: 1223–1234.

23. V. Tang, S. Fu, B.S. Rayner, C.L. Hawkins, 2019, 8-Chloroadenosine induces apoptosis in human coronary artery endothelial cells through the activation of the unfolded protein response, *Redox Biol.* 26: 101274.

24. C. Noyon, T. Roumeguere, C. Delporte, et al., 2017, The presence of modified nucleosides in extracellular fluids leads to the specific incorporation of 5-chlorocytidine into RNA and modulates the transcription and translation, *Mol. Cell Biochem.* 429: 59–71.

25. H. Hayatsu, S.-K. Pan, T. Ukita, 1971, Reaction of sodium hypochlorite with nucleic acids and their constituents, *Chem. Pharm. Bull.* 19: 2189–2192.

26. W. Patton, V. Bacon, A.M. Duffield, et al., 1972, Chlorination studies. I. The reaction of aqueous hypochlorous acid with cytosine, *Biochem. Biophys. Res. Commun.* 48: 880–884.

27. J.P. Gould, J.T. Richards, M.G. Miles, 1984, The kinetics and primary products of uracil chlorination, *Water Res.* 18: 205–212.

28. J.P. Gould, J.T. Richards, M.G. Miles, 1984, The formation of stable organic chloramines during the aqueous chlorination of cytosine and 5-methylcytosine, *Water Res.* 18: 991–999.

29. C.L. Hawkins, M.J. Davies, 2001, Hypochlorite-induced damage to nucleosides: formation of chloramines and nitrogen-centered radicals, *Chem. Res. Toxicol.* 14: 1071–1081.

30. C.L. Hawkins, M.J. Davies, 2002, Hypochlorite-induced damage to DNA, RNA and polynucleotides: formation of chloramines and nitrogen-centered radicals, *Chem. Res. Toxicol.* 15: 83–92.

31. Y. Kawai, H. Morinaga, H. Kondo, et al., 2004, Endogenous formation of novel halogenated 2'-deoxycytidine. Hypohalous acid-mediated DNA modification at the site of inflammation, *J. Biol. Chem.* 279: 51241–51249.

32. W.A. Prutz, 1998, Interactions of hypochlorous acid with pyrimidine nucleotides, and secondary reactions of chlorinated pyrimidines with GSH, NADH, and other substrates, *Arch. Biochem. Biophys.* 349: 183–191.

33. W.A. Prutz, 1999, Consecutive halogen transfer between various functional groups induced by reaction of hypohalous acids: NADH oxidation by halogenated amide groups, *Arch. Biochem. Biophys.* 371: 107–114.

34. D.I. Pattison, M.J. Davies, 2005, Kinetic analysis of the role of histidine chloramines in hypochlorous acid mediated protein oxidation, *Biochemistry* 44: 7378–7387.

35. C. Bernofsky, B.M. Bandara, O. Hinojosa, S.L. Strauss, 1990, Hypochlorite-modified adenine nucleotides: structure, spin-trapping, and formation by activated guinea pig polymorphonuclear leukocytes, *Free Rad. Res. Comms.* 9: 303–315.

36. C.L. Hawkins, D.I. Pattison, M.J. Davies, 2002, Reaction of protein chloramines with DNA and nucleosides: evidence for the formation of radicals, protein-DNA cross-links and DNA fragmentation, *Biochem. J.* 365: 605–615.

37. M. Whiteman, A. Jenner, B. Halliwell, 1999, 8-Chloroadenine: a novel product formed from hypochlorous acid-induced damage to calf thymus DNA, *Biomarkers* 4: 303–310.

38. M. Whiteman, H.S. Hong, A. Jenner, B. Halliwell, 2002, Loss of oxidized and chlorinated bases in DNA treated with reactive oxygen species: implications for assessment of oxidative damage in vivo, *Biochem. Biophys. Res. Commun.* 296: 883–889.

39. M. Masuda, T. Suzuki, M.D. Friesen, et al., 2001, Chlorination of guanosine and other nucleosides by hypochlorous acid and myeloperoxidase of activated human neutrophils. Catalysis by nicotine and trimethylamine, *J. Biol. Chem.* 276: 40486–40496.

40. J.P. Henderson, J. Byun, J.W. Heinecke, 1999, Molecular chlorine generated by the myeloperoxidase-hydrogen peroxide- chloride system of phagocytes produces 5-chlorocytosine in bacterial RNA, *J. Biol. Chem.* 274: 33440–33448.

41. Q. Jiang, B.C. Blount, B.N. Ames, 2003, 5-Chlorouracil, a marker of DNA damage from hypochlorous acid during inflammation. A gas chromatography-mass spectrometry assay, *J. Biol. Chem.* 278: 32834–32840.

42. T. Suzuki, M. Masuda, M.D. Friesen, B. Fenet, H. Ohshima, 2002, Novel products generated from 2'-deoxyguanosine by hypochlorous acid or a myeloperoxidase-H$_2$O$_2$-Cl$^-$ system: identification of diimino-imidazole and amino-imidazolone nucleosides, *Nucleic Acids Res.* 30: 2555–2564.

43. M. Whiteman, A. Jenner, B. Halliwell, 1997, Hypochlorous acid-induced base modifications in isolated calf thymus DNA, *Chem. Res. Toxicol.* 10: 1240–1246.

44. J. Son, B. Pang, J.L. McFaline, K. Taghizadeh, P.C. Dedon, 2008, Surveying the damage: the challenges of developing nucleic acid biomarkers of inflammation, *Mol. Biosyst.* 4: 902–908.

45. H.J. Chen, S.W. Row, C.L. Hong, 2002, Detection and quantification of 5-chlorocytosine in DNA by stable isotope dilution and gas chromatography/negative ion chemical ionization/mass spectrometry, *Chem. Res. Toxicol.* 15: 262–268.

46. J.I. Kang Jr., A. Burdzy, P.F. Liu, L.C. Sowers, 2004, Synthesis and characterization of oligonucleotides containing 5-chlorocytosine, *Chem. Res. Toxicol.* 17: 1236–1244.

47. J.I. Kang, L.C. Sowers, 2008, Examination of hypochlorous acid-induced damage to cytosine residues in a CpG dinucleotide in DNA, *Chem. Res. Toxicol.* 21: 1211–1218.

48. H. Parker, A.M. Albrett, A.J. Kettle, C.C. Winterbourn, 2012, Myeloperoxidase associated with neutrophil extracellular traps is active and mediates bacterial killing in the presence of hydrogen peroxide, J. Leukocyte Biol. 91: 369–376.

49. V. Papayannopoulos, 2018, Neutrophil extracellular traps in immunity and disease, Nat. Rev. Immunol. 18: 134–147.

50. A. Haegens, J.H. Vernooy, P. Heeringa, B.T. Mossman, E.F. Wouters, 2008, Myeloperoxidase modulates lung epithelial responses to proinflammatory agents, Eur. Respir. J. 31: 252–260.

51. G. Yogalingam, A.R. Lee, D.S. Mackenzie, et al., 2017, Cellular uptake and delivery of myeloperoxidase to lysosomes promote lipofuscin degradation and lysosomal stress in retinal cells, J. Biol. Chem. 292: 4255–4265.

52. W.A. Prutz, 1998, Reactions of hypochlorous acid with biological substrates are activated catalytically by tertiary amines, Arch. Biochem. Biophys. 357: 265–273.

53. C. Bernofsky, 1991, Nucleotide chloramines and neutrophil-mediated cytotoxicity, FASEB J. 5: 295–300.

54. N. Shishido, S. Nakamura, M. Nakamura, 2000, Dissociation of DNA double strand by hypohalous acids, Redox Rep. 5: 243–247.

55. C. Suquet, J.J. Warren, N. Seth, J.K. Hurst, 2010, Comparative study of HOCl-inflicted damage to bacterial DNA ex vivo and within cells, Arch. Biochem. Biophys. 493: 135–142.

56. W.A. Prutz, 1996, Hypochlorous acid interactions with thiols, nucleotides, DNA, and other biological substrates, Arch. Biochem. Biophys. 332: 110–120.

57. P.A. Kulcharyk, J.W. Heinecke, 2001, Hypochlorous acid produced by the myeloperoxidase system of human phagocytes induces covalent cross-links between DNA and protein, Biochemistry 40: 3648–3656.

58. S.M. Morris, 1993, The genetic toxicology of 5-fluoropyrimidines and 5-chlorouracil, Mutat. Res. 297: 39–51.

59. O. Santos, L.M. Perez, T.V. Briggle, D.A. Boothman, S.B. Greer, 1990, Radiation, pool size and incorporation studies in mice with 5-chloro-2'-deoxycytidine, Int. J. Rad. Oncol. Biol. Phys. 19: 357–365.

60. J.T. Hale, J.C. Bigelow, L.A. Mathews, J.J. McCormack, 2002, Analytical and pharmacokinetic studies with 5-chloro-2'-deoxycytidine, Biochem. Pharmacol. 64: 1493–1502.

61. B.C. Pal, R.B. Cumming, M.F. Walton, R.J. Preston, 1981, Environmental pollutant 5-chlorouracil is incorporated in mouse-liver and testes DNA, Mutat. Res. 91: 395–401.

62. H. Yu, R. Eritja, L.B. Bloom, M.F. Goodman, 1993, Ionization of bromouracil and fluorouracil stimulates base mispairing frequencies with guanine, J. Biol. Chem. 268: 15935–15943.

63. C.H. Kim, A. Darwanto, J.A. Theruvathu, J.L. Herring, L.C. Sowers, 2010, Polymerase incorporation and miscoding properties of 5-chlorouracil, Chem. Res. Toxicol. 23: 740–748.

64. A. Sassa, N. Kamoshita, T. Matsuda, et al., 2013, Miscoding properties of 8-chloro-2'-deoxyguanosine, a hypochlorous acid-induced DNA adduct, catalysed by human DNA polymerases, Mutagenesis 28: 81–88.

65. L.E. Dillehay, L.H. Thompson, A.V. Carrano, 1984, DNA-strand breaks associated with halogenated pyrimidine incorporation, Mutat. Res. 131: 129–136.

66. E. Michishita, T. Kurahashi, K. Suzuki, et al., 2002, Changes in nuclear matrix proteins during the senescence-like phenomenon induced by 5-chlorodeoxyuridine in HeLa cells, Exp. Gerenol. 37: 885–890.

67. E. Michishita, N. Matsumura, T. Kurahashi, et al., 2002, 5-halogenated thymidine analogues induce a senescence-like phenomenon in HeLa cells, Biosci. Biotechnol. Biochem. 66: 877–879.

68. V. Valinluck, P.F. Liu, J.I. Kang Jr., A. Burdzy, L.C. Sowers, 2005, 5-halogenated pyrimidine lesions within a CpG sequence context mimic 5-methylcytosine by enhancing the binding of the methyl-CpG-binding domain of methyl-CpG-binding protein 2 (MeCP2), Nucleic Acids Res. 33: 3057–3064.

69. V. Valinluck, L.C. Sowers, 2007, Endogenous cytosine damage products alter the site selectivity of human DNA maintenance methyltransferase DNMT1, Cancer Res. 67: 946–950.

70. V.V. Lao, J.L. Herring, C.H. Kim, et al., 2009, Incorporation of 5-chlorocytosine into mammalian DNA results in heritable gene silencing and altered cytosine methylation patterns, Carcinogenesis 30: 886–893.

71. V. Tang, J. Macer-Wright, S.L. Fu, B. Rayner, C. Hawkins, 2017, A role for chlorinated nucleosides in the promotion of inflammation and endothelial dysfunction in atherosclerosis? Free Radic. Biol. Med. 108: S30.

72. E. Rozengurt, W.D. Stein, N.M. Wigglesworth, 1977, Uptake of nucleosides in density-inhibited cultures of 3T3 cells, *Nature* 267: 442–444.

73. R. Marz, R.M. Wohlhueter, P.G. Plagemann, 1979, Purine and pyrimidine transport and phosphoribosylation and their interaction in overall uptake by cultured mammalian cells. A re-evaluation, *J. Biol. Chem.* 254: 2329–2338.

74. R.R. Cummins, D. Balinsky, 1980, Activities of some enzymes of pyrimidine and DNA synthesis in a rat transplantable hepatoma and human primary hepatomas, in cell lines derived from these tissues, and in human fetal liver, *Cancer Res.* 40: 1235–1239.

75. K. Balakrishnan, C.M. Stellrecht, D. Genini, et al., 2005, Cell death of bioenergetically compromised and transcriptionally challenged CLL lymphocytes by chlorinated ATP, *Blood* 105: 4455–4462.

76. C.M. Stellrecht, M. Ayres, R. Arya, V. Gandhi, 2010, A unique RNA-directed nucleoside analog is cytotoxic to breast cancer cells and depletes cyclin E levels, *Breast Cancer Res. Treat.* 121: 355–364.

77. C.M. Stellrecht, C.O. Rodriguez, M. Ayres, V. Gandhi, 2003, RNA-directed actions of 8-chloro-adenosine in multiple myeloma cells, *Cancer Res.* 63: 7968–7974.

78. V. Gandhi, W. Chen, M. Ayres, et al., 2002, Plasma and cellular pharmacology of 8-chloro-adenosine in mice and rats, *Cancer Chemother. Pharmacol.* 50: 85–94.

79. G. Tortora, F. Ciardiello, S. Pepe, et al., 1995, Phase I clinical study with 8-chloro-cAMP and evaluation of immunological effects in cancer patients, *Clin. Cancer Res.* 1: 377–384.

80. M.L. Brandon, L. Mi, W. Chaung, G. Teebor, R.J. Boorstein, 2000, 5-chloro-2'-deoxyuridine cytotoxicity results from base excision repair of uracil subsequent to thymidylate synthase inhibition, *Mutat. Res.* 459: 161–169.

81. K. Fujikawa, H. Yakushiji, Y. Nakabeppu, et al., 2002, 8-chloro-dGTP, a hypochlorous acid-modified nucleotide, is hydrolyzed by hMTH1, the human MutT homolog, *FEBS Lett.* 512: 149–151.

82. R.W. Pero, Y. Sheng, A. Olsson, C. Bryngelsson, M. Lund Pero, 1996, Hypochlorous acid/N-chloramines are naturally produced DNA repair inhibitors, *Carcinogenesis* 17: 13–18.

83. T. Lindahl, R.D. Wood, 1999, Quality control by DNA repair, *Science* 286: 1897–1905.

84. M.T. Morgan, M.T. Bennett, A.C. Drohat, 2007, Excision of 5-halogenated uracils by human thymine DNA glycosylase. Robust activity for DNA contexts other than CpG, *J. Biol. Chem.* 282: 27578–27586.

85. D.P. Turner, S. Cortellino, J.E. Schupp, et al., 2006, The DNA N-glycosylase MED1 exhibits preference for halogenated pyrimidines and is involved in the cytotoxicity of 5-iododeoxyuridine, *Cancer Res.* 66: 7686–7693.

86. C.L. Simms, H.S. Zaher, 2016, Quality control of chemically damaged RNA, *Cell Mol. Life Sci.* 73: 3639–3653.

87. H. Sierakowska, R.R. Shukla, Z. Dominski, R. Kole, 1989, Inhibition of pre-mRNA splicing by 5-fluoro-, 5-chloro-, and 5-bromouridine, *J. Biol. Chem.* 264: 19185–19191.

88. J.B. Dennison, K. Balakrishnan, V. Gandhi, 2009, Preclinical activity of 8-chloroadenosine with mantle cell lymphoma: roles of energy depletion and inhibition of DNA and RNA synthesis, *Br. J. Haematol.* 147: 297–307.

89. V. Gandhi, M. Ayres, R.G. Halgren, et al., 2001, 8-chloro-cAMP and 8-chloro-adenosine act by the same mechanism in multiple myeloma cells, *Cancer Res.* 61: 5474–5479.

90. J.H. Han, Y.H. Ahn, K.Y. Choi, S.H. Hong, 2009, Involvement of AMP-activated protein kinase and p38 mitogen-activated protein kinase in 8-Cl-cAMP-induced growth inhibition, *J. Cell Physiol.* 218: 104–112.

91. C.M. Stellrecht, H.V. Vangapandu, X.F. Le, W. Mao, S. Shentu, 2014, ATP directed agent, 8-chloro-adenosine, induces AMP activated protein kinase activity, leading to autophagic cell death in breast cancer cells, *J. Hematol. Oncol.* 7: 23.

92. A. Mangerich, C.G. Knutson, N.M. Parry, et al., 2012, Infection-induced colitis in mice causes dynamic and tissue-specific changes in stress response and DNA damage leading to colon cancer, *Proc. Natl. Acad. Sci. U.S.A.* 109: E1820–1829.

93. C.G. Knutson, A. Mangerich, Y. Zeng, et al., 2013, Chemical and cytokine features of innate immunity characterize serum and tissue profiles in inflammatory bowel disease, *Proc. Natl. Acad. Sci. U.S.A.* 110: E2332–2341.

CHAPTER SIX

Reactivity of Peroxidase Oxidants with Lipids: The Generation of Biologically Important Modified Lipids

Daniel P. Pike and David A. Ford
Saint Louis University School of Medicine

CONTENTS

ABBREVIATIONS

2-BrFALD:	2-Bromofatty aldehyde
2-BrHA:	2-Bromohexadecanoic acid
2-BrHDA:	2-Bromohexadecanal
2-BrHDyA:	Alkyne-modified 2-BrHDA
2-BrODA:	2-Bromooctodecanal
2-ClAdA:	2-Chloroadipic acid
2-ClDCA:	2-Chlorodicarboxylic acid
2-ClFA:	2-Chlorofatty acid
2-ClFALD:	2-Chlorofatty aldehyde
2-ClFOH:	2-Chlorofatty alcohol
2-ClHA:	2-Chlorohexanoic acid
2-ClHDA:	2-Chlorohexadecanal
2-ClHOH:	2-Chlorohexadecanol
2-ClHyA:	Alkyne-modified 2-ClFA

2-ClOA:	2-Chlorooctodecanoic acid
2-ClODA:	2-Chlorooctadecanal
2-ClODEA:	2-Chlorooctadecenal
2-ClOOH:	2-Chlorooctadecanol
2-ClPA:	2-Chloropalmitic acid
2-IFALD:	2-Iodofatty aldehyde
2-IHDA:	2-Iodohexadecanal
2-IHOH:	2-Iodohexadecanol
2-IODA:	2-Iodooctadecanal
6-IDL:	6-Iodo-5-hydroxy-eicosatrienoic delta lactone
ARDS:	Acute respiratory distress syndrome
BALF:	Bronchoalveolar lavage fluid
BMVEC:	Brain microvascular endothelial cell
DCFDA:	Dichlorofluorescin diacetate
eNOS:	Endothelial nitric oxide synthase

DOI: 10.1201/9781003212287-8

EPO:	Eosinophil peroxidase
ESI-MS/MS:	Electrospray ionization–tandem mass spectrometry
FALD-GSH:	Fatty aldehyde-glutathione
FALDH:	Fatty aldehyde dehydrogenase
GC:	Gas chromatography
GSH:	Glutathione
HCAEC:	Human coronary artery endothelial cell
HDA-GSH:	Hexadecanal-glutathione
HDL:	High-density lipoprotein
HETE:	Hydroxyeisosatetraenoic acid
HOCl:	Hypochlorous acid
HODE:	Hydroxyoctadecadienoic acid
HOSCN:	Hypothiocyanous acid
HOX:	Hypohalous acid
LC:	Liquid chromatography
LDL:	Low-density lipoprotein
LPC:	Lysophosphatidycholine
LPE:	Lysophosphatidylethanolamine
LPO:	Lactoperoxidase
MAPK:	Mitogen-activated protein kinase
MMI:	Methimazole
MPO:	Myeloperoxidase
MS:	Mass spectrometry
NET:	Neutrophil extracellular trap
NICI:	Negative ion chemical ionization
ODA-GSH:	Octadecanal-glutathione
PA:	Palmitic acid
PC:	Phosphatidylcholine
PE:	Phosphatidylethanolamine
PFB:	Pentafluorobenzyl
PMA:	Phorbol-myristate acetate

PPAR:	Peroxisome proliferator-activated receptor
PS:	Phosphatidylserine
RCS:	Reactive chlorinating species
S1P:	Sphingosine-1-phosphate
SPC:	Sphingosylphosphorylcholine
TPO:	Thyroid peroxidase
vWF:	Von Willebrand factor

INTRODUCTION

This chapter provides an overview of lipid products from reactions of peroxidase-generated oxidants with lipids. In general, nucleophilic sites within lipids donate electrons to peroxidase-generated hypohalous acids, leading to lipid halogenation. This chapter will focus on the formation of 2-haloaldehydes through reaction with the vinyl ether bond of plasmalogen glycerophospholipids; the formation of halohydrins through reaction with alkenes within aliphatic chains; and the modification of polar head groups of amine-containing lipid classes. A scheme of these reactions is shown in Figure 6.1 using plasmenylethanolamine with linoleic acid esterified to the sn-2 position of the glycerol backbone as an example lipid target. Chlorinated, brominated, and iodinated lipids have all been identified in mammals, including humans, and they appear to have important roles in physiologic and pathophysiologic processes. The production of these halogenated lipids by leukocytes under inflammatory conditions suggests they have potential to serve as both biomarkers and mediators of human disease.

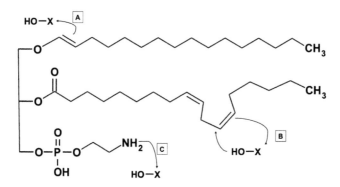

Figure 6.1 Overview of peroxidase-dependent modifications on lipids. 16:0/18:2 plasmenylethanolamine is shown as example lipid target of hypohalous acid HOX. (a) The reaction with the plasmalogen vinyl ether bond, which leads to the liberation of the aliphatic chain as 2-halofatty aldehyde. (b) The reaction with alkenes in aliphatic chains, producing halohydrins. (c) The formation of haloamines using the primary amine in the ethanolamine headgroup of this plasmenylethanolamine species.

PRODUCTION OF 2-CHLOROFATTY ALDEHYDE AND ITS METABOLITES

Plasmalogens are a class of membrane glycerophospholipids in which the aliphatic chain at the sn-1 position is attached to the glycerol backbone through a vinyl ether bond. Choline and ethanolamine are the predominant polar head group moieties of plasmalogens. Plasmalogens are enriched in the phospholipid pools of endothelial cells, leukocytes, smooth muscle cells, cardiac muscle cells, and neurons, while hepatocytes contain little plasmalogen but secrete plasmalogens associated with lipoproteins [1–7]. The molecular structure inferred by the plasmalogen vinyl ether bond is important in multiple biological functions. The bond permits tighter aliphatic packing in plasma membranes, and subsequently, lipid rafts have high plasmalogen content [8–11]. The vinyl ether bond also reacts with free radicals and reactive oxygen species, such as peroxyl radical, UV radiation, and metal ions, suggesting that plasmalogens play a protective role by serving as a sink for these reactive oxygen species, resulting in the production of nonhalogenated intermediates such as hexadecanal and hexadecenal that can be converted into fatty acids including palmitic and palmitoleic acids, respectively [12–18].

In contrast, vinyl ether bond targeting by reactive chlorinating species results in the production of the pro-inflammatory family of 2-chlorofatty aldehyde (2-ClFALD) and its various metabolites. Myeloperoxidase (MPO)-derived HOCl targets the vinyl ether bond, liberating the sn-1 aliphatic chain as 2-ClFALD [19–21]. HOCl preferentially targets the plasmalogen vinyl ether bond rather than other unsaturated moieties in phospholipid aliphatic chains [22]. Two primary species of 2-ClFALD are produced by leukocytes: 2-chlorohexadecanal (2-ClHDA) and 2-chlorooctadecanal (2-ClODA), the 16 and 18 carbon length species, respectively [20,21]. 2-Chlorooctadecenal (2-ClODEA) has also been identified [23]. While leukocytes appear to be the primary source of 2-ClFALD, these lipid species also are generated in transcellular reactions of HOCl with endothelial plasmalogens [20]. It is important to note that the MPO-mediated chlorination of plasmalogens also produces unsaturated lysophosphatidycholine (LPC) and lysophosphatidylethanolamine (LPE) species, which are themselves capable of further HOCl-mediated reaction to chlorohydrins (see the next section) [21]. In addition to targeting of plasmalogens by HOCl, it has been shown that chlorine gas exposure leads to elevated levels of 2-ClFALD and its metabolites in a peroxidase-independent manner [19,24].

2-ClFALD has a variety of metabolic fates, which are shown in Figure 6.2. The aldehyde

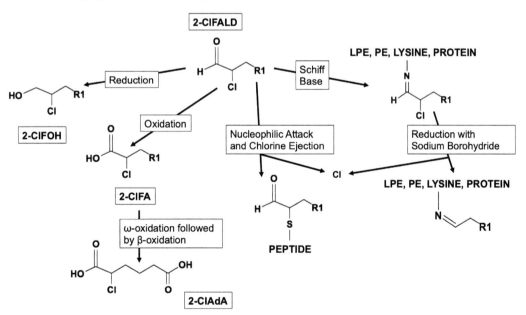

Figure 6.2 2-ClFALD and its metabolites.

functional group of 2-ClFALD forms Schiff base adducts with primary amines, including those in the polar head groups of phosphatidylethanolamines (PEs) and LPEs, lysine, and presumably, proteins [25,26]. Alternatively, the α-chlorinated carbon of 2-ClFALD can undergo nucleophilic attack by sulfhydryl residues on small peptides such as glutathione, expelling the chlorine atom in the process [27]. In contrast to 2-ClFALD, non-halogenated fatty aldehyde (FALD) is not targeted by glutathione [27]. 2-ClFALD can also react with aromatic compounds in an electrophilic aromatic substitution reaction [28]. In enzymatically mediated metabolism, 2-ClFALD can be reduced to 2-chlorofatty alcohol (2-ClFOH) or oxidized by fatty aldehyde dehydrogenase (FALDH) to 2-chlorofatty acid (2-ClFA) [29–31].

While the metabolism of 2-ClFOH has yet to be fully explored, that of 2-ClFA has been investigated. 2-ClFA can be esterified into and stored in complex lipid pools, and it can be metabolized in hepatocytes for clearance, in a process regulated by the peroxisome proliferator-activated receptor (PPAR)-α [32,33]. 2-ClFA enhances PPAR-α expression at the transcriptional level, suggesting that 2-ClFA upregulates its own metabolism [33]. The chlorine atom on the α-carbon prevents β-oxidation from the α-end. However, 2-ClFA is ω-oxidized to a 2-chlorodicarboxylic acid (2-ClDCA). This 2-ClDCA can undergo β-oxidation from the ω-end. Through this process, multiple shorter chain length species of 2-ClDCAs are generated, ultimately resulting in 2-chloroadipic acid (2-ClAdA) production. 2-ClAdA is likely removed from blood by the renal proximal tubule organic acid transporter and is excreted in urine [32].

DETECTION AND QUANTIFICATION OF 2-CLFALD AND METABOLITES

2-ClFALD and its metabolites are detected and quantified using specific mass spectrometry (MS) techniques, which are amenable to the chlorinated lipid functional group. In general, lipids are extracted in the presence of stable isotope internal standards and detected by either gas chromatography (GC)/MS or liquid chromatography (LC)/MS, dependent on the analyte of interest [34,35].

2-ClFALD can be detected by GC paired with negative ion chemical ionization (NICI). Prior to GC/MS, detection is enhanced by derivatizing 2-ClFALD to its pentafluorobenzyl (PFB) oxime

derivative [19,36]. The NICI of the PFB oxime of 2-ClFALD leads to signature fragmentation and ion production. Selected ion monitoring (SIM) of fragmentation products are employed to detect the 2-ClFALD species. 2-ClHDA, 2-ClODA, and 2-ClODEA can be detected and quantified using SIM of the structurally informative fragments m/z 288, 316, and 314, respectively [19,20,23]. In a cell-free model, 2-ClFALD has been detected in low-density lipoprotein (LDL) treated with MPO-derived reactive chlorinating species (RCS) [21]. The requirement of MPO to produce 2-ClFALD was established in human leukocytes, and 2-ClFALD has also been detected in infarcted rat myocardium, in the brains of LPS-injected rats, and human atherosclerotic tissue [20,21,23,37–39].

2-ClFA is also detected using mass spectrometry techniques. Using electrospray ionization–tandem mass spectrometry (ESI-MS/MS), these 2-ClFA carboxylic acids can be detected in negative ion mode following LC. MS/MS exploiting selected reaction monitoring (SRM) is used for 2-chlorohexanoic acid (2-ClHA) and 2-chlorooctodecanoic acid (2-ClOA) detection with transitions of m/z 289 → 253 and m/z 317 → 281, respectively [29]. 2-ClFA is significantly more stable than its aldehyde precursor, and it can be detected in a wider variety of biological samples, including human plasma [27,30,32,40–43]. 2-ClFA esterified in complex lipid pools can also be detected by the same methods used for the detection of free 2-ClFA following release of the esterified 2-ClFA by base hydrolysis [34,35,43]

Studies employing MS techniques demonstrated that rat liver microsomes and HepG2 cells metabolize 2-ClFA to 2-chlorodicarboxylic acids leading to 2-ClAdA production [32]. The final catabolic product, 2-ClAdA, can be detected and quantified using ESI-MS/MS with an SRM of 179 → 143 (loss of HCl) [32]. 2-ClAdA is detectable in both rat and human urine, with an increase in 2-ClAdA levels seen in the urine of LPS-exposed rats [32,33].

Additional metabolites of 2-ClFALD including 2-ClFOH, Schiff base adducts, and adducts with glutathione (GSH) are also quantified using MS techniques. Following 2-ClFOH derivatization to the PFB ester with PFB chloride, subsequent NICI-GC/MS can monitor 2-chlorohexadecanol (2-ClHOH), d_4-2-ClHOH, and 2-chlorooctadecanol (2-ClOOH) using SIMs of m/z 470, 474, and 498, respectively [29]. 2-ClFOH has been detected in phorbol ester-stimulated human neutrophils as well as in 2-ClFALD-treated human coronary artery endothelial cells (HCAECs) and brain microvascular endothelial cells (BMVECs) [29–31]. ESI-MS/MS can be used to detect the Schiff base adducts between 2-ClFALD and PE/LPEs in HCAECs [26]. Finally, the 2-ClFALD modification of glutathione can be detected using ESI-MS/MS. The resulting adducts, hexadecanal-glutathione (HDA-GSH) and octadecanal-glutathione (ODA-GSH), have characteristic SRMs of 546 → 399 and 574 → 427. Both adducts are detected in stimulated human neutrophils and in the plasma of K/BxN mice, a murine arthritis model in which neutrophils play a critical role in the progressive inflammation in the joints [27,44]. Additionally, 2-ClFA levels are elevated in the plasma of these K/BxN mice [27]. The concentrations of 2-ClFALD and its various metabolites present in different animal models of disease and in human biological samples are shown in Table 6.1.

BIOLOGICAL EFFECTS AND SIGNALING PATHWAYS OF 2-CLFALD AND ITS METABOLITES

Due to the dependence of leukocytes and MPO on the production of 2-ClFALD and its metabolites, it is unsurprising that this family of chlorinated lipids appears to play a role in inflammation. This includes a number of pro-inflammatory effects on endothelial cells and on leukocytes themselves. 2-ClFALD is a potent mediator of neutrophil chemotaxis [20]. Both 2-ClFALD and 2-ClFA induce COX-2 mRNA expression in HCAECs, while 2-ClFALD also decreases levels of the protein inhibitor IκB, an important step in order to propagate the pervasive NF-κB-mediated inflammatory processes [45,46]. In BMVECs, another endothelial cell line, 2-ClHDA impairs metabolic activity through mitochondrial membrane dysfunction, ultimately increasing hydroxyl and

TABLE 6.1
Concentration of 2-ClFALD and its metabolites in various biological samples

Lipid species	Species	Tissue	Concentration	Reference
2-ClFALD	Human	Stimulated neutrophils	35 pmol/10^6 cells	[20]
		Stimulated monocytes	6.9 pmol/10^6 cells	[21]
		Atherosclerotic aorta	2.1 pmol/nmol inorganic phosphate	[37]
	Rat	Infarcted heart	4.5 pmol/μmol inorganic phosphate	[38]
		Heart with pericarditis	1.3 pmol/μmol inorganic phosphate	[38]
2-ClFA	Human	Unstimulated neutrophils	1.2 pmol/10^6 cells	[30]
		Stimulated neutrophils	13 pmol/10^6 cells	[30]
		Healthy plasma	0.9 pmol/mL	
		Systemic lupus erythematosus plasma	1.1 pmol/mL	[41]
		Sepsis with neutropenia plasma	0.8 pmol/mL	[42]
		Sepsis without neutropenia plasma	1.9 pmol/mL	[42]
	Rat	Healthy plasma	0.5 pmol/mL	[32]
		LPS-administered plasma	3.2 pmol/mL	[32]
		Sepsis plasma	5.3 pmol/mL	[43]
	Mice	Control BALF	0.01 pmol/mL	[30]
		Sendai-virus exposed BALF	0.05 pmol/mL	[30]
		Control plasma	0.8 pmol/mL	[27,30]
		Sendai-virus exposed plasma	1.4 pmol/mL	[30]
		K/BxN arthritis model plasma	1.8 pmol/mL	[27]
2-ClFOH	Human	Stimulated neutrophils	2.3 pmol/10^6 cells	[30]
FALD-GSH	Mice	Healthy plasma	0.02 pmol/mL	[27]
		K/BxN arthritis model plasma	0.1 pmol/mL	[27]

peroxyl reactive species production, as measured by dichlorofluorescin diacetate (DCFDA) [31]. This was corroborated in hCMEC/D3 brain endothelial cells [25].

2-ClFALD also interferes with endothelial barrier integrity in BMVECs, decreasing barrier resistance and altering tight junction protein localization. Administration of 2-ClFALD directly into the carotids of rats increases blood–brain barrier permeability. The mitogen-activated protein kinase (MAPK) pathways appear to be involved in this dysregulation, as 2-ClFALD treatment leads to phosphorylation of MAPK cascade targets, including JNK1/2, p38, and ERK1/2, while inhibitors of these pathways alleviate the barrier dysfunction [47]. Some of these effects are abrogated by phloretin, a polyphenol compound, which forms a covalent adduct with 2-ClFALD [28,31]. 2-ClFALD also causes microcirculatory changes including enhanced leukocyte rolling and adhesion and permeability barrier loss in vivo in the mesentery [48]. It should also be noted that the sensitivity of endothelium to 2-ClFALD also depends on the vascular bed. In particular, renal endothelium was less responsive to 2-ClFALD-elicited changes compared with pulmonary and coronary beds, suggesting that protein interactions, signaling pathways, or endothelial storage granules targeted by chlorinated lipids may be quite different in the array of vascular beds in the human [49]. Furthermore, if 2-ClFALD is injurious to vascular beds during inflammation, this may indicate that chlorinated lipids may not be as deleterious in the kidney compared with other organs. This concept is supported by the finding that chlorinated lipid levels associate with ARDS in human sepsis but not acute kidney injury [42].

In Langendorff-perfused heart studies, 2-ClFALD was shown to have significant effects on cardiac and pulmonary physiology. 2-ClFALD decreases left ventricular pressure, heart rate, and coronary perfusion [38]. Conversely, 2-ClFALD appears to have no effects on vascular smooth muscle cell viability or migration [50]. However, it should be noted that the potential of 2-ClFALD reacting with thiols in cell culture media or in vivo may explain investigations that fail to show changes elicited by 2-ClFALD [50]. 2-ClFALD in MPO-modified high-density lipoproteins (HDL) inhibits endothelial nitric oxide biosynthesis by decreasing endothelial nitric oxide synthase (eNOS) at the mRNA and protein levels and altering the enzyme's

localization in endothelial cells [39]. Intranasal delivery of 2-ClFALD inhibits aortic vasodilation in response to acetylcholine, which is an eNOS-mediated process [24]. Intranasal 2-ClFALD also increases methacholine-induced airway resistance and protein content in the bronchoalveolar lavage fluid (BALF) [24].

Similarly, 2-ClFA has pro-inflammatory properties on leukocytes and endothelial cells. In human monocytic THP-1 cells, 2-ClFA induces apoptosis, likely by driving ER stress through the production of reactive oxygen species, such as hydrogen peroxide. The addition of antioxidants or silencing CHOP using siRNA prevents 2-ClFA-induced apoptosis [40]. Additionally, 2-ClFA induces neutrophils to expel their DNA and form neutrophil extracellular traps (NETs) (Figure 6.3). 2-ClFA rescues the NET-forming capabilities of MPO-deficient mouse neutrophils. These findings suggest that 2-ClFA is critical for MPO-dependent NET formation [51]. It should however be appreciated that NET formation is quite diverse in terms of triggers, pathways, and types (e.g. suicidal and vital), and the MPO-dependent pathway for NET formation is not universal [52]. In hCMEC/D3 brain endothelial cells, 2-ClFA increases procaspase cleavage and IL-6 and IL-8 expression [53].

Studies using HCAECs suggest a second pathway of chlorinated lipid-induced endothelial barrier dysregulation. 2-ClFA localizes with Weibel–Palade bodies, the storage granules of endothelial cells, and 2-ClFA induces release of their contents, including von Willebrand factor (vWF), P-selectin, and angiopoietin-2 (Ang-2) (Figure 6.4). 2-ClFA also induces the physiological consequences of the release of these compounds, namely platelet adherence, leukocyte adherence, and decreased barrier resistance [54]. The other product of MPO-mediated degradation of plasmalogens, unsaturated lysophopholipids, also induces HCAEC P-selectin surface expression [21]. In vivo, superfusion of 2-ClFA on rat mesenteric vasculature increases leukocyte rolling and adhesion, platelet adherence, mast cell activation, and albumin leakage [48]. Additionally, a recent study indicated that 2-ClFA induces permeability in rat kidney microvasculature in vivo and in human gut epithelial cells in vitro [43].

Like 2-ClFALD, intranasal delivery of 2-ClFA inhibits aortic vasodilation in response to acetylcholine, methacholine-induced airway resistance, and BALF protein content [24]. Finally, a study

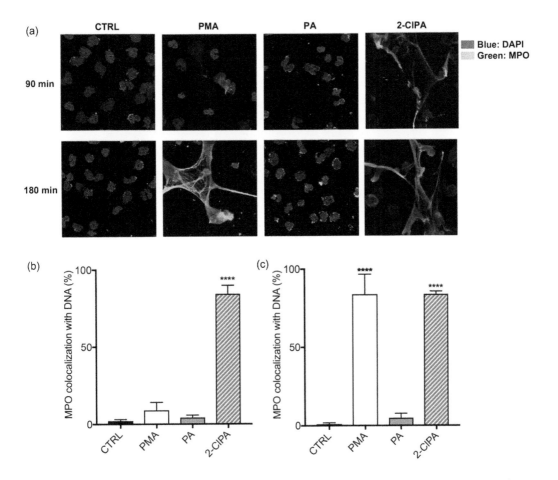

Figure 6.3 2-ClFA induces neutrophils to release their DNA as extracellular traps. Human neutrophils were isolated from peripheral blood and treated with either 0.1% ethanol (CTRL), 100 nM phorbol-myristate acetate (PMA), 10 μM palmitic acid (PA), or 10 μM 2-chloropalmitic acid (2-ClPA) for either 90 or 180 min. (a) Cells were visualized using immunofluorescence targeted for MPO and DAPI. Quantitation of percentage of MPO co-localized with DNA is shown at 90 min (b) and 180 min (c). This data was originally published in the *Journal of Lipid Research*. Palladino E.N.D., et al. 2-Chlorofatty acids: lipid mediators of neutrophil extracellular trap formation. J. Lipid Res. 2018; 59:1424–1424. © 2018 Palladino et al.

involving a large sepsis patient cohort found that the 2-ClFA concentrations in the plasma at day of admission to ICU significantly associate with the future development of acute respiratory distress syndrome (ARDS) and 30-day mortality [42].

Exactly how 2-ClFALD and its metabolites elicit their biological effects is a current area of great interest. Taking advantage of click chemistry techniques, several groups have designed 2-ClFALD and 2-ClFA analogs with ω-terminal alkyne functional groups [25,53,54]. This allows for rapid and specific chemical interactions with azide moieties attached to a reporter. This tool was used for the subcellular localization of these chlorinated lipid species and is also being used to interrogate protein-binding interactions. Using mass spectrometry proteomic approaches, 2-ClFALD was found to modify tight junction-associated proteins, suggesting one possible mechanistic route for the 2-ClFALD-mediated endothelial barrier dysfunction [25].

Whether or not other 2-ClFALD metabolites affect additional biological or biochemical pathways remains to be determined. For example, while the PPAR-α-mediated catabolism of 2-ClFA leads to excretion of 2-ClAdA in the urine, 2-ClAdA itself may have deleterious effects. Similarly, glutathione may sequester 2-ClFALD, but the FALD-GSH (fatty aldehyde-glutathione) adduct may have its own toxic properties. What is clear is that 2-ClFALD and its metabolites affect multiple biochemical and physiological

Marker	2-ClHyA	DAPI	Merge	

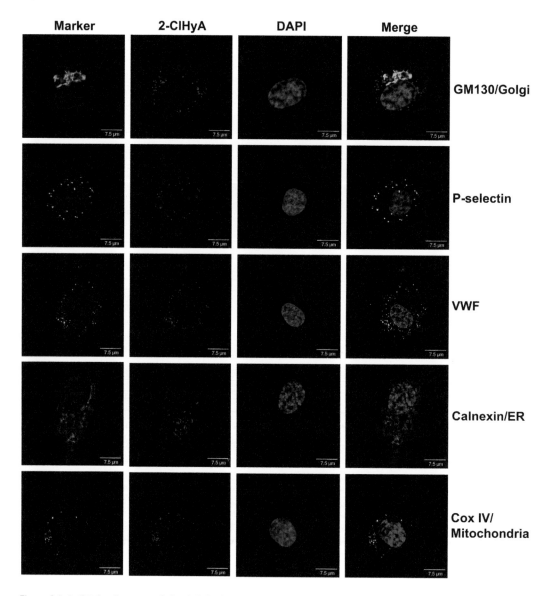

Figure 6.4 2-ClFA localizes to Weibel–Palade bodies in endothelial cells. HCAECs were treated with 10 μM alkyne-modified 2-ClFA (2-ClHyA) for 30 min. Using an azide-TAMRA reporter, localization of the 2-ClFA is shown in red. Co-localization with various proteins is shown in green. This data was originally published in the *Journal of Lipid Research*. Hartman C.L., et al. 2-Chlorofatty acids induce Weibel–Palade body mobilization. *J. Lipid Res.* 2018; 59:113–122. © 2018 Hartman et al.

processes, and further investigation into their production, mechanisms of action, and methods of clearance is critical.

Both 2-ClFALD and 2-ClFA appear to have significant pro-inflammatory roles, as both induce permeability and COX-2 expression in endothelial cells, and both result in the accumulation of intracellular hydrogen peroxide in leukocytes [40,45–47,54]. When superfused onto rat mesenteric vessels, both drive leukocyte rolling and adhesion and a decrease in barrier function [48].

However, it remains to be seen whether the aldehyde and the acid are eliciting these effects through the same mechanisms. For example, 2-ClFALD seems to mediate endothelial permeability in BMVECs through activation of the MAPK cascade and in HCAECs through a mechanism independent of localization to the Weibel–Palade body, while 2-ClFA localizes to and induces Weibel–Palade body mobilization in HCAECs [47,49,54]. However, some important points must be made: these mechanisms are not mutually exclusive, and as mentioned, different endothelial cell lines respond to chlorinated lipids in different manners [49]. Finally, due to the reactivity of 2-ClFALD compared with 2-ClFA, it is likely that the effects of 2-ClFALD are limited to the sites of 2-ClFALD generation, while 2-ClFA is more likely to have direct consequences distally. Much more work needs to be done to fully delineate the mechanisms and importance of the inflammatory processes caused by these chlorinated lipids.

PRODUCTION OF CHLOROHYDRINS

In addition to the plasmalogen vinyl ether bond, MPO-produced HOCl can react with alkenes of unsaturated fatty acyl constituents, leading to chlorohydrin formation. Multiple chlorohydrins produced from targeting a di- or polyunsaturated fatty acyl constituent are unstable, decomposing to epoxides [55,56]. Fatty acid chlorohydrins have been identified in cell-free systems using both unsaturated fatty acids and HDL particles as lipid substrate [55,57]. Oleic, linoleic, and arachidonic chlorohydrins have been the most frequently examined species [55,58].

Cholesterol also contains an alkene bond, and various isomers of cholesterol chlorohydrins have been detected as a result of targeting cholesterol present in HDL, LDL, and red blood cell membrane [58–61]. MPO-derived HOCl can modify cholesterol in a variety of different ways, forming epoxides, hydroxy-cholesterols, and a dichlorinated sterol, in addition to chlorohydrins [58]. Cholesterol chlorohydrin formation can also occur by reacting with other HOCl-modified biomolecules; it does not require HOCl directly. Primary monochloramines, which are themselves products of MPO-derived chlorination, can in turn react with cholesterol yielding chlorohydrins, albeit not as effectively as HOCl [61].

Phosphatidylcholine (PC) acyl chains are targeted by HOCl yielding chlorohydrins [56,58, 62,63]. Additionally, PC-chlorohydrins produced from polyunsaturated PC molecular species have an increased propensity to degrade to LPCs. This effect is most pronounced in PCs containing arachidonic or docosohexaenoic acid, which have four and six double bonds, respectively [62,64]. Finally, unsaturated sphingolipids can also form chlorohydrins [65,66].

Some insights into the mechanisms of chlorohydrin formation have been made. In comparison to MPO-RCS generating system, a neutral-to-acidic pH is required for chlorohydrin production mediated directly by HOCl [61,62]. This evidence, in addition to the fact that dichlorinated sterols have been detected, led Hazen et al. to suggest that molecular chlorine gas is the actual chlorinating agent, not HOCl [61]. HOCl, protons, and chloride ion are in equilibrium with Cl_2 and water, so molecular chlorine gas is present following MPO activity. This indirect involvement of HOCl in chlorohydrin formation is also supported by studies showing that the hydroxyl group of PC chlorohydrins (and bromohydrins, see below) was derived from the buffer, not HOCl itself [67].

DETECTION AND QUANTIFICATION OF CHLOROHYDRINS

Much like the detection of 2-ClFALD and its metabolites, mass spectrometry techniques are the method of choice to detect and quantify the peroxidase-derived chlorohydrins. Because of the wide variety of lipid species that become chlorohydrins, the specific spectrometric and chromatographic methods have the potential to vary significantly depending on the species of interest. However, one commonality between the chlorohydrin mass spectra is that any peaks representing chlorine-containing species should display a characteristic doublet two mass units apart in a 3:1 ratio, reflecting the natural abundance of the chlorine isotopes, ^{35}Cl and ^{37}Cl. Similarly, any dichlorinated molecular species should display a triplet peak pattern in a 9:6:1 ratio. As a note, this isotopic effect on the mass spectra also applies to 2-ClFALD and its metabolites; however, the SIMs and SRMs described above for ^{35}Cl.

Cholesterol chlorohydrins and dichlorocholesterol can be detected and quantified using GC/MS or product ion scanning for m/z 367 using ESI-MS/MS [60,61]. The fatty acid chlorohydrins are typically derivatized using bis-trimethylsilyltrifluoroacetamide prior to analysis, and GC/MS and SIM monitoring can be used for detection and quantitation [55,68]. Oleic acid monochlorohydrin, linoleic acid monochlorohydrin, and linoleic acid bischlorohydrin can be monitored using m/z 463, 461, and 585, respectively [61,68]. The PC chlorohydrins have been detected using matrix-assisted laser desorption/ionization–time of flight (MALDI-TOF) mass spectrometry [56,67].

The alkene bond leading to chlorohydrin production is less reactive than many other host tissue targets of HOCl including the vinyl ether bond of plasmalogens [69]. Accordingly, it is most likely that chlorohydrins will only be found in biological samples under conditions of excessive HOCl production. LPC chlorohydrins have been observed in human atherosclerotic tissue, and oleic and linoleic acid chlorohydrins were detected in a rat model of acute pancreatitis [22,70]. Excitingly, oleic acid chlorohydrin was also detected in the plasma of human acute pancreatitis patients. In a follow-up to this study, it was found that oleic acid chlorohydrin in patient plasma is a prognostic indicator for pancreatitis severity [68].

BIOLOGICAL EFFECTS AND SIGNALING PATHWAYS OF CHLOROHYDRINS

The discovery that plasma levels of oleic acid chlorohydrin could be an important early biomarker in stratifying acute pancreatitis patients suggested they may also mediate disease [68,70]. Early cell-based assays identified a plethora of chlorohydrin-induced effects. Chlorohydrins cause cell death by necrosis at high concentrations and apoptosis at lower concentrations [71–73]. Although necrosis was found in endothelial cells, other studies in red blood cells indicate a potential pathway to explain the necrosis findings. Chlorohydrins affect membrane dynamics and morphology, and fatty acid, cholesterol, and PC chlorohydrins can lyse cells [74,75].

Chlorohydrin-induced apoptosis could occur through a variety of different mechanisms. PC chlorohydrins cause a decrease in intracellular ATP levels in HL60 and U937 cell lines [72,76]. They also cause an increase in endothelial cell caspase activity, as well as an increase in both intracellular superoxide anion production in endothelial cells and luminol-detected undefined reactive oxygen species in leukocytes [73,77]. In an ApoE knockout mouse ex vivo model, PC chlorohydrin treatment of artery segments increased leukocyte adhesion [72,77]. This adherence appears to be P-selectin mediated, and interestingly, statin treatment abrogates the effect [77]. Another ex vivo model demonstrated that linoleic acid monochlorohydrins decrease guinea pig papillary muscle contractile tension [78]. Finally, in conjunction with the in vivo model of acute peritonitis in rats, intraperitoneal injection of oleic acid chlorohydrin leads

to an increase in multiple inflammatory signals, including TNF-α and IL-1β expression in macrophages, plasma IL-6 concentration, and lung and white adipose tissue MPO activity [70].

OTHER MPO-MEDIATED LIPID MODIFICATIONS

In addition to 2-ClFALD and chlorohydrin formation, MPO can modify lipids through other mechanisms: primarily, phospholipid head group modification and lipid peroxidation. PEs and phosphatidylserines (PSs) have head groups with accessible primary amines. These primary amines can react directly with HOCl to form PE-chloramine and PS-chloramine [69,79]. These monochloramine species can also be chlorinated again to dichlorinated species [80,81]. Both the PE-dichloramine and the PS-monochloramine can degrade to form N-centered radicals, which in turn promote lipid peroxidation (discussed below) [79,80]. Alternatively, PS-monochloramines can degrade into phosphatidylglycoaldehydes, and PS-dichloramines degrade into phosphonitriles [80,81].

MPO can also indirectly modify phospholipid head groups through modification by MPO-derived oxidative products. One example previously described is Schiff base adducts of PE and 2-ClFALD [26]. The primary amines of PE and PS can also form Schiff base adducts with p-hydroxyphenyl-acetaldehyde (pHA), an MPO-oxidized product of tyrosine, and these species have been detected in atherosclerotic lesions [82,83]. Head group modification of phospholipids by MPO may play an important role in altering membrane dynamics, signaling pathways, and accessibility to protein-binding partners.

The other major MPO-derived lipid modifications include oxidation and peroxidation mechanisms, as demonstrated by the fact that MPO$^{-/-}$ mice have decreased levels of many lipid (per)oxidation products, including F2-isoprostanes, hydroxyeisosatetraenoic acids (HETEs), hydroxyoctadecadienoic acids (HODEs), and oxidized acyl chains in phosphatidylcholine species following inflammation [84–88]. MPO promotes lipid (per)oxidation through HOCl reactions or indirectly through the generation of a variety of free radical species [89–94]. For example, MPO-generated tyrosine radicals can induce lipid peroxidation, as can radicals formed from the degradation of chloramines, which themselves were previously created from the MPO modification of free amino acids, protein-associated amino acids, and phospholipid headgroups [79,95,96]. MPO-generated hypothiocyanous acid (HOSCN) also promotes lipid peroxidation; however, HOSCN does not generate thiocyanohydrins [63,97,98]. Discussion of all of the biological consequences of lipid (per)oxidation products is beyond the scope of this chapter; however, they have been implicated in a multiple pro- and anti-inflammatory process [99–102]. Finally, reactive nitrogen species produced by MPO can also induce lipid peroxidation and nitration [103–107]. Formation of nitrated lipids has typically been attributed to peroxynitrite as the reactive nitrogen species [108]. However, since MPO produces reactive nitrogen species, it is likely that MPO has a substantial role in the generation of nitrated lipids [109,110].

Peroxidase-generated oxidants also modify sphingolipids including the production of sphingolipid-chlorohydrins [65,66]. Sphingomyelin, a lipid particularly enriched in neural tissue, reacts with HOCl to form a chloramine [66]. MPO has been suggested to be involved in brain sphingolipid metabolism following LPS administration [111]. Other sphingolipids, such as sphingosine-1-phosphate (S1P) and sphingosylphosphorylcholine (SPC), can react with MPO-derived RCS to degrade into 2-hexadecenal (non-chlorinated) and a nitrile-containing species [65].

PRODUCTION OF 2-BROMOFATTY ALDEHYDE AND BROMOHYDRINS

Just as HOCl can react with plasmalogens to create 2-ClFALD, peroxidase-generated HOBr can release 2-bromofatty aldehyde (2-BrFALD), the major species being 2-bromohexadecanal and 2-bromooctodecanal (2-BrHDA and 2-BrODA) [112]. 2-BrFALD is produced by both MPO and eosinophil peroxidase (EPO); however, the likelihood of generating 2-BrFALD or 2-ClFALD is a consequence of the availability of bromide ion and the relative specificities of these enzymes for oxidizing either chloride or bromide [112–114]. In neutrophils at equimolar concentrations of chloride and bromide, MPO preferentially produces 2-BrFALD over 2-ClFALD by an order of magnitude, while at physiologic concentrations (chloride >10^4 greater than bromide), MPO produces both 2-BrFALD and 2-ClFALD at near equal levels [112,115]. At these same physiologic concentrations, EPO almost exclusively produces 2-BrFALD [113].

In another parallel to 2-ClFALD, the α-carbon on 2-BrFALD can undergo nucleophilic attack by sulfhydryl groups, including those in glutathione [116]. This leads to the formation of the FALD-GSH adduct, and in fact, 2-BrFALD is much more likely to contribute to FALD-GSH adduct production than 2-ClFALD. As the adduct formation results in halide expulsion from the aldehyde, this is presumably due to bromide's improved ability to act as a leaving group compared with chloride [116]. 2-BrFALD can also react with proteins via sulfhydryl modification, and it appears to more robustly modify proteins than 2-ClFALD [116] (Figure 6.5). Unlike 2-ClFALD, metabolism of peroxidase-generated 2-BrFALD to 2-bromofatty acid (2-BrFA) has not been observed. This is likely due to the flux of 2-BrFALD to GSH and protein adducts consuming 2-BrFALD prior to oxidation. It should however be noted that 2-BrFA has been detected in animal models of bromine gas exposure [117].

Peroxidases can also brominate unsaturated fatty acids into bromohydrins [118]. Oleic, linoleic, and arachidonic acid bromohydrins are produced in cell-free systems with MPO supplemented with sodium bromide, and oleic acid bromohydrin has been detected following HOBr treatment of LDL [118,119]. In addition, peroxidase-generated bromamines can produce bromohydrins. Bromamines are produced by HOBr brominating primary amines, such as those present in taurine, ethanolamine, and the headgroup of PE [120]. Unsaturated acyl chains in phospholipids can also form bromohydrins, and these are formed more readily than their chlorinated analogues [121]. As with chloride, human peroxidase-mediated oxidation of bromide can lead to modification of multiple different lipid species.

DETECTION AND QUANTIFICATION OF BROMINATED LIPIDS

MS techniques are used in the detection and quantification of brominated lipids. Bromine exists as naturally occurring isotopes with molecular weights of 79 and 81 in an equal ratio, so mass spectrometry analyses of singly brominated compounds display doublet peaks separated by 2 amu. The PFB oxime derivatives of 2-BrFALD species can be detected with NICI-GC [113]. The characteristic fragmentation products of 2-BrHDA and 2-BrODA have m/z's of 332 and 360, respectively.

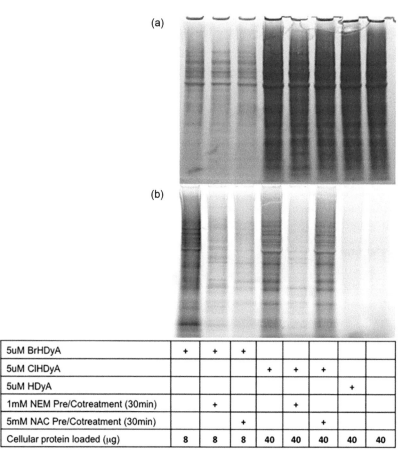

5uM BrHDyA	+	+	+					
5uM ClHDyA				+	+	+		
5uM HDyA							+	
1mM NEM Pre/Cotreatment (30min)		+			+			
5mM NAC Pre/Cotreatment (30min)			+			+		
Cellular protein loaded (μg)	8	8	8	40	40	40	40	40

Figure 6.5 2-BrHDA reacts with proteins more readily than 2-ClHDA. THP-1 cells were pretreated with or without 1 mM NEM or 5 mM NAC for 30 min and then treated with either the alkyne-modified 2-BrHDA (BrHDyA) or 2-ClHDA (ClHDyA) for 30 min at 37°C. Azide-TAMRA reporter was clicked to cell protein and visualized in Panel B. Panel A shows Coomassie blue total protein stain. This data was originally published in the *Journal of Lipid Research*. Duerr M.A., et al. Bromofatty aldehyde derived from bromine exposure and myeloperoxidase and eosinophil peroxidase modify GSH and protein. J. Lipid Res. 2018; 59:696–705. © 2018 Duerr et al.

Since the halide atom is expelled from the α-carbon during nucleophilic attack by the thiol group in glutathione, the FALD-GSH adduct is identical regardless of whether it was created by either 2-ClFALD or 2-BrFALD. Therefore, the same ESI-MS/MS techniques discussed earlier can be used to detect and quantitate the FALD-GSH adduct [27,116]. Fatty acid bromohydrins can also be detected using ESI-MS. Depending on the degree of unsaturation in the fatty acid reactant, multiple bromohydrins can be formed from peroxidase-produced HOBr. Linoleic acid, for example, with two degrees of unsaturation, can form either a monobromohydrin or a bisbromohydrin. Bisbromohydrin species display a triplet pattern in a 1:2:1 ratio, reflecting the isotopic distribution of bromine [118].

BIOLOGICAL EFFECTS AND SIGNALING PATHWAYS OF BROMINATED LIPIDS

Compared with chlorinated lipids, less is known about the biological and physiological effects of brominated lipids. While 2-BrFALD is a chemotactic agent for neutrophils and inhibits THP-1 cell viability more than 2-ClHDA [113,116], the mechanisms responsible for these properties have not been determined. Recently, it was demonstrated that murine myocardium displays histological changes similar to severe myocardial ischemia when treated with intraventricular injection of 2-BrHDA [117]. Investigations are ongoing in these studies to determine the mechanisms responsible for the severe myocardial phenotype, which may be mediated via protein modification, since

2-BrHDA reacts with protein thiol groups much more robustly than 2-ClHDA [116].

It should be noted that 2-bromohexadecanoic acid (2-BrHA) has long been known to inhibit fatty acid oxidation [122–126]. Therefore, it is possible that one direct effect of brominated lipid production is inhibition of fatty acid metabolism. However, as mentioned above, peroxidase-generated production of 2-BrHA has not been detected in biological samples. It is possible that in instances of bromine gas exposure, when 2-BrFA has been detected, 2-BrHA could inhibit fatty acid metabolism.

PRODUCTION OF IODINATED LIPIDS

2-Iodofatty aldehyde (2-IFALD) was the first halogenated lipid discovered to be liberated from plasmalogens. 2-IFALD was discovered in studies with horse, dog, and rat thyroid slices, presumably from the thyroid peroxidase (TPO)-mediated oxidation of iodide [127]. This previously unknown iodinated lipid was characterized using NMR, and subsequent experiments using plasmalogen-rich phospholipid pools and lactoperoxidase (LPO) supplemented with iodide demonstrated the necessity of the plasmalogens in the production of this new lipid [127,128]. The predominant 2-IFALD species are 2-iodohexadecanal (2-IHDA) and 2-iodooctadecanal (2-IODA) [128]. Dog thyrocytes can convert 2-IHDA into the iodinated fatty alcohol, 2-iodohexadecanol (2-IHOH) [128]. 2-Iodofatty acid has not yet been identified or detected.

Other iodinated lipid species can be produced in cell-free peroxidase systems supplemented with iodide and in thyroid slices or thyrocytes, presumably by TPO. One major compound is 6-iodo-5-hydroxy-eicosatrienoic delta lactone (6-IDL). 6-IDL is formed by the peroxidase-mediated iodination of arachidonic acid and has been found in LPO, EPO, and MPO cell-free systems and thyroid slices [129,130]. In addition, docosahexaenoic acid can also be converted into an iodo-lactone in similar systems [131]. Finally, iodohydrin production has been documented in a cell-free system using unsaturated phosphatidylcholines as a substrate [63].

DETECTION AND QUANTIFICATION OF IODINATED LIPIDS

2-IHDA can be detected by GC/MS techniques, similar to other peroxidase-derived halogenated fatty aldehydes. Following derivatization to the

PFB oxime, NICI-GC reveals a characteristic peak at m/z 434, representing the oxime's loss of iodide [128]. The loss of iodine can also be seen in the gas chromatography–mass spectra of 6-IDL, which has a characteristic peak of m/z 303 [129,130]. In addition to mass spectrometry techniques, iodinated lipids can by studied by taking advantage of a property unique to iodine among the halogens – a relatively stable radioisotope. Labeling with ^{125}I allows easy tracking of lipid pools enriched with iodide, and this technique was crucial in the identification and characterization of both 2-IHDA and 6-IDL [127–130].

BIOLOGICAL EFFECTS AND SIGNALING PATHWAYS OF IODINATED LIPIDS

The thyroid has long been known to regulate thyroid hormone production in response to increasing iodine concentration, known as the Wolff–Chaikoff effect [132]. The mechanism of this autoregulation still is not fully understood, and many effects of 2-IHDA on the thyroid and thyroid cells suggest that 2-IHDA could play a role in this physiological phenomenon. Early studies found that 2-IHDA inhibits thyroid NADPH oxidase-mediated H_2O_2 production and thyroglobulin iodination [133,134]. 2-IHDA also inhibits thyroid adenylyl cyclase and cAMP production [135,136]. These inhibitory effects occur in the presence of methimazole (MMI), a TPO inhibitor, while the analogous inhibitory effects of iodide are prevented by MMI, suggesting that the autoregulatory effects of 2-IHDA are downstream of TPO-mediated oxidation of iodide [134]. Later studies identified more autoregulatory effects of 2-IHDA on thyroid cells, including prevention of iodide uptake and decreased mRNA expression of thyroid-specific genes, such as TPO [137].

By inhibiting the TPO-mediated iodide oxidation and subsequent production of thyroid hormone, MMI induces goiter growth. 2-IHDA prevents goiter growth and causes goiter involution, even more efficiently than iodide [136]. One potential mechanism through which 2-IHDA could exert its antiproliferative effects on thyroid cells is through cell cycle regulation. 2-IHDA treatment of thyroid cells leads to a lower proportion of cells in S phase and decreased intracellular cyclin levels [138], which could potentially be mediated by an increase of the micro-RNAs let7f and 138, which themselves were shown to inhibit thyroid proliferation [139].

It is unclear if 6-IDL can be produced by TPO activity in the absence of exogenous arachidonic acid supplementation. Endogenous 6-IDL has only been detected in a patient with Graves' disease (hyperthyroidism) treated with high doses of iodide [140]. However, if it is endogenously produced in thyroid tissue, 6-IDL has also been found to inhibit iodide uptake and organification, rat goiter growth, and thyroid cell proliferation [141–144]. Through effects on proliferation and autoregulation of thyroid cells, it appears that the TPO-produced iodinated lipids could play a significant role in thyroid homeostasis and, therefore, mammalian physiology and metabolism.

CONCLUSION

The field of halogenated lipids produced by peroxidases is evolving. Their presence following leukocyte activation coupled with the development of sensitive detection methods has led to recent exciting studies investigating their production as biomarkers of inflammation, such as 2-ClFA in sepsis and oleic acid chlorohydrin in pancreatitis [42,68]. These recent works represent great steps toward clinical utility of these modified lipids, but further verification is required. For example, plasma 2-ClFA levels and oleic acid chlorohydrin levels need to be examined by independent groups. Multicenter studies of the utility of these biomarkers are also needed to assess potential differences in socioeconomic communities. It is possible that other halogenated lipids may prove to be valuable biomarkers of disease. Additionally, the role of halogenated lipids as mediators of disease needs to be investigated in detail as halogenated lipid-mediated mechanisms may provide new targets for therapy. Directing future studies at determining signaling pathways, identifying potential receptors, and understanding protein modifications represents new frontiers that likely will provide insights for the development of novel therapeutics.

REFERENCES

1. R.V. Dorman, H. Dreyfus, L. Freysz, L.A. Horrocks, 1976, Ether lipid content of phosphoglycerides from the retina and brain of chicken and calf, Biochim. Biophys. Acta. 486: 55–59.

2. R.W. Gross, 1984, High plasmalogen and arachidonic acid content of canine myocardial sarcolemma: a fast atom bombardment mass spectroscopic and gas chromatography-mass spectroscopic characterization, Biochemistry 23: 158–165.

3. R.W. Gross, 1985, Identification of plasmalogen as the major phospholipid constituent of cardiac sarcoplasmic reticulum, Biochemistry 24: 1662–1668.

4. J.A. Post, A.J. Verkleij, B. Roelofsen, J.A. Op de Kamp, 1988, Plasmalogen content and distribution in the sarcolemma of cultured neonatal rat myocytes, FEBS Lett. 240: 78–82.

5. E.J. Murphy, L. Joseph, R. Stephens, L.A. Horrocks, 1992, Phospholipid composition of cultured human endothelial cells, Lipids 27: 150–153.

6. D.A. Ford, R.W. Gross, 1989, Plasmenylethanolamine is the major storage depot for arachidonic acid in rabbit vascular smooth muscle and is rapidly hydrolyzed after angiotensin II stimulation, Proc. Natl. Acad. Sci. U.S.A. 86: 3479–3483.

7. J.E. Vance, 1990, Lipoproteins secreted by cultured rat hepatocytes contain the antioxidant 1-alk-1-enyl-2-acylglycerophosphoethanolamine, Biochim. Biophys. Acta. 1045: 128–134.

8. X.L. Han, R.W. Gross, 1990, Plasmenylcholine and phosphatidylcholine membrane bilayers possess distinct conformational motifs, Biochemistry 29: 4992–4996.

9. L.J. Pike, X. Han, K.N. Chung, R.W. Gross, 2002, Lipid rafts are enriched in arachidonic acid and plasmenylethanolamine and their composition is independent of caveolin-1 expression: a quantitative electrospray ionization/mass spectrometric analysis, Biochemistry 41: 2075–2088.

10. X.L. Han, R.W. Gross, 1991, Alterations in membrane dynamics elicited by amphiphilic compounds are augmented in plasmenylcholine bilayers, Biochim. Biophys. Acta. 1069: 37–45.

11. X.L. Han, R.W. Gross, 1991, Proton nuclear magnetic resonance studies on the molecular dynamics of plasmenylcholine/cholesterol and phosphatidylcholine/cholesterol bilayers, Biochim. Biophys. Acta. 1063: 129–136.

12. B. Engelmann, 2004, Plasmalogens: targets for oxidants and major lipophilic antioxidants, Biochem. Soc. Trans. 32: 147–150.

13. J.M. Dean, I.J. Lodhi, 2018, Structural and functional roles of ether lipids, *Prot. Cell* 9: 196–206.

14. R.A. Zoeller, A.C. Lake, N. Nagan, et al., 1999, Plasmalogens as endogenous antioxidants: somatic cell mutants reveal the importance of the vinyl ether, *Biochem. J.* 338: 769–776.

15. W.B. Rizzo, D.A. Craft, A.L. Dammann, M.W. Phillips, 1987, Fatty alcohol metabolism in cultured human fibroblasts. Evidence for a fatty alcohol cycle, *J. Biol. Chem.* 262: 17412–17419.

16. D. Reiss, K. Beyer, B. Engelmann, 1997, Delayed oxidative degradation of polyunsaturated diacyl phospholipids in the presence of plasmalogen phospholipids in vitro, *Biochem. J.* 323: 807–814.

17. D. Hahnel, T. Huber, V. Kurze, K. Beyer, B. Engelmann, 1999, Contribution of copper binding to the inhibition of lipid oxidation by plasmalogen phospholipids, *Biochem. J.* 340: 377–383.

18. R.A. Zoeller, O.H. Morand, C.R. Raetz, 1988, A possible role for plasmalogens in protecting animal cells against photosensitized killing, *J. Biol. Chem.* 263: 11590–11596.

19. C.J. Albert, J.R. Crowley, F.F. Hsu, A.K. Thukkani, D.A. Ford, 2001, Reactive chlorinating species produced by myeloperoxidase target the vinyl ether bond of plasmalogens: identification of 2-chlorohexadecanal, *J. Biol. Chem.* 276: 23733–23741.

20. A.K. Thukkani, F.F. Hsu, J.R. Crowley, et al., 2002, Reactive chlorinating species produced during neutrophil activation target tissue plasmalogens: production of the chemoattractant, 2-chlorohexadecanal, *J. Biol. Chem.* 277: 3842–3849.

21. A.K. Thukkani, C.J. Albert, K.R. Wildsmith, et al., 2003, Myeloperoxidase-derived reactive chlorinating species from human monocytes target plasmalogens in low density lipoprotein, *J. Biol. Chem.* 278: 36365–36372.

22. M.C. Messner, C.J. Albert, F.-F. Hsu, D.A. Ford, 2006, Selective plasmenylcholine oxidation by hypochlorous acid: formation of lysophosphatidylcholine chlorohydrins, *Chem. Phys. Lipids* 144: 34–44.

23. A. Ullen, G. Fauler, H. Kofeler, et al., 2010, Mouse brain plasmalogens are targets for hypochlorous acid-mediated modification in vitro and in vivo, *Free Radic. Biol. Med.* 49: 1655–1665.

24. D.A. Ford, J. Honavar, C.J. Albert, et al., 2016, Formation of chlorinated lipids post-chlorine gas exposure, *J. Lipid Res.* 57: 1529–1540.

25. C. Nusshold, A. Ullen, N. Kogelnik, et al., 2016, Assessment of electrophile damage in a human brain endothelial cell line utilizing a clickable alkyne analog of 2-chlorohexadecanal, *Free Radic. Biol. Med.* 90: 59–74.

26. K.R. Wildsmith, C.J. Albert, F.F. Hsu, J.L. Kao, D.A. Ford, 2006, Myeloperoxidase-derived 2-chlorohexadecanal forms Schiff bases with primary amines of ethanolamine glycerophospholipids and lysine, *Chem. Phys. Lipids* 139: 157–170.

27. M.A. Duerr, R. Aurora, D.A. Ford, 2015, Identification of glutathione adducts of alpha-chlorofatty aldehydes produced in activated neutrophils, *J. Lipid Res.* 56: 1014–1024.

28. A. Ullen, C. Nusshold, T. Glasnov, et al., 2015, Covalent adduct formation between the plasmalogen-derived modification product 2-chlorohexadecanal and phloretin, *Biochem. Pharmacol.* 93: 470–481.

29. K.R. Wildsmith, C.J. Albert, D.S. Anbukumar, D.A. Ford, 2006, Metabolism of myeloperoxidase-derived 2-chlorohexadecanal, *J. Biol. Chem.* 281: 16849–16860.

30. D.S. Anbukumar, L.P. Shornick, C.J. Albert, et al., 2010, Chlorinated lipid species in activated human neutrophils: lipid metabolites of 2-chlorohexadecanal, *J. Lipid Res.* 51: 1085–1092.

31. A. Ullen, G. Fauler, E. Bernhart, et al., 2012, Phloretin ameliorates 2-chlorohexadecanal-mediated brain microvascular endothelial cell dysfunction in vitro, *Free Radic. Biol. Med.* 53: 1770–1781.

32. V.V. Brahmbhatt, C.J. Albert, D.S. Anbukumar, et al., 2010, {Omega}-oxidation of {alpha}-chlorinated fatty acids: identification of {alpha}-chlorinated dicarboxylic acids, *J. Biol. Chem.* 285: 41255–41269.

33. E.N. Palladino, W.Y. Wang, C.J. Albert, et al., 2017, Peroxisome proliferator-activated receptor-alpha accelerates alpha-chlorofatty acid catabolism, *J. Lipid Res.* 58: 317–324.

34. B.K. Wacker, C.J. Albert, B.A. Ford, D.A. Ford, 2013, Strategies for the analysis of chlorinated lipids in biological systems, *Free radic. Biol. Med.* 59: 92–99.

35. W.Y. Wang, C.J. Albert, D.A. Ford, 2013, Approaches for the analysis of chlorinated lipids, *Anal. Biochem.* 443: 148–152.

36. F.F. Hsu, S.L. Hazen, D. Giblin, et al., 1999, Mass spectrometric analysis of pentafluorobenzyl oxime derivatives of reactive biological aldehydes2, *Int. J. Mass Spectr.* 185–187: 795–812.

37. A.K. Thukkani, J. McHowat, F.F. Hsu, et al., 2003, Identification of alpha-chloro fatty aldehydes and unsaturated lysophosphatidylcholine molecular species in human atherosclerotic lesions, *Circulation* 108: 3128–3133.

38. A.K. Thukkani, B.D. Martinson, C.J. Albert, G.A. Vogler, D.A. Ford, 2005, Neutrophil-mediated accumulation of 2-ClHDA during myocardial infarction: 2-ClHDA-mediated myocardial injury, *Am. J. Physiol. Heart Circ. Physiol.* 288: H2955–2964.

39. G. Marsche, R. Heller, G. Fauler, et al., 2004, 2-chlorohexadecanal derived from hypochlorite-modified high-density lipoprotein-associated plasmalogen is a natural inhibitor of endothelial nitric oxide biosynthesis, *Arterioscler. Thromb. Vasc. Biol.* 24: 2302–2306.

40. W.Y. Wang, C.J. Albert, D.A. Ford, 2014, Alpha-chlorofatty acid accumulates in activated monocytes and causes apoptosis through reactive oxygen species production and endoplasmic reticulum stress, *Arterioscler. Thromb. Vasc. Biol.* 34: 526–532.

41. M.A. Mahieu, C.P. Guild, C.J. Albert, et al., 2014, Alpha-chlorofatty Acid and coronary artery or aorta calcium scores in women with systemic lupus erythematosus. A pilot study, *J. Rheumatol.* 41: 1834–1842.

42. N.J. Meyer, J.P. Reilly, R. Feng, et al., 2017, Myeloperoxidase-derived 2-chlorofatty acids contribute to human sepsis mortality via acute respiratory distress syndrome, *JCI Insight* 2: e96432.

43. D.P. Pike, M.J. Vogel, J. McHowat, et al., 2020, 2-Chlorofatty acids are biomarkers of sepsis mortality and mediators of barrier dysfunction in rats, *J. Lipid Res.* 61: 1115–1127.

44. B.T. Wipke, P.M. Allen, 2001, Essential role of neutrophils in the initiation and progression of a murine model of rheumatoid arthritis, *J. Immunol.* 167: 1601–1608.

45. M.C. Messner, C.J. Albert, D.A. Ford, 2008, 2-Chlorohexadecanal and 2-chlorohexadecanoic acid induce COX-2 expression in human coronary artery endothelial cells, *Lipids* 43: 581–588.

46. Q. Zhang, M.J. Lenardo, D. Baltimore, 2017, 30 years of NF-κB: A blossoming of relevance to human pathobiology, *Cell* 168: 37–57.

47. A. Ullen, E. Singewald, V. Konya, et al., 2013, Myeloperoxidase-derived oxidants induce blood-brain barrier dysfunction in vitro and in vivo, *PLoS One* 8: e64034.

48. H. Yu, M. Wang, D. Wang, et al., 2019, Chlorinated lipids elicit inflammatory responses in vitro and in vivo, *Shock* 51: 114–122.

49. J. McHowat, S. Shakya, D.A. Ford, 2020, 2-Chlorofatty aldehyde elicits endothelial cell activation, *Front. Physiol.* 11: 460.

50. F.H. Greig, L. Hutchison, C.M. Spickett, S. Kennedy, 2015, Differential effects of chlorinated and oxidized phospholipids in vascular tissue: implications for neointima formation, *Clin. Sci.* 128: 579–592.

51. E.N.D. Palladino, L.A. Katunga, G.R. Kolar, D.A. Ford, 2018, 2-Chlorofatty acids: Lipid mediators of neutrophil extracellular trap formation, *J. Lipid Res.* 59: 1424–1432.

52. S. Boeltz, P. Amini, H.J. Anders, et al., 2019, To NET or not to NET: current opinions and state of the science regarding the formation of neutrophil extracellular traps, *Cell Death Differ.* 26: 395–408.

53. E. Bernhart, N. Kogelnik, J. Prasch, et al., 2018, 2-Chlorohexadecanoic acid induces ER stress and mitochondrial dysfunction in brain microvascular endothelial cells, *Redox Biol.* 15: 441–451.

54. C.L. Hartman, M.A. Duerr, C.J. Albert, et al., 2018, 2-Chlorofatty acids induce Weibel-Palade body mobilization, *J. Lipid Res.* 59: 113–122.

55. C.C. Winterbourn, J.J. van den Berg, E. Roitman, F.A. Kuypers, 1992, Chlorohydrin formation from unsaturated fatty acids reacted with hypochlorous acid, *Arch. Biochem. Biophys.* 296: 547–555.

56. J. Arnhold, A.N. Osipov, H. Spalteholz, O.M. Panasenko, J. Schiller, 2001, Effects of hypochlorous acid on unsaturated phosphatidylcholines, *Free Radic. Biol. Med.* 31: 1111–1119.

57. U. Panzenboeck, S. Raitmayer, H. Reicher, et al., 1997, Effects of reagent and enzymatically generated hypochlorite on physicochemical and metabolic properties of high density lipoproteins, *J. Biol. Chem.* 272: 29711–29720.

58. J.J. van den Berg, C.C. Winterbourn, F.A. Kuypers, 1993, Hypochlorous acid-mediated modification of cholesterol and phospholipid: analysis of reaction products by gas chromatography-mass spectrometry, *J. Lipid Res.* 34: 2005–2012.

59. J.W. Heinecke, W. Li, D.M. Mueller, A. Bohrer, J. Turk, 1994, Cholesterol chlorohydrin synthesis by the myeloperoxidase-hydrogen peroxide-chloride system: potential markers for lipoproteins oxidatively damaged by phagocytes, *Biochemistry* 33: 10127–10136.

60. A.C. Carr, J.J. van den Berg, C.C. Winterbourn, 1996, Chlorination of cholesterol in cell membranes by hypochlorous acid, *Arch. Biochem. Biophys.* 332: 63–69.

61. S.L. Hazen, F.F. Hsu, K. Duffin, J.W. Heinecke, 1996, Molecular chlorine generated by the myeloperoxidase-hydrogen peroxide-chloride system of phagocytes converts low density lipoprotein cholesterol into a family of chlorinated sterols, *J. Biol. Chem.* 271: 23080–23088.

62. O.M. Panasenko, H. Spalteholz, J. Schiller, J. Arnhold, 2003, Myeloperoxidase-induced formation of chlorohydrins and lysophospholipids from unsaturated phosphatidylcholines, *Free Radic. Biol. Med.* 34: 553–562.

63. H. Spalteholz, K. Wenske, J. Arnhold, 2005, Interaction of hypohalous acids and heme peroxidases with unsaturated phosphatidylcholines, *BioFactors* 24: 67–76.

64. J. Arnhold, A.N. Osipov, H. Spalteholz, O.M. Panasenko, J. Schiller, 2002, Formation of lysophospholipids from unsaturated phosphatidylcholines under the influence of hypochlorous acid, *Biochim. Biophys. Acta.* 1572: 91–100.

65. V.V. Brahmbhatt, F.F. Hsu, J.L. Kao, E.C. Frank, D.A. Ford, 2007, Novel carbonyl and nitrile products from reactive chlorinating species attack of lysosphingolipid, *Chem. Phys. Lipids* 145: 72–84.

66. C. Nusshold, M. Kollroser, H. Kofeler, et al., 2010, Hypochlorite modification of sphingomyelin generates chlorinated lipid species that induce apoptosis and proteome alterations in dopaminergic PC12 neurons in vitro, *Free Radic. Biol. Med.* 48: 1588–1600.

67. H. Spalteholz, K. Wenske, O.M. Panasenko, J. Schiller, J. Arnhold, 2004, Evaluation of products upon the reaction of hypohalous acid with unsaturated phosphatidylcholines, *Chem. Phys. Lipids* 129: 85–96.

68. E. de-Madaria, X. Molero, L. Bonjoch, et al., 2018, Oleic acid chlorohydrin, a new early biomarker for the prediction of acute pancreatitis severity in humans, *Ann. Intensive Care* 8: 1.

69. O. Skaff, D.I. Pattison, M.J. Davies, 2008, The vinyl ether linkages of plasmalogens are favored targets for myeloperoxidase-derived oxidants: a kinetic study, *Biochemistry* 47: 8237–8245.

70. N. Franco-Pons, J. Casas, G. Fabrias, et al., 2013, Fat necrosis generates proinflammatory halogenated lipids during acute pancreatitis, *Ann. Surgery* 257: 943–951.

71. M.C. Vissers, A.C. Carr, C.C. Winterbour, 2001, Fatty acid chlorohydrins and bromohydrins are cytotoxic to human endothelial cells, *Redox Rep.* 6: 49–55.

72. G. Dever, C.L. Wainwright, S. Kennedy, C.M. Spickett, 2006, Fatty acid and phospholipid chlorohydrins cause cell stress and endothelial adhesion, *Acta Biochim Polon.* 53: 761–768.

73. A. Robaszkiewicz, G. Bartosz, A.R. Pitt, et al., 2014, HOCl-modified phosphatidylcholines induce apoptosis and redox imbalance in HUVEC-ST cells, *Arch Biochem. Biophys.* 548: 1–10.

74. A.C. Carr, M.C. Vissers, N.M. Domigan, C.C. Winterbourn, 1997, Modification of red cell membrane lipids by hypochlorous acid and haemolysis by preformed lipid chlorohydrins, *Redox Rep.* 3: 263–271.

75. A. Robaszkiewicz, F.H. Greig, A.R. Pitt, et al., 2010, Effect of phosphatidylcholine chlorohydrins on human erythrocytes, *Chem. Phys. Lipids* 163: 639–647.

76. G. Dever, L.J. Stewart, A.R. Pitt, C.M. Spickett, 2003, Phospholipid chlorohydrins cause ATP depletion and toxicity in human myeloid cells, *FEBS Lett.* 540: 245–250.

77. G.J. Dever, R. Benson, C.L. Wainwright, S. Kennedy, C.M. Spickett, 2008, Phospholipid chlorohydrin induces leukocyte adhesion to ApoE-/- mouse arteries via upregulation of P-selectin, *Free Radic. Biol. Med.* 44: 452–463.

78. H. Iwase, Y. Yamada, H. Uemura, et al., 1997, Effect of monochlorohydrins of linoleic acid on guinea-pig cardiac papillary muscles, *Biochem Biophys. Res. Commun.* 231: 295–298.

79. D.I. Pattison, C.L. Hawkins, M.J. Davies, 2003, Hypochlorous acid-mediated oxidation of lipid components and antioxidants present in low-density lipoproteins: absolute rate constants, product analysis, and computational modeling, *Chem. Res. Toxicol.* 16: 439–449.

80. Y. Kawai, H. Kiyokawa, Y. Kimura, et al., 2006, Hypochlorous acid-derived modification of phospholipids: characterization of aminophospholipids as regulatory molecules for lipid peroxidation, *Biochemistry* 45: 14201–14211.

81. J. Flemmig, H. Spalteholz, K. Schubert, S. Meier, J. Arnhold, 2009, Modification of phosphatidylserine by hypochlorous acid, *Chem. Phys. Lipids* 161: 44–50.

82. S.L. Hazen, J. Heller, F.F. Hsu, A. d'Avignon, J.W. Heinecke, 1999, Synthesis, isolation, and characterization of the adduct formed in the

reaction of p-hydroxyphenylacetaldehyde with the amino headgroup of phosphatidylethanolamine and phosphatidylserine, *Chem. Res. Toxicol.* 12: 19–27.

83. J.I. Heller, J.R. Crowley, S.L. Hazen, et al., 2000, p-hydroxyphenylacetaldehyde, an aldehyde generated by myeloperoxidase, modifies phospholipid amino groups of low density lipoprotein in human atherosclerotic intima, *J. Biol. Chem.* 275: 9957–9962.

84. T. Stelmaszynska, E. Kukovetz, G. Egger, R.J. Schaur, 1992, Possible involvement of myeloperoxidase in lipid peroxidation, *Int. J. Biochem.* 24: 121–128.

85. S.M. Sepe, R.A. Clark, 1985, Oxidant membrane injury by the neutrophil myeloperoxidase system. I. Characterization of a liposome model and injury by myeloperoxidase, hydrogen peroxide, and halides, *J. Immunol.* 134: 1888–1895.

86. R. Zhang, M.L. Brennan, Z. Shen, et al., 2002, Myeloperoxidase functions as a major enzymatic catalyst for initiation of lipid peroxidation at sites of inflammation, *J. Biol. Chem.* 277: 46116–46122.

87. L. Kubala, K.R. Schmelzer, A. Klinke, et al., 2010, Modulation of arachidonic and linoleic acid metabolites in myeloperoxidase-deficient mice during acute inflammation, *Free Radic. Biol. Med.* 48: 1311–1320.

88. E.A. Podrez, M. Febbraio, N. Sheibani, et al., 2000, Macrophage scavenger receptor CD36 is the major receptor for LDL modified by monocyte-generated reactive nitrogen species, *J. Clin. Invest.* 105: 1095–1108.

89. O.M. Panasenko, J. Arnhold, J. Schiller, K. Arnold, V.I. Sergienko, 1994, Peroxidation of egg yolk phosphatidylcholine liposomes by hypochlorous acid, *Biohim. Biophys. Acta.* 1215: 259–266.

90. O.M. Panasenko, S.A. Evgina, R.K. Aidyraliev, V.I. Sergienko, Y.A. Vladimirov, 1994, Peroxidation of human blood lipoproteins induced by exogenous hypochlorite or hypochlorite generated in the system of "myeloperoxidase+H_2O_2+Cl⁻", *Free Radic. Biol. Med.* 16: 143–148.

91. O.M. Panasenko, S.A. Evgina, E.S. Driomina, et al., 1995, Hypochlorite induces lipid peroxidation in blood lipoproteins and phospholipid liposomes, *Free Radic. Biol. Med.* 19: 133–140.

92. O.M. Panasenko, J. Arnhold, A. Vladimirov Yu, K. Arnhold, V.I. Sergienko, 1997, Hypochlorite-induced peroxidation of egg yolk phosphatidylcholine is mediated by hydroperoxides, *Free Radic. Res.* 27: 1–12.

93. O.M. Panasenko, J. Arnhold, J. Schiller, 1997, Hypochlorite reacts with an organic hydroperoxide forming free radicals, but not singlet oxygen, and thus initiates lipid peroxidation, *Biochemistry* 62: 951–959.

94. S. Miyamoto, G.R. Martinez, D. Rettori, et al., 2006, Linoleic acid hydroperoxide reacts with hypochlorous acid, generating peroxyl radical intermediates and singlet molecular oxygen, *Proc. Natl. Acad. Sci. U.S.A.* 103: 293–298.

95. L.J. Hazell, M.J. Davies, R. Stocker, 1999, Secondary radicals derived from chloramines of apolipoprotein B-100 contribute to HOCl-induced lipid peroxidation of low-density lipoproteins, *Biochem. J.* 339: 489–495.

96. M.L. Savenkova, D.M. Mueller, J.W. Heinecke, 1994, Tyrosyl radical generated by myeloperoxidase is a physiological catalyst for the initiation of lipid peroxidation in low density lipoprotein, *J. Biol. Chem.* 269: 20394–20400.

97. M. Exner, M. Hermann, R. Hofbauer, et al., 2004, Thiocyanate catalyzes myeloperoxidase-initiated lipid oxidation in LDL, *Free Radic. Biol. Med.* 37: 146–155.

98. F.O. Ismael, J.M. Proudfoot, B.E. Brown, et al., 2015, Comparative reactivity of the myeloperoxidase-derived oxidants HOCl and HOSCN with low-density lipoprotein (LDL): Implications for foam cell formation in atherosclerosis, *Arch. Biochem. Biophys.* 573: 40–51.

99. A.R. Brash, 1999, Lipoxygenases: occurrence, functions, catalysis, and acquisition of substrate, *J. Biol. Chem.* 274: 23679–23682.

100. A. Ayala, M.F. Munoz, S. Arguelles, 2014, Lipid peroxidation: production, metabolism, and signaling mechanisms of malondialdehyde and 4-hydroxy-2-nonenal, *Oxid. Med. Cell. Longevity* 2014: 360438.

101. R. Mashima, T. Okuyama, 2015, The role of lipoxygenases in pathophysiology; new insights and future perspectives, *Redox Biol.* 6: 297–310.

102. M.M. Gaschler, B.R. Stockwell, 2017, Lipid peroxidation in cell death, *Biochem. Biophys. Res. Commun.* 482: 419–425.

103. J. Byun, D.M. Mueller, J.S. Fabjan, J.W. Heinecke, 1999, Nitrogen dioxide radical generated by the myeloperoxidase-hydrogen peroxide-nitrite system promotes lipid peroxidation of low density lipoprotein, *FEBS Lett.* 455: 243–246.

104. S.L. Hazen, R. Zhang, Z. Shen, et al., 1999, Formation of nitric oxide-derived oxidants by myeloperoxidase in monocytes: pathways for

monocyte-mediated protein nitration and lipid peroxidation in vivo, Circ. Res. 85: 950–958.

105. E.A. Podrez, D. Schmitt, H.F. Hoff, S.L. Hazen, 1999, Myeloperoxidase-generated reactive nitrogen species convert LDL into an atherogenic form in vitro, J. Clin. Invest. 103: 1547–1560.

106. V.A. Kostyuk, T. Kraemer, H. Sies, T. Schewe, 2003, Myeloperoxidase/nitrite-mediated lipid peroxidation of low-density lipoprotein as modulated by flavonoids, FEBS Lett. 537: 146–150.

107. D. Schmitt, Z. Shen, R. Zhang, et al., 1999, Leukocytes utilize myeloperoxidase-generated nitrating intermediates as physiological catalysts for the generation of biologically active oxidized lipids and sterols in serum, Biochemistry 38: 16904–16915.

108. B.A. Freeman, V.B. O'Donnell, F.J. Schopfer, 2018, The discovery of nitro-fatty acids as products of metabolic and inflammatory reactions and mediators of adaptive cell signaling, Nitric Oxide 77: 106–111.

109. J.P. Eiserich, S. Baldus, M.L. Brennan, et al., 2002, Myeloperoxidase, a leukocyte-derived vascular NO oxidase, Science 296: 2391–2394.

110. J.P. Eiserich, M. Hristova, C.E. Cross, et al., 1998, Formation of nitric oxide-derived inflammatory oxidants by myeloperoxidase in neutrophils, Nature 391: 393–397.

111. M. Goeritzer, E. Bernhart, I. Plastira, et al., 2020, Myeloperoxidase and septic conditions disrupt sphingolipid homeostasis in murine brain capillaries in vivo and immortalized human brain endothelial cells in vitro, Int. J. Mol. Sci. 21: 1143.

112. C.J. Albert, J.R. Crowley, F.F. Hsu, A.K. Thukkani, D.A. Ford, 2002, Reactive brominating species produced by myeloperoxidase target the vinyl ether bond of plasmalogens: disparate utilization of sodium halides in the production of alpha-halo fatty aldehydes, J. Biol. Chem. 277: 4694–4703.

113. C.J. Albert, A.K. Thukkani, R.M. Heuertz, et al., 2003, Eosinophil peroxidase-derived reactive brominating species target the vinyl ether bond of plasmalogens generating a novel chemoattractant, alpha-bromo fatty aldehyde, J. Biol. Chem. 278: 8942–8950.

114. E.L. Thomas, P.M. Bozeman, M.M. Jefferson, C.C. King, 1995, Oxidation of bromide by the human leukocyte enzymes myeloperoxidase and eosinophil peroxidase. Formation of bromamines, J. Biol. Chem. 270: 2906–2913.

115. W. Wu, M.K. Samoszuk, S.A. Comhair, et al., 2000, Eosinophils generate brominating oxidants in allergen-induced asthma, J. Clin. Invest. 105: 1455–1463.

116. M.A. Duerr, E.N.D. Palladino, C.L. Hartman, et al., 2018, Bromofatty aldehyde derived from bromine exposure and myeloperoxidase and eosinophil peroxidase modify GSH and protein, J. Lipid Res. 59: 696–705.

117. S. Ahmad, J.X. Masjoan Juncos, A. Ahmad, et al., 2019, Bromine inhalation mimics ischemia-reperfusion cardiomyocyte injury and calpain activation in rats, Am. J. Physiol. Heart Circ. Physiol. 316: H212–223.

118. A.C. Carr, C.C. Winterbourn, J.J. van den Berg, 1996, Peroxidase-mediated bromination of unsaturated fatty acids to form bromohydrins, Arch. Biochem. Biophys. 327: 227–233.

119. A.C. Carr, E.A. Decker, Y. Park, B. Frei, 2001, Comparison of low-density lipoprotein modification by myeloperoxidase-derived hypochlorous and hypobromous acids, Free Radic. Biol. Med. 31: 62–72.

120. A.C. Carr, J.J. van den Berg, C.C. Winterbourn, 1998, Differential reactivities of hypochlorous and hypobromous acids with purified Escherichia coli phospholipid: formation of haloamines and halohydrins, Biochim. Biophys. Acta. 1392: 254–264.

121. O.M. Panasenko, T. Vakhrusheva, V. Tretyakov, H. Spalteholz, J. Arnhold, 2007, Influence of chloride on modification of unsaturated phosphatidylcholines by the myeloperoxidase/hydrogen peroxide/bromide system, Chem. Phys. Lipids 149: 40–51.

122. J.F. Chase, P.K. Tubbs, 1972, Specific inhibition of mitochondrial fatty acid oxidation by 2-bromopalmitate and its coenzyme A and carnitine esters, Biochem. J. 129: 55–65.

123. J.F. Chase, P.K. Tubbs, 1969, Conditions for the self-catalysed inactivation of carnitine acetyltransferase. A novel form of enzyme inhibition, Biochem. J. 111: 225–235.

124. J.F. Chase, P.K. Tubbs, 1970, Specific alkylation of a histidine residue in carnitine acetyltransferase by bromoacetyl-L-carnitine, Biochem. J. 116: 713–720.

125. B.M. Raaka, J.M. Lowenstein, 1979, Inhibition of fatty acid oxidation by 2-bromooctanoate. Evidence for the enzymatic formation of 2-bromo-3-ketooctanoyl coenzyme A and the inhibition of 3-ketothiolase, J. Biol. Chem. 254: 6755–6762.

126. R.A. Coleman, P. Rao, R.J. Fogelsong, E.S. Bardes, 1992, 2-Bromopalmitoyl-CoA and 2-bromopalmitate: promiscuous inhibitors of membrane-bound enzymes, *Biochim. Biophys. Acta.* 1125: 203–209.

127. A. Pereira, J.C. Braekman, J.E. Dumont, J.M. Boeynaems, 1990, Identification of a major iodolipid from the horse thyroid gland as 2-iodo-hexadecanal, *J. Biol. Chem.* 265: 17018–17025.

128. V. Panneels, P. Macours, H. Van den Bergen, et al., 1996, Biosynthesis and metabolism of 2-iodohexadecanal in cultured dog thyroid cells, *J. Biol. Chem.* 271: 23006–23014.

129. J.M. Boeynaems, W.C. Hubbard, 1980, Transformation of arachidonic acid into an iodolactone by the rat thyroid, *J. Biol. Chem.* 255: 9001–9004.

130. J. Turk, W.R. Henderson, S.J. Klebanoff, W.C. Hubbard, 1983, Iodination of arachidonic acid mediated by eosinophil peroxidase, myeloperoxidase and lactoperoxidase. Identification and comparison of products, *Biochim. Biophys. Acta* 751: 189–200.

131. J.M. Boeynaems, J.T. Watson, J.A. Oates, W.C. Hubbard, 1981, Iodination of docosahexaenoic acid by lactoperoxidase and thyroid gland in vitro: formation of an Iodolactone, *Lipids* 16: 323–327.

132. K. Markou, N. Georgopoulos, V. Kyriazopoulou, A.G. Vagenakis, 2001, Iodine-induced hypothyroidism, *Thyroid* 11: 501–510.

133. R. Ohayon, J.M. Boeynaems, J.C. Braekman, et al., 1994, Inhibition of thyroid NADPH-oxidase by 2-iodohexadecanal in a cell-free system, *Mol. Cell. Endocrinol.* 99: 133–141.

134. V. Panneels, H. Van den Bergen, C. Jacoby, et al., 1994, Inhibition of H_2O_2 production by iodoaldehydes in cultured dog thyroid cells, *Mol. Cell. Endocrinol.* 102: 167–176.

135. V. Panneels, J. Van Sande, H. Van den Bergen, et al., 1994, Inhibition of human thyroid adenylyl cyclase by 2-iodoaldehydes, *Mol. Cell. Endocrinol.* 106: 41–50.

136. L. Thomasz, R. Oglio, D.T. Rivandeira, et al., 2010, Inhibition of goiter growth and of cyclic AMP formation in rat thyroid by 2-iodohexadecanal, *Mol. Cell. Endocrinol.* 317: 141–147.

137. L.E. Rossich, L. Thomasz, J.P. Nicola, et al., 2016, Effects of 2-iodohexadecanal in the physiology of thyroid cells, *Mol. Cell. Endocrinol.* 437: 292–301.

138. L. Thomasz, K. Coulonval, L. Salvarredi, et al., 2015, Inhibitory effects of 2-iodohexadecanal on FRTL-5 thyroid cells proliferation, *Mol. Cell. Endocrinol.* 404: 123–131.

139. L.A. Salvarredi, L. Thomasz, L.E. Rossich, et al., 2015, 2-Iodohexadecanal inhibits thyroid cell growth in part through the induction of let-7f microRNA, *Mol. Cell. Endocrinol.* 414: 224–232.

140. A. Dugrillon, W.M. Uedelhoven, M.A. Pisarev, G. Bechtner, R. Gartner, 1994, Identification of delta-iodolactone in iodide treated human goiter and its inhibitory effect on proliferation of human thyroid follicles, *Hormone Metabol. Res.* 26: 465–469.

141. G.D. Chazenbalk, R.M. Valsecchi, L. Krawiec, et al., 1988, Thyroid autoregulation. Inhibitory effects of iodinated derivatives of arachidonic acid on iodine metabolism, *Prostaglandins* 36: 163–172.

142. L. Krawiec, G.D. Chazenbalk, S.A. Puntarulo, et al., 1988, The inhibition of PB125I formation in calf thyroid caused by 14-iodo-15-hydroxy-eicosatrienoic acid is due to decreased H_2O_2 availability, *Hormone Metabol. Res.* 20: 86–90.

143. M.A. Pisarev, G.D. Chazenbalk, R.M. Valsecchi, et al., 1988, Thyroid autoregulation. Inhibition of goiter growth and of cyclic AMP formation in rat thyroid by iodinated derivatives of arachidonic acid, *J. Endocrinol. Invest.* 11: 669–674.

144. A. Dugrillon, G. Bechtner, W.M. Uedelhoven, P.C. Weber, R. Gartner, 1990, Evidence that an iodolactone mediates the inhibitory effect of iodide on thyroid cell proliferation but not on adenosine $3'$, $5'$-monophosphate formation, *Endocrinology* 127: 337–343.

CHAPTER SEVEN

Roles of Myeloperoxidase in the Oxidation of Apolipoproteins: Interest of Monitoring Myeloperoxidase Oxidation of Apolipoproteins A-1 and B-100 to Improve the Estimation of Lipoprotein Quality in Cardiovascular Diseases

Catherine Coremans
Université Libre de Bruxelles

Karim Zouaoui Boudjeltia
ISPPC CHU de Charleroi

Pierre Van Antwerpen and Cédric Delporte
Université Libre de Bruxelles

CONTENTS

ABBREVIATIONS

ABCA1:	ATP-binding cassette A1 receptor
apoA-1:	Apolipoprotein A-1
apoB-100:	Apolipoprotein B-100
CAD:	Coronary artery disease
Cl-Tyr:	3-Chloro-tyrosine
HDL:	High-density lipoprotein
H_2O_2:	Hydrogen peroxide
HOCl:	Hypochlorous acid
LCAT:	Lecithin–cholesterol acyltransferase
LDL:	Low-density lipoprotein
Mox-HDL:	Myeloperoxidase-modified high-density lipoprotein
Mox-LDL:	Myeloperoxidase-modified low-density lipoprotein
MPO:	Myeloperoxidase
NO_2-Tyr:	3-Nitro-tyrosine
NOX:	NADPH oxidase
RCT:	Reverse cholesterol transport
SR-B1:	Scavenger receptor class B type 1

EVIDENCE OF MYELOPEROXIDASE IMPACT IN CARDIOVASCULAR DISEASE

Atherosclerosis develops as a result of a set of dysfunctions including inflammation, oxidative stress, loss of endothelial function

DOI: 10.1201/9781003212287-9

and disruption of the renin–angiotensin system [1]. The concomitant presence of dyslipidemia enables the lipid accumulation in the vascular wall. This chronic inflammatory disease occurs in specific arterial regions where shear stress abnormalities appear. It begins with the deficiency of endothelium function [2]. The synthesis of inflammatory mediators initiates the production of oxidized *low- and high-density lipoproteins* (LDLs, HDLs), which contribute in turn to the production of inflammatory species [3]. The oxidation of LDLs also promotes the formation of foam cells by accumulation of LDL-derived cholesterol in macrophages [4]. Among mechanisms of oxidation of lipoproteins, myeloperoxidase (MPO) oxidation is believed to be one of the most relevant oxidation processes. Indeed, enzymatically active MPO is extensively expressed in atherosclerotic lesions, and its involvement in atherosclerotic plaque progression has been well established [5]. MPO and its derived oxidants have pro-atherogenic properties [6]. In addition to lipoprotein oxidation, MPO promotes endothelial dysfunction, endothelial cell apoptosis and thrombosis and may contribute to plaque destabilization [6–9].

Numerous clinical studies have assessed the level of MPO in healthy volunteers and in patients with elevated cardiovascular risk. Of the 20 studies assessed by Teng et al. [6], the majority highlights a positive association between MPO concentration and coronary artery disease (CAD). In nearly all these studies, determination of MPO was performed from collected venous blood, except for one study where authors collected blood samples from abdominal aorta and coronary arteries [10]. The interest in such specific blood sampling lies in the fact that the highest concentrations of MPO are localized in atheromatous plaque rather than in general circulation [11].

While MPO can reach plasma concentrations up to 40 ng/mL in the healthy state, elevated MPO levels (>350 ng/mL) are observed in patients with significant increased of cardiovascular risk [11–13]. MPO correlates with increases in cerebral aneurysms when comparing MPO levels between aneurysm tissue and femoral arterial tissue from the same individuals [14]. In stable CAD, inflammation increases MPO concentration in blood and induces a decrease of apolipoprotein A-1 (apoA-1) and HDL levels. It is suggested that MPO level itself, associated with measurement of MPO/HDL and MPO/apoA-1 ratios, can differentiate among CAD patients and identifies those with higher risk of acute coronary syndrome and stroke [15]. Therefore, circulating MPO concentration correlates not only with the presence of coronary disease but also with disease severity [6]. Recently, an active precursor of MPO (pro-MPO) has been detected in the circulation, and its level increases in cardiovascular disease (CVD) patients [16]. Pro-MPO has similar enzymatic properties to MPO, with a chlorination activity about 70% compared with mature MPO. Not all the pro-MPO reach the mature form, and some can be localized in azurophilic granules [17].

A higher MPO concentration in plasma indicates the activation of neutrophils and macrophages prior cardiovascular events. However, MPO is also potentially able to predict major adverse coronary events, such as myocardial infarction [18]. It is suggested that MPO may be a marker of vulnerable plaque in asymptomatic patients [6,19]. In addition to this short-term prediction, there is evidence for MPO predicting cardiovascular mortality in patients with CAD. Concerning non-CAD patients, the utility of MPO in predicting cardiovascular mortality remains unclear [6].

The fact that MPO supports initiation and development of CVD suggests the possible atheroprotective effect of MPO deficiency [20]. While the frequency of infections does not increase in individuals with genetic MPO deficiency, the absence of hypochlorous acid (HOCl) formation leads to lower LDL oxidation and may reduce cardiovascular events. When comparing MPO-deficient individuals with a control group, cardiovascular events are statistically less frequent among the MPO-deficient individuals [20]. Other studies regarding MPO genetics state that some genotypes are associated with an increase of CAD [21,22].

Studying MPO can provide information to extend the prognosis obtained with traditional markers. Due to its pro-inflammatory properties, MPO is both a marker and key contributor to vascular inflammation [23]. Strong evidence suggests that MPO measurement may improve CVD risk estimation, even if standardization of sampling and laboratory guidelines are necessary before using MPO in routine clinical practice [24]. The inconsistency of enzyme-linked immunosorbent assays (ELISA) used to measure MPO makes it difficult to quantitatively compare studies [6]. However, the study of products of MPO activity seems promising. In this context, degradation of lipoprotein quality due to MPO oxidation has to be investigated in order to fully understand the impact of MPO in atherosclerosis and to provide biomarkers with multiple purposes. This MPO-dependent oxidation of lipoproteins is discussed in the following sections.

PATHOPHYSIOLOGY OF MPO IN ATHEROSCLEROSIS

MPO plays a key role among the actors of the oxidation processes during atherosclerosis. This enzyme can produce strong antimicrobial oxidative species and can be found in azurophilic granules of neutrophils and, to a lesser extent, in monocytes [25]. MPO is active in the extracellular medium by degranulation of neutrophils after activation of an intracellular signaling pathway [26]. The degranulation allows the secretory granules to secrete their contents extracellularly, which releases MPO among the granular contents [27] and also forms part of the neutrophil extracellular trap (NET). This large, extracellular, web-like structure is composed of cytosolic and granule proteins that are assembled on a scaffold of decondensed chromatin [27,28]. Its physiological function is to protect against infection, but it can contribute to tissue injury in noninfectious disease states. During the early stages of atherosclerosis, NET promotes inflammation by increasing monocyte recruitment and triggering macrophages to release reactive oxygen species and pro-inflammatory cytokines [29]. Therefore, MPO is considered as a specific marker of the activation and degranulation of polymorphonuclear neutrophils [30].

The neutrophils and monocytes migrate during atherosclerotic process through the endothelium of the vascular wall [31]. This infiltration allows MPO to be localized in both lumen and intima of vessels. The presence of MPO has been reported in nonmyeloid cell types, such as endothelial cells [26]. Endothelial cells can bind and internalize MPO, with an increase of intracellular oxidant production [32]. An endogenous expression of active MPO in these cells has been described, with likely a function related to angiogenesis and vascular repair in vivo [33,34].

MPO is catalytically active in the presence of hydrogen peroxide (H_2O_2). When a neutrophil is activated, nicotinamide adenine dinucleotide phosphate oxidase (Nox or NADPH oxidase) produces the superoxide anion ($O_2{}^{\bullet-}$) in the phagosome, from an oxygen molecule using NADPH. Superoxide anions undergo dismutation, spontaneously or via the action of superoxide dismutase [35], by consuming protons and forming H_2O_2 [36], the substrate for MPO. Nox are a family of enzyme complexes with several subunits, which can be distinguished according to their location. Smooth muscle cells contain Nox 1 and Nox 4, endothelial cells express mainly Nox 2 and Nox 4 [37], while macrophages strongly express Nox 2 [38]. As Nox is expressed on endothelial cells, endothelial cells are capable of generating H_2O_2 at the luminal surface [39] (Figure 7.1). The oxidation

Colocalization of MPO and Nox on endothelial cell surface

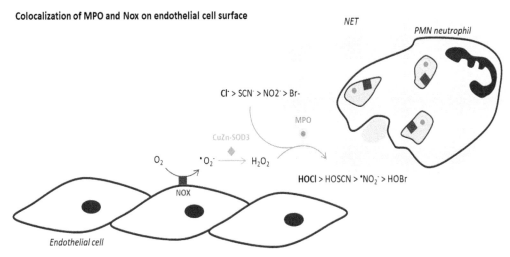

Figure 7.1 Oxidative reaction chain of Nox, SOD and MPO around endothelial cells. The simultaneous presence of Nox and MPO in the extracellular medium allows the activation of extracellular MPO to oxidize extracellular targets. Hypochlorous acid is the most abundant final oxidant agent.

of LDLs by MPO (leading to the so-called Mox-LDL) can also occur at the surface of endothelial cells and will not therefore be limited to the sub-endothelial space [40]. Whether at the luminal surface of the vessel or at the subendothelial space, MPO and lipoproteins will be found together in atherosclerotic lesions.

MPO AND DYSFUNCTIONAL-PROATHEROGENIC LIPOPROTEINS

The oxidation of amino acid residues by MPO leads to the formation of oxidized lipoproteins referred as Mox-LDL and Mox-HDL. Complexes of MPO with other lipoproteins have been reported, but the focus of this chapter will be on HDLs and LDLs [41]. In the healthy state, HDLs carry an excess of cholesterol from the body tissues to the liver where the molecule will be degraded. HDL is the smallest and densest of the lipoproteins because it contains a high proportion of proteins [42]. This heterogeneous lipoprotein family is composed of several subclasses, which are dependent on density, size, shape and lipid and protein composition [43]. The metabolic cycle of HDL begins with the expression of apoA-1 by the liver, which is incorporated in preβ-HDL particles. Going through different stages of composition, HDL eventually takes the form of HDL2-rich cholesteryl ester, to be excreted.

Several types of apolipoproteins can be found on the HDL surface, including apolipoproteins A, C, D, E and L. ApoA-1 represents 75% of the protein content of HDLs and allows the interaction between HDL and receptors/transporters [44]. ApoA-1 also activates lecithin–cholesterol acyltransferase (LCAT), which converts free cholesterol into cholesteryl esters during the metabolism of HDL. Its interaction with ATP-binding cassette A1 (ABCA1) is essential to mediate the efflux of cholesterol from macrophages to lipid-poor apoA-1 [45]. This reverse cholesterol transport (RCT) has a key role in reducing atheroma. When macrophages under the vascular endothelium assimilate (M)ox-LDL and increase their lipid content, HDL can reverse this pro-atherogenic trend by removing cholesterol from the vessel wall. Even if LDLs are considered as "bad cholesterol," this lipoprotein nonetheless is essential for directing the cholesterol synthesized in the liver or received from food, to the body cells to be incorporated in membranes or used for hormone synthesis. LDL is derived from other low-density lipoproteins (very low and intermediate density lipoproteins), and its composition is less complex than HDL. LDL has on its surface only one apolipoprotein, apolipoprotein B-100 (apoB-100), which allows the cellular recognition of LDL by the LDL receptor (LDLr) [46]. This family of lipoproteins consists of particles varying in size and density. Small dense LDL particles are considered to be more pro-atherogenic than large LDL particles [47].

The conversion of LDL into Mox-LDL generates a more atherogenic form within the artery wall, which is taken up and accumulates in macrophages [6]. Mox-LDL has been reported to co-localize with MPO on the luminal side of the endothelial layer and in the thickened intima [48,49]. In the development of atheromatous plaque, this accumulation of Mox-LDLs in macrophages results in the formation of foam cells. LDL oxidation with HOCl promotes a high uptake of the modified lipoproteins by macrophages [50]. This increased uptake is due to interaction between Mox-LDLs and the macrophage class B scavenger receptors CD36 and SR-BI [51]. For example, exposure of mouse macrophages to Mox-LDLs induces increased intracellular concentrations of cholesterol and cholesteryl esters [52]. The endocytosis of Mox-LDLs by macrophages is also known to partially inactivate lysosomal enzymes, which further promotes the enrichment of intracellular lipids [6,53,54].

In addition to promoting lipid uptake, Mox-LDLs can also promote pro-inflammatory responses from monocytes and endothelial cells and hence further contribute to the development and progression of atherosclerosis [6,55]. Endothelial cells are stimulated to release chemokines such as interleukin-8 to induce a chemotactic migration of neutrophils to the endothelium of the vascular wall [3,56]. MPO itself is known to modulate nitric oxide (NO·)-dependent signaling processes during inflammation (see Chapter 13), with Mox-LDL shown to decrease NO· synthesis by endothelial cells and enhance vascular endothelial dysfunction [57,58]. The migration of Mox-LDL into the subendothelial space will be further promoted owing to an increase in endothelial permeability and the adherence of leukocytes. Mox-LDLs activate the respiratory burst in macrophages and neutrophils in order to maintain H_2O_2 generation [59] and also induce secretion of tumor necrosis factor alpha (TNF-α) by monocytes [3]. Furthermore, Mox-LDL has effects on platelet function by increasing the sensitivity of platelets to low levels of agonists [60]. It may cause irreversible aggregation of platelets and during atherosclerotic plaque rupture, leading to thrombus formation [61].

Oxidation of LDL adversely impacts HDL metabolism by inhibiting the activity of LCAT. This enzyme is essential for HDL maturation by mediating esterification of HDL-associated cholesterol before hepatic uptake. In case of loss of LCAT activity, the antiatherogenic reverse cholesterol transport pathway of HDL can be altered [62]. The anti-atherosclerotic effect of HDL can also be impaired when HDL is modified by MPO and its associated oxidants, as a result of the formation of Mox-HDL and a loss of cholesterol reverse transport [48].

The initial evidence for the formation of Mox-HDL came from studies showing the co-localization of HOCl-modified proteins with apoA-1 in human plaques and endothelial cells from atherosclerotic lesions, detectable even in the early stages of the disease [48]. Thus, this apoA-1 was found to be enriched in 3-nitro-tyrosine (NO_2-Tyr) and 3-chloro-tyrosine (Cl-Tyr), which are the markers of MPO activity [63]. The level of Cl-Tyr on apoA-1 is reported to be inversely proportional to its capacity to collect cholesterol from foam cells [64,65]. Indeed, HDL or lipid-free apoA-1 exposed to HOCl is less able to remove cholesterol from cells by the cell membrane transporter ABCA1 [66]. From a clinical point of view, the level of Cl-Tyr in apoA-1 is higher in patients with CAD than in healthy volunteers [64]. In addition, the content of MPO-modified apoA-1 in aortic lesions is correlated with the severity of the disease [67].

By regarding functional areas of apoA-1, such as binding site of MPO or the protein moiety responsible for LCAT activation, residues other than Tyr have been selected as specific markers for Mox-HDL, particularly Met and Trp, as outlined below. For example, differences between control subjects and patients with stable CAD or acute coronary syndrome have been established in relation to the presence of Cl-Tyr (at Tyr192) and the oxidation of Met (at Met 148) of apoA-1 [68]. The residue of Trp 72 also seems to be promising as a biomarker, since it is the subject of a multitude of studies that highlighted its importance in cholesterol efflux [44,68–71]. It must be noted that cholesterol efflux capacity is not completely dependent on levels of functional apoA-1 [72]. Extraction of

cholesterol from the human body is also impaired by the competition between Mox-HDL and native HDL to interact with the scavenger receptor B-1 (SR-B1) in the liver. Mox-HDL can also inhibit platelet activation via this scavenger receptor [73].

Furthermore, it is well established that Mox-HDL possesses pro-inflammatory characteristics. The antiapoptotic activity of HDL on endothelial cells is inhibited with MPO modification, notably by losing its capacity to inhibit caspase activation and to activate endothelial NO$^{•}$ synthase activity. In addition, Mox-HDL induces the expression of vascular cell adhesion molecule 1 in endothelial cells and promotes migration and extravasation of leukocytes across the vascular endothelium. These pro-inflammatory activities are related to the loss of interaction with SR-B1 [74].

Even if low HDL levels are associated with increased cardiovascular risk, the beneficial effects of HDL are maintained only if HDL is functional. For now, it is not possible to differentiate functional from dysfunctional HDLs in patients with high MPO activity. It is therefore necessary to monitor the quality of lipoproteins by developing new methods in order to complete the classic quantification. Mass spectrometry and immunological methods are still under investigation, as to which is able to provide the most reliable and convenient way to assess Mox-HDLs and Mox-LDLs in patients with CVDs.

ACTIVITY OF MPO ON LIPOPROTEINS

The interest in MPO activity in atherosclerotic lesions centers predominantly on the modification made to the protein moiety of lipoproteins via the MPO/H_2O_2/(pseudo)halide oxidative system [75]. The major oxidants produced by MPO and involved in lipoprotein modifications are hypochlorous acid (HOCl), hypothiocyanous acid (HOSCN), peroxynitrite and hypobromous acid (HOBr) [76,77]. In vivo, proteins are the major targets of MPO oxidants as their kinetic reactivity is typically more favorable for proteins, free amino acids and amino compounds, followed by antioxidants, lipids and nucleic acids [78].

The highly cationic character of MPO (pI > 10) enables its binding to electronegative molecules or surfaces such as the endothelial wall [8,79,80]. After intraluminal release from neutrophils, MPO binds to the vessel wall, where it accumulates along the endothelium and is transcytosed to the subendothelial space [8]. Furthermore, MPO rapidly adsorbs at the surface of lipoproteins and has a strong interaction with the protein moiety, owing to the anionic characteristic of lipoproteins [81,82].

The enzyme can associate and/or bind to the external and anionic parts of various apolipoproteins. The NH_2-$\beta\alpha$1 domain of apoB-100 from LDL has been characterized as suitable for MPO interaction. Currently, the only peptide able to form a complex with MPO identified in vitro is [445]EQIQDDCTGDED[456] [83]. Investigations are still ongoing concerning the exact binding sites of MPO on apoB-100, as it is a large protein with 4,536 amino acid residues [84]. It is likely that apoB-100 can bind more than one MPO and that LDL is the preferred target of MPO compared with HDL [41,81]. Whereas the binding site of MPO on apoA-1 from HDL was determined to be between residues Ala 190 and Leu 203 of the protein sequence of 245 amino acids [63].

In early studies, it was postulated that peroxidation of the lipoprotein lipid moiety was the initial step of a chain reaction leading to the transformation of the protein moiety. However, a study of LDL oxidation by HOCl shows the preferential oxidation of amino acid residues of apoB-100 compared with lipidic peroxidation. While Lys residues are quantitatively the major target, lipid oxidation is less favored than protein oxidation on comparing the amounts of lipid hydroperoxides, cholesterol or fatty acid oxidation products formed [52]. It was shown that after the initial oxidation of the protein moiety such as at Lys residues, the production of chloramines and their subsequent decomposition to radicals initiate the lipid peroxidation [85].

Once bound on apolipoproteins, MPO oxidation occurs predominantly on the protein moieties such as apoB-100 in LDL and apoA-1 in HDL. As the major oxidant produced, HOCl is produced locally and reacts with amino acids [86]. Depending on the reactivity of the amino acids with HOCl, there is a disparity among the targeted residues. First, sulfur amino acids such as free Cys or Met are oxidized ($k \sim 10^8$ $M^{-1}s^{-1}$) [6]. Cys residues contain a free thiol group and are the most easily oxidized site in protein. Cys residues are one of the first targeted residues by MPO modification, unless they are already involved in disulfide bridge [87]. Met residues are more accessible and are highly oxidizable,

making methionine sulfoxide (ox-Met) a major oxidation product of HOCl in biological media [88]. The ability of sulfur compounds to moderate MPO activity is frequently highlighted, and Met has been postulated to act as a sacrificial antioxidant against protein oxidation [89].

The reactivity of HOCl with other nucleophiles, including Trp and terminal amines, occurs at k-values of $\sim 10^4$–10^5 $M^{-1}s^{-1}$ [6]. With HOCl, Lys and His become chloramines that can oxidize other compounds [90]. Lys and His residues are sensitive to MPO oxidation but are not selectively targeted. Indeed, they can be found in patients in hemodialysis, with a high MPO activity, as well in healthy volunteers without cardiovascular risk [91]. Some amino acids are less reactive with HOCl, such as Tyr, but nevertheless their oxidation is significant (Figure 7.2). In this case, the products of their reaction are considered as hallmarks of inflammatory tissue injury and are detected during inflammation. Cl-Tyr is the first residue to have been described as a specific product of MPO oxidation [92]. Tyrosine is modified on the phenol containing side chain to result in the formation of chlorinated derivatives (Cl-Tyr and 3,5-di-chloro-tyrosine). Nitrated derivatives (e.g. NO_2Tyr) have also been observed, formed by consumption of nitric oxide by reactive species, when HOCl reacts with nitrite (NO_2^-) or peroxynitrite ($ONOO^-$) in nitrous species.

Oxidation of Trp is a good compromise between sensitivity and specificity to MPO oxidation. Its reactivity with HOCl is more rapidly than that of Tyr ($k \sim 44$ $M^{-1}s^{-1}$), and some Trp residues seem particularly sensitive to MPO oxidation [44,86]. Trp can be modified by MPO on its indole ring side chain. The benzene portion can be mono- or doubly oxidized (5-mono or 5,7-dihydroxytryptophan) and the pyrrole moiety can be monooxidized (2-oxo-tryptophan in equilibrium with 2-hydroxy-tryptophan). Besides hydroxytryptophans, N-formyl-kynurenine and kynurenine forms can also be produced [93].

Hazen et al. (1997) [92] identified Cl-Tyr as a "molecular fingerprint" for MPO-catalyzed oxidation, present in multiple proteins isolated from human atherosclerotic lesions and highly abundant in LDLs. Indeed, MPO is the only known human enzyme able to produce HOCl that chlorinates Tyr. The formation of Cl-Tyr is not the only product of MPO activity, for both LDL and HDL. For example, concerning MPO-modified

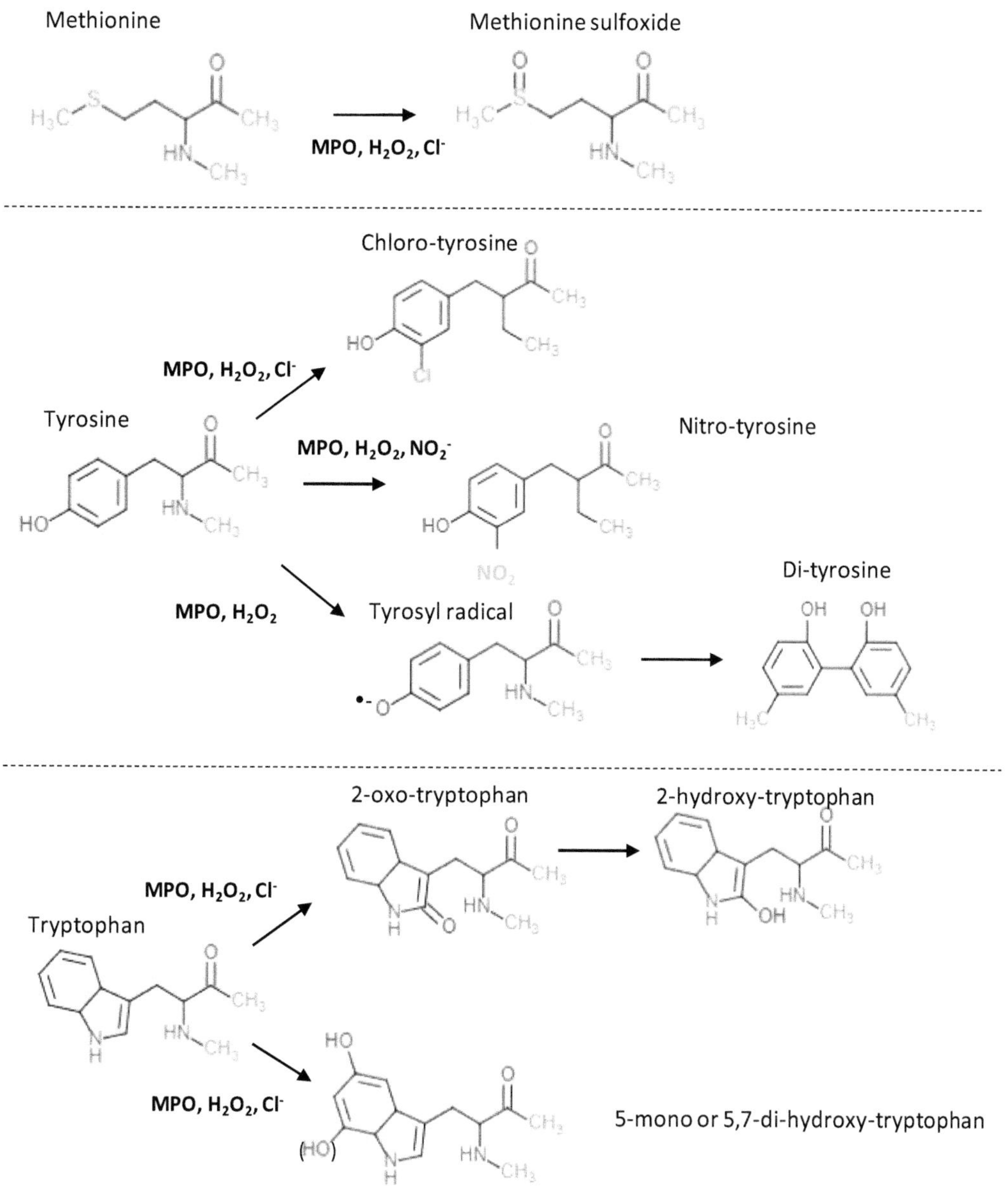

Figure 7.2 Major modifications involving MPO on methionine, tyrosine and tryptophan residues.

(Mox-)HDL, Trp 72 and Tyr 192 are reported to most clinically relevant modifications of apoA-1 and considered as a the marker of atherosclerotic activity of MPO and HDL dysfunction [94–98].

Modifications of Apolipoprotein A-1

Bergt et al. (2000) [95] have demonstrated that modifications of lipid-free apoA-1 lead to the loss of apoA-1 Met residues, consistent with the high sensitivity of Met to the MPO/H$_2$O$_2$/Cl$^-$ system. Mass spectrometry identifies five tryptic fragments consistent with the formation of Met sulfoxide for three fragments and chlorination of other residues [99]. Using model peptides, Bergt et al. (2004) [100] also reported that Lys residues are involved in the regiospecific formation of Cl-Tyr by MPO through HOCl, in a YXXK/KXXY peptide motif by intermediate production of chloramine. The local secondary structure is also a key factor controlling the reactivity of protein-bound amino acids. The helical wheel representation of amphipathic helices predicts that Tyr and Lys residues in the YXXK and KXXY motif lie next to each other on the same face of the α-helix. Bergt suggests a single Tyr residue (Tyr 192), to be the major site of chlorination by HOCl and resides in the YXXK motif [100].

Shao et al. (2005) [96] compared both chlorination and nitration of apoA-1. If Tyr 192 is the single major target in lipid-free apoA-1 for nitration, the presence of lipid seems to modify the accessibility of Tyr 192 to the aqueous environment and can reduce its nitration level. Therefore, lipid-poor apoA-1, the biologically active ligand for ATP-binding cassette A1 receptor (ABCA1), was postulated to be the major target for nitration in the artery wall and the primary target for oxidation [96]. When Tyr 192 is chlorinated, the ability of apoA-1 to promote ABCA1-dependent cholesterol efflux is impaired. In contrast, nitration of Tyr 192 had little impact on this biological function [96]. Zheng et al. (2005) [65] have shown that plasma levels of NO_2Tyr and Cl-Tyr in apoA-1 are higher in patients with CAD than in healthy subjects, suggesting their clinical relevance. Chlorination of Tyr residues of apoA-1, either in endogenous plasma or after MPO-induced modification in vitro, is associated with the specific loss of ABCA1-induced cholesterol acceptor activity (see also above) [65,69].

In order to determine whether oxidative modifications of apoA-1 Tyr residues are responsible for the MPO-mediated inactivation of cholesterol acceptor activity, Peng et al. (2005) [70] made recombinant apoA-1 by substituting seven Tyr residues with Phe. Compared with native apoA-1, the recombinant protein was equally susceptible to dose-dependent MPO-mediated loss of ABCA1-dependent cholesterol acceptor activity. Thus, Tyr chlorination is not required either for MPO-mediated loss of the cholesterol acceptor activity of apoA-1 nor for lipid-binding activity. It is noteworthy that MPO also targeted apoA-1 Trp and Lys residues. In 2008, Peng et al. [101] tested different modifications of apoA-1 residues to evaluate their impact on apoA-1 activities. The Lys modification by MPO seemed to have a modest influence on apoA-1 function, since reductive methylation of Lys primary amine groups into tertiary amines decreases the reactivity with HOCl, but did not lead to protection of apoA-1 function. The substitution of Met and Try residues (with among

them mutation of Trp 72) by using recombinant human apoA-1 proves to be more functionally important. Thus, the Met residues in apoA-1 seem to play a protective role by scavenging oxidants [102]. The four Trp residues studied (cf Table 7.1) were replaced by Phe. This variant was competent for physiological lipidation by cellular ABCA1 and was equally competent compared with wild-type apoA-1 in terms of its ability to interact with lipids. However, the ABCA1-dependent cholesterol acceptor activity of wild-type apoA-1 was inhibited by MPO oxidation while the variant maintained its activity even with a high concentration of H_2O_2. The result was the same with HOCl treatment. The lipid-binding activity of the variant apoA-1 is also resistant to MPO-mediated inhibition. However, this variant was more susceptible to MPO-induced cross-linking with the loss of α-helical content in the apoA-1 structure.

Huang et al. (2014) [44] have developed a high-affinity monoclonal antibody specifically recognizing apoA-1/HDL modified by the MPO/H_2O_2/Cl⁻ system. They demonstrated that the oxindolyl alanine residue (2-OH-Trp) corresponding to Trp 72 of apoA-1 is the immunogenic epitope. ApoA-1 in the blood circulation shows little 2-OH-Trp 72, but 20% of the apoA-1 in atherosclerotic plaque contained this modified Trp 72. This modified apoA-1 was characterized as being low in lipids, devoid of cholesterol acceptor activity and having a potent pro-inflammatory activity on endothelial cells [44]. In addition, the biogenesis of HDL was impaired. In clinical settings, high levels of oxTrp 72-apoA-1 have been associated with an increased risk of CVD [44]. Huang concludes that circulating levels of 2-OH-Trp 72-apoA1 can be used to monitor pro-atherogenic process in the artery wall [44].

More recently, incorporation of site-specific oxTrp (including Trp 72) into apoA-1 has been performed [71]. By using genetic code expansion technology, noncanonical amino acid 5-hydroxytryptophan (5-OH-Trp) has been inserted at position 72 in recombinant human apoA-1. A significant impairment of in vitro cholesterol acceptor activity and in vivo HDL biogenesis function was observed with recombinant apoA-1 compared with wild-type apoA-1. However, site-specific incorporation of 5-OH-Trp at amino acid position 72 does not make apoA-1 pro-inflammatory, compared with MPO-modified apoA-1, which includes a large amount of 2-OH-Trp as described above.

TABLE 7.1
Summary of interesting modified residues on apoA-I

Reference	Tested condition	Modification	Modified residues
Bergt 2000 [99]	ApoA-1 and HDL treated with MPO/H_2O_2/Cl⁻	Chlorophenylalanine Methionine sulfoxide	Phe 57, Phe 71 Met 86, Met 112, Met 148
Bergt 2004 [100]	HDL treated with HOCl (80:1, mol/mol, oxidant/HDL particle)	Chlorotyrosine	Tyr 192, Tyr 236, Tyr 29, Tyr 18, Tyr 100, Tyr 115, Tyr 166
Shao 2005 [96]	ApoA-1 treated with MPO/H_2O_2/NO_2^- or ONOO⁻	Nitrotyrosine	Tyr 192, Tyr 18, Tyr 29, Tyr 236, Tyr 100, Tyr 115, Tyr 166
		Nitrotyrosine, Methionine sulfoxide	Met 112 and Tyr 115 (single peptide)
	HDL treated with MPO/H_2O_2/Cl⁻ or HOCl	Chlorotyrosine	Tyr 192
	HDL treated with MPO/H_2O_2/NO_2^-	Nitrotyrosine	Tyr 18, Tyr 29, Tyr 236, Tyr 100
	HDL treated with ONOO⁻		Tyr 192, Tyr 18, Tyr 29, Tyr 236, Tyr 115, Tyr 166
Zheng 2005 [65]	HDL treated with MPO/H_2O_2 (<50 μM)/NO_2^-	Nitrotyrosine	Tyr 192, Tyr 166
	HDL treated with MPO/H_2O_2 (<100 μM)/NO_2^-		Tyr 192, Tyr 166, Tyr 29, Tyr 236
	HDL treated with 100 μM peroxynitrite		Tyr 166, Tyr 18, Tyr 236
	HDL treated with MPO/H_2O_2 (<50 μM)/Cl⁻	Chlorotyrosine	Tyr 192, Tyr 166
	HDL treated with MPO/H_2O_2 (<100 μM)/Cl⁻		Tyr 192, Tyr 166, Tyr 29, Tyr 236
	HDL treated with 100 μM HOCl		Tyr 192, Tyr 166, Tyr 29, Tyr 236
	ApoA-1 in vivo	Nitrotyrosine	Tyr 192, Tyr 166
		Chlorotyrosine	Tyr 166
Shao 2006 [115]	ApoA-1 treated with MPO/H_2O_2/Cl⁻	Chlorotyrosine Methionine sulfoxide	Tyr 192
Peng 2008 [101]	ApoA-1 isolated from human atheroma tissue	Monohydroxytryptophan	Trp 8, Trp 50, Trp 72, Trp 108,
		Dihydroxytryptophan	Trp 108
		Methionine sulfoxide	Met 48, Met 112
		2-Aminoadipic acid	Lysine
Huang 2014 [44]	ApoA-1 isolated from human atheroma tissue	Oxidized tryptophan	Trp 72

Modifications of Apolipoprotein B-100

If apoA-1 is a well-characterized MPO-modified protein, MPO-dependent modifications of apoB-100 still need to be studied further. Early studies by Yang et al. [103] in 1999 described the formation of 2,4-dinitrophenylhydrazine (DNPH)-reactive modifications of apoB-100 following exposure of LDL to MPO in vitro. A major tryptic peptide was highlighted and characterized as VELEVPQLSFILK, corresponding to amino acid residues 53–66 on apoB-100, and mass spectrometry indicated formation of a Met sulfoxide. It was the first study to demonstrate that modifications in addition to aldehydes and ketones are formed during LDL oxidation by MPO-derived oxidants. These data also suggested a direct interaction of the LDL particle with the active site of MPO. They identified 14 tryptic peptides by using LDL oxidized by HOCl. They succeeded in determining oxidized Cys (Cys 61/185/234/451/4190/3734/3890), Lys (Lys 120), Trp (Trp 1114/1210/1893/3567) and Met (Met 3569) [104]. Most of these peptides are located on the LDL surface. They noted that previous experiments with LDL oxidized by copper provided good experimental insights into the chemistry of LDL oxidations but were not relevant in vivo. Following these results, they studied selective in vitro oxidations of apoB-100 by MPO [105]. Two tryptic peptides were highlighted, determined by amino acids 1–14 (EEEMLENVSLVCPK) and 53–66 (VELEVPQLCSFILK). They described previously the linkage of these peptides by a disulfide bond between their Cys residues in native LDL [106]. They proposed that the modification of Met 4 was a selective oxidation by MPO.

Some residues have been identified depending on their location and their functional area on apoB-100. The LDL receptor-binding domain of apoB-100 is an important functional site [107]. In order to determine the mutation responsible of familial defective apoB-100, Boren et al. (1998) analyzed LDL receptor-binding site in apoB-100 [108] (Figure 7.2). By using bacteriophage clone technology and producing transgenic mice with mutant apo-B protein, they identified a domain (residues 3,359–3,369) with a significant functionality in receptor binding. Besides the first mutation in apoB-100 being identified and characterized, p.(Arg3527Gln), Fernández-Higuero et al. (2015) [109] analyzed the structure of two recent pathogenic apoB-100 variants that have been described: p.(Arg1164Thr) and p.(Gln4494del), which showed impaired LDL receptor (LDLr) binding capacity and diminished LDL uptake. Therefore, it could be interesting to investigate and monitor residues that can be targeted by MPO activity, such as Trp or Met residues. The evaluation of the impact of their modification on the interaction between LDL and LDLr could provide clarifications about pro-atherogenic LDL.

Hamilton et al. (2008) [110] revealed specific modifications (nitration and oxidation) in the apoB-100 moiety of in vivo LDL, such as Tyr 103/413/666/2524/3490/3791/4088 and Phe 3965. Tyrosine nitration and lipid peroxidation seemed to disturb the phospholipid belt of LDL and hydrophobic stacking of aromatic amino acids in the lipid core. This disturbance was postulated to induce α-helices to adopt a new conformation leading to protein unfolding, which may contribute to more atherogenic LDLs.

Chakraborty et al. (2010) identified a typical footprint of MPO-modified apoB-100 [111]. By inducing modification of apoB-100 with peroxynitrite, HOCl and other reactive species such as hydroxyl radicals, they have characterized different modified amino acids [112]. Tyr 583 and Trp 2524 were oxidized by hydroxyl radicals and peroxynitrite. Tyr 144, Tyr 276, Tyr 4451 and Tyr 4509 were oxidized by hydroxyl radicals and HOCl. Tyr 3295 was oxidized by all three oxidants. This suggests a common mechanism of oxidation related to early events in atherosclerosis. However, their attempt to quantify relative oxidation of specific amino acid residues in apoB-100 revealed that this dataset was not optimal for quantitative assessments due to variations in the retention times of the peptides. At high HOCl treatment of 1:10 (HOCl:protein, m/m), two oxidations – Tyr 3139 and Trp 3153 – were observed in the LDL receptor-binding region of apoB-100. Moreover, the analysis of Trp 4369 was relevant to modifications that occur in familial hypercholesterolemia. Indeed, Boren et al. (1998) proposed that the carboxyl terminus of apoB-100 interacts with Arg 3500 to permit normal interaction between LDL and LDLr. The loss of Arg at this site destabilizes this interaction, resulting in receptor-binding defective LDL [108]. Therefore, oxidation of residues such as Trp 4369, located near the binding site of LDL, could modify interaction between receptors and apoB-100. These oxidations could alter LDLr binding and prove major players in early events in atherosclerotic plaque formation.

We investigated the interaction of MPO with native and modified LDLs and revealed oxidative modifications on apoB-100 in vitro (by HOCl or MPO/H_2O_2/Cl$^-$ system) and in vivo (Table 7.2) [113]. Altogether, more than 97 peptides containing modified residues could be identified. Depending on the oxidation system used, differences were observed between the chemical HOCl reagent and the HOCl generated by the MPO/H_2O_2/Cl$^-$ system, as the field of action of HOCl produced by MPO is dependent on its adsorption zone (Figure 7.3). To confirm the results obtained in vitro, LDLs isolated from patients at high cardiovascular risk were also analyzed and principle residues of interest were highlighted. Among the peptide residues

TABLE 7.2
Summary of interesting modified residues on apoB-100 from literature

Tested conditions	Modifications	Modified residues	Reference
LDL oxidized by HOCl	oxCys	Cys61/185/234/451/4190/3734/3890	[104]
	oxLys	Lys120	
	oxTrp	Trp1114/1210/1893/3567	
	oxMet	Met3569	
ApoB-100 in vitro by MPO	oxMet4	[1]EEEMLENVSLVCPK[14]	[105]
LDL in vivo	oxTy	Tyr 103/413/666/2524/3490/3791/4088	[110]
	oxPhe	Phe 3965	
Hydroxyl radical and peroxynitrite	oxTy	Tyr 583 and Trp 2524	[111]
	oxTrp		
Hydroxyl radical and HOCl	oxTy	Tyr 144, Tyr 276, Tyr 4451 and Tyr 4509	
Hydroxyl radical and peroxynitrite and HOCl	oxTy	Tyr 3295	
HOCl	oxTyr	Tyr 3139 and Trp 3153	
	oxTrp		
	oxTrp	Trp 4369	
Patients and volunteers	oxMet	Met 4/4192	[91]
	oxTrp	Trp 1114/3536	
Patient only	oxMet	Met 2499	
	oxTrp	Trp 2894/3606	
	Cl-Tyr	Tyr 76/102/125/749	
	dioxTrp	Trp 4369	

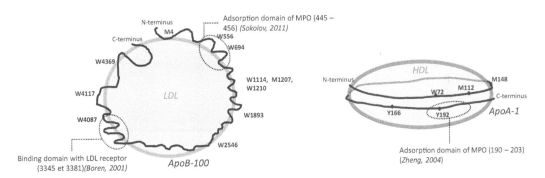

Figure 7.3 MPO modifications of interest in apolipoprotein B-100 (LDL) and A-1 (HDL) involved in biological modification of lipoproteins. Functional domains on these proteins such as adsorption are of MPO or binding area with receptor.

sensitive to oxidation of the MPO were Met 4/4192 and Trp 1114/3536. These modified residues are also observed in healthy volunteers but to a lesser extent, making them nonspecific. More specific residues, whose changes were only observed in patients, have been highlighted, such as oxidized Met 2499, Trp 2894/3606, Cl-Tyr 76/102/125/749 and dihydroxy-Trp 4369.

It has also been pointed out in the literature that HOCl, added as a reagent, does not completely mimic the enzymatic activity of the MPO/H_2O_2/Cl system [114]. Indeed, the MPO activity could be underestimated, because of its specific interaction with apoB-100, which modifies its conformation and its enzymatic activity. Indeed, the chlorinating activity of MPO increases when it adsorbs at the surface of LDLs, resulting in local structural changes [91]. Furthermore, Sokolov et al. (2010) [41] suggested that MPO interacted more strongly with LDL than with HDL.

In summary, oxidized residues of apo-A1 and apoB-100 are present in patients with cardiovascular risk or diseases, and further researches are needed to investigate the clinical relevance of their deleterious effects *in vivo*. Moreover, MPO plasma concentration is correlated to cardiovascular risk, and its activity is likely linked to oxidation, chlorination and nitration of lipoproteins, such as LDL and HDL. Therefore, and in addition to studying classical risk factors to assess cardiovascular risk, evaluation of causal factors of atherosclerosis such as MPO-oxidized apoB-100 and apoA-1 could bring additional information to better assess the cardiovascular risk.

CONCLUSION

In this chapter, the impact of MPO activity on lipoprotein oxidation has been discussed in the context of CVD. MPO produces Mox-LDLs and Mox-HDLs principally by targeting the protein moieties to impair the physiological roles of these lipoproteins and to promote atherosclerosis and more generally CVD. Indeed, Mox-LDLs have a higher pro-atherogenic properties than native LDLs, and Mox-HDLs lose the antiatherogenic properties of HDLs (lipid poor apoA-1 particles). They both contribute to the maintenance of the inflammatory disease. While researchers have investigated the modifications present on both Mox-LDLs and Mox-HDLs, the role of several modifications on the physiopathology is still unclear and remains a key topic to investigate. Furthermore, it would be interesting to monitor modifications on LDLs/HDLs in large cohort patients for a future better risk assessment of CVD in patients.

REFERENCES

1. K. Husain et al. 2015. Inflammation, oxidative stress and renin angiotensin system in atherosclerosis. *World J. Biol. Chem.* 6: 209–217.
2. P. Libby et al. 2010. Inflammation in Atherosclerosis. *Circ. J.* 74: 213–220.
3. K. Z. Boudjeltia et al. 2006. Triggering of inflammatory response by myeloperoxidase-oxidized LDL. *Biochem. Cell Biol.* 84: 805–812.
4. R. Ganesan et al. 2018. Oxidized LDL phagocytosis during foam cell formation in atherosclerotic plaques relies on a PLD2–CD36 functional interdependence. *J. Leukoc. Biol.* 103: 867–883.
5. A. Daugherty et al. 1994. Myeloperoxidase, a catalyst for lipoprotein oxidation, is expressed in human atherosclerotic lesions. *J. Clin. Invest.* 94: 437–444.
6. N. Teng et al. 2017. The roles of myeloperoxidase in coronary artery disease and its potential implication in plaque rupture. *Redox Rep.* 22: 51–73.
7. V. Loria et al. 2008. Myeloperoxidase: A new biomarker of inflammation in ischemic heart disease and acute coronary syndromes. *Mediators Inflamm.* 2008: 135625.
8. K. Manchanda et al. 2018. MPO (Myeloperoxidase) reduces endothelial glycocalyx thickness dependent on its cationic charge. *Arterioscler. Thromb. Vasc. Biol.* 38: 1859–1867.
9. B. S. Rayner, D. T. Love, and C. L. Hawkins 2014. Comparative reactivity of myeloperoxidase-derived oxidants with mammalian cells. *Free Radic. Biol. Med.* 71: 240–255.
10. A. Alipour et al. 2013. Trans-vessel gradient of myeloperoxidase in coronary artery disease. *Eur. J. Clin. Invest.* 43: 920–925.
11. A. Trentini et al. 2020. Development, optimization and validation of an absolute specific assay for active myeloperoxidase (MPO) and its application in a clinical context: Role of MPO specific activity in coronary artery disease. *Clin. Chem. Lab. Med.* 58: 1749–1758.
12. T. J. Mocatta et al. 2007. Plasma concentrations of myeloperoxidase predict mortality after myocardial infarction. *J. Am. Coll. Cardiol.* 49: 1993–2000.
13. T. Franck et al. 2009. A new easy method for specific measurement of active myeloperoxidase in human biological fluids and tissue extracts. *Talanta* 80: 723–729.
14. Y. Chu et al. 2015. Myeloperoxidase is increased in human cerebral aneurysms and increases formation and rupture of cerebral aneurysms in mice. *Stroke* 46: 1651–1656.
15. E. Kimak et al. 2018. Myeloperoxidase level and inflammatory markers and lipid and lipoprotein parameters in stable coronary artery disease. *Lipids Health Dis.* 17: 71.
16. I. S. Khalilova et al. 2018. A myeloperoxidase precursor, promyeloperoxidase, is present in human plasma and elevated in cardiovascular disease patients. *PLoS One* 13: e0192952.
17. W. M. Nauseef 2018. Biosynthesis of human myeloperoxidase. *Arch. Biochem. Biophys.* 642: 1–9.

18. B. U. Goldmann et al. 2009. Neutrophil activation precedes myocardial injury in patients with acute myocardial infarction. *Free Radic. Biol. Med.* 47: 79–83.

19. W. H. W. Tang et al. 2011. Plasma myeloperoxidase predicts incident cardiovascular risks in stable patients undergoing medical management for coronary artery disease. *Clin. Chem.* 57: 33–39.

20. D. Kutter et al. 2000. Consequences of total and subtotal myeloperoxidase deficiency: Risk or benefit ? *Acta Haematol.* 104: 10–15.

21. B. Nikpoor et al. 2001. A functional myeloperoxidase polymorphic variant is associated with coronary artery disease in French-Canadians. *Am. Heart J.* 142: 336–339.

22. F. W. Asselbergs et al. 2004. Myeloperoxidase polymorphism related to cardiovascular events in coronary artery disease. *Am. J. Med.* 116: 429–430.

23. S. Baldus et al. 2003. Myeloperoxidase serum levels predict risk in patients with acute coronary syndromes. *Circulation* 108: 1440–1445.

24. R. K. Schindhelm et al. 2009. Myeloperoxidase: A useful biomarker for cardiovascular disease risk stratification? *Clin. Chem.* 55: 1462–1470.

25. F. R. Tavora et al. 2009. Monocytes and neutrophils expressing myeloperoxidase occur in fibrous caps and thrombi in unstable coronary plaques. *BMC Cardiovasc. Disord.* 9: 27.

26. L. Vanhamme et al. 2018. The other myeloperoxidase: Emerging functions. *Arch. Biochem. Biophys.* 649: 1–14.

27. V. Papayannopoulos 2017. Neutrophil extracellular traps in immunity and disease. *Nat. Rev. Immunol.* 18: 134–147.

28. V. Brinkmann et al. 2004. Neutrophil extracellular traps kill bacteria. *Science* 303: 1532–1535.

29. T. Josefs et al. 2020. Neutrophil extracellular traps promote macrophage inflammation and impair atherosclerosis resolution in diabetic mice. *JCI Insight* 5: e134796.

30. A. H. B. Wu 2005. Markers for early detection of cardiac diseases. *Scand. J. Clin. Lab. Invest.* 65: 112–121.

31. A. Warnatsch et al. 2015. Neutrophil extracellular traps license macrophages for cytokine production in atherosclerosis. *Science* 349: 316–320.

32. J. J. Yang et al. 2001. Internalization of proteinase 3 is concomitant with endothelial cell apoptosis and internalization of myeloperoxidase with generation of intracellular oxidants. *Am. J. Pathol.* 158: 581–592.

33. G. La Rocca et al. 2009. Oxidative stress induces myeloperoxidase expression in endocardial endothelial cells from patients with chronic heart failure. *Basic Res. Cardiol.* 104: 307–320.

34. A. Khalil et al. 2018. Myeloperoxidase promotes tube formation, triggers ERK1/2 and Akt pathways and is expressed endogenously in endothelial cells. *Arch. Biochem. Biophys.* 654: 55–69.

35. B. H. J. Bielski and A. O. Allen 1977. Mechanism of the disproportionation of superoxide radicals. *J. Phys. Chem.* 81: 1048–1050.

36. S. J. Klebanoff et al. 2013. Myeloperoxidase: A front-line defender against phagocytosed microorganisms. *J. Leukoc. Biol.* 93: 185–198.

37. H. Li, S. Horke, and U. Förstermann 2014. Vascular oxidative stress, nitric oxide and atherosclerosis. *Atherosclerosis* 237: 208–219.

38. D. Sorescu et al. 2002. Superoxide production and expression of Nox family proteins in human atherosclerosis. *Circulation* 105: 1429–1435.

39. J. A. Holland, L. M. Ziegler, and J. W. Meyer 1996. Atherogenic levels of low-density lipoprotein increase hydrogen peroxide generation in cultured human endothelial cells: Possible mechanism of heightened endocytosis. *J. Cell. Physiol.* 166: 144–151.

40. K. Zouaoui Boudjeltia et al. 2004. Oxidation of low density lipoproteins by myeloperoxidase at the surface of endothelial cells: An additional mechanism to subendothelium oxidation. *Biochem. Biophys. Res. Commun.* 325: 434–438.

41. A. V. Sokolov et al. 2010. Identification and properties of complexes formed by myeloperoxidase with lipoproteins and ceruloplasmin. *Chem. Phys. Lipids* 163: 347–355.

42. L. Yetukuri et al. 2010. Composition and lipid spatial distribution of HDL particles in subjects with low and high HDL-cholesterol. *J. Lipid Res.* 51: 2341–2351.

43. A. Kontush et al. 2015. Structure of HDL: Particle subclasses and molecular components. *Handb. Exp. Pharmacol.* 224: 3–51.

44. Y. Huang et al. 2014. An abundant dysfunctional apolipoprotein A1 in human atheroma. *Nat. Med.* 20: 193–203.

45. G.-J. Zhao et al. 2012. The interaction of ApoA-I and ABCA1 triggers signal transduction pathways to mediate efflux of cellular lipids. *Mol. Med.* 18: 149–158.

46. J. F. Oram 2003. HDL Apolipoproteins and ABCA1. *Arterioscler. Thromb. Vasc. Biol.* 23: 720–727.

47. K. R. Feingold and C. Grunfeld 2000. Introduction to lipids and lipoproteins. MDText. com, Inc. https://www.ncbi.nlm.nih.gov/books/NBK305896/.

48. E. Malle et al. 2006. Myeloperoxidase-mediated oxidation of high-density lipoproteins: Fingerprints of newly recognized potential proatherogenic lipoproteins. *Arch. Biochem. Biophys.* 445: 245–255.

49. N. Moguilevsky et al. 2004. Monoclonal antibodies against LDL progressively oxidized by myeloperoxidase react with ApoB-100 protein moiety and human atherosclerotic lesions. *Biochem. Biophys. Res. Commun.* 323: 1223–1228.

50. L. J. Hazell and R. Stocker 1993. Oxidation of low-density lipoprotein with hypochlorite causes transformation of the lipoprotein into a high-uptake form for macrophages. *Biochem. J.* 290: 165–172.

51. G. Marsche et al. 2003. Class B scavenger receptors CD36 and SR-BI are receptors for hypochlorite-modified low density lipoprotein. *J. Biol. Chem.* 278: 47562–47570.

52. L. J. Hazell, J. J. M. van den Berg, and R. Stocker 1994. Oxidation of low-density lipoprotein by hypochlorite causes aggregation that is mediated by modification of lysine residues rather than lipid oxidation. *Biochem. J.* 302: 297–304.

53. W. Li et al. 1998. Uptake of oxidized LDL by macrophages results in partial lysosomal enzyme inactivation and relocation. *Arterioscler. Thromb. Vasc. Biol.* 18: 177–184.

54. A. C. Carr 2001. Hypochlorous acid-modified low-density lipoprotein inactivates the lysosomal protease cathepsin B: Protection by ascorbic and lipoic acids. *Redox Rep.* 6: 343–349.

55. R. Stocker and J. F. Keaney 2004. Role of oxidative modifications in atherosclerosis. *Physiol. Rev.* 84: 1381–1478.

56. C. Woenckhaus et al. 1998. Hypochlorite-modified LDL: Chemotactic potential and chemokine induction in human monocytes. *Clin. Immunol. Immunopathol.* 86: 27–33.

57. J. P. Eiserich et al. 2002. Myeloperoxidase, a leukocyte-derived vascular NO oxidase. *Science* 296: 2391–2394.

58. A. I. Abdo et al. 2017. Low-density lipoprotein modified by myeloperoxidase oxidants induces endothelial dysfunction. *Redox Biol.* 13: 623–632.

59. T. Nguyen-Khoa et al. 1999. Oxidized low-density lipoprotein induces macrophage respiratory burst via its protein moiety: A novel pathway in atherogenesis? *Biochem. Biophys. Res. Commun.* 263: 804–809.

60. J. A. M. Relou et al. 2003. Low-density lipoprotein and its effect on human blood platelets. *Cell. Mol. Life Sci.* 60: 961–971.

61. L. G. Coleman et al. 2004. LDL oxidized by hypochlorous acid causes irreversible platelet aggregation when combined with low levels of ADP, thrombin, epinephrine, or macrophage-derived chemokine (CCL22). *Blood* 104: 380–389.

62. M. R. McCall et al. 2001. LDL modified by hypochlorous acid is a potent inhibitor of lecithin-cholesterol acyltransferase activity. *Arterioscler. Thromb. Vasc. Biol.* 21: 1040–1045.

63. L. Zheng et al. 2004. Apolipoprotein A-I is a selective target for myeloperoxidase-catalyzed oxidation and functional impairment in subjects with cardiovascular disease. *J. Clin. Invest.* 114: 529–541.

64. S. Pennathur et al. 2004. Human atherosclerotic intima and blood of patients with established coronary artery disease contain high density lipoprotein damaged by reactive nitrogen species. *J. Biol. Chem.* 279: 42977–42983.

65. L. Zheng et al. 2005. Localization of nitration and chlorination sites on apolipoprotein A-I catalyzed by myeloperoxidase in human atheroma and associated oxidative impairment in. *J. Biol. Chem.* 280(1): 38–47.

66. C. Bergt et al. 2004. The myeloperoxidase product hypochlorous acid oxidizes HDL in the human artery wall and impairs ABCA1-dependent cholesterol transport. *Proc. Natl. Acad. Sci. U.S.A.* 101: 13032–13037.

67. G. Pankhurst et al. 2003. Characterization of specifically oxidized apolipoproteins in mildly oxidized high density lipoprotein. *J. Lipid Res.* 44: 349–355.

68. B. Shao et al. 2014. Humans with atherosclerosis have impaired ABCA1 cholesterol efflux and enhanced high-density lipoprotein oxidation by myeloperoxidase. *Circ. Res.* 114: 1733–1742.

69. B. Shao et al. 2006. Myeloperoxidase impairs ABCA1-dependent cholesterol efflux through methionine oxidation and site-specific tyrosine chlorination of apolipoprotein A-I. *J. Biol. Chem.* 281: 9001–9004.

70. D.-Q. Peng et al. 2005. Tyrosine modification is not required for myeloperoxidase-induced loss of apolipoprotein A-I functional activities. *J. Biol. Chem.* 280: 33775–33784.

71. M. Zamanian-Daryoush et al. 2020. Site-specific 5-hydroxytryptophan incorporation into apolipoprotein A-I impairs cholesterol efflux activity and high-density lipoprotein biogenesis. *J. Biol. Chem.* 295: 4836–4848.

72. A. V Khera et al. 2011. Cholesterol efflux capacity, high-density lipoprotein function, and atherosclerosis. *N. Engl. J. Med.* 364: 127–135.

73. M. Valiyaveettil et al. 2008. Oxidized high-density lipoprotein inhibits platelet activation and aggregation via scavenger receptor BI. *Blood* 111: 1962–1971.

74. A. Urundhati et al. 2009. Modification of high density lipoprotein by myeloperoxidase generates a pro-inflammatory particle. *J. Biol. Chem.* 284: 30825–30835.

75. E. Malle et al. 2000. Immunohistochemical evidence for the myeloperoxidase/H_2O_2/halide system in human atherosclerotic lesions. *Eur. J. Biochem.* 267: 4495–4503.

76. M. J. Davies 2011. Myeloperoxidase-derived oxidation: Mechanisms of biological damage and its prevention. *J. Clin. Biochem. Nutr.* 48: 8–19.

77. C. N. Koyani et al. 2015. Myeloperoxidase scavenges peroxynitrite: A novel anti-inflammatory action of the heme enzyme. *Arch. Biochem. Biophys.* 571: 1–9.

78. D. I. Pattison, C. L. Hawkins, and M. J. Davies 2009. What are the plasma targets of the oxidant hypochlorous acid? A kinetic modeling approach. *Chem. Res. Toxicol.* 22: 807–817.

79. A. L. P. Chapman et al. 2013. Ceruloplasmin is an endogenous inhibitor of myeloperoxidase. *J. Biol. Chem.* 288: 6465–6477.

80. E. M. Daphna et al. 1998. Association of myeloperoxidase with heparin: Oxidative inactivation of proteins on the surface of endothelial cells by the bound enzyme. *Mol. Cell. Biochem.* 183(1–2): 55–61.

81. A. C. Carr et al. 2000. Myeloperoxidase binds to low-density lipoprotein: Potential implications for atherosclerosis. *FEBS Lett.* 487: 176–180.

82. C. Delporte et al. 2013. Low-density lipoprotein modified by myeloperoxidase in inflammatory pathways and clinical studies. *Mediators Inflamm.* 2013: 971579.

83. A. V Sokolov et al. 2011. Revealing binding sites for myeloperoxidase on the surface of human low density lipoproteins. *Chem. Phys. Lipids* 164: 49–53.

84. C. Cladaras et al. 1986. The complete sequence and structural analysis of human apolipoprotein B-100: Relationship between apoB-100 and apoB-48 forms. *EMBO J.* 5: 3495–3507.

85. L. J. Hazell, M. J. Davies, and R. Stocker 1999. Secondary radicals derived from chloramines of apolipoprotein B-100 contribute to HOCl-induced lipid peroxidation of low-density lipoproteins. *Biochem. J.* 339: 489–495.

86. E. Malle et al. 2006. Modification of low-density lipoprotein by myeloperoxidase-derived oxidants and reagent hypochlorous acid. *Biochem. Biophys. Acta* 1761: 392–415.

87. A. C. Carr et al. 2001. Comparison of low-density lipoprotein modification by myeloperoxidase-derived hypochlorous and hypobromous acids. *Free Radic. Biol. Med.* 31: 62–72.

88. Y. Aratani 2018. Myeloperoxidase: Its role for host defense, inflammation, and neutrophil function. *Arch. Biochem. Biophys.* 640: 47–52.

89. M. Tien 1999. Myeloperoxidase-catalyzed oxidation of tyrosine. *Arch. Biochem. Biophys.* 367: 61–66.

90. D.I. Pattison and M.J. Davies 2006. Reactions of myeloperoxidase-derived oxidants with biological substrates: Gaining chemical insight into human inflammatory diseases. *Curr. Med. Chem.* 13: 3271–3290.

91. C. Delporte et al. 2014. Impact of myeloperoxidase-LDL interactions on enzyme activity and subsequent posttranslational oxidative modifications of apoB-100. *J. Lipid Res.* 55: 747–757.

92. S. L. Hazen and J. W. Heinecke 1997. 3-Chlorotyrosine, a specific marker of myeloperoxidase-catalyzed oxidation, is markedly elevated in low density lipoprotein isolated from human atherosclerotic intima. *J. Clin. Invest.* 99: 2075–2081.

93. E. L. Finley et al. 1998. Identification of tryptophan oxidation products in bovine α-crystallin. *Protein Sci.* 7: 2391–2397.

94. E. A. Podrez, H. M. Abu-Soud, and S. L. Hazen 2000. Myeloperoxidase-generated oxidants and atherosclerosis. *Free Radic. Biol. Med.* 28: 1717–1725.

95. C. Bergt et al. 1999. Hypochlorite modification of high density lipoprotein: Effects on cholesterol efflux from J774 macrophages. *FEBS Lett.* 452: 295–300.

96. B. Shao et al. 2005. Tyrosine 192 in apolipoprotein A-I is the major site of nitration and chlorination by myeloperoxidase, but only chlorination markedly impairs. *J. Biol. Chem.* 280: 5983–5993.

97. J. W. Heinecke 1998. Oxidants and antioxidants in the pathogenesis of atherosclerosis: Implications for the oxidized low density lipoprotein hypothesis. *Atherosclerosis* 141: 1–15.

98. J. W. Heinecke 1999. Mass spectrometric quantification of amino acid oxidation products in proteins: Insights into pathways that promote LDL oxidation in the human artery wall. *FASEB J.* 13: 1113–1120.

99. C. Bergt et al. 2000. Reagent or myeloperoxidase-generated hypochlorite affects discrete regions in lipid-free and lipid-associated human apolipoprotein A-I. *Biochem. J.* 346: 345–354.

100. C. Bergt et al. 2004. Lysine residues direct the chlorination of tyrosines in YXXK motifs of apolipoprotein A-I when hypochlorous acid oxidizes high density lipoprotein. *J. Biol. Chem.* 279: 7856–7866.

101. C. S. Moran et al. 2014. Osteoprotegerin deficiency limits angiotensin II-induced aortic dilatation and rupture in the apolipoprotein E-knockout mouse. *Arterioscler. Thromb. Vasc. Biol.* 34: 2609–2616.

102. B. Garner et al. 1998. Oxidation of high density lipoproteins. II. Evidence for direct reduction of lipid hydroperoxides by methionine residues ff apolipoproteins AI and AII. *J Biol Chem.* 273: 6088–6095.

103. C. Y. Yang et al. 1989. Structure of apolipoprotein B-100 of human low density lipoproteins. *Arterioscler. Thromb. Vasc. Biol.* 9: 96–108.

104. C. Y. Yang et al. 1997. Oxidative modifications of apoB-100 by exposure of low density lipoproteins to HOCl in vitro. *Free Radic. Biol. Med.* 23: 82–89.

105. C. Y. Yang et al. 2001. Selective oxidation in vitro by myeloperoxidase of the N-terminal amine in apolipoprotein B-100. *J. Lipid Res.* 42:1891–1896.

106. C. Y. Yang et al. 1990. Isolation and characterization of sulfhydryl and disulfide peptides of human apolipoprotein B-100. *Proc. Natl. Acad. Sci. U.S.A.* 87: 5523–5527.

107. R. Milne et al. 1989. The use of monoclonal antibodies to localize the low density lipoprotein receptor-binding domain of apolipoprotein B. *J. Biol. Chem.* 264: 19754–19760.

108. J. Borén et al. 1998. Identification of the low density lipoprotein receptor-binding site in apolipoprotein B100 and the modulation of its binding activity by the carboxyl terminus in familial defective Apo-B100. *J. Clin. Invest.* 101: 1084–1093.

109. J. A. Fernández-Higuero et al. 2015. Structural analysis of APOB variants, p.(Arg3527Gln), p.(Arg1164Thr) and p.(Gln4494del), causing Familial Hypercholesterolaemia provides novel insights into variant pathogenicity. *Sci Rep* 5: 18184.

110. R. T. Hamilton et al. 2008. LDL protein nitration: Implication for LDL protein unfolding. *Arch. Biochem. Biophys.* 479: 1–14.

111. S. Chakraborty, Y. Cai, and M. A. Tarr 2010. Mapping oxidations of apolipoprotein B-100 in human low-density lipoprotein by liquid chromatography–tandem mass spectrometry. *Anal. Biochem.* 404: 109–117.

112. S. Chakraborty, Y. Cai, and M. A. Tarr 2014. In vitro oxidative footprinting provides insight into apolipoprotein B-100 structure in low density lipoprotein. *Proteomics* 14: 2614–2622.

113. C. Delporte et al. 2011. Optimization of apolipoprotein-B-100 sequence coverage by liquid chromatography-tandem mass spectrometry for the future study of its posttranslational modifications. *Anal. Biochem.* 411: 129–138.

114. G. Marsche et al. 2008. Hypochlorite-modified high-density lipoprotein acts as a sink for myeloperoxidase in vitro. *Cardiovasc. Res.* 79: 187–194.

115. B. Shao et al. 2006. Myeloperoxidase impairs ABCA1-dependent cholesterol efflux through methionine oxidation and site-specific tyrosine chlorination of apolipoprotein A-I. *J. Biol. Chem.* 281: 9001–9004.

CHAPTER EIGHT

Global Profiling of Cell Responses to (Pseudo)Hypohalous Acids

Joshua D. Chandler
Emory University
Children's Healthcare of Atlanta

CONTENTS

(PSEUDO)HYPOHALOUS ACIDS (HOX): CHEMISTRY, BIOLOGY, AND POTENTIAL FOR REDOX SIGNALING

Reactive species are generated by cells in response to diverse stimuli including pathogen and danger signals, nutrient abundance, toxicants (including excess beneficial molecules), physical stressors, oxygen tension, and developmental cues [1–8]. Because aerobes use oxygen as the terminal electron acceptor in cellular respiration, there is constant risk of univalent oxygen reduction to form superoxide radical anion, the reactive oxygen species (ROS) that gives rise to a number of other ROS including hydrogen peroxide and hydroxyl radical [9]. Additionally, cells actively coordinate ROS production by a variety of mechanisms [6,10,11]. ROS such as hydrogen peroxide can regulate processes such as metabolism, receptor signaling, and wound healing [12–14]. Signaling occurs by reaction of the ROS with one or more biological molecules, frequently protein-bound cysteine thiols, to elicit a coordinated response [6,8,15,16]. Redox signaling generally operates below the concentrations of ROS that elicit cytotoxicity [17].

Less attention has been paid to the (pseudo)hypohalous acids (HOX) in redox signaling compared with hydrogen peroxide. HOXs are a diverse group of ROS generated from the reduction of hydrogen peroxide by specific peroxidases. In mammals, HOXs include hypochlorous acid (HOCl), hypothiocyanous acid (HOSCN), hypobromous acid (HOBr), and hypoiodous acid (HOI). HOX are produced by the chordata peroxidases myeloperoxidase (MPO), eosinophil peroxidase (EPO), lactoperoxidase (LPO), and thyroid peroxidase and also by peroxidasins (Figure 8.1; HOI and thyroid peroxidase not shown) [18,19]. HOX production is limited by substrate concentration and peroxidase selectivity [20–22]. Under physiological conditions, chloride can be oxidized to HOCl solely by MPO, bromide can be oxidized to HOBr by MPO, EPO, and peroxidasin, and (*pseudo*halide) thiocyanate can be oxidized to HOSCN by each of the aforementioned peroxidases as well as LPO [23,24].

For a given HOX, there may be homeostatic, beneficially adaptive, and pathological signaling

DOI: 10.1201/9781003212287-10

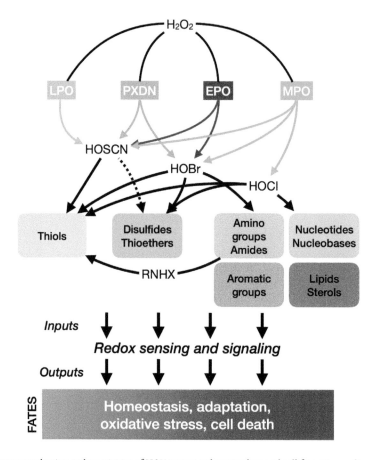

Figure 8.1 Divergent production and reactivities of HOX impact redox signaling and cell fate. Mammalian peroxidases including the chordata peroxidases (LPO, EPO, and MPO) and peroxidasin (PXDN) catalyze the reduction of hydrogen peroxide (H_2O_2) via a (pseudo)halide 2-electron donor, including thiocyanate, bromide, or chloride (not shown), to create (pseuo)hypohalous acids (HOX), e.g., HOSCN, HOBr, and HOCl. All peroxidases shown can produce HOSCN; all but LPO can produce HOBr; and only MPO can produce HOCl under physiological conditions. Increasing concentrations of thiocyanate drive production of HOSCN at the expense of other HOXs (not shown). HOXs diverge in reactivity with biological molecules in metabolites, proteins, and lipid membranes, including thiols, disulfides, thioethers, amino groups, amides, nucleobases, nucleosides and nucleotides, aromatic groups, lipids, and sterols (list not exhaustive). HOSCN is selective in reactivity, tending to oxidize thiols and reacting less rapidly (dashed arrow) with disulfides and thioethers, while HOCl and HOBr are promiscuous oxidants that react rapidly with many functional groups. Some by-products of HOCl and HOBr reaction with amino groups (i.e., halamines; RNHX) are also reactive toward more nucleophilic species, particularly thiols. The extent of HOX reactions with biological molecules acts as input to redox sensing and signaling, which may elicit a number of outputs such as adaptations in metabolism, gene/protein expression, and/or facile repair of the perturbed redox steady state by dedicated enzymes. These events influence the fate of the cell to return to homeostasis, adapt through the rearrangement of metabolism and phenotype, or develop oxidative stress and potentially to undergo cell death.

pathways that occur in the range of concentrations leading up to cytotoxicity, with concentration ranges calibrated to each HOX according to its reactivity (*vide infra*). This is analogous to hydrogen peroxide, which exerts a range of effects as its local concentration increases or decreases [17]. Although HOXs are associated with inflammatory sequelae, wherein local concentrations might be quite high, low steady-state HOX exposure could occur in bodily compartments where they are regularly generated (e.g., steady-state concentrations of HOSCN ranging from 35 to 65 μM have been reported in saliva [25]). More evidence is needed to determine whether redox signals from specific HOX diverge or overlap with those of hydrogen peroxide (and each other). From a physiological perspective, HOX-based signaling may be limited to specific tissue environs, requiring the presence of appropriate peroxidases to function.

Chordata peroxidases and peroxidasins are selective for thiocyanate, which also reacts with other HOX to replace them with HOSCN [20,21]. Thiocyanate abundance is highly variable between bodily compartments and individuals, so that this substrate greatly influences which HOXs are produced in vivo [26–28]. Thiocyanate ranges from 10^{-7} to 10^{-2} M in various bodily compartments and is generally highest in secretory fluids such as saliva, airway lining fluid, and tears [26]. (Compare with approximately 10^{-1} M for chloride, 10^{-5} M for bromide, and $<10^{-6}$ M for iodide.) Environmental factors that increase cyanide exposure, such as vegetable consumption (especially of crucifers) and smoking, increase bodily thiocyanate via the detoxification of cyanide by sulfurtransferases (e.g., rhodanese) [26,28,29]. Thiocyanate has been associated with improved pulmonary and cardiovascular outcomes in clinical and animal studies of inflammatory and infectious diseases [30–35], indicating that HOSCN elicits specific cellular responses that may be more beneficial compared with other HOX [36–40]. Different mechanisms of redox signaling of HOSCN and HOCl, the predominant HOX at inflammatory sites [27,28], might account for such differences. Tissue compartments with higher exposure to certain HOX, such as HOBr in basement membranes, HOI in thyroid, and HOSCN in secretory mucosae [25,41–44], may have specialized redox and metabolic adaptations to contend with increased exposure to those oxidants.

HOXs have striking differences in reactivity in terms of both potential reaction partners and comparative rates of reactions (Figure 8.1) [29,45–50]. HOX reactivities are defined by differences in their steady-state reduction potentials, which control which molecules can donate electrons to them, and their pK_a's, which regulate HOX partitioning between the more reactive acid form and less reactive conjugate base ([OX]$^-$) [23,28,51]. HOCl and HOBr are stronger oxidants than HOSCN and HOI, and decreased protonation of HOSCN at physiological pH further limits its reactivity [28]. These relative constraints on HOSCN indicate that it might act on a narrow subset of sensitive targets to elicit its physiological effects [28,29,52].

As an arm of the innate immune system, HOXs are weaponized by neutrophils and monocytes (which both produce MPO); eosinophils (which produce EPO); and mucosal epithelium (which produces LPO) [53–57]. Recognition of the relationship of HOX and immunity has led to extensive research into their effectiveness against different microbes and to their potential involvement in off-target damage. For example, there is mounting evidence from clinical studies that MPO-derived HOCl causes tissue damage associated with, and possibly causative in, lung function decline in cystic fibrosis [58–62]. Large amounts of MPO are expressed by developing neutrophils (approximately 5% of cellular protein) [63], accumulating in primary (azurophilic) granules during bone marrow development, after which expression of genes encoding granule proteins ceases [53,64]. Neutrophils are the first responders to inflammatory sites and secrete MPO into their phagolysosomes or extracellularly (i.e., exocytosis or extracellular trap release) [65]. MPO is expressed in lesser amounts by monocytes and rapidly decreases as these cells develop into macrophages unless GM-CSF is present [53,66]. MPO secreted by leukocytes can bind cellular macromolecules and form associations with other cells [67,68], potentially altering where and how the HOX can elicit redox signals.

HOXs are also involved in metabolism. HOI is essential in the iodination of thyroid hormones T_3 and T_4 [43], HOBr is required for the formation of sulfilimine cross-linkages in the extracellular matrix [69], and HOSCN is catalytically detoxified by mammalian thioredoxin reductases (TrxRs) and modulates the activity of several enzymes [37,70,71]. HOSCN can alter cellular metabolism by reacting with redox-active glycolytic enzymes, promoting altered carbon flux through glycolysis to generate increased reducing equivalents [72].

Although the promiscuity of HOCl and HOBr makes the potential for finely tuned signaling less obvious, lower doses of HOCl can induce Nrf2 in lung epithelial cells, and chlor-/bromamines (primary metabolites of HOCl/HOBr) have potent cell signaling effects including suppression of cytokine release [73–76]. The Escherichia coli transcriptional activator RclR functions as a specific HOCl sensor [77]. Metabolites and proteins may further dictate signaling of HOCl and HOBr via more selective secondary products, such as halamines (Figure 8.1) [77–79].

Taken together, these studies indicate that HOXs elicit specific redox signals distinct from hydrogen peroxide and other ROS (Figure 8.1). Distinguishing the signaling mechanisms of HOX from other ROS and from each other is crucial to understanding their effects in health and disease.

However, with such a large number of potential reactions and few opportunities for direct measurement of HOX in vivo, this is a difficult subject to study. Most studies to date have focused on a limited number of biomarkers specific to certain HOX, but this misses the full range of reaction products connecting HOX to pathways of metabolism and redox signaling. To address this challenge, carefully designed experiments capable of sensitive global profiling of cellular responses to HOX are needed.

NON-TARGETED GLOBAL APPROACHES TO ELUCIDATE DIVERGENT REDOX SIGNALING OF HOX

To date, most knowledge about HOX in biology has been derived from reductionist experiments, concerned with discrete constituents of biological systems to explain complex organismal phenomena. Empowered by molecular biology, reductionism has resulted in numerous breakthroughs in the life sciences. However, wider implementation of global approaches could greatly improve scientific understanding of the roles of HOX in biology. In a global framework, groups of genes and their products (and byproducts) coordinate biological responses as a community with dynamic relationships [80]. From this perspective, coordinated alteration of a molecular pathway may be more important than a single large change in one component. Elucidating the full gene, protein and metabolite networks that are responsive to specific HOX would enhance understanding of their respective roles in biological systems. This can be accomplished by using so-called "-omics" techniques (e.g., genomics, transcriptomics, proteomics, metabolomics, lipidomics) to measure as many of the relevant molecules (i.e., genes, mRNA transcripts, proteins, metabolites, lipids) as possible. At the time of this writing, only a handful of studies have relied on "-omics" techniques to study HOX (vide infra).

"-Omics" techniques enable the study of large numbers of biological variables, typically from hundreds to tens of thousands [81]. Advances in technology, including cloud computing and open-source systems biology, have made "-omics" data interpretation more accessible in recent years [82,83]. In addition to being broad in scope, several "-omics" methods, such as those that use nucleotide sequencing or high-resolution mass spectrometry, do not require a priori knowledge of a biological molecule to detect and quantify it. Once such "known unknowns" are recognized, researchers may use existing data and additional experiments to learn more about them [84,85]. This offers the exciting potential to discover new molecules not previously considered, such as splice variants, posttranslational modifications (PTMs), and novel metabolites.

The remainder of this chapter places emphasis on metabolomics and redox proteomics, as these methods capture the functional components of cells that most often serve as the direct interface with HOX. However, genetic responses (such as changes in mRNA expression covered by transcriptomics) are also major players in responses to HOX and merit brief mention here. Several "-omics" studies of genetic responses to one or more HOX have been published. Gene expression profiling has shown that lung epithelial cells induce Nrf2 activity after HOCl exposure in an epidermal growth factor receptor (EGFR)- and mitogen-activated protein kinase (MAPK)-independent manner [76]. Transcriptomics of Pseudomonas aeruginosa, a clinically relevant human lung and burn wound pathogen, exposed to HOCl, HOBr, and HOSCN, revealed global separation of genetic and protein aggregation responses to all three oxidants, with HOSCN-exposed cells diverging from HOCl- and HOBr-exposed cells [86]. HOSCN had the most impact on genes controlling antibiotic resistance and susceptibility, while HOCl and HOBr had the largest impact on genes involved in heat shock responses [86]. Critically, this study showed overall more differences than similarities among the differentially expressed gene targets and protein aggregates of HOX (comparing HOSCN vs. HOCl/HOBr) [86]. Gene expression profiling has also been used to show the dose dependence of RAW 264.7 macrophage-like cell transcriptional responses, with antioxidant responses at lower doses giving way to heat shock and DNA damage response genes at higher doses [87], resembling the dose dependence observed for the redox signaling of hydrogen peroxide [17]. Thus, understanding genetic responses will be key to elucidating the redox signaling of HOX.

THE METABOLOME: INTERFACE OF HOX WITH ENERGY, STRUCTURE, AND FUNCTION

Metabolites, including carbohydrates, organic acids, amino acids, biogenic amines, nucleobases, nucleosides, nucleotides, vitamins, lipids, and other small molecules, govern cell biology [88,89]. Metabolites are derived from diet, microbiome, endogenous metabolism, and exposure to environmental compounds [90]. Metabolites provide chemical and electrical energy, serve as building blocks for macromolecules (and a means of interconversion of these building blocks), and enable waste removal from cells. Metabolites may also act as signaling molecules [91–98]. Disruption of critical metabolic reactions radiates to other metabolite pools until redundant pathways converge to reinforce homeostasis. Cells may respond to stress with metabolic rewiring, thereby altering metabolic flux.

Most metabolomics experiments measure metabolite abundances, which indicate the net result of synthesis, degradation, and transport. Due to redundant inputs and outputs, metabolite abundances alone are not sufficient to establish which steps in a pathway have been disrupted. For this reason, stable isotopologues of suspected metabolic precursors are often used in experiments to trace metabolite flux down to the level of individual atoms [99].

Several metabolites are redox-active, regulating the intracellular redox status of cells and subcellular compartments. These include reduced and oxidized forms of glutathione (γ-glutamyl-cysteinyl-glycine; GSH), cysteine, methionine, selenomethionine, nicotinamide adenine dinucleotide (NAD^+), and nicotinamide adenine dinucleotide phosphate ($NADP^+$). Selenocysteine is another redox-active species, but is very low abundance as a free amino acid in vivo due to its rapid incorporation into proteins [100]. Many of the aforementioned metabolites are poised to react with some or all of the HOXs (Figure 8.1).

Sulfur- and selenium-containing metabolites are generally strong nucleophiles that rapidly react with HOX [101], often playing critical roles in maintaining cellular functions [81]. These include GSH, cysteine, methionine, coenzyme A and seleno- analogues, and exogenous sulfur species from diet and microbes including ergothioneine, mycothiol, bacillithiol [102–104]. Notably, low-molecular-weight thiols (GSH and cysteine) are the only metabolites that are major targets of HOSCN [49], though selenomethionine can also undergo rapid reactions with HOSCN [50]. Reactions of all HOX with sulfur- and selenium-containing metabolites involve 2-electron oxidation, which is often reversible and repaired by dedicated enzymes [105–107].

HOCl and HOBr also react with nitrogen-containing metabolites, forming chlor- and bro-mamines, respectively [79,108–110]. Chlor-/bromamine formation causes a cascade of further reactions, including halogen transfer, Schiff base formation, and production of reactive protein carbonyls [110–112]. HOCl and HOBr also react with nucleotides and nucleobases [113–115], hexosamines [116], sterols [117,118], and double bonds in lipids (e.g., the vinyl ether bond of plasmalogens, forming halofatty acids) [119,120]. Thus, there are many entry points of HOX into the metabolome by direct reactions and many potential products. Increased methionine sulfoxide and glutathione sulfonamide in cystic fibrosis are evidence that HOCl and/or HOBr are associated with and possibly causal in pathogenesis of this disease [60–62]. Many products of metabolite reactions with HOX are also reactive molecules, including halamines, reactive carbonyls, and halogenated lipids [79,110,119,121,122].

Several groups have directly examined the impact of one or more HOXs on cellular metabolism and bioenergetics. LPO-derived HOSCN has been shown to inhibit glucose transport, promote leakage of glucose, amino acids, and minerals, and limit glucose-stimulated metabolism in multiple bacteria [123–125]. HOSCN limits cystine uptake in Streptococcus agalactiae, but cystine in excess of growth requirements can confer resistance to the oxidant, likely due to its role in GSH and protein synthesis [126]. HOSCN inhibits several enzymes critical to bacterial metabolism such as urease in Helicobacter pylori and low-molecular-weight thioredoxin reductase (L-TrxR) in E. coli [37,127]. In mammalian cells, sublethal doses of HOSCN inhibit glycolysis in J774A.1 macrophage-like cells [72], a cell line previously shown to be sensitive to HOSCN-mediated cell death [128]. HOSCN ($\geq 10\,\mu$M) decreased lactate secretion and depleted intracellular ATP and NADH at higher doses, but NADPH and total NADP(H) were increased by HOSCN exposure, and glucose transport was unaffected [72]. Altered metabolic flux of glucose in response to HOSCN occurred in conjunction with oxidation of glyceraldehyde 3-phosphate dehydrogenase (GAPDH), aldolase, and triosephosphate isomerase, which is similar to multiple observations from hydrogen peroxide-exposed cells that also increased pentose phosphate pathway activity after GAPDH became oxidized [129–131]. This could in turn provide increased reducing equivalents for TrxR-mediated HOSCN removal [37]. In a separate study using J774A.1 cells with HOSCN concentrations ≥50 μM, Love et al. observed that decreased ATP production following HOSCN is associated with mitochondrial cytochrome oxidation and increased mitochondrial permeability, while 100 μM HOSCN increased the capacity of the cells to utilize palmitate for mitochondrial respiration [132]. Notably, the steady-state HOSCN concentration in human saliva is similar to the concentrations that elicited these effects [25,44]. It is possible that the impact of HOSCN on metabolism of cells found in secretory environs, which may be constantly exposed to the oxidant in vivo, is quite different from cells in other environments.

As promiscuous oxidants, HOCl and HOBr may impact cellular metabolism in a number of ways. Halogenation of a metabolite both clears it from the pool and creates a new species that might inhibit a metabolic enzyme. Halogenation of amino groups creates a number of potent, interconvertible reactive species [73–75]. Adenosine chlorination forms 8-chloroadenosine (8-ClAd), which is incorporated into ATP (as 8-ClATP) by J774A.1 macrophage-like cells [133]. 8-ClAd inhibited lactate release after prolonged incubation, and high doses (50 μM) increased proton leak, maximal respiratory capacity, and spare respiratory capacity of these cells [133]. At lower doses (4–16 μM) of 8-ClAd in human coronary artery endothelial cells (HCAEC), which also incorporated 8-ClAd into 8-ClATP, there were no significant changes to mitochondrial function, but glycolysis and lactate release were inhibited [134]. HOBr can oxidize deoxyribonucleosides, which can lead to their uptake by cells and incorporation into DNA (in the case of deoxycytidine) and miscoding by DNA polymerases (in the case of deoxyguanosine and potentially for deoxyuridine derived from deoxycytidine) [115,135].

HOCl and HOBr also react with lipids to disrupt fatty acid metabolism, necessitating ω-hydroxylation, multistep oxidation of the alcohol to carboxylic acid, and reverse-directional β-oxidation, yielding 2-chloroadipic acid in the case of HOCl [119]. Halogenated lipids, derived from membrane plasmalogens, promote their own removal via agonism of peroxisome proliferator-activated receptor (PPAR)-α; however, the accumulation of modified fatty acids can occur and cause cellular dysfunction in myeloid and endothelial cells [119]. Bromo- and chloroaldehydes are also reactive with GSH and protein nucleophiles [136]. Free and total 2-chloropalmitic acid and 2-chlorostearic acid are associated with increased risk of acute respiratory distress syndrome development in patients with sepsis and promote vascular leak and neutrophil adherence to endothelial cells [137].

Taken together, existing studies provide an important foundation for future research into metabolic effects of HOX exposure. Importantly, multiple mechanisms appear to converge on glycolytic sensing of oxidative stress, similar to hydrogen peroxide (vide supra). However, HOCl and HOBr appear to induce a number of additional changes that may more broadly disrupt metabolism. More research is needed to determine the full extent of metabolic impact of each HOX, including which species are impacted, what species are generated by the exposure, and the effects of those changes to the metabolic landscape on cell function.

APPLICATIONS OF METABOLOMICS IN STUDIES OF HOX

Improvements in the accuracy and resolving power of modern mass spectrometers have enabled coverage of hundreds to thousands of metabolites in routine experiments [138–140]. High-resolution, accurate mass spectrometry has seen use in recent studies of HOX biology and biochemistry, including quantification of thiocyanate in breath condensate [141], determination of novel LPO oxidation products (i.e., evidence of novel hyposelenocyanous acid) [142], and non-targeted metabolomics of cystic fibrosis bronchoalveolar lavage fluid to reveal correlations of MPO and methionine sulfoxide with pediatric lung disease [62]. High resolving power in mass spectrometry confers the significant advantage of discriminating isotopologues with the same nominal masses, e.g., sulfur-34, oxygen-18, and double occurrence of carbon-13 [143]. Unit resolution mass spectrometers, generally operated in tandem MS experiments for compound identification, remain critical workhorse instruments for metabolite detection and quantification and can sensitively assay dozens to hundreds of metabolites in a single experiment [144–146]. However, unit resolution instruments are not as well equipped for discovery metabolomics due to their low resolving power.

Orthogonal information combined with mass spectrometry improves confidence in the annotation of mass spectra to specific small molecules and biological interpretation. Compound separations by gas or liquid chromatography enhance assay sensitivity and are also critical for accurate metabolite identification [85,147]. MS/MS has proven crucial for identifying the structural makeup of known and novel metabolites [148,149]. Complementary advances in nuclear magnetic resonance (NMR) technology to service metabolomics have also been projected [150]. Both MS and NMR benefit from the use of stable isotopologues (e.g., carbon-13) for compound detection; MS for standardization, enrichment, and metabolic flux; and NMR for signal enrichment of magnetic nuclei. To validate metabolomic studies,

functional measures of metabolism such as the Seahorse XF Analyzer and enzyme assays are also important.

In general, metabolomics experiments require metabolism to be quenched, metabolites extracted from macromolecules, and subsequently measured and identified based on reproducible characteristics in detection, fragmentation, and/or separation (varying by technique; Figure 8.2). Some limitations to consider in metabolomics experiments include whether a method is biased in favor of specific compounds and compound classes (e.g., chromatographic and spectrometric limitations) and/or higher abundance species; whether metabolic quenching is sufficiently rapid to preserve species of interest [151]; whether sample derivatization is

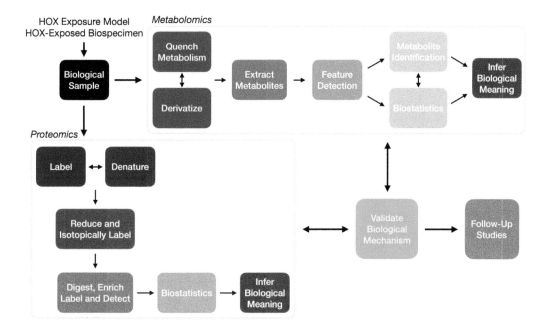

Figure 8.2 Schematic overview of parallel metabolomic and redox proteomic workflows to profile global cellular responses to HOX exposure. An exposure model is employed and/or HOX-exposed biospecimens are procured to produce biological samples. In metabolomics, metabolism is quenched rapidly, and derivatization reagents are applied if needed for redox stabilization, metabolite detection, or tagging. Metabolites are extracted and detected by methods such as high-resolution mass spectrometry. Metabolite detection often begins at the feature level, with discernible biological peaks recorded before an identity has been ascertained. Detected features can be analyzed for relationships to important study variables ("Biostatistics") before or after metabolite identities are determined, and biological inferences are made. In the (redox) proteomics approach, depicted here based on a general workflow for the analysis of redox state of protein cysteines, proteins are redox labeled to preserve the redox state of target modifications, e.g., the cysteine thiol. Once isolated, proteins can be reduced to unmask target PTMs for labeling and further denature proteins for digestion. Proteins are digested to peptides, then peptides that have been labeled are enriched. Biostatistical methods are used to determine which proteins' redox poise is affected by the study variables and biological meaning is inferred. Both workflows can suggest mechanisms underlying the observations that need to be validated by conducting additional experiments. Each approach can complement the other as orthogonal techniques to study the effect of HOX on global metabolism. Novel findings will often suggest follow-up studies designed to test newly generated hypotheses derived from the global approach.

necessary (e.g., to preserve metabolite redox state) [152]; and how much unwanted signal variation and assay noise can be mitigated. Authentic internal standards added prior to assay address a number of these issues at once.

In non-targeted metabolomics, it is typically impossible to have an internal standard for every compound that could be observed. In this case, limited standards can be used to monitor assay performance, or whole cells and organisms can be isotopically labeled and their lysates used as standards [153–156]. However, the latter solution is imperfect if trying to compare a labeled organism with a different organism or the same organism from significantly different genetic or environmental conditions. Stable isotopes also have important applications in metabolic flux determination [99], and the inherent challenge of global metabolic labeling in mammalian cells has been used to discern the origin of metabolites in culture [157]. Stable isotopic labeling has also been used to trace oxygen atoms originating from HOCl and other oxidants [158]. When internal standards for quantification are not feasible, a flexible alternative approach is to use consistently measured reference materials with known quantities of metabolites to perform reference calibration [159].

In mass spectrometry, a single chemical gives rise to multiple convoluted spectra, consisting of adducts, isotopes, in-source fragments, and other features that are not always easily accounted for [160]. For this reason, it can be helpful to group unidentified features in untargeted metabolomics according to their retention time and correlation across study samples [161]. This approach decreases the odds of type II error, i.e., a false negative resulting from overly stringent multiple comparisons adjustment [162].

Most metabolomics experiments lack spatial resolution, reporting the bulk concentrations of metabolites. If desired, this can be addressed by preparing sections of sample or by subcellular fractionation [163,164]. MS imaging has been applied to tissues and single cells and can be combined with higher-resolution imaging modalities [165,166]. At the macroscopic level, rapid evaporative ionization MS of lipids has been used to intraoperatively identify tumors with high accuracy [167]. Tuning spatially resolved techniques to products of HOX could aid in elucidating the localization of HOX in tissue pathology.

THE REDOX PROTEOME: A MAJOR PLAYER IN HOX-DEPENDENT REDOX SIGNALING

Proteins are major targets of HOX owing to their enrichment of sulfur, nitrogen, and carbon nucleophiles found in amino acids and peptide backbones. Proteomics experiments detect as many proteins in a biological system as possible, by quantifying either digested peptides or intact proteins. Flexible sample preparation and enrichment techniques can be used to focus on specific functional groups, PTM, or protein–protein interactions. Redox proteomics, focused on redox-active residues of proteins [6,168,169], has obvious relevance to studies of HOX. Redox proteomics has the potential to both establish direct protein targets of HOX and discover (mal)adaptive signaling mechanisms in response to the oxidants. The latter approach could also be conducted with regard to protein abundance or other important PTMs such as phosphorylation or glycosylation [168].

As a highly nucleophilic amino acid with an array of redox PTMs, cysteine is a natural subject of redox proteomics [6]. Protein cysteines determine structure and serve in catalytic and regulatory roles [168]. Cysteine thiol (RSH), disulfide (RSSR), and sulfenic acid (RSOH) are central redox states of this amino acid in proteins [170]. When RSOH is reduced by a protein or small molecule RSH, an RSSR is formed, while cysteine persulfidation (RSS$^-$) occurs when RSOH reacts with hydrogen sulfide [6]. RSOH can also become sequentially oxidized to sulfinic (RSO$_2$H) and sulfonic acids (RSO$_3$H), thiosulfonates (RS[O]$_2$SR), and sulfen- and sulfonamides (RSNRR′ and RS[O]$_2$NRR′, respectively) [6]. Several modifications, including S-nitrosylation, Michael adduction, and coordination of cations, do not require an RSOH intermediate [15,168]. Cysteine can also react with a range of natural products and toxicants, serving as an interface with the exposome [102,171–175].

HOXs react with protein RSH to form sulfenyl (pseudo)halide intermediates (RSX; e.g., sulfenyl chloride or sulfenyl thiocyanate), which are rapidly hydrolyzed to RSOH and the corresponding (pseudo)halide [6]. RSSRs may also be nucleophiles in reactions with HOX, resulting in sequential oxidation and bond cleavage [176,177]. Protein structure, localization, and orthogonal modifications confer selective reactivity to the 214,000 cysteines encoded in the redox proteome [106,178,179]. Due to differences in reactivity, it is reasonable to expect HOCl, HOBr, and HOSCN interact with selective subsets of the cysteine proteome. HOCl and HOSCN result in aggregation of different subsets of proteins in *P. aeruginosa*, mediated in part by polyphosphate synthesis [86].

There are several studies demonstrating significant impact of HOX on the redox proteome of various organisms. Under HOCl stress, *Bacillus* species and *Staphylococcus aureus* undergo extensive bacillithiolation of antioxidant, metabolism, and chaperone proteins [171]. GAPDH represents a large fraction of total bacillithiolated proteins following HOCl exposure, which protects it from irreversible inactivation [180]. Mycothiolation in *Mycobacterium smegmatis* is similarly protective against HOCl oxidation of antioxidant and metabolic proteins, and absence of mycothiol exacerbates cysteine proteome oxidation by HOCl [102]. Radioisotopic carbon-14 from HOS^{14}CN was detectible in isolated GAPDH and creatinine kinase, and HOSCN treatment of J774A.1 mouse macrophage-like cells led to increased RSOH staining in extracted proteomes using the probe DAz-2 [181]. J774A.1 exposure to HOSCN increased reversible oxidation of 18 proteins, including several involved in glycolysis, antioxidant/redox signaling, cytoskeleton, and chaperone functions [72]. Oxidation of glycolytic proteins was associated with inhibition of glycolysis and increased pentose-phosphate pathway activity (*vide supra*) [72]. Comparative studies of the effects of different HOX on cellular redox proteomes will help to elucidate the divergent mechanisms of these oxidants.

APPLICATIONS OF REDOX PROTEOMICS IN STUDIES OF HOX

Methods to study cysteine redox proteomics often begin by "locking" RSH with an alkylating agent, then reduce redox PTMs of interest, and alkylate these with a different tag (Figure 8.2) [170]. The choice of reducing agent will influence which PTMs are unmasked, with varying selectivity [182]. Alkylating agents are also varied in mechanism: N-ethylmaleimide is a Michael acceptor that reversibly alkylates RSH to form a racemic mixture, while iodoacetmide and other S_N2 reagents follow a non-chiral, irreversible reaction [183–185]. (Mechanism of reversibility of the cysteine Michael adduct illustrated in Ref. [183].) Both are capable of off-target modifications and side reactions. To study RSOH, experimenters may prioritize *in situ* alkylation with specific probes (e.g., dimedone) first, as traditional alkylating agents may also react with RSOH [186,187]. Irreversible modifications are usually not detected in these methods without taking an alternative approach to specifically label them [188]. Ultimately, two or more redox states (such as reduced, RSH, vs. all reversibly oxidized cysteines) are discriminated simultaneously by MS [182,189,190]. Because they do not impact chromatography or ionization efficiency, stable isotopologues are ideal for this purpose [191,192].

An important goal in redox proteomics is detecting a large enough yield of cysteinyl peptides to develop a robust model of redox networks. More depth of coverage increases the potential to discover key interactions that drive redox networks. Xiao et al. recently reported alkylation of cysteine residues with phosphate-linked tags, dramatically increasing coverage of reactive cysteine residues by over an order of magnitude and enabling more comprehensive redox proteome analysis [193]. This study reported mouse organ-specific and age-dependent redox protein networks and revealed a frequent selection of arginine residues associated with redox active cysteines throughout the mouse proteome [193]. Gel-based methods have also been used to analyze protein cysteines [171,194]. Redox-modified proteins can be separated in a gel via redox-induced dimerization and/or by introducing high-molecular-weight tags [194–196].

Methionine is another sulfur-containing, nucleophilic residue in proteins that regulates folding, function, protein–protein interactions, and oxidative stress [197–200]. *E. coli* with 40% protein methionine replaced by norleucine have equal fitness at resting state compared with control cells, but are more vulnerable to HOCl, hydrogen peroxide, and ionizing radiation [198]. Methionine is especially vulnerable to oxidation by HOCl and HOBr, while HOSCN does not oxidize methionine at rapid rates *in vivo* [45,48,49]. Selenomethionine (which *does* react efficiently with HOSCN [50]) can be randomly incorporated into proteins in place of methionine as exposure and absorption are increased [100]. Methionine and selenomethionine oxidation by HOX causes addition of an oxygen atom in place of an electron lone pair, creating a chiral oxide that is reduced back stereoselectively via dedicated enzymes [201,202]. Selenomethionine selenoxide can be reduced directly by glutathione and thioredoxin reductase (similar to the GSH peroxidase mimetic, ebselen) [203,204]. The redox state of protein methionine in humans is a biomarker of oxidative stress [205]. Reduced protein methionines can be labeled by oxaziridine reagents to introduce a clickable tag [206]. A limitation of this technique is that some methionine is oxidized instead of being conjugated [206]. Nonetheless, such a method could be invaluable for gaining insights into the impact of HOX on the methionine proteome.

Studies of chlorotyrosine and bromotyrosine in proteins are advantageous due to their specificity for HOCl and HOBr, respectively. However, the overall frequency of these modifications is quite low [58]. Chloro- and bromotyrosine are also considered irreversible, but free chloro- and bromotyrosine can be dehalogenated (generating 4-hydroxyphenylacetic acid) in mammals [207,208]. Tyrosine chlorination can be site-directed by neighboring amino acids to regulate protein function, as in the case of cholesterol efflux by apolipoprotein A-I [200]. HOCl (purified or generated by MPO) creates chlorotyrosines on human fibronectin, which enhances heparin binding and increases human coronary artery smooth muscle cell proliferation [209]. Bromotyrosine is enriched in basement membranes of human and mouse kidneys and is decreased >85% if peroxidasin is knocked out [41]. Native bromination of tyrosine-1485 on α2-collagen IV is conserved in normal humans and mice [41].

Bulk chloro-/bromotyrosines from digested proteins can be recovered using methanesulfonic acid, minimizing the risk of artifactual halogenation posed by HCl and HBr [210]. Site-specific chlorotyrosine can be detected on MS instrumentation with unit resolution via MS/MS/MS (MS^3), first fragmenting tryptic peptides, then selecting the chlorotyrosine-derived fragment for discrimination from MS^2-level isobars [211]. Increased accuracy of modern MS instrumentation facilitates detection of chlorotyrosine in proteins without MS^3, and false matches could be discriminated based on the chlorine-specific mass defect [212]. Nybo et al. reported that replacing standard trichloroacetic acid/acetone precipitation of proteins with buffer exchange and witholding alkylating agents decreased artifactual chlorination of basement membrane proteins, while increasing sensitivity to chlorotyrosine [213]. This study raises the question of whether chlorination (and bromination) events have been underrepresented in studies using standard protein isolation methods. Continued research into tyrosine chlorination and bromination

is likely to be of major importance to understanding the impact of HOCl and HOBr in in vivo studies and may reveal new mechanisms of protein functional modulation by alterations in critical tyrosine residues.

INTEGRATING "-OMICS" DATA TO CONTEXTUALIZE HOX REDOX BIOLOGY

"-Omics" approaches are a powerful way to study cellular responses to HOX. However, none of these methods is all-encompassing. "-Omics" data can be contextualized to other data within a study to more clearly resolve biological information [82,214,215]. Determining relationships across datasets can elucidate the meaning of variables of interest, e.g., the impact of inflammatory myeloid cells on lung metabolites [216]. Redox proteomics, metabolomics, and analysis of metabolic fluxes provide highly complementary information, and their combination can highlight physiological, pathological, and toxicological mechanisms in complex systems [131,193,217,218].

A relevant example of how protein and metabolite data complement each other is oxidation of GAPDH by HOSCN and increased synthesis of NADP(H) [72]. A redox metabolic network could regulate these mechanisms, integrating several published observations. For example, HOSCN oxidizes GAPDH [72], which in turn inhibits glycolysis and increases glucose flux through the pentose phosphate pathway [72,129–131]. Increasing NADPH from the oxidative phase of the pathway provides reducing equivalents to TrxR, which maintains thioredoxin (Trx) in its reduced state, Trx-(SH)$_2$ [219], and metabolizes HOSCN [37]. Trx-(SH)$_2$ can regenerate GAPDH activity [220] and promote GAPDH expression [221]. Selective inhibition of the Trx system by auranofin increases GAPDH oxidation [178], while siRNA directed against Trx1 inhibits GAPDH activity (but also increases glycolytic flux, measured via a tritiated tracer) [218]. A speculated redox metabolic network based on these observations (Figure 8.3) illustrates the point that experimental designs to jointly leverage metabolomics and redox proteomics could rapidly enhance our understanding of the role(s) of HOX in biological systems.

CONCLUSIONS

Chordata peroxidases and peroxidasins are major players in redox biology, producing HOXs that exist at the interfaces of immunity, inflammation,

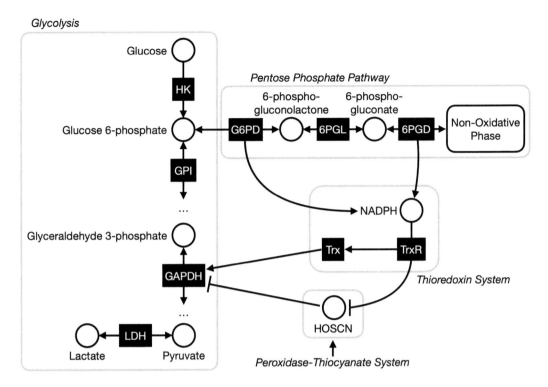

Figure 8.3 Speculated redox metabolic network: counter-regulation of glycolytic flux by the Trx system and HOSCN. The depicted redox metabolic network was inferred and constructed based on multiple observations in the scientific literature [34,64,120–122, 162,199–202], to illustrate a plausible relationship of HOX with redox protein-regulated metabolism. Proteins are depicted as black rectangles, and metabolites as open circles. Arrows indicate the flow of metabolites or electrons (in the case of NADPH → Trx and Trx → GAPDH), while perpendicular lines indicate oxidative inhibition (HOSCN and GAPDH) or reductive clearance (TrxR and HOSCN). Bidirectional arrows indicate reversible reactions. Ellipses indicate one or more additional metabolic steps that have not been depicted for brevity. In the illustration, HOSCN inhibition of GAPDH decreases glycolytic flux of glucose to pyruvate and lactate and increases pentose phosphate pathway activity, generating NADPH. The activity of HOSCN is opposed by TrxR (which catalytically reduces HOSCN) and Trx (which restores oxidatively inactivated GAPDH), which are maintained by NADPH from the pentose phosphate pathway. The redox metabolic circuit places HOSCN and the Trx system as opposing forces to fine-tune glycolytic flux and pentose phosphate pathway in HOSCN-exposed cells. New abbreviations: 6PGD, 6-phosphogluconate dehydrogenase; 6PGL, 6-phosphogluconolactonase; G6PD, glucose 6-phosphate dehydrogenase; GPI, glucose phosphate isomerase; HK, hexokinase; LDH, lactate dehydrogenase.

physiology, and metabolism. Thus, HOXs are of great importance in human health and disease. Key to resolving the role(s) HOXs play in vivo is understanding how they elicit oxidant-specific portfolios of redox signaling. The rapid reactivity of HOX and their partially overlapping arrays of reactants make this a very complex issue. However, advances in specific and sensitive molecular measurements, steady improvements in computing power and cloud computing, and an active systems biology research community are making powerful "-omics" approaches ever more accessible to researchers. Importantly, global approaches also enable scientists to consider how parts of a biological system form networks (and what happens when those networks rearrange).

Functional validation studies, e.g., using metabolic tracers and activity assays, remain essential to rigorously evaluate study conclusions.

Researchers studying the redox biology of HOX have predominantly used reductionist methods to date. These researchers have collectively produced a foundation of knowledge on which the scientific field is poised to expand by increasing adoption of "-omics" methods. Metabolomics and redox proteomics have dual relevancy to cell function and reactivity with HOX, enabling deep molecular profiling of oxidant reactivity and cell biology. "-Omics" methods are well suited for researchers studying HOX exposure and can be excellent tools to gain a global view of cellular responses to these oxidants.

REFERENCES

1. H. Sies, C. Berndt, D.P. Jones, 2017, Oxidative Stress, *Annu. Rev. Biochem.* 86: 715–748.

2. H. Sies, 2017, Hydrogen peroxide as a central redox signaling molecule in physiological oxidative stress: Oxidative eustress, *Redox Biol.* 11: 613–619.

3. D.P. Jones, H. Sies, 2015, The redox code, *Antioxid. Redox Signal.* 23: 734–746.

4. H. Sies, 2014, Role of metabolic H_2O_2 generation: Redox signaling and oxidative stress, *J. Biol. Chem.* 289: 8735–8741.

5. Y. Nisimoto, B.A. Diebold, D. Cosentino-Gomes, J.D. Lambeth, 2014, Nox4: A hydrogen peroxide-generating oxygen sensor, *Biochemistry* 53: 5111–5120.

6. Y.-M. Go, J.D. Chandler, D.P. Jones, 2015, The cysteine proteome, *Free Radic. Biol. Med.* 84: 227–245.

7. G.P. Sorescu, 2004, Bone morphogenic protein 4 produced in endothelial cells by oscillatory shear stress induces monocyte adhesion by stimulating reactive oxygen species production from a nox1-based NADPH oxidase, *Circ. Res.* 95: 773–779.

8. Y.M. Janssen-Heininger, B.T. Mossman, N.H. Heintz, et al., 2008, Redox-based regulation of signal transduction: Principles, pitfalls, and promises, *Free Radic. Biol. Med.* 45: 1–17.

9. I. Fridovich, 1983, Superoxide radical: An endogenous toxicant, *Annu. Rev. Pharmacol. Toxicol.* 23: 239–257.

10. C.C. Winterbourn, 2008, Reconciling the chemistry and biology of reactive oxygen species, *Nat. Chem. Biol.* 4: 278–286.

11. B.M. Babior, R.S. Kipnes, J.T. Curnutte, 1973, Biological defense mechanisms. The production by leukocytes of superoxide, a potential bactericidal agent, *J. Clin. Invest.* 52: 741–744.

12. N.R. Love, Y. Chen, S. Ishibashi, et al., 2013, Amputation-induced reactive oxygen species are required for successful Xenopus tadpole tail regeneration, *Nat. Cell Biol.* 15: 222–228.

13. H. Lei, A. Kazlauskas, 2014, A reactive oxygen species-mediated, self-perpetuating loop persistently activates platelet-derived growth factor receptor, *Mol. Cell Biol.* 34: 110–122.

14. H.R. Molavian, M. Kohandel, S. Sivaloganathan, 2016, High concentrations of H_2O_2 make aerobic glycolysis energetically more favorable for cellular respiration, *Front. Physiol.* 7: 362.

15. N. Gould, P.T. Doulias, M. Tenopoulou, K. Raju, H. Ischiropoulos, 2013, Regulation of protein function and signaling by reversible cysteine S-nitrosylation, *J. Biol. Chem.* 288: 26473–26479.

16. C.C. Winterbourn, 2013, The biological chemistry of hydrogen peroxide, *Methods Enzymol.* 528: 3–25.

17. H. Sies, D.P. Jones, 2020, Reactive oxygen species (ROS) as pleiotropic physiological signalling agents, *Nat. Rev. Mol. Cell Biol.* 21: 363–383.

18. M. Zámocký, S. Hofbauer, I. Schaffner, et al., 2015, Independent evolution of four heme peroxidase superfamilies, *Arch. Biochem. Biophys.* 574: 108–119.

19. M.J. Davies, C.L. Hawkins, D.I. Pattison, M.D. Rees, 2008, Mammalian heme peroxidases: From molecular mechanisms to health implications, *Antioxid. Redox Signal.* 10: 1199–1234.

20. J.C. Van Dalen, W.M. Whitehouse, C.C. Winterbourn, J.A. Kettle, 1997, Thiocyanate and chloride as competing substrates for myeloperoxidase, *Biochem. J.* 327: 487–492.

21. M. Paumann-Page, R.-S. Katz, M. Bellei, et al., 2017, Pre-steady-state kinetics reveal the substrate specificity and mechanism of halide oxidation of truncated human peroxidasin 1, *J. Biol. Chem.* 292: 4583–4592.

22. P.G. Furtmuller, U. Burner, C. Obinger, 1998, Reaction of myeloperoxidase compound I with chloride, bromide, iodide, and thiocyanate, *Biochemistry* 37: 17923–17930.

23. J. Arnhold, E. Monzani, P.G. Furtmüller, et al., 2006, Kinetics and thermodynamics of halide and nitrite oxidation by mammalian heme peroxidases, *Eur. J. Inorg. Chem.* 2006: 3801–3811.

24. C.J. van Dalen, A.J. Kettle, 2001, Substrates and products of eosinophil peroxidase, *Biochem. J.* 358: 233–239.

25. K.M. Pruitt, J. Tenovuo, B. Mansson-Rahemtulla, P. Harrington, D.C. Baldone, 1986, Is thiocyanate peroxidation at equilibrium in vivo? *Biochim. Biophys. Acta* 870: 385–391.

26. J.D. Chandler, B.J. Day, 2012, Thiocyanate: A potentially useful therapeutic agent with host defense and antioxidant properties, *Biochem. Pharmacol.* 84: 1381–1387.

27. P.E. Morgan, D.I. Pattison, J. Talib, et al., 2011, High plasma thiocyanate levels in smokers are a key determinant of thiol oxidation induced by myeloperoxidase, *Free Radic. Biol. Med.* 51: 1815–1822.

28. J.D. Chandler, B.J. Day, 2015, Biochemical mechanisms and therapeutic potential of pseudohalide thiocyanate in human health, *Free Radic. Res.* 49: 695–710.

29. D.I. Pattison, M.J. Davies, C.L. Hawkins, 2012, Reactions and reactivity of myeloperoxidase-derived oxidants: Differential biological effects of hypochlorous and hypothiocyanous acids, *Free Radic. Res.* 46: 975–995.

30. J.D. Chandler, E. Min, J. Huang, et al., 2015, Antiinflammatory and antimicrobial effects of thiocyanate in a cystic fibrosis mouse model, *Am. J. Respir. Cell Mol. Biol.* 53: 193–205.

31. P.E. Nedoboy, P.E. Morgan, T.J. Mocatta, et al., 2014, High plasma thiocyanate levels are associated with enhanced myeloperoxidase-induced thiol oxidation and long-term survival in subjects following a first myocardial infarction, *Free Radic. Res.* 48: 1256–1266.

32. J.D. Chandler, E. Min, J. Huang, D.P. Nichols, B.J. Day, 2013, Nebulized thiocyanate improves lung infection outcomes in mice, *Br. J. Pharmacol.* 169: 1166–1177.

33. P.E. Morgan, R.P. Laura, R.A. Maki, W.F. Reynolds, M.J. Davies, 2015, Thiocyanate supplementation decreases atherosclerotic plaque in mice expressing human myeloperoxidase, *Free Radic. Res.* 49: 743–749.

34. D. Lorentzen, L. Durairaj, A.A. Pezzulo, et al., 2011, Concentration of the antibacterial precursor thiocyanate in cystic fibrosis airway secretions, *Free Radic. Biol. Med.* 50: 1144–1150.

35. W.M. Malisoff, D. Marine, 1936, Prevention of atherosclerosis in rabbits. I. Administration of potassium thiocyanate, *Exp. Biol. Med.* 35: 356–358.

36. M.M. Lloyd, M.A. Grima, B.S. Rayner, et al., 2013, Comparative reactivity of the myeloperoxidase-derived oxidants hypochlorous acid and hypothiocyanous acid with human coronary artery endothelial cells, *Free Radic. Biol. Med.* 65: 1352–1362.

37. J.D. Chandler, D.P. Nichols, J.A. Nick, R.J. Hondal, B.J. Day, 2013, Selective metabolism of hypothiocyanous acid by mammalian thioredoxin reductase promotes lung innate immunity and antioxidant defense, *J. Biol. Chem.* 288: 18421–18428.

38. G.E. Conner, C. Wijkstrom-Frei, S.H. Randell, V.E. Fernandez, M. Salathe, 2007, The lactoperoxidase system links anion transport to host defense in cystic fibrosis, *FEBS Lett.* 581: 271–278.

39. P. Moskwa, D. Lorentzen, K.J. Excoffon, et al., 2007, A novel host defense system of airways is defective in cystic fibrosis, *Am. J. Respir. Crit. Care Med.* 175: 174–183.

40. Y. Xu, S. Szep, Z. Lu, 2009, The antioxidant role of thiocyanate in the pathogenesis of cystic fibrosis and other inflammation-related diseases, *Proc. Natl. Acad. Sci. U.S.A.* 106: 20515–20519.

41. C. He, W. Song, T.A. Weston, et al., 2020, Peroxidasin-mediated bromine enrichment of basement membranes, *Proc. Natl. Acad. Sci. U.S.A.* 117: 15827–15836.

42. B. Bathish, M. Paumann-Page, L.N. Paton, A.J. Kettle, C.C. Winterbourn, 2020, Peroxidasin mediates bromination of tyrosine residues in the extracellular matrix, *J. Biol. Chem.* 295: 12697–12705.

43. H.R. Chung, 2014, Iodine and thyroid function, *Ann. Pediatr. Endocrinol. Metabol.* 19: 8.

44. H. Below, R. Baguhl, W. Gessner, et al., 2018, Specific and robust ion chromatographic determination of hypothiocyanite in saliva samples, *Anal. Bioanal. Chem.* 410: 2739–2749.

45. D.I. Pattison, M.J. Davies, 2001, Absolute rate constants for the reaction of hypochlorous acid with protein side chains and peptide bonds, *Chem. Res. Toxicol.* 14: 1453–1464.

46. D.I. Pattison, M.J. Davies, 2006, Reactions of myeloperoxidase-derived oxidants with biological substrates: Gaining chemical insight into human inflammatory diseases, *Curr. Med. Chem.* 13: 3271–3290.

47. C. Storkey, M.J. Davies, D.I. Pattison, 2014, Reevaluation of the rate constants for the reaction of hypochlorous acid (HOCl) with cysteine, methionine, and peptide derivatives using a new competition kinetic approach, *Free Radic. Biol. Med.* 73: 60–66.

48. D.I. Pattison, M.J. Davies, 2004, Kinetic analysis of the reactions of hypobromous acid with protein components: Implications for cellular damage and use of 3-bromotyrosine as a marker of oxidative stress, *Biochemistry* 43: 4799–4809.

49. O. Skaff, D.I. Pattison, M.J. Davies, 2009, Hypothiocyanous acid reactivity with low-molecular-mass and protein thiols: Absolute rate constants and assessment of biological relevance, *Biochem. J.* 422: 111–117.

50. O. Skaff, D.I. Pattison, P.E. Morgan, et al., 2012, Selenium-containing amino acids are targets for myeloperoxidase-derived hypothiocyanous acid: Determination of absolute rate constants and implications for biological damage, *Biochem. J.* 441: 305–316.

51. P. Nagy, G.N. Jameson, C.C. Winterbourn, 2009, Kinetics and mechanisms of the reaction of hypothiocyanous acid with 5-thio-2-nitrobenzoic acid and reduced glutathione, *Chem. Res. Toxicol.* 22: 1833–1940.

52. T.J. Barrett, C.L. Hawkins, 2012, Hypothiocyanous acid: Benign or deadly? *Chem. Res. Toxicol.* 25: 263–273.

53. S.J. Klebanoff, 2005, Myeloperoxidase: Friend and foe, *J. Leukoc. Biol.* 77: 598–625.

54. S. Klebanoff, W. Clem, R. Luebke, 1966, The peroxidase-thiocyanate-hydrogen peroxide antimicrobial system, *Biochim. Biophys. Acta* 117: 63–72.

55. A.L.P. Chapman, M.B. Hampton, R. Senthilmohan, C.C. Winterbourn, A.J. Kettle, 2002, Chlorination of bacterial and neutrophil proteins during phagocytosis and killing of *Staphylococcus aureus*, *J. Biol. Chem.* 277: 9757–9762.

56. J.N. Green, A.J. Kettle, C.C. Winterbourn, 2014, Protein chlorination in neutrophil phagosomes and correlation with bacterial killing, *Free Radic. Biol. Med.* 77: 49–56.

57. C. Wijkstrom-Frei, S. El-Chemaly, R. Ali-Rachedi, et al., 2003, Lactoperoxidase and human airway host defense, *Am. J. Respir. Cell. Mol. Biol.* 29: 206–212.

58. E. Thomson, S. Brennan, R. Senthilmohan, et al., 2010, Identifying peroxidases and their oxidants in the early pathology of cystic fibrosis, *Free Radic. Biol. Med.* 49: 1354–1360.

59. A.J. Kettle, R. Turner, C.L. Gangell, et al., 2014, Oxidation contributes to low glutathione in the airways of children with cystic fibrosis, *Eur. Respir. J.* 44: 122–129.

60. N. Dickerhof, J.F. Pearson, T.S. Hoskin, et al., 2017, Oxidative stress in early cystic fibrosis lung disease is exacerbated by airway glutathione deficiency, *Free Radic. Biol. Med.* 113: 236–243.

61. N. Dickerhof, R. Turner, I. Khalilova, et al., 2017, Oxidized glutathione and uric acid as biomarkers of early cystic fibrosis lung disease, *J. Cystic Fibrosis* 16: 214–221.

62. J.D. Chandler, C. Margaroli, H. Horati, et al., 2018, Myeloperoxidase oxidation of methionine associates with early cystic fibrosis lung disease, *Eur. Respir. J.* 52: 1801118.

63. S.J. Klebanoff, A.J. Kettle, H. Rosen, C.C. Winterbourn, W.M. Nauseef, 2013, Myeloperoxidase: A front-line defender against phagocytosed microorganisms, *J. Leukoc. Biol.* 93: 185–198.

64. U. Gullberg, N. Bengtsson, E. Bülow, et al., 1999, Processing and targeting of granule proteins in human neutrophils, *J. Immunol. Methods* 232: 201–210.

65. C. Margaroli, R. Tirouvanziam, 2016, Neutrophil plasticity enables the development of pathological microenvironments: Implications for cystic fibrosis airway disease, *Mol. Cell. Pediatr.* 3: 38.

66. S. Sugiyama, Y. Okada, G.K. Sukhova, et al., 2001, Macrophage myeloperoxidase regulation by granulocyte macrophage colony-stimulating factor in human atherosclerosis and implications in acute coronary syndromes, *Am. J. Pathol.* 158: 879–891.

67. V.L. Shepherd, J.R. Hoidal, 1990, Clearance of neutrophil-derived myeloperoxidase by the macrophage mannose receptor, *Am. J. Respir. Cell. Mol. Biol.* 2: 335–340.

68. G. Yogalingam, A.R. Lee, D.S. Mackenzie, et al., 2017, Cellular uptake and delivery of myeloperoxidase to lysosomes promote lipofuscin degradation and lysosomal stress in retinal cells, *J. Biol. Chem.* 292: 4255–4265.

69. A.S. McCall, C.F. Cummings, G. Bhave, et al., 2014, Bromine is an essential trace element for assembly of collagen IV scaffolds in tissue development and architecture, *Cell* 157: 1380–1392.

70. R. Fabrini, A. Bocedi, S. Camerini, et al., 2014, Inactivation of human salivary glutathione transferase P1-1 by hypothiocyanite: A posttranslational control system in search of a role, *PLoS One* 9: e112797.

71. N.L. Cook, C.H. Moeke, L.I. Fantoni, D.I. Pattison, M.J. Davies, 2016, The myeloperoxidase-derived oxidant hypothiocyanous acid inhibits protein tyrosine phosphatases via oxidation of key cysteine residues, *Free Radic. Biol. Med.* 90: 195–205.

72. D.T. Love, T.J. Barrett, M.Y. White, et al., 2016, Cellular targets of the myeloperoxidase-derived oxidant hypothiocyanous acid (HOSCN) and its role in the inhibition of glycolysis in macrophages. *Free Radic. Biol. Med.* 94: 88–98.

73. J. Marcinkiewicz, M. Mak, M. Bobek, et al., 2005, Is there a role of taurine bromamine in inflammation? Interactive effects with nitrite and hydrogen peroxide, *Inflamm. Res.* 54: 42–49.

74. A. Kanayama, J.-I. Inoue, Y. Sugita-Konishi, M. Shimizu, Y. Miyamoto, 2002, Oxidation of IκBα at methionine 45 is one cause of taurine chloramine-induced inhibition of NF-κB activation, *J. Biol. Chem.* 277: 24049–24056.

75. E. Park, G. Schuller-Levis, M.R. Quinn, 1995, Taurine chloramine inhibits production of nitric oxide and TNF-alpha in activated RAW 264.7 cells by mechanisms that involve transcriptional and translational events, J. Immunol. 154: 4778–4784.

76. L. Zhu, J. Pi, S. Wachi, et al., 2008, Identification of Nrf2-dependent airway epithelial adaptive response to proinflammatory oxidant-hypochlorous acid challenge by transcription profiling, Am. J. Physiol. Lung Cell. Mol. Physiol. 294: L469–L477.

77. B.W. Parker, E.A. Schwessinger, U. Jakob, M.J. Gray, 2013, The RclR protein is a reactive chlorine-specific transcription factor in Escherichia coli, J. Biol. Chem. 288: 32574–32584.

78. A.V. Peskin, C.C. Winterbourn, 2001, Kinetics of the reactions of hypochlorous acid and amino acid chloramines with thiols, methionine, and ascorbate, Free Radic. Biol. Med. 30: 572–579.

79. A.V. Peskin, C.C. Winterbourn, 2003, Histamine chloramine reactivity with thiol compounds, ascorbate, and methionine and with intracellular glutathione, Free Radic. Biol. Med. 35: 1252–1260.

80. R.K. Delker, R.S. Mann, 2017, From reductionism to holism: Toward a more complete view of development through genome engineering, Adv. Exp. Med. Biol. 1016: 45–74.

81. K.K. Dennis, Y.M. Go, D.P. Jones, 2019, Redox systems biology of nutrition and oxidative stress, J. Nutr. 149: 553–565.

82. L.G. Gardinassi, J. Xia, S.E. Safo, S. Li, 2017, Bioinformatics tools for the interpretation of metabolomics data, Curr. Pharmacol. Rep. 3: 374–383.

83. K. O'Shea, B.B. Misra, 2020, Software tools, databases and resources in metabolomics: Updates from 2018 to 2019, Metabolomics 16: 36.

84. S. Li, Y. Park, S. Duraisingham, et al., 2013, Predicting network activity from high throughput metabolomics, PLoS Comput. Biol. 9: e1003123.

85. E.L. Schymanski, J. Jeon, R. Gulde, et al., 2014, Identifying small molecules via high resolution mass spectrometry: Communicating confidence, Environ. Sci. Technol. 48: 2097–2098.

86. B. Groitl, J.-U. Dahl, J.W. Schroeder, U. Jakob, 2017, Pseudomonas aeruginosa defense systems against microbicidal oxidants, Mol. Microbiol. 106: 335–350.

87. C.G. Woods, J. Fu, P. Xue, et al., 2009, Dose-dependent transitions in Nrf2-mediated adaptive response and related stress responses to hypochlorous acid in mouse macrophages, Toxicol. Appl. Pharmacol. 238: 27–36.

88. O. Fiehn, 2002, Metabolomics – The link between genotypes and phenotypes, Plant Mol. Biol. 48: 155–171.

89. G.J. Patti, O. Yanes, G. Siuzdak, 2012, Innovation: Metabolomics: The apogee of the omics trilogy, Nat. Rev. Mol. Cell. Biol. 13: 263–269.

90. S.M. Rappaport, 2011, Implications of the exposome for exposure science, J. Expos. Sci. Environ. Epidemiol. 21: 5–9.

91. C.E. Heim, M.E. Bosch, K.J. Yamada, et al., 2020, Lactate production by Staphylococcus aureus biofilm inhibits HDAC11 to reprogramme the host immune response during persistent infection, Nat. Microbiol. 5: 1271–1284.

92. A. Fu, J.C. Alvarez-Perez, D. Avizonis, et al., 2020, Glucose-dependent partitioning of arginine to the urea cycle protects beta-cells from inflammation, Nat. Metab. 2: 432–446.

93. J. Zhang, J. Muri, G. Fitzgerald, et al., 2020, Endothelial lactate controls muscle regeneration from ischemia by inducing M2-like macrophage polarization, Cell Metabol. 31: 1136–1153.

94. M.P. Murphy, L.A.J. O'Neill, 2018, Krebs Cycle Reimagined: The emerging roles of succinate and itaconate as signal transducers, Cell 174: 780–784.

95. D. Olagnier, A.M. Brandtoft, C. Gunderstofte, et al., 2018, Nrf2 negatively regulates STING indicating a link between antiviral sensing and metabolic reprogramming, Nat. Commun. 9: 3506.

96. E.L. Mills, D.G. Ryan, H.A. Prag, et al., 2018, Itaconate is an anti-inflammatory metabolite that activates Nrf2 via alkylation of KEAP1, Nature 556: 113–117.

97. E.T. Chouchani, V.R. Pell, E. Gaude, et al., 2014, Ischaemic accumulation of succinate controls reperfusion injury through mitochondrial ROS, Nature 515: 431–435.

98. D. Zhang, Z. Tang, H. Huang, et al., 2019, Metabolic regulation of gene expression by histone lactylation, Nature 574: 575–580.

99. C. Jang, L. Chen, J.D. Rabinowitz, 2018, Metabolomics and Isotope Tracing, Cell 173: 822–837.

100. R.F. Burk, K.E. Hill, 2015, Regulation of selenium metabolism and transport, Annu. Rev. Nutr. 35: 109–134.

101. L. Carroll, M.J. Davies, D.I. Pattison, 2015, Reaction of low-molecular-mass organoselenium compounds (and their sulphur analogues) with inflammation-associated oxidants, Free Radic. Res. 49: 750–767.

102. M. Hillion, J. Bernhardt, T. Busche, et al., 2017, Monitoring global protein thiol-oxidation and protein S-mycothiolation in *Mycobacterium smegmatis* under hypochlorite stress, *Sci. Rep.* 7: 1195.

103. B.M. Cumming, K.C. Chinta, V.P. Reddy, A.J.C. Steyn, 2018, Role of ergothioneine in microbial physiology and pathogenesis, *Antioxid. Redox Signal.* 28: 431–444.

104. N. Dickerhof, L. Paton, A.J. Kettle, 2020, Oxidation of bacillithiol by myeloperoxidase-derived oxidants, *Free Radic. Biol. Med.* 158: 74–83.

105. A. Meister, M.E. Anderson, 1983, Glutathione, *Annu. Rev. Biochem.* 52: 711–760.

106. Y.M. Go, D.P. Jones, 2013, Thiol/disulfide redox states in signaling and sensing, *Crit. Rev. Biochem. Mol. Biol.* 48: 173–181.

107. G.H. Kwak, K.Y. Hwang, H.Y. Kim, 2012, Analyses of methionine sulfoxide reductase activities towards free and peptidyl methionine sulfoxides, *Arch. Biochem. Biophys.* 527: 1–5.

108. A.L. Chapman, O. Skaff, R. Senthilmohan, A.J. Kettle, M.J. Davies, 2009, Hypobromous acid and bromamine production by neutrophils and modulation by superoxide, *Biochem. J.* 417: 773–781.

109. R. Senthilmohan, A.J. Kettle, 2006, Bromination and chlorination reactions of myeloperoxidase at physiological concentrations of bromide and chloride, *Arch. Biochem. Biophys.* 445: 235–244.

110. A.V. Peskin, R.G. Midwinter, D.T. Harwood, C.C. Winterbourn, 2005, Chlorine transfer between glycine, taurine, and histamine: Reaction rates and impact on cellular reactivity, *Free Radic. Biol. Med.* 38: 397–405.

111. C.L. Hawkins, 2020, Hypochlorous acid-mediated modification of proteins and its consequences, *Essays Biochem.* 64: 75–86.

112. S.L. Hazen, A. D'Avignon, M.M. Anderson, F.F. Hsu, J.W. Heinecke, 1998, Human neutrophils employ the myeloperoxidase-hydrogen peroxide-chloride system to oxidize α-amino acids to a family of reactive aldehydes, *J. Biol. Chem.* 273: 4997–5005.

113. B.W. Griffin, R. Haddox, 1985, Chlorination of NADH: Similarities of the HOCl-supported and chloroperoxidase-catalyzed reactions, *Arch. Biochem. Biophys.* 239: 305–309.

114. J.L. Macer-Wright, N.R. Stanley, N. Portman, et al., 2019, A role for chlorinated nucleosides in the perturbation of macrophage function and promotion of inflammation, *Chem. Res. Toxicol.* 32: 1223–1234.

115. J.P. Henderson, J. Byun, M.V. Williams, et al., 2001, Bromination of deoxycytidine by eosinophil peroxidase: A mechanism for mutagenesis by oxidative damage of nucleotide precursors, *Proc. Natl. Acad. Sci. U.S.A.* 98: 1631–1636.

116. C.L. Hawkins, M.J. Davies, 1998, Degradation of hyaluronic acid, poly- and mono-saccharides, and model compounds by hypochlorite: Evidence for radical intermediates and fragmentation, *Free Radic. Biol. Med.* 24: 1396–1410.

117. S.L. Hazen, F.F. Hsu, K. Duffin, J.W. Heinecke, 1996, Molecular chlorine generated by the myeloperoxidase-hydrogen peroxide-chloride system of phagocytes converts low density lipoprotein cholesterol into a family of chlorinated sterols, *J. Biol. Chem.* 271: 23080–23088.

118. A.C. Carr, J.J. van den Berg, C.C. Winterbourn, 1996, Chlorination of cholesterol in cell membranes by hypochlorous acid, *Arch. Biochem. Biophys.* 332: 63–69.

119. E.N.D. Palladino, C.L. Hartman, C.J. Albert, D.A. Ford, 2018, The chlorinated lipidome originating from myeloperoxidase-derived HOCl targeting plasmalogens: Metabolism, clearance, and biological properties, *Arch. Biochem. Biophys.* 641: 31–38.

120. C.J. Albert, J.R. Crowley, F.F. Hsu, A.K. Thukkani, D.A. Ford, 2002, Reactive brominating species produced by myeloperoxidase target the vinyl ether bond of plasmalogens: Disparate utilization of sodium halides in the production of halo fatty aldehydes, *J. Biol. Chem.* 277: 4694–4703.

121. A.K. Thukkani, J. McHowat, F.-F. Hsu, et al., 2003, Identification of α-chloro fatty aldehydes and unsaturated lysophosphatidylcholine molecular species in human atherosclerotic lesions, *Circulation* 108: 3128–3133.

122. C.L. Hartman, M.A. Duerr, C.J. Albert, et al., 2018, 2-Chlorofatty acids induce Weibel-Palade body mobilization, *J. Lipid Res.* 59: 113–122.

123. V.M. Marshall, B. Reiter, 1980, Comparison of the antibacterial activity of the hypothiocyanite anion towards Streptococcus lactis and *Escherichia coli*, *J. Gen. Microbiol.* 120: 513–516.

124. M.N. Mickelson, 1977, Glucose transport in *Streptococcus agalactiae* and its inhibition by lactoperoxidase-thiocyanate-hydrogen peroxide, *J. Bacteriol.* 132: 541–548.

125. M.N. Mickelson, 1979, Antibacterial action of lactoperoxidase-thiocyanate-hydrogen peroxide on *Streptococcus agalactiae*, *Appl. Environ. Microbiol.* 38: 821–826.

126. M.N. Mickelson, A.J. Anderson, 1984, Cystine antagonism of the antibacterial action of lactoperoxidase-thiocyanate-hydrogen peroxide on *Streptococcus agalactiae*, *Appl. Environ. Microbiol.* 47: 338–342.

127. K. Shin, K. Yamauchi, S. Teraguchi, H. Hayasawa, I. Imoto, 2002, Susceptibility of *Helicobacter pylori* and its urease activity to the peroxidase-hydrogen peroxide-thiocyanate antimicrobial system, *J. Med. Microbiol.* 51: 231–237.

128. M.M. Lloyd, D.M. van Reyk, M.J. Davies, C.L. Hawkins, 2008, Hypothiocyanous acid is a more potent inducer of apoptosis and protein thiol depletion in murine macrophage cells than hypochlorous acid or hypobromous acid, *Biochem. J.* 414: 271–280.

129. T. Hildebrandt, J. Knuesting, C. Berndt, B. Morgan, R. Scheibe, 2015, Cytosolic thiol switches regulating basic cellular functions: GAPDH as an information hub? *Biol. Chem.* 396: 523–537.

130. A. Kuehne, H. Emmert, J. Soehle, et al., 2015, Acute activation of oxidative pentose phosphate pathway as first-line response to oxidative stress in human skin cells, *Mol. Cell.* 59: 359–371.

131. J. van der Reest, S. Lilla, L. Zheng, S. Zanivan, E. Gottlieb, 2018, Proteome-wide analysis of cysteine oxidation reveals metabolic sensitivity to redox stress, *Nat. Commun.* 9: 1581.

132. D.T. Love, C. Guo, E.I. Nikelshparg, et al., 2020, The role of the myeloperoxidase-derived oxidant hypothiocyanous acid (HOSCN) in the induction of mitochondrial dysfunction in macrophages, *Redox Biol.* 36: 101602.

133. J.L. Macer-Wright, I. Sileikaite, B.S. Rayner, C.L. Hawkins, 2020, 8-Chloroadenosine alters the metabolic profile and downregulates antioxidant and DNA damage repair pathways in macrophages, *Chem. Res. Toxicol.* 33: 402–413.

134. V. Tang, S. Fu, B.S. Rayner, C.L. Hawkins, 2019, 8-Chloroadenosine induces apoptosis in human coronary artery endothelial cells through the activation of the unfolded protein response, *Redox Biol.* 26: 101274.

135. A. Sassa, T. Ohta, T. Nohmi, M. Honma, M. Yasui, 2011, Mutational specificities of brominated DNA adducts catalyzed by human DNA polymerases, *J. Mol. Biol.* 406: 679–686.

136. M.A. Duerr, E.N.D. Palladino, C.L. Hartman, et al., 2018, Bromofatty aldehyde derived from bromine exposure and myeloperoxidase and eosinophil peroxidase modify GSH and protein, *J. Lipid Res.* 59: 696–705.

137. N.J. Meyer, J.P. Reilly, R. Feng, et al., 2017, Myeloperoxidase-derived 2-chlorofatty acids contribute to human sepsis mortality via acute respiratory distress syndrome, *JCI Insight* 2: e96432.

138. S. Eliuk, A. Makarov, 2015, Evolution of orbitrap mass spectrometry instrumentation, *Annu. Rev. Anal. Chem.* 8: 61–80.

139. M. Ghaste, R. Mistrik, V. Shulaev, 2016, Applications of fourier transform ion cyclotron resonance (FT-ICR) and orbitrap based high resolution mass spectrometry in metabolomics and lipidomics, *Int. J. Mol. Sci.* 17: 816.

140. P. Barbier Saint Hilaire, U.M. Hohenester, B. Colsch, et al., 2018, Evaluation of the high-field orbitrap fusion for compound annotation in metabolomics, *Anal. Chem.* 90: 3030–3035.

141. J.D. Chandler, H. Horati, D.I. Walker, et al., 2018, Determination of thiocyanate in exhaled breath condensate, *Free Radic. Biol. Med.* 126: 334–340.

142. B.J. Day, P.E. Bratcher, J.D. Chandler, et al., 2020, The thiocyanate analog selenocyanate is a more potent antimicrobial pro-drug that also is selectively detoxified by the host, *Free Radic. Biol. Med.* 146: 324–332.

143. R. Nakabayashi, K. Saito, 2017, Ultrahigh resolution metabolomics for S-containing metabolites, *Curr. Opin. Biotechnol.* 43: 8–16.

144. S. Becker, L. Kortz, C. Helmschrodt, J. Thiery, U. Ceglarek, 2012, LC-MS-based metabolomics in the clinical laboratory, *J. Chromatogr. B Analyt. Technol. Biomed. Life. Sci.* 883–884: 68–75.

145. A. Teleki, R. Takors, 2019, Quantitative profiling of endogenous metabolites using hydrophilic interaction liquid chromatography-tandem mass spectrometry (HILIC-MS/MS), *Methods Mol. Biol.* 1859: 185–207.

146. T. Cajka, O. Fiehn, 2016, Toward merging untargeted and targeted methods in mass spectrometry-based metabolomics and lipidomics, *Anal. Chem.* 88: 524–545.

147. T.M. Annesley, 2003, Ion suppression in mass spectrometry, *Clin. Chem.* 49: 1041–1044.

148. R.A. Quinn, A.V. Melnik, A. Vrbanac, et al., 2020, Global chemical effects of the microbiome include new bile-acid conjugations, *Nature* 579: 123–129.

149. A.T. Aron, E.C. Gentry, K.L. McPhail, et al., 2020, Reproducible molecular networking of untargeted mass spectrometry data using GNPS, *Nat. Protoc.* 15: 1954–1991.

150. D.S. Wishart, 2019, NMR metabolomics: A look ahead, J. Magn. Reson. 306: 155–161.

151. W. Lu, X. Su, M.S. Klein, et al., 2017, Metabolite measurement: Pitfalls to avoid and practices to follow, Annu. Rev. Biochem. 86: 277–304.

152. J.M. Johnson, F.H. Strobel, M. Reed, J. Pohl, D.P. Jones, 2008, A rapid LC-FTMS method for the analysis of cysteine, cystine and cysteine/cystine steady-state redox potential in human plasma, Clin. Chim. Acta 396: 43–48.

153. N.G. Mahieu, X. Huang, Y. Chen, Jr., G.J. Patti, 2014, Credentialing features: A platform to benchmark and optimize untargeted metabolomic methods, Anal. Chem. 86: 9583–9589.

154. M.R. Mashego, L. Wu, J.C. Van Dam, et al., 2004, MIRACLE: Mass isotopomer ratio analysis of U-13C-labeled extracts. A new method for accurate quantification of changes in concentrations of intracellular metabolites, Biotechnol. Bioeng. 85: 620–628.

155. C.S. Clendinen, G.S. Stupp, B. Wang, T.J. Garrett, A.S. Edison, 2016, (13)C Metabolomics: NMR and IROA for Unknown Identification, Curr. Metabolomics 4: 116–120.

156. G.S. Stupp, C.S. Clendinen, R. Ajredini, et al., 2013, Isotopic ratio outlier analysis global metabolomics of caenorhabditis elegans, Anal. Chem. 85: 11858–11865.

157. N. Grankvist, J.D. Watrous, K.A. Lagerborg, et al., 2018, Profiling the metabolism of human cells by deep (13)C labeling, Cell. Chem. Biol. 25: 1419–1427.

158. N. Rios, R. Radi, B. Kalyanaraman, J. Zielonka, 2020, Tracking isotopically labeled oxidants using boronate-based redox probes, J. Biol. Chem. 295: 6665–6676.

159. K.H. Liu, M. Nellis, K. Uppal, et al., 2020, Reference standardization for quantification and harmonization of large-scale metabolomics, Anal. Chem. 92: 8836–8844.

160. N.G. Mahieu, G.J. Patti, 2017, Systems-level annotation of a metabolomics data set reduces 25000 features to fewer than 1000 unique metabolites, Anal. Chem. 89: 10397–10406.

161. C.D. Broeckling, F.A. Afsar, S. Neumann, A. Ben-Hur, J.E. Prenni, 2014, RAMClust: A novel feature clustering method enables spectral-matching-based annotation for metabolomics data, Anal. Chem. 86: 6812–6817.

162. M. Vinaixa, S. Samino, I. Saez, et al., 2012, A guideline to univariate statistical analysis for LC/MS-based untargeted metabolomics-derived data, Metabolites 2: 775–795.

163. N. Garg, M. Wang, E. Hyde, et al., 2017, Three-dimensional microbiome and metabolome cartography of a diseased human lung, Cell Host Microbe. 22: 705–716.e4.

164. W.D. Lee, D. Mukha, E. Aizenshtein, T. Shlomi, 2019, Spatial-fluxomics provides a subcellular-compartmentalized view of reductive glutamine metabolism in cancer cells, Nat. Commun. 10: 1351.

165. R.M. Caprioli, 2019, Imaging mass spectrometry: A perspective, J. Biomol. Tech. 30: 7–11.

166. M.E. Duenas, J.J. Essner, Y.J. Lee, 2017, 3D MALDI mass spectrometry imaging of a single cell: Spatial mapping of lipids in the embryonic development of zebrafish, Sci. Rep. 7: 14946.

167. J. Balog, L. Sasi-Szabo, J. Kinross, et al., 2013, Intraoperative tissue identification using rapid evaporative ionization mass spectrometry, Sci. Transl. Med. 5: 194ra93.

168. Y.M. Go, D.P. Jones, 2013, The redox proteome, J. Biol. Chem. 288: 26512–26520.

169. J. Yang, K.S. Carroll, D.C. Liebler, 2016, The expanding landscape of the thiol redox proteome, Mol. Cell Proteomics 15: 1–11.

170. C.E. Paulsen, K.S. Carroll, 2013, Cysteine-mediated redox signaling: Chemistry, biology, and tools for discovery, Chem. Rev. 113: 4633–4679.

171. B.K. Chi, A.A. Roberts, T.T.T. Huyen, et al., 2013, S-Bacillithiolation protects conserved and essential proteins against hypochlorite stress in firmicutes bacteria, Antioxid. Redox Signal. 18: 1273–1295.

172. V.V. Loi, N.T.T. Huyen, T. Busche, et al., 2019, Staphylococcus aureus responds to allicin by global S-thioallylation – Role of the Brx/BSH/YpdA pathway and the disulfide reductase MerA to overcome allicin stress, Free Radic. Biol. Med. 139: 55–69.

173. Y.M. Go, D.P. Jones, 2014, Redox biology: Interface of the exposome with the proteome, epigenome and genome, Redox Biol. 2: 358–360.

174. Y.H. Jan, D.E. Heck, A.C. Dragomir, et al., 2014, Acetaminophen reactive intermediates target hepatic thioredoxin reductase, Chem. Res. Toxicol. 27: 882–894.

175. S.M. Rappaport, H. Li, H. Grigoryan, W.E. Funk, E.R. Williams, 2012, Adductomics: Characterizing exposures to reactive electrophiles, Toxicol. Lett. 213: 83–90.

176. M. Karimi, B. Crossett, S.J. Cordwell, D.I. Pattison, M.J. Davies, 2020, Characterization of disulfide (cystine) oxidation by HOCl in a model peptide:

Evidence for oxygen addition, disulfide bond cleavage and adduct formation with thiols, *Free Radic. Biol. Med.* 154: 62–74.

177. M. Karimi, M.T. Ignasiak, B. Chan, et al., 2016, Reactivity of disulfide bonds is markedly affected by structure and environment: Implications for protein modification and stability, *Sci. Rep.* 6: 38572.

178. Y.M. Go, J.R. Roede, D.I. Walker, et al., 2013, Selective targeting of the cysteine proteome by thioredoxin and glutathione redox systems, *Mol. Cell Proteomics* 12: 3285–3296.

179. C.C. Winterbourn, M.B. Hampton, 2008, Thiol chemistry and specificity in redox signaling, *Free Radic. Biol. Med.* 45: 549–561.

180. M. Imber, N.T.T. Huyen, A.J. Pietrzyk-Brzezinska, et al., 2018, Protein S-bacillithiolation functions in thiol protection and redox regulation of the glyceraldehyde-3-phosphate dehydrogenase GAP in staphylococcus aureus under hypochlorite stress, *Antioxid. Redox Signal.* 28: 410–430.

181. T.J. Barrett, D.I. Pattison, S.E. Leonard, et al., 2012, Inactivation of thiol-dependent enzymes by hypothiocyanous acid: Role of sulfenyl thiocyanate and sulfenic acid intermediates, *Free Radic. Biol. Med.* 52: 1075–1085.

182. B. McDonagh, G.K. Sakellariou, M.J. Jackson, 2014, Application of redox proteomics to skeletal muscle aging and exercise, *Biochem. Soc. Trans.* 42: 965–970.

183. D. Lin, S. Saleh, D.C. Liebler, 2008, Reversibility of covalent electrophile-protein adducts and chemical toxicity, *Chem. Res. Toxicol.* 21: 2361–2369.

184. C.A. Evans, 2019, Reducing complexity? Cysteine reduction and S-alkylation in proteomic workflows: Practical considerations, *Methods Mol. Biol.* 1977: 83–97.

185. P.G. Hains, P.J. Robinson, 2017, The impact of commonly used alkylating agents on artifactual peptide modification, *J. Proteome Res.* 16: 3443–3447.

186. J. Yang, V. Gupta, K.A. Tallman, et al., 2015, Global, in situ, site-specific analysis of protein S-sulfenylation, *Nat. Protoc.* 10: 1022–1037.

187. J.A. Reisz, E. Bechtold, S.B. King, L.B. Poole, C.M. Furdui, 2013, Thiol-blocking electrophiles interfere with labeling and detection of protein sulfenic acids, *FEBS J.* 280: 6150–6161.

188. S. Akter, L. Fu, Y. Jung, et al., 2018, Chemical proteomics reveals new targets of cysteine sulfinic acid reductase, *Nat. Chem. Biol.* 14: 995–1004.

189. L.I. Leichert, F. Gehrke, H.V. Gudiseva, et al., 2008, Quantifying changes in the thiol redox proteome upon oxidative stress in vivo, *Proc. Natl. Acad. Sci. U.S.A.* 105: 8197–8202.

190. K. Araki, H. Kusano, N. Sasaki, et al., 2016, Redox sensitivities of global cellular cysteine residues under reductive and oxidative stress, *J. Proteome Res.* 15: 2548–2559.

191. M. Sethuraman, M.E. McComb, H. Huang, et al., 2004, Isotope-coded affinity tag (ICAT) approach to redox proteomics: Identification and quantitation of oxidant-sensitive cysteine thiols in complex protein mixtures, *J. Proteome Res.* 3: 1228–1233.

192. M.E. Albertolle, T.T.N. Phan, A. Pozzi, F.P. Guengerich, 2018, Sulfenylation of human liver and kidney microsomal cytochromes p450 and other drug-metabolizing enzymes as a response to redox alteration, *Mol. Cell Proteomics* 17: 889–900.

193. H. Xiao, M.P. Jedrychowski, D.K. Schweppe, et al., 2020, A quantitative tissue-specific landscape of protein redox regulation during aging, *Cell* 180: 968–983.e24.

194. L.B. Poole, C.M. Furdui, S.B. King, 2020, Introduction to approaches and tools for the evaluation of protein cysteine oxidation, *Essays Biochem.* 64: 1–17.

195. L.A.G. van Leeuwen, E.C. Hinchy, M.P. Murphy, E.L. Robb, H.M. Cocheme, 2017, Click-PEGylation – A mobility shift approach to assess the redox state of cysteines in candidate proteins, *Free Radic. Biol. Med.* 108: 374–382.

196. J.R. Roede, Y.M. Go, D.P. Jones, 2012, Redox equivalents and mitochondrial bioenergetics, *Methods Mol. Biol.* 810: 249–280.

197. E.J. Walker, J.Q. Bettinger, K.A. Welle, J.R. Hryhorenko, S. Ghaemmaghami, 2019, Global analysis of methionine oxidation provides a census of folding stabilities for the human proteome, *Proc. Natl. Acad. Sci. U.S.A.* 116: 6081–6090.

198. S. Luo, R.L. Levine, 2009, Methionine in proteins defends against oxidative stress, *FASEB J.* 23: 464–472.

199. D. Johnson, J. Travis, 1979, The oxidative inactivation of human alpha-1-proteinase inhibitor. Further evidence for methionine at the reactive center, *J. Biol. Chem.* 254: 4022–4026.

200. B. Shao, M.N. Oda, C. Bergt, et al., 2006, Myeloperoxidase impairs ABCA1-dependent cholesterol efflux through methionine oxidation and site-specific tyrosine chlorination of apolipoprotein A-I, *J. Biol. Chem.* 281: 9001–9004.

201. B.C. Lee, D.T. Le, V.N. Gladyshev, 2008, Mammals reduce methionine-S-sulfoxide with MsrA and are unable to reduce methionine-R-sulfoxide, and this function can be restored with a yeast reductase, *J. Biol. Chem.* 283: 28361–28369.

202. Z. Péterfi, L. Tarrago, V.N. Gladyshev, 2016, Practical guide for dynamic monitoring of protein oxidation using genetically encoded ratiometric fluorescent biosensors of methionine sulfoxide, *Methods* 109: 149–157.

203. L. Carroll, D.I. Pattison, S. Fu, et al., 2017, Catalytic oxidant scavenging by selenium-containing compounds: Reduction of selenoxides and N-chloramines by thiols and redox enzymes, *Redox Biol.* 12: 872–882.

204. A. Müller, E. Cadenas, P. Graf, H. Sies, 1984, A novel biologically active seleno-organic compound—1, *Biochem. Pharmacol.* 33: 3235–3239.

205. S. Suzuki, Y. Kodera, T. Saito, et al., 2016, Methionine sulfoxides in serum proteins as potential clinical biomarkers of oxidative stress, *Sci. Rep.* 6: 38299.

206. S. Lin, X. Yang, S. Jia, et al., 2017, Redox-based reagents for chemoselective methionine bioconjugation, *Science* 355: 597–602.

207. A.R. Mani, S. Ippolito, J.C. Moreno, T.J. Visser, K.P. Moore, 2007, The metabolism and dechlorination of chlorotyrosine in vivo, *J. Biol. Chem.* 282: 29114–29121.

208. A.R. Mani, J.C. Moreno, T.J. Visser, K.P. Moore, 2016, The metabolism and de-bromination of bromotyrosine in vivo, *Free Radic. Biol. Med.* 90: 243–251.

209. T. Nybo, H. Cai, C.Y. Chuang, et al., 2018, Chlorination and oxidation of human plasma fibronectin by myeloperoxidase-derived oxidants, and its consequences for smooth muscle cell function, *Redox Biol.* 19: 388–400.

210. C.L. Hawkins, P.E. Morgan, M.J. Davies, 2009, Quantification of protein modification by oxidants, *Free Radic. Biol. Med.* 46: 965–988.

211. L. Mouls, E. Silajdzic, N. Haroune, C.M. Spickett, A.R. Pitt, 2009, Development of novel mass spectrometric methods for identifying HOCl-induced modifications to proteins, *Proteomics* 9: 1617–1631.

212. K. Tveen-Jensen, A. Reis, L. Mouls, A.R. Pitt, C.M. Spickett, 2013, Reporter ion-based mass spectrometry approaches for the detection of non-enzymatic protein modifications in biological samples, *J. Proteomics* 92: 71–79.

213. T. Nybo, M.J. Davies, A. Rogowska-Wrzesinska, 2019, Analysis of protein chlorination by mass spectrometry, *Redox Biol.* 26: 101236.

214. B.B. Misra, C.D. Langefeld, M. Olivier, L.A. Cox, 2019, Integrated omics: Tools, advances, and future approaches, *J. Mol. Endocrinol.* 62: R21–R45.

215. K. Uppal, C. Ma, Y.-M. Go, D.P. Jones, 2018, xMWAS: A data-driven integration and differential network analysis tool, *Bioinformatics* 34: 701–702.

216. J.D. Chandler, X. Hu, E.-J. Ko, et al., 2019, Low-dose cadmium potentiates lung inflammatory response to 2009 pandemic H1N1 influenza virus in mice, *Environ. Int.* 127: 720–729.

217. Y.M. Go, J.R. Roede, M. Orr, Y. Liang, D.P. Jones, 2014, Integrated redox proteomics and metabolomics of mitochondria to identify mechanisms of cd toxicity, *Toxicol. Sci.* 139: 59–73.

218. M.J. Lopez-Grueso, R. Gonzalez-Ojeda, R. Requejo-Aguilar, et al., 2019, Thioredoxin and glutaredoxin regulate metabolism through different multiplex thiol switches, *Redox Biol.* 21: 101049.

219. A. Holmgren, 1985, Thioredoxin, *Annu. Rev. Biochem.* 54: 237–271.

220. H. Yan, M.F. Lou, M.R. Fernando, J.J. Harding, 2006, Thioredoxin, thioredoxin reductase, and alpha-crystallin revive inactivated glyceraldehyde 3-phosphate dehydrogenase in human aged and cataract lens extracts, *Mol. Vis.* 12: 1153–1159.

221. M. Kontou, R.D. Will, C. Adelfalk, et al., 2004, Thioredoxin, a regulator of gene expression, *Oncogene* 23: 2146–2152.

PART THREE

Peroxidases in Innate Immunity

CHAPTER NINE

Myeloperoxidase and Immune Cell Recruitment and Activation

Martin Mollenhauer

Clinic III for Internal Medicine, Department of Cardiology, University of Cologne

Anna Klinke

Herz- und Diabeteszentrum NRW, Universitätsklinik der Ruhr-Universität Bochum

CONTENTS

ABBREVIATIONS

Akt:	Protein kinase B
aMPO:	Catalytically active MPO
ANCA:	Anti-neutrophil cytoplasmic autoantibody
CCL:	CC-chemokine ligand
CXCL:	C-X-C motif ligand
ECs:	Endothelial cell
ERK1/2:	Extracellular signal-related kinases 1 and 2
HOCl:	Hypochlorous acid
HOSCN:	Hypothiocyanous acid
ICAM-1:	Intercellular adhesion molecule-1
IL:	Interleukin
iMPO:	Catalytically inactive MPO
LPS:	Lipopolysaccharide
MIP-1α:	Macrophage inflammatory protein-1α
NE:	Neutrophil elastase
NETs:	Neutrophil extracellular traps
NF-κB:	Nuclear factor kappaB
NO:	Nitric oxide
Nrf2:	Nuclear factor erythroid-2-related factor 2
oxHDL:	Oxidized high-density lipoprotein
oxLDL:	Oxidized low-density lipoprotein
p38MAPK:	p38 mitogen-activated protein kinase
PMN:	Polymorphonuclear neutrophil
PR3:	Proteinase 3
ROS:	Reactive oxygen species
TNF-α:	Tumor necrosis factor-α
VCAM-1:	Vascular adhesion molecule-1

DOI: 10.1201/9781003212287-12

INTRODUCTION

Myeloperoxidase (MPO) serves as an important element of host defense, which is mainly attributed to the microbicidal activity of MPO-derived reactive species. However, MPO also modulates the function of innate immune cells, an effect, which is caused either by MPO independently of its catalytic activity or by generation of reactive species and varies dependent on their type and concentration. These properties contribute to MPO's role in host defense, in a way that leukocyte recruitment, release of neutrophil extracellular traps (NETs), leukocyte cytokine and reactive oxygen species (ROS) release and phagocytosis are affected. At the same time, this characteristic modulates MPO's pro-inflammatory properties. It can amplify leukocyte-dependent damage of host tissue either during host defense or under conditions of sterile inflammation such as ischemia and reperfusion or low-grade chronic inflammation. The mechanisms and consequences of MPO's interaction with innate immune cells appear to be highly diverse. Dependent on the effector molecules, their concentration and the surrounding conditions, pro-inflammatory as well as inhibitory properties have been described. This chapter will focus on MPO's role in innate immune cell activation and recruitment with respect to the responsible molecules, the affected cells and the functional consequences.

MPO ACTIVATES INNATE IMMUNE CELLS

MPO-Dependent Effects Mediated by Receptor Binding

It was demonstrated that MPO, independent of its catalytic activity, provokes cytokine secretion, in particular the release of tumor necrosis factor (TNF)-α, and an enhanced respiratory burst of resident alveolar or peritoneal macrophages [1–4]. This effect was induced by catalytically active as well as by recombinant inactive or isolated, inactivated MPO and was suggested to result from binding of MPO to the mannose receptor on macrophages (Figure 9.1). The authors observed that the MPO–mannose receptor interaction led to an exacerbation of experimental arthritis [2,3]. Enhanced bactericidal activity and phagocytosis of *Candida albicans* by macrophages were also associated to this interaction [5,6]. Others identified the leukocyte integrin CD11b/CD18

to serve as a receptor for MPO. MPO binding to CD11b/CD18 on polymorphonuclear neutrophils (PMNs) induced activation of certain intracellular signaling cascades: Extracellular signal-related kinases 1 and 2 (ERK1/2) and protein kinase B (Akt) were activated, which prolonged PMN life span and consequently augmented experimental lung inflammation [7]. Moreover, p38 mitogen-activated protein kinase (MAPK) activation led to augmented CD11b/CD18 surface expression and release of ROS by PMN [8] (Figure 9.1, Table 9.1).

MPO-Dependent Effects Mediated by Reactive Species

Innate immune intracellular signaling is furthermore provoked by MPO-derived hypohalogenous acids. In high concentrations, hypochlorous acid (HOCl) and hypobromous acid (HOBr) are cytotoxic. In in vitro studies, the cytotoxic concentration is dependent on the assay media; protein- and amino-acid-free or -low buffers avoid scavenging effects, which take place in full serum containing cell culture media. This needs to be taken into account when comparing concentration-dependent effects described in the literature. Viability of monocyte-derived macrophages or a macrophage cell line was significantly reduced after exposure to HOCl or HOBr [9,10]. Interestingly, hypothiocyanous acid (HOSCN), which more selectively oxidizes thiols compared with HOCl and HOBr, was most potent in inducing apoptosis and necrosis in macrophages, in part via reaction with thiol residues of mitochondrial proteins [9] (Figure 9.1, Table 9.1). Moreover, proteins involved in energy metabolism of macrophages are modified by HOSCN, which can also lead to cell death [11]. Immune cells harbor a variety of protective molecules to resist a certain level of oxidative stress. Glutathione is important to prevent HOCl-induced cytotoxicity in macrophages [10]. Similarly, HOCl-modified taurine, i.e. taurine chloramine (TauCl), attenuated activation of nuclear factor "kappa-light-chain-enhancer" of activated B-cells (NF-κB) in LPS- and interferon-γ-stimulated macrophages [12] and bacteria-exposed PMN [13] and reduced subsequent cytokine secretion (Table 9.1). It appears that HOCl can even induce antioxidative signaling. In a macrophage cell line, HOCl stimulated the expression and subsequent antioxidative signaling of nuclear factor erythroid 2-related factor 2 (Nrf2) [14,15], an effect that

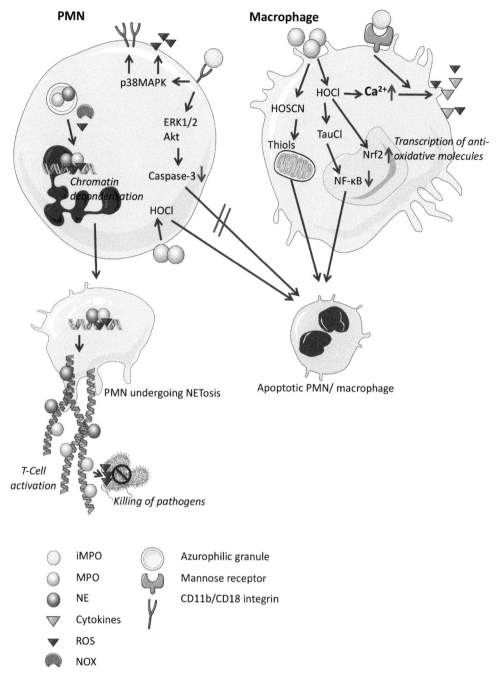

PMN

Macrophage

p38MAPK

ERK1/2
Akt

Caspase-3

Chromatin decondensation

HOCl

HOSCN

HOCl → **Ca²⁺**↑

TauCl

Thiols

Nrf2

Transcription of anti-oxidative molecules

NF-κB

PMN undergoing NETosis

Apoptotic PMN/ macrophage

T-Cell activation

Killing of pathogens

○ iMPO
◔ MPO
● NE
▽ Cytokines
▼ ROS
◓ NOX

○ Azurophilic granule
⨆ Mannose receptor
Y CD11b/CD18 integrin

Figure 9.1 Schematic demonstration of MPO-dependent mechanisms of leukocyte activation. MPO binds to mannose receptors and CD11b/CD18 integrins, which induces intracellular signalling cascades leading to cytokine and ROS release, surface molecule expression or delay of apoptosis. HOCl and HOSCN exert proapoptotic effects. Intracellular MPO translocates together with NE to the nucleus leading to chromatin decondensation and finally to NETosis. NET-bound MPO contributes to killing of pathogens and priming of T cells. Abbreviations: Akt, protein kinase B; EC, endothelial cell; ERK1/2, extracellular signal-related kinases 1 and 2; iMPO, catalytically inactive MPO; HOCl, hypochlorous acid; HOSCN, hypothiocyanous acid; ICAM-1, intercellular adhesion molecule-1; NE, neutrophil elastase; NETosis, release of neutrophil extracellular traps; NFκB, nuclear factor kappa-light-chain-enhancer of activated B-cells; NOX, NADPH-oxidase; p38MAPK, p38 mitogen-activated protein kinase; PMN, polymorphonuclear neutrophil; ROS, reactive oxygen species; SMC, smooth muscle cells; VCAM-1, vascular adhesion molecule-1; TauCl, taurine chloramine. Figures are based on http://www.servier.com.

TABLE 9.1

Effects of MPO and MPO-derived molecules on immune cells and ECs affecting immune cell activation and recruitment

Effector molecule/ condition	Target/mechanism	Cell species	Effect	Reference
Effects of catalytically inactive MPO				
iMPO	Mannose receptor binding	Macrophages	Cytokine release ↑	[1–4]
iMPO	Mannose receptor binding	Macrophages	Bactericidal activity, C. albicans phagocytosis ↑	[5,6]
iMPO	CD11b/CD18 binding, Erk1/2, Akt activation	PMN	Prolongation of life span	[7]
iMPO	CD11b/CD18 binding, p38MAPK activation	PMN	ROS release, CD11b/CD18 expression ↑	[8]
iMPO	Glycocalyx, electrostatic interaction	Leukocytes	Attraction ↑	[63]
iMPO	Glycocalyx, electrostatic interaction	ECs	Leukocyte recruitment ↑	[63]
iMPO	-	ECs	Cytokine and ROS release ↑	[78]
iMPO	Actin cytoskeleton rearrangements, elasticity, cytosolic Ca^{2+}↑	Platelets	Agonist-induced aggregation ↑	[95]
Effects of catalytically active MPO				
aMPO	Calpain activation	ECs	VCAM-1 ↑	[86]
aMPO	PMN-NET binding	T-cells	Priming ↑	[58]
Effects of HOCl				
HOCl	Nrf2 activation	Macrophages	Anti-oxidative molecule expression ↑	[14,15]
HOCl	Cytosolic Ca^{2+}↑	Macrophages	Cytokine, ROS release ↑	[16]
HOCl	-	Macrophages	Cytokine release ↑	[15]
HOCl	-	PMN	Apoptosis ↑	[38]
HOCl	Synergy with NE	PMN	Histone H4 degradation, NETosis ↑	[54]
HOCl	Mac-1 receptor activation	DC	Infl. activation ↓, CD86, IL-12, IL-23 ↓	[106]
HOCl	NO oxidation	DC	Glycolysis, maturation ↓	[108]
HOCl	Peptide/glycoprotein oxidation	Macrophages	Phagocytosis ↑	[110]
HOCl	Oxidation of plasma fibronectin	ECs	Adherence ↓, proliferation ↓, ECM synthesis ↓	[85]
HOCl	NO oxidation	Platelets	P-selectin, PECAM-1 ↑	[96]
Effects of HOSCN				
HOSCN	Oxidation of metabolic regulators	Macrophages	Apoptosis, necrosis ↑	[11]

(*Continued*)

TABLE 9.1 (*Continued*)
Effects of MPO and MPO-derived molecules on immune cells and ECs affecting immune cell activation and recruitment

Effector molecule/ condition	Target/mechanism	Cell species	Effect	Reference
HOSCN	Oxidation of thiols	Macrophages	Apoptosis, necrosis ↑	[9]
HOSCN	p38MAPK, NF-κB activation	ECs	E-selectin, ICAM-1, VCAM-1 ↑	[66]
Effects of MPO-modified lipoproteins				
MPOoxHDL	NF-κB activation	ECs	VCAM-1 ↑	[83]
MPOoxLDL	-	ECs	P-selectin ↑	[87]
HOCloxLDL	-	PMN	ROS release, adhesion, chemotaxis ↑	[88–90]
Effects of MPO-modified taurine				
Taurine chloramine	NF-κB activation ↓	PMN, macrophages	Cytokine secretion ↓ Apoptosis ↑	[12,13,39]
Effects of MPO deficiency and inhibition				
MPO-inhibitor/ MPO-deficiency	NF-κB, p38MAPK, Erk1/2 activity ↑	PMN	Zymosan-induced cytokine secretion, CD11b/CD18 expression ↑	[17–20]
MPO-deficiency	-	PMN	LPS-induced CXCL1, MIP-1α ↓ IL-6, IL-10, CCL5, TNF-α ↑	[22]
MPO-deficiency	-	PMN	LPS-induced apoptosis ↓	[41]
MPO-inhibitor	-	PMN	PR3-ANCA-induced degranulation, ROS release, NETosis ↓	[23]

disappeared with increasing HOCl concentrations. Nevertheless, cytokine and ROS release of macrophages was induced by HOCl [15,16], which was in part associated with increased concentrations of cytosolic calcium (Figure 9.1). Interestingly, M1-polarized macrophages were more susceptible to HOCl stimulation than M2-polarized [16].

Activation of Innate Immune Cells during MPO Deficiency or MPO Inhibition

A number of studies tested the role of MPO for activation of innate immune cells using PMN from MPO knockout ($Mpo^{-/-}$) mice or treated with a pharmacological MPO inhibitor. Dependent on the activating agent, contrasting results were obtained. Stimulation of PMN or macrophages with zymosan, which binds to toll-like receptor 2 (TLR2), complement receptor 3 and dectin-1, provoked activation of NF-κB and ERK1/2, the secretion of cytokines and the expression of CD11b/ CD18 integrins, which was more pronounced in cells isolated from $Mpo^{-/-}$ mice or treated with an MPO inhibitor compared with wild-type (WT) cells without MPO inhibition [17–20] (Table 9.1). Similar results were obtained with *C. albicans* stimulation [21]. In accordance, local zymosan treatment induced more severe PMN infiltration to the lungs of $Mpo^{-/-}$ compared with WT mice [17] (Figure 9.2). The authors suggested that hydrogen peroxide (H_2O_2) might be the main mediator of PMN activation upon zymosan exposure, which is depleted when MPO is present [17,18]. In contrast, upon LPS instillation, lung PMN and macrophage infiltration were markedly less pronounced in $Mpo^{-/-}$ compared with WT mice with significantly lower levels of cytokines in $Mpo^{-/-}$ mice [22]. However, in vitro stimulation of PMN with the

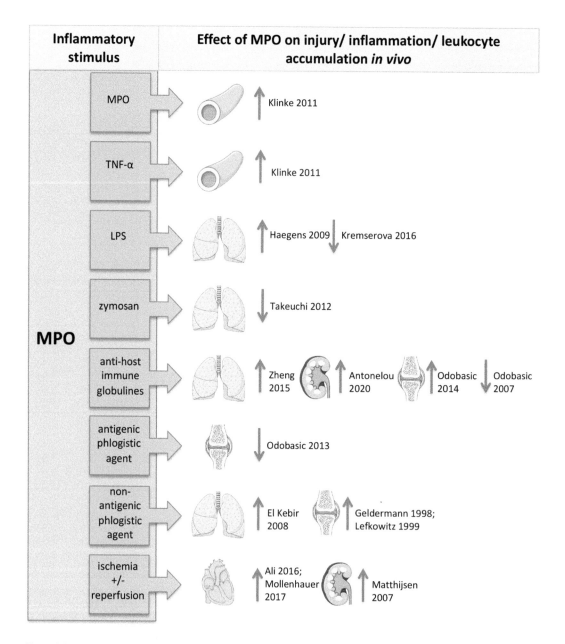

Inflammatory stimulus	Effect of MPO on injury/ inflammation/ leukocyte accumulation *in vivo*
MPO	↑ Klinke 2011
TNF-α	↑ Klinke 2011
LPS	↑ Haegens 2009 ↓ Kremserova 2016
zymosan	↓ Takeuchi 2012
anti-host immune globulines	↑ Zheng 2015 ↑ Antonelou 2020 ↑ Odobasic 2014 ↓ Odobasic 2007
antigenic phlogistic agent	↓ Odobasic 2013
non-antigenic phlogistic agent	↑ El Kebir 2008 ↑ Geldermann 1998; Lefkowitz 1999
ischemia +/- reperfusion	↑ Ali 2016; Mollenhauer 2017 ↑ Matthijsen 2007

Figure 9.2 MPO-dependent inflammation and host injury *in vivo*. MPO modulated leukocyte recruitment, inflammation and/or host tissue injury in different *in vivo* models. The left column depicts the inflammatory stimuli that were used, organ symbols reflect host organ that was examined. Figures are based on http://www.servier.com.

TLR4 ligand LPS showed that cytokine expression was lower for CXCL1 and macrophage inflammatory protein (MIP)-1α but higher for interleukin (IL)-6, CCL-5, IL-10 and TNF-α in MPO-deficient PMN [22]. This suggests that the *in vivo* findings may not only be mediated by MPO's effects on the innate immune cells but may involve effects on endothelial integrity as well, as discussed in following sections. In *vitro* treatment of PMN with cytokines or proteinase 3 (PR3) anti-neutrophil cytoplasmic autoantibody (PR3-ANCA) led to degranulation, NETosis and ROS release, which was lower when MPO was pharmacologically inhibited [23] (Table 9.1).

MPO AFFECTS INNATE IMMUNE CELL APOPTOSIS

Mature PMN have the shortest blood half-live span of all leukocytes of a few days [24,25]. If not activated and recruited, they get destroyed within the liver, spleen and bone marrow (BM) [26–30]. Under inflammatory conditions, they can leave the blood stream and infiltrate the surrounding tissues, where their life span can be prolonged, as their apoptosis and necrosis are modulated by inflammatory mediators [30–32]. PMN apoptosis is a process of tightly controlled cell death, which is crucial in particular for the resolution of inflammatory processes. During apoptosis, PMN are ideally packed into apoptotic bodies, which allows recognition and uptake by phagocytes such as macrophages and dendritic cells [33]. The proper removal of dying PMN not only prevents over-excessive oxidative damage to surrounding healthy tissue, it also excites further immune modulatory effects, e.g. on macrophages in terms of cytokine release [34,35].

Therefore, malfunction of apoptotic processes in PMN has been closely linked to the development of severe diseases. For example, the attenuation of PMN apoptosis, thus postponing the resolution of inflammation, is a mechanism leading to severe septic symptoms in patients [36,37]. Given its high abundance in PMN and the known effects of ROS in apoptosis regulation, several studies investigated the influence of MPO on PMN apoptosis and its related role in inflammation. Both, pro- and antiapoptotic functions of MPO have been reported.

Proapoptotic effects of MPO have been linked to HOCl and HOSCN. It was demonstrated that MPO-deficient PMN showed delayed apoptosis rates upon stimulation with phorbol myristate acetate (PMA) or PMA together with H_2O_2 (Table 9.1). This effect could be reversed by additional treatment with either MPO or HOCl in vitro. [38]. Another study related proapoptotic effects of HOCl to the formation of TauCl. In the neutrophil HL-60 cell line, it was demonstrated that TauCl induced apoptosis in the presence of TNF-α and that H_2O_2-induced apoptosis was mediated by MPO's catalytic activity. It was suggested that TauCl prevented antiapoptotic NF-κB activation and reduced expression of the NF-κB target gene FLICE inhibitory protein short form (FLIPS) [39]. As mentioned in the section above, MPO-derived HOSCN was more effective in inducing apoptosis in macrophages than HOCl or HOBr, which was linked to HOSCN-specific oxidation of thiol groups of mitochondrial membrane proteins [9] (Figure 9.1). In vivo, BM transplantation in mice resulted in pronounced lung neutrophilia due to reduced PMN apoptosis in recipients of MPO-deficient BM subsequently leading to their early death [40]. The importance of MPO for PMN apoptosis could be further confirmed in a model of LPS-induced lung inflammation. Herein, $Mpo^{-/-}$ mice showed elevated infiltration of PMN and increased levels of the proinflammatory chemokine CCL5 in bronchoalveolar lavage fluids and a decreased rate of PMN apoptosis characterized by enhanced phosphatidylserine surface expression [41].

In contrast to these findings, a recent study disclosed an antiapoptotic role of MPO in PMN, which was mediated by binding to CD11b/CD18 integrins [7] (Figure 9.1). MPO treatment of isolated human PMN resulted in increased survival and suppressed apoptosis in vitro, an effect, which was blocked by a CD11b antibody, but not by MPO inhibition. Similarly, intravenous MPO injection in rats prevented PMN apoptosis. This could be further confirmed in a mouse model of carrageenan-induced lung injury: intravenous MPO treatment rescued PMN from apoptosis by preventing mitochondrial dysfunction and subsequent activation of caspase-3 via elevated integrin CD11b/CD18 signaling. Although the mechanism had not been fully revealed, MPO-integrin binding led to transient activation of ERK1/2 and Akt, inducing phosphorylation (Ser112 and Ser136) of the Bcl-2-antagonist of cell death (BAD). With this, MPO induced prolonged PMN survival resulting in intensified acute lung injury and attenuated the resolution of lung inflammation [7,42] (Figure 9.2).

Further studies may unravel the complex role of MPO for innate immune cell apoptosis. It may be relevant to discriminate between catalytic and non-catalytic functions. Proapoptotic effects have been mainly reported for HOCl, TauCl and HOSCN. These results were further underlined by in vivo studies in MPO-deficient animals indicating reduced PMN apoptosis in acute lung injury models. Antiapoptotic effects of MPO have been linked to the MPO protein itself. However, in vivo findings of leukocyte accumulation need to be carefully interpreted, as MPO's impact on apoptosis and on recruitment of leukocytes may be intermingled. Furthermore, the type of the inflammatory stimulus, (e.g. LPS- vs. carrageenan-induced lung injury) and subsequent different MPO levels and different levels of leukocyte activation at the site of inflammation might be of relevance. Moreover, the specific effects of MPO on PMN apoptosis may be dependent on the exposure time, the condition of the isolated cells and may differ between acute and chronic experimental settings.

MPO INDUCES NEUTROPHIL NETOSIS

NETosis of PMN is a specific way of cell death creating NETs at sites of inflammation, i.e. release of "net"-like structures into the extracellular space within minutes to hours after activation. These NETs are composed of decondensed chromatin and bound cytosolic factors, e.g. MPO and neutrophil elastase (NE) [43]. Initially, NETosis had been described as a mechanism of PMN to trap and bind pathogens, thereby inhibiting their further spreading and, in limited cases, to provide antimicrobial killing in the initial phase of inflammation [43]. Moreover, recent studies indicated that NET release and NET-bound factors also contribute to the progression of sterile inflammatory conditions such as cancer, atherosclerosis [44] and ischemia and reperfusion [45]. Regulation of NETosis is dependent on cellular ROS production with activation of the nicotinamide adenine dinucleotide phosphate oxidase (NOX) playing an important role [46,47].

During NETosis, PMN undergo major subcellular changes in three different stages defined by stability and localization of the chromatin within the cell and finally by cellular lysis [48]. In this regard, MPO exerts a dual role in the regulation of NETosis by being an essential part of (i) chromatin remodeling during NET formation and, after NET release, (ii) killing of pathogens by the production of oxidants and subsequent activation of other inflammatory cells [48]. It was described that shortly after PMN activation, NE is translocated to the nucleus. Thereafter, MPO escapes the azurophilic granules and co-localizes with the DNA, thereby synergistically enhancing chromatin decondensation (Figure 9.1). Although the molecular mechanisms are not fully understood, binding of NE to the DNA had been identified to be a major mechanism in histone degradation, especially in cleavage of histone H4. In this regard, MPO did not show direct effects on histone degradation alone but had strong synergistic effects together with NE in chromatin decondensation

independently of its catalytic activity in PMA-activated PMN [49] (Table 9.1).

Other studies reported that HOCl induced NET formation in human PMN [46]. This mechanism could be further confirmed when pharmacological MPO inhibition was performed, which disturbed NET formation in PMA-activated PMN [50]. It was furthermore observed that PMN isolated from human donors with complete MPO deficiency did not form NETs after stimulation with PMA or opsonized *C. albicans* subsequently resulting in impaired fungicidal activity. Interestingly, in this study pharmacological MPO inhibition delayed NET formation in MPO-competent PMN, but treatment with activated, MPO-competent PMN or MPO-derived histamine chloramines did not restore NET formation in MPO-deficient PMN, indicating that MPO acts cell autonomously in NETosis induction [51].

Mechanistic investigations revealed that, besides the importance of the overall pH value, NOX- and MPO-derived ROS, but not mitochondrial ROS, are important mediators of NET release [52]. It appears that intracellular or even intragranular localization of the important mediators is required [53], since inhibition of intragranular MPO activity or neutralization of intragranular MPO-derived ROS significantly inhibited NET formation. In accordance with the study published by Metzler et al. [51], extracellular MPO supplementation did not rescue NET formation in complete MPO-deficient PMN and extracellular ROS depletion did not inhibit PMA-induced NET formation, which identified intragranular MPO as a specific regulator of NETosis induction [54]. Consequently, the contribution of MPO on NETosis depends on the type of stimulus and its subsequent production of ROS in this process. NETosis induction by PMA, a strong stimulator of NOX activity, requires MPO for NET release, whereas other, e.g. bacterial PMN activation by *P. aeruginosa* or PMN activation with the calcium (Ca^{2+}) ionophore ionomycin, induced NET release independently of MPO in PMN [55] indicating different pathways of NETosis induction [56].

Besides these endogenous effects of MPO, there is evidence that NET-bound MPO is involved in the killing of pathogens. Catalytically active MPO is released in high amounts during NETosis and can produce HOCl in the presence of its substrate H_2O_2, which resulted in the killing of pathogens such as *S. aureus in vitro* [57]. Interestingly, human PMN-derived NETs can prime T cells by NET-to-cell contact via reduction of their activation threshold and expression of CD25 and CD69, indicating a link between innate and adaptive immune responses, where MPO might be involved [58].

MPO AFFECTS LEUKOCYTE RECRUITMENT

Recruitment of leukocytes from the blood stream to the vascular endothelium and subsequent infiltration of the vessel wall and surrounding tissue is an essential part of inflammation. While indispensable for host defense, this mechanism is mainly detrimental under conditions of sterile inflammation, where it importantly contributes to tissue damage. Leukocyte recruitment comprises a well-orchestrated multistep process initiated by margination of leukocytes to the endothelium followed by capture and rolling. This is mediated by P-, E- and L-selectins on ECs, which interact with leukocyte selectin ligands. During rolling, endothelium-bound cytokines induce leukocyte activation with conformational change of their β2-integrins, which bind to EC adhesion molecules intercellular cell adhesion molecule (ICAM)-1 and vascular cell adhesion molecule (VCAM)-1. Upon firm adhesion, leukocytes migrate along the endothelium before they transmigrate and move through the tissue directed by a gradient of chemokines [59,60]. A number of experimental studies provide evidence that MPO is involved in the recruitment of leukocytes. It was shown that PMN infiltration was markedly attenuated in *Mpo*$^{-/-}$ mice upon myocardial ischemia and ischemia followed by reperfusion (I/R) [61], upon renal I/R [62], in a model of acute LPS-induced lung inflammation [22] and of acute scrotal inflammation [63]. In a murine model of nephrotoxic nephritis, MPO inhibition significantly reduced glomerular macrophage infiltration [23]. Similarly, MPO inhibition reduced infiltration of PMN and monocytes to ischemic myocardium in mice [64] and reduced pulmonary PMN infiltration in a model of immune complex-induced pulmonary vasculitis [65]. Furthermore, intraperitoneal [66], intra-arterial and intrahepatic [63] injection and mesenteric superfusion [67] using MPO or MPO-derived species induced significant leukocyte recruitment (Figure 9.2). While various mechanisms have been unraveled, it is yet unclear which molecules or intermediates are mainly responsible for the observed effects on the vascular wall and on EC integrity and leukocyte function.

MPO-Dependent Leukocyte Recruitment via Modulation of the Vascular Endothelium

MPO binds to the vascular endothelium and is transcytosed to the subendothelial space [68,69]. It was estimated that local extracellular MPO concentrations under inflammatory conditions can be high, up to the millimolar range [70]. It is well known that MPO importantly contributes to the development of endothelial dysfunction, which is described in detail in Chapter 13 of this book. Dysfunctional or inflamed endothelium implies abatement of its repulsive and increase of its adhesive properties toward leukocytes. Thus, MPO's impact on endothelial function, not least by the reduction of nitric oxide bioavailability, is likely to be an important component of leukocyte recruitment. However, the mechanisms of MPO-dependent leukocyte recruitment are diverse. By in vivo experiments, it was demonstrated that MPO modulates endothelial integrity independently of its catalytic activity, but dependent on its cationic charge [63]. MPO leads to a collapse of the negatively charged endothelial glycocalyx, which facilitates leukocyte margination [63,71] (Figure 9.3). Similar effects had been described before for other cationic proteins such as azurocidin and PR3 [72–74], and electrostatic interactions are known to be involved in PMN recruitment [75–77]. Interestingly, hepatic leukocyte infiltration was more pronounced following intraportal injection of a catalytically inactive MPO variant compared with active MPO [63]. Similarly, recombinant catalytically inactive MPO was shown to activate cultured ECs and stimulate their release of IL-6, IL-8 and ROS, which was observed to a minor extent for recombinant active MPO in that study [78] (Table 9.1). In this regard, it is a matter of discussion, whether MPO's catalytic activity can even diminish leukocyte recruitment. It is assumed that ROS can oxidatively modify cell surface receptors and thus block the recruitment process [78,79].

MPO's cytotoxic properties may contribute to dysfunction or "non-responsiveness" of leukocytes and ECs. Furthermore, given that H_2O_2 is an important regulator of leukocyte recruitment [80], its consumption by MPO may attenuate recruitment. Thus, it is supposed that, whereas catalytically active MPO induces a fast and massive EC activation, inactive MPO is responsible for a slow but steady response, as it was seen for ROS

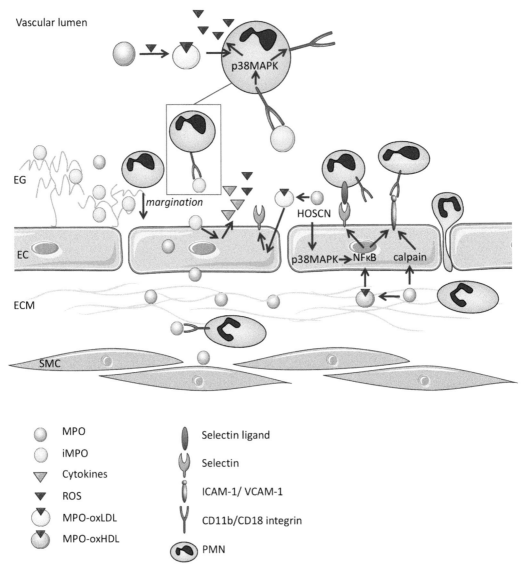

Figure 9.3 Schematic demonstration of MPO-dependent mechanisms of leukocyte recruitment. MPO binds to the EG and leads to its collapse via electrostatic interactions, which facilitates leukocyte margination and interaction with ECs. In ECs, MPO, independent of its catalytic activity, leads to the release of cytokines and ROS and via HOSCN to expression of surface receptors. MPO-modified HDL and LDL also induce surface molecule expression. In PMN MPO binding to CD11b/ CD18 integrins provokes ROS release and further integrin expression. ROS release is also induced by MPO-modified LDL. Abbreviations: EG, endothelial glycocalyx; EC, endothelial cell; iMPO, catalytically inactive MPO; HOCl, hypochlorous acid; HOSCN, hypothiocyanous acid; ICAM-1, intercellular adhesion molecule-1; NFκB, nuclear factor kappa-light-chain-enhancer of activated B-cells; oxHDL, oxidized high-density lipoprotein; oxLDL, oxidized low-density lipoprotein; p38MAPK, p38 mitogen-activated protein kinase; PMN, polymorphonuclear neutrophil; ROS, reactive oxygen species; SMC, smooth muscle cells; VCAM-1, vascular adhesion molecule-1. Figures are based on http://www.servier.com.

release by ECs in vitro [78]. It is difficult to estimate the proportion of MPO that gets inactivated in the extracellular milieu, but in vitro observations demonstrated that it may be a relevant fraction [81]. HOCl itself inactivates MPO, and other factors like exhausting of MPO's substrates may contribute to cessation of catalytic activity [82]. However, anti-inflammatory effects, including reduction of leukocyte recruitment exerted by application of MPO inhibitors in vivo [23,64,65], challenge the concept that inactive MPO is the main responsible agent. In a murine model of acute immune-complex-induced vasculitis, it was demonstrated that upon MPO inhibition, while pulmonary MPO activity was decreased, total MPO accumulation was increased, and at the same time PMN infiltration was significantly reduced [65] (Figure 9.2). This supports the notion that MPO's catalytic activity plays a significant role for leukocyte recruitment.

Concerning MPO-derived reactive species, only HOSCN, but not HOCl, which is the main MPO-derived oxidant under physiological conditions, induced upregulation of E-selectin, ICAM-1 and VCAM-1 on cultured ECs and stimulated PMN and eosinophil adherence [66] (Figure 9.3, Table 9.1). This effect was mediated by activation of p38 MAPK and subsequently NF-κB [83]. Stimulation of PMN adhesion mediated by NF-κB activation in ECs could be induced by HOCl only with lethal concentrations [84]. In contrast, only HOCl, but not HOSCN, modified plasma fibronectin leading to endothelial disintegrity [85]. A subcellular endothelial target that has been identified recently is the protease calpain, which was activated by MPO leading to increased VCAM-1 expression and enhanced leukocyte adhesion to aortic segments [86]. Apart from MPO and MPO-derived reactive molecules, oxidatively modified biomolecules exert pro-inflammatory effects. High-density lipoprotein (HDL), which was exposed to the MPO-hydrogen peroxide-chloride system, provoked activation of cultured ECs via activation of NF-κB with subsequent VCAM-1 expression [87]. Similarly, phospholipid chlorohydrin, which can be formed by a reaction of HOCl with unsaturated fatty acyl chains of low-density lipoproteins (LDL), was observed to upregulate the endothelial expression of P-selectin and enhance leukocyte adhesion to arterial segments [88] (Figure 9.3).

MPO-Dependent Leukocyte Recruitment via Modulation of the Leukocyte

As it is described above in this chapter, a multitude of studies demonstrate MPO-mediated activation of different leukocyte subpopulations, which may also enhance their recruitment. Activation and increased endothelial adhesion of leukocytes in a MPO-dependent manner have been demonstrated for HOCl-modified LDL, which induced superoxide release of PMN or splenocytes [88,89]. In addition, HOCl-modified LDL exerted chemotactic effects on PMN [90]. Apart from these effects,

which are dependent on MPO's catalytic activity, MPO binds to PMN via CD11b/CD18 integrins, which does not only lead to their activation [8] but also mediates their adhesion [91] (Figure 9.3). Electrostatic interactions of MPO with the anionic PMN glycocalyx have also been demonstrated to mediate their motility and convey MPO chemokine-like properties [63].

In aggregate, MPO itself, MPO-derived reactive species and MPO-modified biomolecules are responsible for leukocyte adhesion and modification of the vascular endothelium promoting leukocyte recruitment and thus accounting for MPO's important role in host defense on the one hand and its pro-inflammatory properties on the other.

MPO AFFECTS PLATELET FUNCTION

Platelets have been originally described as the major effector cell type for hemostasis and thrombosis. Furthermore, they link pro-thrombotic and pro-inflammatory processes by expressing various inflammatory surface receptors and secretory peptides after activation. By secretion of various cytokines such as IL-1β, CCL5, PDGF or MIP-1α, platelets not only activate ECs, thereby contributing to leukocyte recruitment, but they also directly bind to leukocytes and modulate their activation [92,93]. Vice versa, molecules released by PMN have been shown to activate platelets, and treatment of platelets with MPO-derived ROS resulted in a marked increase of platelet activation and peptide secretion in vitro [94]. MPO directly binds to platelets and retains its catalytic activity. Recent studies indicate that MPO does not directly act as an agonist for platelets, but rather "primes" platelets susceptible for agonist- (e.g. ADP) dependent activation [95,96]. In this regard, MPO reorganizes the actin cytoskeleton of activated platelets, thereby increasing their elasticity and inducing cytosolic Ca^{2+} entry [95]. MPO furthermore catabolizes NO within platelets and induces the expression of specific surface receptors such as P-selectin and PECAM-1 [96] (Figure 9.4).

The role of MPO in platelet aggregation is still not fully understood. MPO alone did not induce aggregation of naive platelets nor did it increase attachment to naive or stimulated ECs [96]. Furthermore, although PMN-derived MPO-containing NETs were able to activate platelets, pharmacological inhibition of MPO did not show effects in this regard [97]. In vivo investigations demonstrated that

Platelet

Dendritic cell

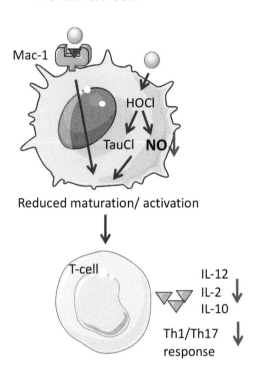

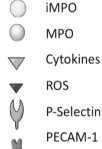

◯	iMPO
◔	MPO
▽	Cytokines
▼	ROS
Ψ	P-Selectin
▮	PECAM-1

Figure 9.4 Schematic demonstration of MPO-dependent mechanisms of platelet and dendritic cell activation. In platelets, MPO reorganizes the cellular actin cytoskeleton and oxidizes cellular NO, thereby increasing the expression of surface receptors and priming the cells for further activation. In dendritic cells, MPO attenuates maturation and activation by binding to the inhibitory surface receptor Mac-1, by formation of TauCl and by NO oxidation. This delays subsequent T-cell activation and the release of pro-inflammatory cytokines. Abbreviations: Ca^{2+}, calcium ion; NO, nitric oxide; Mac-1, macrophage-1 antigen; HOCl, hypochlorous acid; TauCl, taurine chloramine; IL-, Interleukine; Th, T helper cell; iMPO, catalytically inactive MPO; ROS, reactive oxygen species; PECAM-1, Platelet endothelial cell adhesion molecule 1. Figures are based on http://www.servier.com.

MPO significantly enhanced ADP-induced platelet aggregation [95] and reduced bleeding in a murine model of skin injury [96]. Spontaneous platelet activation by HOCl was elevated in chronic heart failure patients but not in healthy donors [98], further indicating that MPO does not act as a platelet activator per se, but rather as a co-regulating factor under pathological conditions.

MPO REGULATES ADAPTIVE IMMUNITY

Dendritic cells play a key role in regulation of the immune response as specialized antigen-presenting cells. They detect and acquire pathogens within the blood stream and tissues and, after activation, upregulate the expression of several surface receptors and migrate to draining lymph nodes (dLN).

During this process, they lose their pathogen uptake capacity and differentiate into antigen-presenting cells by upregulating the secretion of inflammatory cytokines and the expression of specific surface receptors like major histocompatibility complex (MHC). By presenting antigens to naive CD4$^+$ and CD8$^+$ cells, they link innate and adaptive immunity [99,100]. After activation by inflammatory stimuli, PMN rapidly migrate to the site of inflammation and to dLN, thereby shuttling antigens [101] and regulating DC activation in several ways and mechanisms [100]. In this regard, MPO can get released by PMN in close proximity to DCs during inflammatory processes [102], and several studies investigated its specific effects on DC activation.

Mpo$^{-/-}$ mice showed elevated splenic CD4$^+$ T-cell proliferation, cytokine production and an augmented Th1:Th2 ratio indicating an attenuating role of MPO in regulating adaptive immune responses in a model of glomerulonephritis [103]. However, the extent of renal injury was not altered. In an experimental model of rheumatoid arthritis, suppression of adaptive immunity could also be demonstrated, but disease severity was attenuated by MPO deficiency [104] (Figure 9.2). The mechanism of MPO-mediated DC suppression was further investigated in a study employing Mpo$^{-/-}$ mice, PMN depletion and pharmacological MPO inhibition. It revealed that MPO negatively effects various functions of DCs resulting in enhanced skin delayed-type hypersensitivity and antigen-induced arthritis in Mpo$^{-/-}$ mouse models due to elevated DC-mediated CD4$^+$ T-cell activation [102]. It was suggested that the effect was due to the activation of inhibitory DC surface receptors via MPO-derived ROS (Figure 9.4). There is evidence that MPO binds to and oxidatively activates the Mac-1 receptor on DCs, which inhibits DC maturation [42,105], resulting in reduced IL-12 expression and attenuated Th1 responses [102] (Table 9.1). MPO furthermore attenuated IL-23 and CD86 expression of DCs resulting in reduced Th17 responses and co-stimulatory activation of naive T-cells [106]. Taken together, MPO attenuates DC activation, antigen uptake/processing and migration of DCs to lymph nodes and subsequently inhibits adaptive immune responses with decreased generation of CD4$^+$ T-cells [102].

It was observed that HOCl and to a lesser extend HOBr exerted potent inhibitory effects on DCs. This is in accordance to prior findings indicating that TauCl acts as an inhibitor of DC maturation by reducing the capacity to induce the release of activating cytokines (e.g. IL-2, IL-10) from T cells [107]. DC inhibition depends on the reaction profile of MPO's products, which is supported by the fact that inhibitory effects of HOSCN on DCs were less pronounced compared with HOCl [102]. MPO might furthermore indirectly modulate DC maturation by oxidizing NO, a main regulator of TLR-driven glycolytic upregulation in DCs [108], which reversed the effects of HOCl-mediated DC inhibition in vitro [106] (Figure 9.4). In vivo, HOCl in low doses showed anti-inflammatory properties and reduced cytokine secretion in a murine model of atopic dermatitis in a DC-dependent manner [109]. In contrast, MPO-derived HOCl led to the oxidation of proteins and glycoproteins within the inflammatory sites, thereby enhancing their immunogenicity. This process led to increased pathogen recognition, -uptake and -presentation by DCs and macrophages via mannose receptor, scavenger receptors A (CD204) and CD36 [110], although this might be of minor importance in view of direct inhibitory effects of MPO on DCs.

CONCLUSION

MPO importantly affects innate immune cell activation and recruitment. It directly modulates phagocyte intracellular signaling, cytokine and ROS release, surface molecule expression, apoptosis and NETosis. Furthermore, MPO indirectly influences phagocyte behavior by affecting platelets and ECs. The mechanisms are complex and involve agonistic receptor binding, electrostatic interactions and oxidative modulation of intra- and extracellular biomolecule structure and function. Apart from that, indirect mechanisms like consumption of H_2O_2 may play a role. This can result in stimulation as well as diminution of innate immune cell activity, which highly depends on the type of stimulus and model used. Given that a certain portion of secreted MPO becomes inactivated, it is of importance that MPO exerts a number of effects independently of its catalytic activity.

Furthermore, depending on the availability of MPO's substrates, which are, for example, altered in smokers, concentrations of HOCl and HOSCN vary, which widely differ in their effects on immune cell function. Of note, the consequence of MPO deficiency or pharmacological inhibition depends on the individual conditions, e.g. on the type of model and the innate immune cell-activating agent. It furthermore needs to be considered that effects of intracellular vs. extracellular MPO localization can be substantially different, e.g. for NETosis induction. Moreover, converse findings regarding MPO-dependent innate immune cell accumulation may result from the fact that induction of apoptosis and of recruitment may counteract.

Thus, MPO's role on innate immune cell activation and recruitment is dependent on type and time point of the disease or condition. Importantly, results from studies that applied pharmacological MPO inhibition in different disease animal models point toward the fact that MPO's catalytic activity provokes pro-inflammatory leukocyte activation and recruitment, reinforcing the concept of MPO being a promising therapeutic target. Further research may help to unravel the complex interplay of MPO and immune cell function during host defense and inflammatory diseases.

REFERENCES

1. D.L. Lefkowitz, K. Mills, D. Morgan, S.S. Lefkowitz, 1992, Macrophage activation and immunomodulation by myeloperoxidase, Proc. Soc. Exp. Biol. Med. 199: 204–210.

2. M.P. Gelderman, R. Stuart, D. Vigerust, et al., 1998, Perpetuation of inflammation associated with experimental arthritis: the role of macrophage activation by neutrophilic myeloperoxidase, Mediators Inflamm. 7: 381–389.

3. D.L. Lefkowitz, M.P. Gelderman, S.R. Fuhrmann, et al., 1999, Neutrophilic myeloperoxidase-macrophage interactions perpetuate chronic inflammation associated with experimental arthritis, Clin. Immunol. 91: 145–155.

4. K. Grattendick, R. Stuart, E. Roberts, et al., 2002, Alveolar macrophage activation by myeloperoxidase: a model for exacerbation of lung inflammation, Am. J. Respir. Cell Mol. Biol. 26: 716–722.

5. S.S. Lefkowitz, M.P. Gelderman, D.L. Lefkowitz, N. Moguilevsky, A. Bollen, 1996, Phagocytosis and intracellular killing of Candida albicans by macrophages exposed to myeloperoxidase, J. Infect. Dis. 173: 1202–1207.

6. D.L. Lefkowitz, J.A. Lincoln, S.S. Lefkowitz, A. Bollen, N. Moguilevsky, 1997, Enhancement of macrophage-mediated bactericidal activity by macrophage-mannose receptor-ligand interaction, Immunol. Cell Biol. 75: 136–141.

7. D. El Kebir, L. Jozsef, W. Pan, J.G. Filep, 2008, Myeloperoxidase delays neutrophil apoptosis through CD11b/CD18 integrins and prolongs inflammation, Circ. Res. 103: 352–359.

8. D. Lau, H. Mollnau, J.P. Eiserich, et al., 2005, Myeloperoxidase mediates neutrophil activation by association with CD11b/CD18 integrins, Proc. Natl. Acad. Sci. U.S.A. 102: 431–436.

9. M.M. Lloyd, D.M. van Reyk, M.J. Davies, C.L. Hawkins, 2008, Hypothiocyanous acid is a more potent inducer of apoptosis and protein thiol depletion in murine macrophage cells than hypochlorous acid or hypobromous acid, Biochem. J. 414: 271–280.

10. Y.T. Yang, M. Whiteman, S.P. Gieseg, 2012, Intracellular glutathione protects human monocyte-derived macrophages from hypochlorite damage, Life Sci. 90: 682–688.

11. D.T. Love, T.J. Barrett, M.Y. White, et al., 2016, Cellular targets of the myeloperoxidase-derived oxidant hypothiocyanous acid (HOSCN) and its role in the inhibition of glycolysis in macrophages, Free Radic. Biol. Med. 94: 88–98.

12. M. Barua, Y. Liu, M.R. Quinn, 2001, Taurine chloramine inhibits inducible nitric oxide synthase and TNF-alpha gene expression in activated alveolar macrophages: decreased NF-kappaB activation and IkappaB kinase activity, J. Immunol. 167: 2275–2281.

13. A. Kanayama, J. Inoue, Y. Sugita-Konishi, M. Shimizu, Y. Miyamoto, 2002, Oxidation of Ikappa Balpha at methionine 45 is one cause of taurine chloramine-induced inhibition of NF-kappa B activation, J. Biol. Chem. 277: 24049–24056.

14. J. Pi, Q. Zhang, C.G. Woods, et al., 2008, Activation of Nrf2-mediated oxidative stress response in macrophages by hypochlorous acid, Toxicol. Appl. Pharmacol. 226: 236–423.

15. C.G. Woods, J. Fu, P. Xue, et al., 2009, Dose-dependent transitions in Nrf2-mediated adaptive response and related stress responses to hypochlorous acid in mouse macrophages, Toxicol. Appl. Pharmacol. 238: 27–36.

16. B.S. Rayner, Y. Zhang, B.E. Brown, et al., 2018, Role of hypochlorous acid (HOCl) and other inflammatory mediators in the induction of macrophage extracellular trap formation, Free Radic. Biol. Med. 129: 25–34.

17. K. Takeuchi, Y. Umeki, N. Matsumoto, et al., 2012, Severe neutrophil-mediated lung inflammation in myeloperoxidase-deficient mice exposed to zymosan, Inflamm. Res. 61: 197–205.

18. N. Tateno, N. Matsumoto, T. Motowaki, K. Suzuki, Y. Aratani, 2013, Myeloperoxidase deficiency induces MIP-2 production via ERK activation in zymosan-stimulated mouse neutrophils, *Free Radic. Res.* 47: 376–385.

19. K. Fujimoto, T. Motowaki, N. Tamura, Y. Aratani, 2016, Myeloperoxidase deficiency enhances zymosan phagocytosis associated with up-regulation of surface expression of CD11b in mouse neutrophils, *Free Radic. Res.* 50: 1340–1349.

20. D. Endo, T. Saito, Y. Umeki, K. Suzuki, Y. Aratani, 2016, Myeloperoxidase negatively regulates the expression of proinflammatory cytokines and chemokines by zymosan-induced mouse neutrophils, *Inflamm. Res.* 65: 151–159.

21. M. Homme, N. Tateno, N. Miura, N. Ohno, Y. Aratani, 2013, Myeloperoxidase deficiency in mice exacerbates lung inflammation induced by nonviable *Candida albicans*, *Inflamm. Res.* 62: 981–990.

22. A. Haegens, P. Heeringa, R.J. van Suylen, et al., 2009, Myeloperoxidase deficiency attenuates lipopolysaccharide-induced acute lung inflammation and subsequent cytokine and chemokine production, *J. Immunol.* 182: 7990–7996.

23. M. Antonelou, E. Michaelsson, R.D.R. Evans, et al., 2020, Therapeutic myeloperoxidase inhibition attenuates neutrophil activation, ANCA-mediated endothelial damage, and crescentic GN, *J. Am. Soc. Nephrol.* 31: 350–364.

24. J.T. Dancey, K.A. Deubelbeiss, L.A. Harker, C.A. Finch, 1976, Neutrophil kinetics in man, *J. Clin. Invest.* 58: 705–715.

25. J. Pillay, I. den Braber, N. Vrisekoop, et al., 2010, In vivo labeling with 2H$_2$O reveals a human neutrophil lifespan of 5.4 days, *Blood* 116: 625–627.

26. M.L. Thakur, J.P. Lavender, R.N. Arnot, D.J. Silvester, A.W. Segal, 1977, Indium-111-labeled autologous leukocytes in man, *J. Nucl. Med.* 18: 1014–1021.

27. S.H. Saverymuttu, A.M. Peters, A. Keshavarzian, H.J. Reavy, J.P. Lavender, 1985, The kinetics of 111indium distribution following injection of 111indium labelled autologous granulocytes in man, *Br. J. Haematol.* 61: 675–685.

28. B.T. Suratt, S.K. Young, J. Lieber, et al., 2001, Neutrophil maturation and activation determine anatomic site of clearance from circulation, *Am. J. Physiol. Lung Cell Mol. Physiol.* 281: L913–921.

29. C. Martin, P.C.E. Burdon, G. Bridger, et al., 2003, Chemokines acting via CXCR2 and CXCR4 control the release of neutrophils from the bone marrow and their return following senescence, *Immunity* 19: 583–593.

30. P. Hampson, J. Hazeldine, J.M. Lord, 2013, Neutrophil apoptosis and its induction as a potential treatment for chronic inflammatory disease, *Curr. Opin. Hematol.* 20: 10–15.

31. M.A. Brach, S. deVos, H.J. Gruss, F. Herrmann, 1992, Prolongation of survival of human polymorphonuclear neutrophils by granulocyte-macrophage colony-stimulating factor is caused by inhibition of programmed cell death, *Blood* 80: 2920–2924.

32. K. Wang, D. Scheel-Toellner, S.H. Wong, et al., 2003, Inhibition of neutrophil apoptosis by type 1 IFN depends on cross-talk between phosphoinositol 3-kinase, protein kinase C-delta, and NF-kappa B signaling pathways, *J. Immunol.* 171: 1035–1041.

33. S. Fox, A.E. Leitch, R. Duffin, C. Haslett, A.G. Rossi, 2010, Neutrophil apoptosis: relevance to the innate immune response and inflammatory disease, *J. Innate Immun.* 2: 216–227.

34. V.A. Fadok, D.L. Bratton, A. Konowal, et al., 1998, Macrophages that have ingested apoptotic cells in vitro inhibit proinflammatory cytokine production through autocrine/paracrine mechanisms involving TGF-beta, PGE2, and PAF, *J. Clin. Invest.* 101: 890–898.

35. A.E. Leitch, R. Duffin, C. Haslett, A.G. Rossi, 2008, Relevance of granulocyte apoptosis to resolution of inflammation at the respiratory mucosa, *Mucosal. Immunol.* 1: 350–363.

36. R. Taneja, J. Parodo, S.H. Jia, et al., 2004, Delayed neutrophil apoptosis in sepsis is associated with maintenance of mitochondrial transmembrane potential and reduced caspase-9 activity, *Crit. Care Med.* 32: 1460–1469.

37. A. Paunel-Gorgulu, T. Kirichevska, T. Logters, J. Windolf, S. Flohe, 2012, Molecular mechanisms underlying delayed apoptosis in neutrophils from multiple trauma patients with and without sepsis, *Mol. Med.* 18: 325–335.

38. T. Tsurubuchi, Y. Aratani, N. Maeda, H. Koyama, 2001, Retardation of early-onset PMA-induced apoptosis in mouse neutrophils deficient in myeloperoxidase, *J. Leukoc. Biol.* 70: 52–58.

39. A. Kanayama, Y. Miyamoto, 2007, Apoptosis triggered by phagocytosis-related oxidative stress through FLIPS down-regulation and JNK activation, *J. Leukoc. Biol.* 82: 1344–1352.

40. C. Milla, S. Yang, D.N. Cornfield, et al., 2004, Myeloperoxidase deficiency enhances inflammation after allogeneic marrow transplantation, *Am. J. Physiol. Lung Cell Mol. Physiol.* 287: L706–714.

41. S. Kremserova, T. Perecko, K. Soucek, et al., 2016, Lung neutrophilia in myeloperoxidase deficient mice during the course of acute pulmonary inflammation, *Oxid. Med. Cell. Longev.* 2016: 5219056.

42. D. El Kebir, J.G. Filep, 2013, Modulation of neutrophil apoptosis and the resolution of inflammation through beta2 integrins, *Front. Immunol.* 4: 60.

43. V. Delgado-Rizo, M.A. Martinez-Guzman, L. Iniguez-Gutierrez, et al., 2017, Neutrophil extracellular traps and its implications in inflammation: an overview, *Front. Immunol.* 8: 81.

44. C. Silvestre-Roig, Q. Braster, K. Wichapong, et al., 2019, Externalized histone H4 orchestrates chronic inflammation by inducing lytic cell death, *Nature* 569: 236–240.

45. K. Eghbalzadeh, L. Georgi, T. Louis, et al., 2019, Compromised anti-inflammatory action of neutrophil extracellular traps in PAD4-deficient mice contributes to aggravated acute inflammation after myocardial infarction, *Front. Immunol.* 10: 2313.

46. L.J. Palmer, P.R. Cooper, M.R. Ling, et al., 2012, Hypochlorous acid regulates neutrophil extracellular trap release in humans, *Clin. Exp. Immunol.* 167: 261–268.

47. M.A. Khan, L.M. Philip, G. Cheung, et al., 2018, Regulating NETosis: increasing pH promotes NADPH oxidase-dependent NETosis, *Front. Med. (Lausanne)* 5: 19.

48. E. Neubert, D. Meyer, F. Rocca, et al., 2018, Chromatin swelling drives neutrophil extracellular trap release, *Nat. Commun.* 9: 3767.

49. V. Papayannopoulos, K.D. Metzler, A. Hakkim, A. Zychlinsky, 2010, Neutrophil elastase and myeloperoxidase regulate the formation of neutrophil extracellular traps, *J. Cell Biol.* 191: 677–691.

50. K. Akong-Moore, O.A. Chow, M. von Kockritz-Blickwede, V. Nizet, 2012, Influences of chloride and hypochlorite on neutrophil extracellular trap formation, *PLoS One* 7: e42984.

51. K.D. Metzler, T.A. Fuchs, W.M. Nauseef, et al., 2011, Myeloperoxidase is required for neutrophil extracellular trap formation: implications for innate immunity, *Blood* 117: 953–959.

52. T. Kirchner, S. Moller, M. Klinger, et al., 2012, The impact of various reactive oxygen species on the formation of neutrophil extracellular traps, *Mediators Inflamm.* 2012: 849136.

53. A. Sheshachalam, N. Srivastava, T. Mitchell, P. Lacy, G. Eitzen, 2014, Granule protein processing and regulated secretion in neutrophils, *Front. Immunol.* 5: 448.

54. H. Bjornsdottir, A. Welin, E. Michaelsson, et al., 2015, Neutrophil NET formation is regulated from the inside by myeloperoxidase-processed reactive oxygen species, *Free Radic. Biol. Med.* 89: 1024–1035.

55. H. Parker, M. Dragunow, M.B. Hampton, A.J. Kettle, C.C. Winterbourn, 2012, Requirements for NADPH oxidase and myeloperoxidase in neutrophil extracellular trap formation differ depending on the stimulus, *J. Leukoc. Biol.* 92: 841–849.

56. E.F. Kenny, A. Herzig, R. Kruger, et al., 2017, Diverse stimuli engage different neutrophil extracellular trap pathways, *Elife* 6: e24437.

57. H. Parker, A.M. Albrett, A.J. Kettle, C.C. Winterbourn, 2012, Myeloperoxidase associated with neutrophil extracellular traps is active and mediates bacterial killing in the presence of hydrogen peroxide, *J. Leukoc. Biol.* 91: 369–376.

58. K. Tillack, P. Breiden, R. Martin, M. Sospedra, 2012, T lymphocyte priming by neutrophil extracellular traps links innate and adaptive immune responses, *J. Immunol.* 188: 3150–3159.

59. K. Ley, C. Laudanna, M.I. Cybulsky, S. Nourshargh, 2007, Getting to the site of inflammation: the leukocyte adhesion cascade updated, *Nat. Rev. Immunol.* 7: 678–689.

60. C. Nussbaum, A. Klinke, M. Adam, S. Baldus, M. Sperandio, 2013, Myeloperoxidase: a leukocyte-derived protagonist of inflammation and cardiovascular disease, *Antioxid. Redox Signal.* 18: 692–713.

61. M. Mollenhauer, K. Friedrichs, M. Lange, et al., 2017, Myeloperoxidase mediates postischemic arrhythmogenic ventricular remodeling, *Circ. Res.* 121: 56–70.

62. R.A. Matthijsen, D. Huugen, N.T. Hoebers, et al., 2007, Myeloperoxidase is critically involved in the induction of organ damage after renal ischemia reperfusion, *Am. J. Pathol.* 171: 1743–1752.

63. A. Klinke, C. Nussbaum, L. Kubala, et al., 2011, Myeloperoxidase attracts neutrophils by physical forces, *Blood* 117: 1350–1358.

64. M. Ali, B. Pulli, G. Courties, et al., 2016, Myeloperoxidase inhibition improves ventricular function and remodeling after experimental myocardial infarction, *JACC Basic Transl. Sci.* 1: 633–643.

65. W. Zheng, R. Warner, R. Ruggeri, et al., 2015, PF-1355, a mechanism-based myeloperoxidase inhibitor, prevents immune complex vasculitis and anti-glomerular basement membrane glomerulonephritis, J. Pharmacol. Exp. Ther. 353: 288–298.

66. J.G. Wang, S.A. Mahmud, J. Nguyen, A. Slungaard, 2006, Thiocyanate-dependent induction of endothelial cell adhesion molecule expression by phagocyte peroxidases: a novel HOSCN-specific oxidant mechanism to amplify inflammation, J. Immunol. 177: 8714–8722.

67. M. Suzuki, H. Asako, P. Kubes, et al., 1991, Neutrophil-derived oxidants promote leukocyte adherence in postcapillary venules, Microvasc. Res. 42: 125–138.

68. S. Baldus, J.P. Eiserich, A. Mani, et al., 2001, Endothelial transcytosis of myeloperoxidase confers specificity to vascular ECM proteins as targets of tyrosine nitration, J. Clin. Invest. 108: 1759–1770.

69. C. Tiruppathi, T. Naqvi, Y. Wu, et al., 2004, Albumin mediates the transcytosis of myeloperoxidase by means of caveolae in endothelial cells, Proc. Natl. Acad. Sci. U.S.A. 101: 7699–7704.

70. M.B. Hampton, A.J. Kettle, C.C. Winterbourn, 1998, Inside the neutrophil phagosome: oxidants, myeloperoxidase, and bacterial killing, Blood 92: 3007–3017.

71. K. Manchanda, H. Kolarova, C. Kerkenpass, et al., 2018, MPO (Myeloperoxidase) reduces endothelial glycocalyx thickness dependent on its cationic charge, Arterioscler. Thromb. Vasc. Biol. 38: 1859–1867.

72. A. David, Y. Kacher, U. Specks, I. Aviram, 2003, Interaction of proteinase 3 with CD11b/CD18 (beta2 integrin) on the cell membrane of human neutrophils, J. Leukoc. Biol. 74: 551–557.

73. O. Soehnlein, X. Xie, H. Ulbrich, et al., 2005, Neutrophil-derived heparin-binding protein (HBP/CAP37) deposited on endothelium enhances monocyte arrest under flow conditions, J. Immunol. 174: 6399–6405.

74. O. Soehnlein, L. Lindbom, C. Weber, 2009, Mechanisms underlying neutrophil-mediated monocyte recruitment, Blood 114: 4613–4623.

75. J.I. Gallin, J.R. Durocher, A.P. Kaplan, 1975, Interaction of leukocyte chemotactic factors with the cell surface. I. Chemotactic factor-induced changes in human granulocyte surface charge, J. Clin. Invest. 55: 967–974.

76. J.I. Gallin, 1980, Degranulating stimuli decrease the negative surface charge and increase the adhesiveness of human neutrophils, J. Clin. Invest. 65: 298–306.

77. T.M. Schaack, A. Takeuchi, I. Spilberg, R.H. Persellin, 1980, Alteration of polymorphonuclear leukocyte surface charge by endogenous and exogenous chemotactic factors, Inflammation 4: 37–44.

78. D.L. Lefkowitz, E. Roberts, K. Grattendick, et al., 2000, The endothelium and cytokine secretion: the role of peroxidases as immunoregulators, Cell. Immunol. 202: 23–30.

79. P.M. Bozeman, J.R. Hoidal, V.L. Shepherd, 1988, Oxidant-mediated inhibition of ligand uptake by the macrophage mannose receptor, J. Biol. Chem. 263: 1240–1247.

80. T.R. Hurd, M. DeGennaro, R. Lehmann, 2012, Redox regulation of cell migration and adhesion, Trends Cell. Biol. 22: 107–115.

81. C.C. King, M.M. Jefferson, E.L. Thomas, 1997, Secretion and inactivation of myeloperoxidase by isolated neutrophils, J. Leukoc. Biol. 61: 293–302.

82. C.C. Winterbourn, M.B. Hampton, J.H. Livesey, A.J. Kettle, 2006, Modeling the reactions of superoxide and myeloperoxidase in the neutrophil phagosome: implications for microbial killing, J. Biol. Chem. 281: 39860–39869.

83. T. Rehani, A. Jonas, A. Slungaard, 2010, The major phagocyte peroxidase-derived oxidant HOSCN stimulates gene-specific p38 MAPK-dependent, NF-κb-mediated activation of tissue factor, VCAM-1 and ICAM-1 expression in endothelium, Blood 116: 1481–1481.

84. J.M. Pullar, C.C. Winterbourn, M.C. Vissers, 2002, The effect of hypochlorous acid on the expression of adhesion molecules and activation of NF-kappaB in cultured human endothelial cells, Antioxid, Redox Signal. 4: 5–15.

85. S. Vanichkitrungruang, C.Y. Chuang, C.L. Hawkins, et al., 2019, Oxidation of human plasma fibronectin by inflammatory oxidants perturbs endothelial cell function, Free Radic. Biol. Med. 136: 118–134.

86. Z. Etwebi, G. Landesberg, K. Preston, S. Eguchi, R. Scalia, 2018, Mechanistic role of the calcium-dependent protease calpain in the endothelial dysfunction induced by MPO (Myeloperoxidase), Hypertension 71: 761–770.

87. A. Undurti, Y. Huang, J.A. Lupica, et al., 2009, Modification of high density lipoprotein by myeloperoxidase generates a pro-inflammatory particle, J. Biol. Chem. 284: 30825–30835.

88. G.J. Dever, R. Benson, C.L. Wainwright, S. Kennedy, C.M. Spickett, 2008, Phospholipid chlorohydrin induces leukocyte adhesion to ApoE-/- mouse arteries via upregulation of P-selectin, *Free Radic. Biol. Med.* 44: 452–463.

89. S. Kopprasch, W. Leonhardt, J. Pietzsch, H. Kuhne, 1998, Hypochlorite-modified low-density lipoprotein stimulates human polymorphonuclear leukocytes for enhanced production of reactive oxygen metabolites, enzyme secretion, and adhesion to endothelial cells, *Atherosclerosis* 136: 315–324.

90. C. Woenckhaus, A. Kaufmann, D. Bussfeld, et al., 1998, Hypochlorite-modified LDL: chemotactic potential and chemokine induction in human monocytes, *Clin. Immunol. Immunopathol.* 86: 27–33.

91. M.W. Johansson, M. Patarroyo, F. Öberg, A. Siegbahn, K. Nilsson, 1997, Myeloperoxidase mediates cell adhesion via the α(M)β2 integrin (Mac-1, CD11b/CD18), *J. Cell Sci.* 110: 1133–1139.

92. M. Arman, H. Payne, T. Ponomaryov, A. Brill, 2015, Role of platelets in inflammation, *Thromb. Haemost.* 114: 449–458.

93. A. Margraf, A. Zarbock, 2019, Platelets in inflammation and resolution, *J. Immunol.* 203: 2357–2367.

94. R.A. Clark, S.J. Klebanoff, 1979, Myeloperoxidase-mediated platelet release reaction, *J. Clin. Invest.* 63: 177–183.

95. I.V. Gorudko, A.V. Sokolov, E.V. Shamova, et al., 2013, Myeloperoxidase modulates human platelet aggregation via actin cytoskeleton reorganization and store-operated calcium entry, *Biol. Open* 2: 916–923.

96. H. Kolarova, A. Klinke, S. Kremserova, et al., 2013, Myeloperoxidase induces the priming of platelets, *Free Radic. Biol. Med.* 61: 357–369.

97. O. Elaskalani, N.B. Abdol Razak, P. Metharom, 2018, Neutrophil extracellular traps induce aggregation of washed human platelets independently of extracellular DNA and histones, *Cell Commun. Signal.* 16: 24.

98. A. Mongirdiene, J. Laukaitiene, V. Skipskis, A. Kasauskas, 2019, The effect of oxidant hypochlorous acid on platelet aggregation and dityrosine concentration in chronic heart failure patients and healthy controls, *Medicina (Kaunas)* 55: 198.

99. R.M. Steinman, 2012, Decisions about dendritic cells: past, present, and future, *Annu. Rev. Immunol.* 30: 1–22.

100. S. Schuster, B. Hurrell, F. Tacchini-Cottier, 2013, Crosstalk between neutrophils and dendritic cells: a context-dependent process, *J. Leukoc. Biol.* 94: 671–675.

101. V. Abadie, E. Badell, P. Douillard, et al., 2005, Neutrophils rapidly migrate via lymphatics after Mycobacterium bovis BCG intradermal vaccination and shuttle live bacilli to the draining lymph nodes, *Blood* 106: 1843–1850.

102. D. Odobasic, A.R. Kitching, Y. Yang, et al., 2013, Neutrophil myeloperoxidase regulates T-cell-driven tissue inflammation in mice by inhibiting dendritic cell function, *Blood* 121: 4195–4204.

103. D. Odobasic, A.R. Kitching, T.J. Semple, S.R. Holdsworth, 2007, Endogenous myeloperoxidase promotes neutrophil-mediated renal injury, but attenuates T cell immunity inducing crescentic glomerulonephritis, *J. Am. Soc. Nephrol.* 18: 760–770.

104. D. Odobasic, Y. Yang, R.C. Muljadi, et al., 2014, Endogenous myeloperoxidase is a mediator of joint inflammation and damage in experimental arthritis, *Arthritis Rheumatol.* 66: 907–917.

105. S. Podgrabinska, O. Kamalu, L. Mayer, et al., 2009, Inflamed lymphatic endothelium suppresses dendritic cell maturation and function via Mac-1/ICAM-1-dependent mechanism, *J. Immunol.* 183: 1767–1779.

106. D. Odobasic, A.R. Kitching, S.R. Holdsworth, 2016, Neutrophil-mediated regulation of innate and adaptive immunity: the role of myeloperoxidase, *J. Immunol. Res.* 2016: 2349817.

107. J. Marcinkiewicz, B. Nowak, A. Grabowska, et al., 1999, Regulation of murine dendritic cell functions in vitro by taurine chloramine, a major product of the neutrophil myeloperoxidase-halide system, *Immunology* 98: 371–378.

108. P.M. Thwe, E. Amiel, 2018, The role of nitric oxide in metabolic regulation of dendritic cell immune function, *Cancer Lett.* 412: 236–242.

109. T. Fukuyama, B.C. Martel, K.E. Linder, et al., 2018, Hypochlorous acid is antipruritic and anti-inflammatory in a mouse model of atopic dermatitis, *Clin. Exp. Allergy* 48: 78–88.

110. R. Biedron, M.K. Konopinski, J. Marcinkiewicz, S. Jozefowski, 2015, Oxidation by neutrophils-derived HOCl increases immunogenicity of proteins by converting them into ligands of several endocytic receptors involved in antigen uptake by dendritic cells and macrophages, *PLoS One* 10: e0123293.

CHAPTER TEN

Bactericidal Activity of the Oxidants Derived from Mammalian Heme Peroxidases

Heather L. Shearer, Mark B. Hampton, and Nina Dickerhof
University of Otago

CONTENTS

INTRODUCTION

The halogenation cycle of the four specialist mammalian heme peroxidases enables them to oxidize, with varied efficiency, the halides chloride (Cl^-), bromide (Br^-), iodide (I^-) and the pseudohalide thiocyanate (SCN^-) to their respective hypohalous acids (Figure 10.1). Two of these enzymes, myeloperoxidase (MPO) and lactoperoxidase (LPO), are found in environments where they are able to produce enough hypochlorous acid (HOCl) and hypothiocyanous acid ($HOSCN$), respectively, to contribute to the innate immune system. HOCl, commonly referred to as chlorine bleach, is well known for its broad-spectrum activity against bacteria, fungi and viruses. In this chapter, we discuss what is known about the mechanisms by which HOCl and HOSCN kill bacteria. We focus on bacteria since little mechanistic information is available for other microbes.

Neutrophil Myeloperoxidase

Neutrophils are the most abundant circulating white blood cells in humans. They are quickly recruited to sites of infection via chemoattractants and ingest bacteria into internal vacuoles called phagosomes. The NADPH oxidase multicomponent protein complex is assembled on the phagosomal membrane, enabling transfer of electrons from cytosolic NADPH to phagosomal oxygen to generate superoxide [1]. At the same time, cytoplasmic granules containing antimicrobial and hydrolytic proteins are released into the phagosome. One of the granule constituents is MPO, which constitutes 5% of the neutrophil protein [2]. Superoxide dismutates to hydrogen peroxide (H_2O_2), and MPO can use this H_2O_2 to generate HOCl and HOSCN. Chemical probes and the detection of chlorinated proteins indicate that HOCl is generated within the limited confines of a

DOI: 10.1201/9781003212287-13

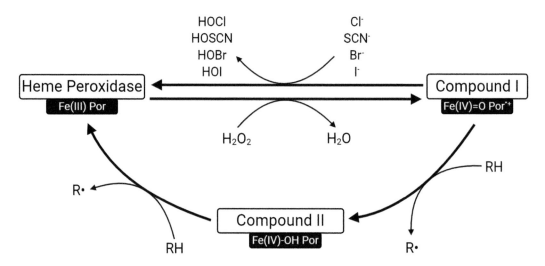

Figure 10.1 General halogenation and peroxidase cycles of mammalian heme peroxidases. Heme peroxidases react with H_2O_2 to form Compound I. Compound I can then oxidize the available halide and pseudohalides Cl^-, SCN^-, Br^- and I^- to form hypohalous acids. Alternatively, Compound I can be reduced to Compound II, resulting in radical species (R·). Compound II is then reduced back to the native enzyme state. The substrate preferences of specific peroxidases are shown in Figure 10.3.

neutrophil phagosome [3–5]. The transport of Cl^- into the phagosomes is important to ensure continued HOCl production [6], but it is not known if enough SCN^- is available to neutrophils to also enable HOSCN production in a phagosome.

MPO activity is not restricted to phagosomes. The contents of neutrophil granules can be released extracellularly through neutrophil degranulation or lysis, the most spectacular of which is during neutrophil extracellular trap (NET) formation (Figure 10.2). NETs are structures comprising neutrophil DNA and proteins that can trap invasive organisms and are thought to contribute to neutrophil antimicrobial activity [7]. Of note, NETs contain substantial quantities of enzymatically active MPO that upon H_2O_2 addition has been shown to kill entrapped bacteria [8].

The main substrate of MPO is considered to be Cl^- due to its high concentration in plasma. However, the preferred substrate of MPO is SCN^-, and at physiological plasma concentrations of Cl^- and SCN^-, up to a quarter of the H_2O_2 will be used by MPO to form HOSCN [9]. Much higher SCN^- concentrations have been reported in lung airway fluid [10], meaning that HOSCN formation will be favored by MPO in this environment (Figure 10.3). While the concentration of Cl^- is maintained in vivo, the concentration of SCN^- in biological fluids can vary greatly with diet and smoking status, with significantly higher SCN^- levels reported in smokers [11–13] and vegans [14].

Secretory Fluid Lactoperoxidase

The enzyme LPO is found in secretory fluids, including saliva and nasal and airway lining fluid, and as such acts as a barrier to bacterial invasion [10,26]. The concentration of LPO in human airway secretions is estimated to be 3–12 µg/mL [10]. Its major substrate, SCN^-, is present at these sites, leading to the formation of HOSCN from available H_2O_2 (Figure 10.3). Sources of extracellular H_2O_2 include the neutrophil NADPH oxidase, epithelial dual oxidase (DUOX) [27] or bacteria themselves [28–31] (Figure 10.4). Unlike the phagocytic NADPH oxidase, which is active for a few minutes during the agonist-stimulated oxidative burst, DUOX generates H_2O_2 continuously [32–34]. The LPO–SCN^-–H_2O_2 enzymatic system has a strong pH dependence with the rate of HOSCN production being maximal at pH 5–6 [35]. In the respiratory tract, where LPO plays an important role in bacterial defense, the pH is estimated to be 6.8 [36–39].

ASSESSMENT OF BACTERICIDAL AND BACTERIOSTATIC ACTIVITY

The antibacterial activity of HOCl and HOSCN is typically assessed by counting the colonies that form on agar plates following oxidant exposure. The inability to form colonies indicates a loss of replicative potential and is a surrogate marker of

MAMMALIAN HEME PEROXIDASES: DIVERSE ROLES IN HEALTH AND DISEASE

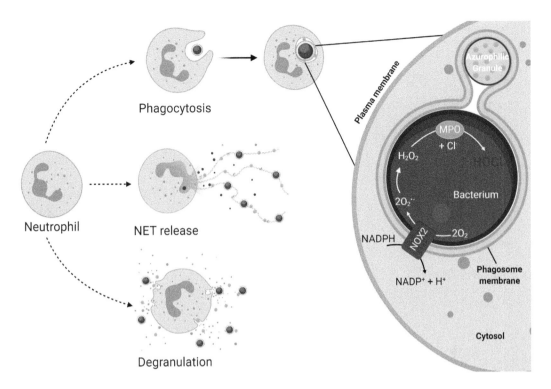

Figure 10.2 Intracellular and extracellular exposures of bacteria to neutrophil MPO. Following phagocytosis, neutrophil granule contents, including MPO (green), are released into the phagosome containing the engulfed bacterium (purple). Superoxide (O_2^-), formed by the NADPH oxidase, is converted to HOCl. Bacteria are also exposed to MPO extracellularly, either when attached to NETs or following degranulation, where the contents of neutrophil granules are released extracellularly.

death. It is important to note that this method cannot distinguish between death that occurs immediately following oxidant exposure and that which occurs as the bacteria are attempting to grow on the nutrient-rich agar plates. Indeed, bacteria have shown improved survival when cultured under anaerobic conditions, indicating that lethal damage occurs as a result of oxidative stress as the bacteria attempt to grow on the agar plates [40]. Bacterial viability can also be assessed using culture-independent techniques, using fluorescent dyes sensitive to properties such as membrane integrity, membrane potential or enzyme activity (reviewed in Ref. [41]). Sublethal oxidative stress can inhibit bacterial growth, with the bacteriostatic activity of HOSCN well recognized. Restricting bacterial growth is useful in impeding colonization and assisting phagocytic cells to clear invasive infections. Bacteriostatic activity is typically measured by introducing the antibacterial agent of choice under conditions where growth can occur, followed by quantifying turbidity of the culture or bacterial colony-forming units.

There are number of methodological factors that can impact assessment of the bactericidal and bacteriostatic activity of oxidants. For oxidants such as HOCl that are rapidly consumed by their targets, efficacy is dependent on the density of bacteria in the system and is best described as an *amount per bacteria* rather than a concentration. Media composition is also critical, as oxidants can quickly react with certain constituents, either removing them from the solution or converting them to other reactive species. For example, adding HOCl to media containing amine groups leads to the formation of secondary chloramines, the bactericidal effect of which might be different from that of HOCl [42]. The high reactivity of HOCl means it is necessary to mix the solution when adding it to bacteria to avoid exposing only a small fraction of bacteria to a high, localized dose. HOSCN is much longer-lived in biological systems than HOCl [43], and therefore, its concentration rather than bacterial density is more important for activity. Exposure time also becomes relevant. Most studies that

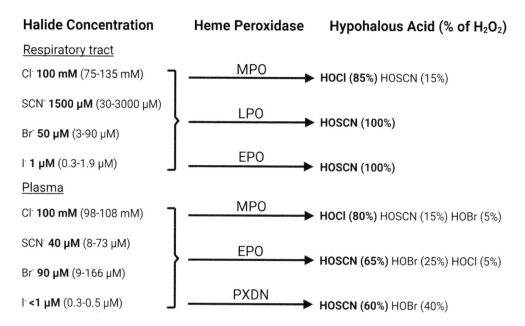

Figure 10.3 The generation of hypohalous acids by the four specialist mammalian peroxidases, MPO, LPO, eosinophil peroxidase (EPO) and peroxidasin (PXDN), in biological fluids. In the respiratory tract, comprising here the airway fluid, nasal fluid and saliva, Cl^- is at much higher concentrations than SCN^-, Br^- and I^- [10,15–23]. In the plasma, while Cl^- levels are the same [20,21], SCN^- and I^- levels are lower and the concentration of Br^- is slightly higher [11–13,23,24]. The concentrations of halides in bold are median values. Hypohalous acid as a percentage of the hydrogen peroxide used by each respective peroxidase was determined using the median halide concentration and the rate constants for the reduction of compound I by the respective halide taken from Ref. [25]. The rate constant for PXDN is from a truncated recombinant human peroxidasin containing peroxidase and Ig domains. Products amounting to less than 1% are not shown. MPO and EPO can oxidize Cl^-, SCN^-, Br^- or I^-, while LPO and PXDN can oxidize SCN^-, Br^- or I^-. The predominant product for each peroxidase is highlighted in bold.

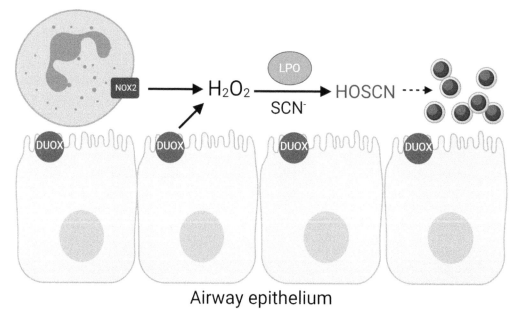

Figure 10.4 LPO-dependent HOSCN generation in the airways. At sites of infection, such as the airways, LPO (orange) is present and will use H_2O_2 generated by epithelial dual oxidase (DUOX) [27], neutrophil NOX2-dependent NADPH oxidase (NOX2) [1] or bacteria [28–31], along with SCN^- from the surrounding environment to generate HOSCN to kill invading pathogens (purple).

have examined bacterial sensitivity to HOSCN used the MPO/LPO-SCN$^-$-H$_2$O$_2$ system, where the actual concentration of HOSCN generated is not measured. HOSCN degrades in aqueous buffers, and the observed antimicrobial activity will depend on how fresh the stock solution is.

BACTERIAL SENSITIVITY TO HYPOCHLOROUS ACID

HOCl, commonly known as chlorine bleach, has been used as a disinfectant since the late 19th century when its use as a medical disinfectant was first recognized [44]. It is now the most common disinfectant in the developed world and is used in medical, industrial and domestic settings. HOCl, a weak acid, is in equilibrium with hypochlorite ($^-$OCl) and molecular chlorine (Cl$_2$) in aqueous solutions, the proportion of which depends on the pH and the concentration of Cl$^-$ [45]. With a pK$_a$ of 7.4, HOCl and $^-$OCl are present at equal proportions under physiological conditions. HOCl is a considerably stronger oxidant than $^-$OCl, and therefore, the bactericidal properties of chlorine bleach are largely attributed to HOCl. To ensure the stability of commercial solutions of chlorine bleach, they are prepared at basic pH, where $^-$OCl predominates.

The majority of research on bacterial killing by reagent HOCl or the MPO-Cl$^-$-H$_2$O$_2$ system has been performed with the Gram-negative bacterium Escherichia coli [46–55]. The efficacy of reagent HOCl in killing other bacteria has also been reported, examples of which are shown in Table 10.1. The dose of HOCl required to kill 50% of the bacteria (LD$_{50}$) ranges from 2.5 nmol/10^8 CFU for Pseudomonas aeruginosa to 91 nmol/10^8 CFU for Mycobacterium smegmatis. Bonvillain et al. compared cystic fibrosis and non-cystic fibrosis pathogens, with resistance to HOCl correlating with clinical pathogenicity [56]. HOCl resistance was highest in P. aeruginosa, followed by Staphylococcus aureus, Burkholderia cepacia, E. coli and Klebsiella pneumoniae. Resistance to H$_2$O$_2$ is much higher than that to HOCl but also varies among bacterial species. B. cepacia, E. coli and S. aureus were killed at lower doses by H$_2$O$_2$ than were K. pneumoniae and P. aeruginosa [56]. Importantly, bacteria survive orders of magnitude more H$_2$O$_2$ than HOCl, so the conversion of H$_2$O$_2$ into HOCl by peroxidases is vital for the innate immune system [56].

The role of HOCl in microbial killing in the neutrophil phagosome is a topic of ongoing debate [57], owing to the observation that individuals with MPO deficiency rarely suffer from persistent infections [58]. Recently, the oxidation

TABLE 10.1

Examples of LD$_{50}$ for killing of different bacteria by HOCl

Bacterium	Strain	Gram	LD$_{50}$ (nmol/10^8 CFU)	Reference
Streptococcus pneumoniae	D39	+	4.7	[a]
	SP264		6	
Pseudomonas aeruginosa	PAO1	−	2.5	[59],[a]
	Clinical isolate		7	[56]
Staphylococcus aureus	USA300	+	6–11	[b]
	Clinical isolate		7	[56]
	502a		7.5–13	[4,63]
Escherichia coli	DH5α	−	3	[56]
Klebsiella pneumoniae	43816, Serotype 2	−	3	[56]
Burkholderia cepacia	Clinical isolate	−	5	[56]
Mycobacterium smegmatis	mc^{2}155	+	91	[93]

Bacteria were treated with HOCl for 10–60 min in PBS or HBSS (pH 7.4), neither of which contains ingredients known to react with HOCl. LD$_{50}$ was determined as the concentration of oxidant necessary to kill 50% of bacteria as determined by counting colony-forming units (CFU).

[a] Shearer et al. (in preparation).

[b] Ashby et al. (in preparation).

of bacterial glutathione was monitored during neutrophil phagocytosis to gauge the exposure of P. aeruginosa to HOCl in the phagosome [59]. The extent of glutathione oxidation in P. aeruginosa recovered from neutrophils was similar to that observed upon exposure to lethal doses of HOCl, indicating that the concentration of HOCl produced in phagosomes is sufficient to kill P. aeruginosa [59]. The LD_{50} of HOCl for P. aeruginosa in this study was 2.3 nmol/10^8 bacteria [59], which is similar to what has been reported for E. coli and K. pneumoniae [56]. This suggests that these bacteria would also be susceptible to HOCl-mediated killing in the neutrophil phagosome. A clinical isolate of P. aeruginosa has been reported to be three times more resistant to HOCl [56], which is likely to extend survival times within the phagosome.

The challenge faced by phagosomal bacteria will be different to that of bacteria treated with a bolus of HOCl. First, HOCl production in the phagosome will be continuous, depending on continued activity of the NADPH oxidase and myeloperoxidase and the availability of chloride [6]. Also, the majority of HOCl generated in the phagosome will react with neutrophil proteins [4,60], so killing may not be the result of HOCl itself. HOCl reacts with amines on amino acids and proteins to generate chloramines (R-NHCl). The reaction of chloramines with ammonia can yield ammonia chloramines, which have been shown to be cytotoxic, owing to their ability to penetrate cell membranes [61]. It has also been proposed that HOCl can form dichloramines, which break down into ammonia monochloramine (NH_2Cl) and ammonia dichloramine ($NHCl_2$), which have bactericidal properties [62]. S. aureus has been shown to have a similar susceptibility to NH_2Cl and $NHCl_2$ as HOCl [62,63]. In contrast, negatively charged taurine chloramine or peptide chloramines were found to be weak antimicrobial agents [62]. Chloramines can be long-lived, resulting in killing of E. coli several hours following HOCl exposure [64], possibly due to slow cell membrane penetration [61].

BACTERIAL TARGETS OF HYPOCHLOROUS ACID AND CHLORAMINES

HOCl is a promiscuous oxidant that can react with virtually all biomolecules [65]. The kinetically preferred targets for HOCl are sulfur-containing amino acid residues, cysteine and methionine and low-molecular-weight thiols [65,66]. HOCl can also react, albeit 10^3–10^4-fold slower, with histidine, lysine and tryptophan side chains on proteins, heme groups, iron–sulfur centers, phospholipid head groups, glycosaminoglycan chains and nucleotides [65,67,68]. The toxicity of HOCl is therefore likely due to reaction with multiple bacterial targets. Indeed, there is evidence for HOCl disrupting many vital cellular processes in bacteria, including metabolic energy balance and respiration [52,67,69–71], substrate transport [52,70,72], DNA and protein synthesis [73,74] and thiol homeostasis [46,59,75,76] (Table 10.2).

Early studies reported a loss of respiration and ATP in E. coli following exposure to HOCl that paralleled cell death [52,69,71]. An inability to import amino acids (leucine, glutamine, proline) and sugars (thiomethylgalactoside, glucose) accompanied HOCl-mediated killing [52,72]. The barrier function of the cell membrane was retained, and the HOCl-sensitive metabolic enzymes aldolase and β-galactosidase remained active in the cytoplasm at bactericidal doses [52,67,71,72]. Consequently, cell death is likely the result of damage to transport and energy-transducing systems located on the inner membrane. A firm link between the loss of inner membrane function and abolishment of bacterial ATP production was established by demonstrating that HOCl inhibits uptake of the respiratory substrate succinate and the activities of complex II and the ATP synthase [49,70,77]. Ammonia chloramine also causes a loss of transport function; however, differences between the two oxidants were observed [72]. With HOCl, inhibition of membrane transport preceded death, indicating it is not a consequence of bacterial death, and transport functions could be completely inhibited by the oxidant. In contrast, transport inhibition tracked with viability loss at low doses of ammonia chloramine, and this oxidant was unable to completely inhibit transport function despite causing a complete loss of viability at higher doses.

The high reactivity of HOCl with iron/sulfur (Fe/S) clusters in ferredoxins and the loss of labile iron and sulfide from HOCl-treated E. coli pointed to Fe/S clusters in complex II as the molecular target for HOCl-induced respiratory loss [67,78,79]. However, the amount of oxidant required to destroy Fe/S clusters exceeded those required to inhibit enzymatic reactions of the dehydrogenase system, leading to the proposal of alternative inactivation sites

TABLE 10.2
Cellular processes affected by exposure of bacteria to HOCl

Cellular process	Effect of HOCl	Bacterial species	Reference
Substrate transport	Inhibition of uptake of glucose and amino acids	E. coli	[52]
	Inhibition of uptake of glutamine, proline, thiomethylgalactoside, leucine[a]	E. coli	[72]
	Inhibition of uptake of glucose, succinate, amino acids	E. coli P. aeruginosa S. lactis	[70]
Energy production	ATP loss	E. coli P. aeruginosa S. lactis	[52,70,71]
	Oxidation of iron-sulfur centers	E. coli	[78,79]
	Inhibition of complex II	E. coli P. aeruginosa	[49,77,80]
	Inhibition of ATP synthase	E. coli	[70]
Protein synthesis and translocation	Inhibition of protein synthesis	E. coli	[73]
	Chlorination of RNA	E. coli	[82]
	Inhibition of protein transport across the inner membrane	E coli	[48]
DNA synthesis	Inhibition of DNA synthesis	E. coli	[73]
	Loss of DNA and membrane interaction	E. coli	[74]
	DNA strand breaks	E. coli	[81]
General protein function	Oxidative unfolding and protein aggregation	E. coli	[83]
	Methionine sulfoxide formation[b]	E. coli	[48]
	Reversible protein thiol modification[b]	E. coli	[75,76]
Thiol homeostasis	General breakdown in thiol redox balance[b]	E.coli	[84]
	Oxidation of mycothiol	M. smegmatis	[93]
	Oxidation of glutathione	E. coli P. aeruginosa[a]	[46,59]
	Oxidation of bacillithiol	S. aureus	[94]

[a] Effect was also observed with chloramines.
[b] Effect was (also) observed in response to HOCl and during phagocytosis in an MPO-dependent manner.

in complex II, including the FAD and cytochrome b556 subunits [49,80]. Damage to succinate-dependent respiration and ATP-producing capacity was also observed in P. aeruginosa and Streptococcus lactis following treatment with bactericidal doses of HOCl [70,80]. While the loss of succinate-dependent respiration was an early event in the oxidative deactivation of the facultative anaerobe E. coli and could not entirely account for oxidative killing, it was closely paralleled by a loss of viability in the obligate aerobe P. aeruginosa [80]. These results highlight the differences in the susceptibility of critical targets between different bacteria.

In addition to metabolic and transport dysfunction, HOCl exposure resulted in a near instant termination of bacterial DNA synthesis, which was accompanied by an inhibition of bacterial growth [73]. One possible explanation for this effect is the modification of membrane structures in a way that prevents the chromosomal origin of replication from binding [74]. Whether the HOCl-induced impairment of the membrane/DNA interaction is a consequence of oxidation of membrane lipid or protein components remains to be investigated. This mechanism is in line with studies on bacterial energy production that concluded that oxidative injury of the cell envelope is sufficient to cause loss of cell viability and precedes modification of cytosolic components. Alternative mechanisms for the disruption of DNA synthesis are damage to the DNA template itself or the inactivation of replication enzymes. Because the DNA repair genes recA and recB were among the protective mechanisms identified to be important for HOCl resistance, DNA strand breaks might also be a consequence of HOCl exposure [81]. RNA, but not DNA, isolated from E. coli exposed to the MPO-Cl$^-$−H$_2$O$_2$ system showed detectable levels of 5-chlorocytosine, indicating that RNA is targeted for chlorination [82]. This might in part contribute to the inhibition of protein synthesis in E. coli exposed to bactericidal doses of HOCl, although DNA synthesis was inhibited to a substantially higher degree than protein synthesis [73].

To gain further insight into the molecular targets underlying HOCl-mediated damage, Rosen et al. monitored the oxidation of methionine residues on bacterial proteins, as oxidation of this amino acid to methionine sulfoxide is among the fastest reactions of HOCl in biological systems [48]. While proteins of the outer membrane and periplasm consumed HOCl and formed methionine sulfoxides, a microbicidal effect was only observed when inner membrane proteins and cytosolic proteins became oxidized [48]. Together with earlier findings, this result pinpointed the inner membrane as the site for the HOCl-inflicted lethal damage. Bacterial methionine was shown to become oxidized not only following treatment with reagent HOCl but also during phagocytosis by human neutrophils in an MPO-dependent manner [48]. Furthermore, pathways for translocating proteins across the inner membrane were identified as a specific target for methionine oxidation [48]. A causal link between methionine oxidation and loss of viability was established by showing that E. coli mutants lacking the repair enzyme, methionine sulfoxide reductase, were more sensitive to killing by HOCl compared with wild type [48]. Also, bacteria deficient in the HOCl-activated molecular chaperone Hsp33, which protects against the unfolding and aggregation of proteins in E. coli treated with HOCl [83], were killed more readily by HOCl [83].

As early as 1979, oxidation of cysteine residues in proteins has been described for E. coli treated with HOCl and chloramines [69]. Recently, a breakdown of bacterial thiol redox balance was

demonstrated to occur during phagocytosis by a neutrophil-like cell line using roGFP2-based fusion probes [84]. Redox-sensitive cysteines can form reversible modifications and act as sites for redox regulation [85]. Using a quantitative redox proteomics technique (OxICAT), Leichert et al. identified that many thiol proteins in E. coli were reversibly oxidized (30%–90%) in response to bacteriostatic, sublethal doses of HOCl [75]. Among the proteins with the highest proportion of oxidized cysteines were enzymes involved in glucose metabolism (glyceraldehyde-3-P-dehydrogenase, 93% oxidized; aconitase B, 68%), antioxidant response (thiol peroxidase AhpC, 63%; thiol peroxidase Tpx, 64%; glutaredoxin C, 64%) and transcription (ribosomal proteins, 63%–67%; elongation factor TU, 61%; transcriptional regulator 62%). Interestingly, one third of the redox-sensitive proteins were encoded by genes that when deleted made the bacteria more sensitive to HOCl stress, consistent with the role of these redox-regulated proteins in protecting E. coli from oxidative stress [75]. Recently, OxICAT was used to monitor the changes in the E. coli proteome during phagocytosis by a neutrophil-like cell line [76]. As with HOCl treatment, the majority of significantly oxidized thiol proteins were from glucose and protein metabolism, while some were involved in stress response and nucleotide metabolism.

One form of reversible thiol modification is S-thiolation, in which a low-molecular-weight thiol (LMWT) forms a disulfide with a protein cysteine that has first been oxidized to a sulfenic acid. This modification prevents further irreversible oxidation of the cysteine. Glutathione is utilized for this purpose in most Gram-negative bacteria, while many Gram-positive bacteria lack glutathione and instead synthesize other LMWTs such as bacillithiol and mycothiol [86–89]. S-thiolated groups can be removed by glutaredoxins, mycoredoxins and bacilliredoxins to restore protein function using the respective LMWT as a cofactor [90–92].

In E. coli, glutathione loss parallels cell death upon treatment with HOCl, and glutathione-deficiency leads to an increased susceptibility to HOCl and chloramines [46]. Similarly, loss of mycothiol and bacillithiol correlates with loss of viability in M. smegmatis and S. aureus, respectively ([93,Ashby et al. [in preparation]]), and strains lacking these LMWTs are more susceptible to HOCl [86,95,96]. While only 6%–7% of bacillithiol forms mixed disulfides with proteins upon exposure to HOCl, collectively these studies point to a protective role of LMTWs against this oxidant in some bacteria [94,97]. In contrast, doses of HOCl that were required to significantly deplete glutathione in *P. aeruginosa* exceeded those needed to kill the bacteria [59]. Furthermore, significant protein glutathionylation was only observed when all bacteria were dead and constituted merely 2% of the total glutathione pool. There are a number of possible reasons for the apparent absence of S-glutathionylation as a protective mechanism in *P. aeruginosa*. It might be that the glutathione recycling machinery is very efficient in these bacteria, making S-glutathionylation difficult to detect until the bacteria and reducing mechanism are completely deactivated. Alternatively, glutathione levels might be low relative to other sensitive targets or other vital constituents possess an exquisite sensitivity to HOCl, as previously shown for the electron transport chain in *P. aeruginosa* [80].

As discussed earlier, it has been proposed that oxidative stress encountered during bacterial recovery contributes to HOCl toxicity [40]. HOCl-mediated inactivation of superoxide dismutase, GSH depletion and the release of free iron are likely to contribute to the increased difficulty of bacteria to grow in oxygen [78].

In summary, HOCl and chloramines can induce cell death by reacting with a multitude of cellular components, with many of the targets located at the inner membrane (Table 10.2). It is worth noting that much of the research in this field was performed over two decades ago. The application of new proteomic and metabolomic methodologies may provide new insight. Also, much of the research on mechanisms of bactericidal activity has come from studies with *E. coli* and to a lesser extent *P. aeruginosa*. Critical targets may vary between species, and future studies could be aimed at elucidating critical targets in Gram-positive bacteria with a particular focus on bacteria posing a threat to human health due to their rapid development of antibiotic resistance such as *S. aureus* and *S. pneumoniae*.

BACTERIAL SENSITIVITY TO HYPOTHIOCYANOUS ACID

HOSCN and the MPO/LPO-SCN$^-$-H$_2$O$_2$ system have been shown to have an antibacterial effect against Gram-positive [28,98–106] and Gram-negative bacteria [10,98,105,107–111]. HOSCN can act as a bacteriostatic agent and/or a bactericidal agent, depending on dose. Responses of bacteria to HOSCN is dependent upon many variables, including bacterial strain, temperature, pH, H$_2$O$_2$/Cl$^-$/SCN$^-$ levels and exposure time. pH is a particularly important factor, as HOSCN has a pK$_a$ of 5.3 and its conjugate base hypothiocyanite (OSCN$^-$) will predominate at physiological pH [112]. As the pH decreases, more will be present as HOSCN, which is the stronger oxidant and has greater ability to penetrate cell membranes [112]. Indeed, HOSCN generated via the MPO- and LPO-SCN$^-$-H$_2$O$_2$ system was significantly more microbicidal to *P. aeruginosa* at pH 6.8, mimicking secreted fluids, than at pH 7.4, mimicking plasma [109].

HOSCN has been shown to act as an effective bacteriostatic and bactericidal agent against many species of bacteria, including *E. coli* [10,105, 107,108,110,113], *S. aureus* [98], *P. aeruginosa* [10,98, 108,110], *B. cepacia* [10], *Haemophilus influenzae* [10] and *Helicobacter pylori* [111]. Screening of 15 bacterial isolates from cystic fibrosis sputum for susceptibility to HOSCN identified differences in killing between bacterial species, with inhibition of 50% of bacterial viability (IC$_{50}$) values ranging from 13 μM/h for *P. aeruginosa* (isolate PA-39) to 1,600 μM/h for methicillin-resistant *S. aureus* (isolate 43) [114].

Seleno-moeities are generally more reactive than their sulfur-containing counterparts [115–117], and a chemical SCN$^-$ analogue, selenocyanate (SeCN$^-$), was able to be utilized by LPO to generate HOSeCN, which was more bactericidal than HOSCN in the LPO-H$_2$O$_2$ system against sensitive and resistant cystic fibrosis isolates [114]. Similar to some oral streptococci, clinical isolates of *P. aeruginosa* with NADPH-dependent HOSCN reductase activity have been found to be more resistant to HOSCN-mediated killing than those without [109].

The bactericidal action of HOSCN on *E. coli* has been shown to be dependent upon oxidant exposure time [107]. Bacterial respiration was inhibited with short exposures, but bacterial recovery was observed once the oxidant was removed. In contrast, longer oxidant exposure resulted in bacterial killing, with respiration inhibition becoming irreversible. In addition, similar to what has been reported for HOCl, the bactericidal effects of HOSCN on *E. coli* cells have been shown to vary depending on oxygen exposure after treatment, with bacteria plated anaerobically, rather than aerobically, surviving oxidant exposure [118].

Much work on HOSCN-mediated antimicrobial effects has been carried out using oral bacteria from the *Streptococcus* genus given their exposure to HOSCN produced in saliva [28,100–102,104,106,118]. Many of these bacteria are catalase-negative and produce H_2O_2 as a part of their normal metabolism. Instead of being bactericidal, HOSCN has as a protective effect in many streptococci, guarding bacteria from H_2O_2- or HOCl-mediated killing [100–102,118]. Resistance to HOSCN-mediated killing in some oral streptococci has been attributed to the presence of NAD(P)H-dependent HOSCN-reductases [28,102,106,119], although these have not been identified in all resistant strains. Additionally, *Aggregatibacter actinomycetemcomitans*, a Gram-negative bacterium that is present in the mouth, has shown HOSCN resistance, with addition of SCN$^-$ to the MPO-Cl$^-$-H_2O_2 system abolishing bactericidal activity [120].

Streptococcus pneumoniae is a commensal bacterium in the nasopharynx but can cause serious infections, including pneumonia [121]. Recent work by Shearer et al. (in preparation) has shown that two lab strains and two lung clinical isolates of *S. pneumoniae* are highly resistant to HOSCN, with the highest dose tested (800 μM) unable to kill. In addition, the addition of SCN$^-$ to a MPO-SCN$^-$-H_2O_2 system protected the bacteria from HOCl-mediated killing. As many bacteria in the *Streptococcus* genus produce their own H_2O_2 [28–31] and survive in SCN$^-$-rich environments, such as the mouth and lungs, their resistance to HOSCN-mediated killing may allow for the bacteria to outcompete other organisms.

BACTERIAL TARGETS OF HYPOTHIOCYANOUS ACID

HOSCN is relatively specific for thiol groups, which are first oxidized to sulfenic acids and can then react undergo further reaction with other thiols [43]. Unlike HOCl, HOSCN does not react with methionine or amine residues. There is some evidence that the MPO-SCN$^-$-H_2O_2 system can promote lipid peroxidation [121,123]. Some of the biological damage observed with HOSCN or the MPO-SCN$^-$-H_2O_2 system might also be mediated through carbamylation of amino groups (i.e. formation of R-NONH$_2$). This modification results from the reaction with cyanate (OCN$^-$), which is formed during the decomposition of HOSCN, or the oxidation of SCN$^-$ by MPO [124,125]. It is worth noting that HOSCN can be secondary

TABLE 10.3

Cellular processes affected by exposure of bacteria to the LPO-SCN$^-$-H_2O_2 system

Cellular process	Effect of HOSCN	Bacterial species	Reference
Substrate transport	Inhibition of glucose uptake	S. agalactiae S. mutans	[128,129]
	Inhibition of valine uptake	E. coli	[113]
Glycolysis	Inhibition of hexokinase	S. cremoris	[106]
	Inhibition glyceraldehyde-3-phosphate dehydrogenase (GAPDH)	S. cremoris S. pyogenes S. sangius S. mitis S. mutans S. salavarius	[102,106,140]
	Inhibition of aldolase	S. cremoris	[106]
Pentose phosphate cycle	Inhibition of 6-Phosphogluconate dehydrogenase	S. cremoris	[106]
Respiration	Inhibition of oxygen uptake	E. coli	[107]
	Failure to establish an electrochemical proton gradient	E. coli	[130]
	Inhibition of respiratory dehydrogenases	E. coli	[132]
pH adaption	Urease inactivation	H. pylori	[111]

oxidant of HOCl, as the latter reacts rapidly with SCN$^-$ to form HOSCN [126].

Given the presence of the antimicrobial LPO-SCN$^-$-H$_2$O$_2$ system in mammalian secretions, early studies explored targets for HOSCN in bacteria found in the mouth and genitourinary system (Table 10.3). In these Gram-positive, facultative anaerobic bacteria, the LPO-SCN$^-$-H$_2$O$_2$ system reversibly inhibited glycolysis and oxygen uptake [102,106]. The ability to recover differed among the *Streptococcus* species [102]. The primary site for inhibition of glycolysis was found to be thiol-sensitive enzymes glyceraldehyde-3-phosphate dehydrogenase (GAPDH), hexokinase and aldolase [102,106,127]. The pentose phosphate pathway was also affected by the LPO-SCN$^-$-H$_2$O$_2$ system through inhibition of 6-phosphogluconate dehydrogenase [106]. Furthermore, glucose transport was shown to be reversibly inhibited [128,129].

In *E. coli*, a loss in membrane transport, oxygen uptake and the ability to generate an electrochemical proton gradient across its inner membrane was observed upon exposure to the LPO-SCN$^-$-H$_2$O$_2$ system [107,113,130] (Table 10.3). A leakage of potassium ions and amino acids indicated damage to the inner membrane, which was more pronounced in *E. coli* than in Gram-positive *S. lactis*, consistent with an increased susceptibility of *E. coli* to killing by the LPO antimicrobial system [131]. To investigate molecular targets for HOSCN in *E. coli*, Thomas and Aune monitored thiol oxidation, which correlated with a loss in respiration and viability [107]. Thiol content, respiration and viability could all be restored after short-term, but not long-term, incubation with the LPO antimicrobial system [107]. Specific respiratory enzymes inhibited in *E. coli* by HOSCN were found to be substrate-specific dehydrogenases, with the most susceptible being succinate dehydrogenase [132]. As with HOCl, recovery was greater if *E. coli* were incubated anaerobically rather than aerobically after the HOSCN challenge suggesting that a compromise in *E. coli* antioxidant defenses contributes in part to HOSCN toxicity [118].

The mechanism of action of HOSCN against *H. pylori* has also been investigated and found to involve the inactivation of its urease activity [111]. This enzyme has an active site cysteine and hydrolyzes urea into ammonia allowing *H. pylori* to survive in the acidic environment of the stomach.

FUTURE DIRECTIONS

HOCl and chloramines can induce bacterial death by reacting with a multitude of cellular constituents. As such, it is virtually impossible for bacteria to develop the resistance that they do for other antimicrobial agents. Indeed, the best strategy for a successful pathogen is to avoid phagocytosis or to impede oxidant generation so that it drops to a level that enables survival [133]. Bacteria have many well-studied defenses that can provide some protection against HOCl, the details of which have been reviewed elsewhere [134,135]. A number of prokaryote transcription factors have redox-sensitive cysteine residues, which upon oxidation upregulate a number of genes encoding proteins that can reduce or degrade oxidized proteins, prevent protein aggregation, chelate redox-active metals and maintain thiol homeostasis [136]. Interestingly, there were different patterns of gene expression in *P. aeruginosa* exposed to HOCl and HOSCN [136]. The mechanism for these differences has not been investigated, but they suggest that sublethal doses of HOCl and HOSCN activate a different combination of transcription factors or other transcriptional regulators in the same bacteria.

Sensitizing bacteria to innate immune system oxidants by compromising bacterial defense systems, particularly thiol systems, holds promise as a novel antimicrobial therapy. In support of this proposal are encouraging studies demonstrating that the colonization of *S. pneumoniae* in mice and the survival of *S. aureus* in human whole blood and neutrophils are decreased if the ability of these bacteria to import, synthesize or recycle their LMWTs is abolished [137–139]. HOSCN is more selective in its reactivity than HOCl, and it appears that species such as oral streptococci can be resistant. It is not clear exactly how this is achieved, though NADPH-dependent thioredoxin reductase activity appears to offer some protection [102,109]. Further examination of genes that promote resistance may reveal new therapeutic strategies to target these bacteria, particularly those that colonize the respiratory tract where the LPO system has a prominent role in innate defense.

ACKNOWLEDGMENTS

We thank Prof. Christine Winterbourn for her critical reading of the chapter. This research was supported by the Health Research Council of New Zealand (15/479). Figures were created with BioRender.com.

REFERENCES

1. C.C. Winterbourn, A.J. Kettle, M.B. Hampton, 2016, Reactive oxygen species and neutrophil function, *Annual Review of Biochemistry* 85: 765–792.

2. J. Schultz, K. Kaminker, 1962, Myeloperoxidase of the leucocyte of normal human blood. I. Content and localization, *Archives of Biochemistry and Biophysics* 96: 465–467.

3. A.M. Albrett, L.V. Ashby, N. Dickerhof, A.J. Kettle, C.C. Winterbourn, 2018, Heterogeneity of hypochlorous acid production in individual neutrophil phagosomes revealed by a rhodamine-based probe, *Journal of Biological Chemistry* 293: 15715–15724.

4. A.L. Chapman, M.B. Hampton, R. Senthilmohan, C.C. Winterbourn, A.J. Kettle, 2002, Chlorination of bacterial and neutrophil proteins during phagocytosis and killing of *Staphylococcus aureus*, *Journal of Biological Chemistry* 277: 9757–9762.

5. Q. Jiang, J.K. Hurst, 1997, Relative chlorinating, nitrating, and oxidizing capabilities of neutrophils determined with phagocytosable probes, *Journal of Biological Chemistry* 272: 32767–32772.

6. C.C. Winterbourn, M.B. Hampton, J.H. Livesey, A.J. Kettle, 2006, Modeling the reactions of superoxide and myeloperoxidase in the neutrophil phagosome implications for microbial killing, *Journal of Biological Chemistry* 281: 39860–39869.

7. V. Brinkmann, U. Reichard, C. Goosmann, et al., 2004, Neutrophil extracellular traps kill bacteria, *Science* 303: 1532–1535.

8. H. Parker, A.M. Albrett, A.J. Kettle, C.C. Winterbourn, 2012, Myeloperoxidase associated with neutrophil extracellular traps is active and mediates bacterial killing in the presence of hydrogen peroxide, *Journal of Leukocyte Biology* 91: 369–376.

9. J.C. Van Dalen, W.M. Whitehouse, C.C. Winterbourn, J.A. Kettle, 1997, Thiocyanate and chloride as competing substrates for myeloperoxidase, *Biochemical Journal* 327: 487–492.

10. C. Wijkstrom-Frei, S. El-Chemaly, R. Ali-Rachedi, et al., 2003, Lactoperoxidase and human airway host defense, *American Journal of Respiratory Cell and Molecular Biology* 29: 206–212.

11. P.E. Morgan, D.I. Pattison, J. Talib, et al., 2011, High plasma thiocyanate levels in smokers are a key determinant of thiol oxidation induced by myeloperoxidase, *Free Radical Biology and Medicine* 51: 1815–1822.

12. P. Nedoboy, P. Morgan, T. Mocatta, et al., 2014, High plasma thiocyanate levels are associated with enhanced myeloperoxidase-induced thiol oxidation and long-term survival in subjects following a first myocardial infarction, *Free Radical Research* 48: 1256–1266.

13. K. Tsuge, M. Kataoka, Y. Seto, 2000, Cyanide and thiocyanate levels in blood and saliva of healthy adult volunteers, *Journal of Health Science* 46: 343–350.

14. A.M. Leung, A. LaMar, X. He, L.E. Braverman, E.N. Pearce, 2011, Iodine status and thyroid function of Boston-area vegetarians and vegans, *The Journal of Clinical Endocrinology & Metabolism* 96: E1303–E1307.

15. E. Thomson, S. Brennan, R. Senthilmohan, et al., 2010, Identifying peroxidases and their oxidants in the early pathology of cystic fibrosis, *Free Radical Biology and Medicine* 49: 1354–1360.

16. D. Lorentzen, L. Durairaj, A.A. Pezzulo, et al., 2011, Concentration of the antibacterial precursor thiocyanate in cystic fibrosis airway secretions, *Free Radical Biology and Medicine* 50: 1144–1150.

17. C.P. Schultz, M.K. Ahmed, C. Dawes, H.H. Mantsch, 1996, Thiocyanate levels in human saliva: quantitation by Fourier transform infrared spectroscopy, *Analytical Biochemistry* 240: 7–12.

18. N. Van Haeringen, F. Ensink, E. Glasius, 1979, The peroxidase-thiocyanate-hydrogenperoxide system in tear fluid and saliva of different species, *Experimental Eye Research* 28: 343–347.

19. Ł. Minarowski, D. Sands, A. Minarowska, et al., 2008, Thiocyanate concentration in saliva of cystic fibrosis patients, *Folia Histochemica et Cytobiologica* 46: 245–246.

20. J. Hull, W. Skinner, C. Robertson, P. Phelan, 1998, Elemental content of airway surface liquid from infants with cystic fibrosis, *American Journal of Respiratory and Critical Care Medicine* 157: 10–14.

21. L. Joris, I. Dab, P.M. Quinton, 1993, Elemental composition of human airway surface fluid in healthy and diseased airways, *American Journal of Respiratory and Critical Care Medicine* 148: 1633–1637.

22. J.J. Smith, S.M. Travis, E.P. Greenberg, M.J. Welsh, 1996, Cystic fibrosis airway epithelia fail to kill bacteria because of abnormal airway surface fluid, *Cell* 85: 229–236.

23. K. Diem, C. Lentner, 1974, *Scientific Tables*, Seventh ed., Ciba-Geigy Limited, Switzerland.

24. J. Holzbecher, D.E. Ryan, 1980, The rapid determination of total bromine and iodine in biological fluids by neutron activation, *Clinical Biochemistry* 13: 277–278.

25. M. Paumann-Page, R.-S. Katz, M. Bellei, et al., 2017, Pre-steady-state kinetics reveal the substrate specificity and mechanism of halide oxidation of truncated human peroxidasin 1, *Journal of Biological Chemistry* 292: 4583–4592.

26. J.D. Chandler, B.J. Day, 2012, Thiocyanate: a potentially useful therapeutic agent with host defense and antioxidant properties, *Biochemical Pharmacology* 84: 1381–1387.

27. A. van der Vliet, 2008, NADPH oxidases in lung biology and pathology: host defense enzymes, and more, *Free Radical Biology and Medicine* 44: 938–955.

28. E. Thomas, K. Pera, K. Smith, A. Chwang, 1983, Inhibition of Streptococcus mutans by the lactoperoxidase antimicrobial system, *Infection and Immunity* 39: 767–778.

29. C.D. Pericone, S. Park, J.A. Imlay, J.N. Weiser, 2003, Factors contributing to hydrogen peroxide resistance in *Streptococcus pneumoniae* include pyruvate oxidase (SpxB) and avoidance of the toxic effects of the Fenton reaction, *Journal of Bacteriology* 185: 6815–6825.

30. C.D. Pericone, K. Overweg, P.W. Hermans, J.N. Weiser, 2000, Inhibitory and bactericidal effects of hydrogen peroxide production by *Streptococcus pneumoniae* on other inhabitants of the upper respiratory tract, *Infection and Immunity* 68: 3990–3997.

31. B. Spellerberg, D.R. Cundell, J. Sandros, et al., 1996, Pyruvate oxidase, as a determinant of virulence in Streptococcus pneumoniae, *Molecular Microbiology* 19: 803–813.

32. H. Fischer, 2009, Mechanisms and function of DUOX in epithelia of the lung, *Antioxidants & Redox Signaling* 11: 2453–2465.

33. T. Decoursey, E. Ligeti, 2005, Regulation and termination of NADPH oxidase activity, *Cellular and Molecular Life Sciences CMLS* 62: 2173–2193.

34. G.E. Conner, C. Wijkstrom-Frei, S.H. Randell, V.E. Fernandez, M. Salathe, 2007, The lactoperoxidase system links anion transport to host defense in cystic fibrosis, *FEBS letters* 581: 271–278.

35. K.M. Pruitt, B. Mansson-Rahemtulla, D.C. Baldone, F. Rahemtulla, 1988, Steady-state kinetics of thiocyanate oxidation catalyzed by human salivary peroxidase, *Biochemistry* 27: 240–245.

36. C. FenolI-Palomares, J. Muñoz-Montagud, V. Sanchiz, et al., 2004, Unstimulated salivary flow rate, pH and buffer capacity of saliva in healthy volunteers, *Revista Espanola de Enfermedades Digestivas* 96: 773–783.

37. D. McShane, J. Davies, M. Davies, et al., 2003, Airway surface pH in subjects with cystic fibrosis, *European Respiratory Journal* 21: 37–42.

38. H. Fischer, J.H. Widdicombe, B. Illek, 2002, Acid secretion and proton conductance in human airway epithelium, *American Journal of Physiology-Cell Physiology* 282: C736–C743.

39. S. Jayaraman, Y. Song, L. Vetrivel, L. Shankar, A. Verkman, 2001, Noninvasive in vivo fluorescence measurement of airway-surface liquid depth, salt concentration, and pH, *The Journal of Clinical Investigation* 107: 317–324.

40. S. Dukan, S. Belkin, D. Touati, 1999, Reactive oxygen species are partially involved in the bacteriocidal action of hypochlorous acid, *Archives of Biochemistry and Biophysics* 367: 311–316.

41. S.S. Kumar, A.R. Ghosh, 2019, Assessment of bacterial viability: a comprehensive review on recent advances and challenges, *Microbiology* 165: 593–610.

42. L.V. Ashby, R. Springer, M.B. Hampton, A.J. Kettle, C.C. Winterbourn, 2020, Evaluating the bactericidal action of hypochlorous acid in culture media, *Free Radical Biology and Medicine* 159: 119–124.

43. D.I. Pattison, M.J. Davies, C.L. Hawkins, 2012, Reactions and reactivity of myeloperoxidase-derived oxidants: differential biological effects of hypochlorous and hypothiocyanous acids, *Free Radical Research* 46: 975–995.

44. W.A. Rutala, D.J. Weber, 1997, Uses of inorganic hypochlorite (bleach) in health-care facilities, *Clinical Microbiology Reviews* 10: 597–610.

45. A.J. Kettle, A.M. Albrett, A.L. Chapman, et al., 2014, Measuring chlorine bleach in biology and medicine, *Biochimica et Biophysica Acta (BBA)-General Subjects* 1840: 781–793.

46. J.A. Chesney, J.W. Eaton, J. Mahoney, 1996, Bacterial glutathione: a sacrificial defense against chlorine compounds, *Journal of Bacteriology* 178: 2131–2135.

47. R.M. Rakita, B.R. Michel, H. Rosen, 1990, Differential inactivation of *Escherichia coli* membrane dehydrogenases by a myeloperoxidase-mediated antimicrobial system, *Biochemistry* 29: 1075–1080.

48. H. Rosen, S.J. Klebanoff, Y. Wang, et al., 2009, Methionine oxidation contributes to bacterial killing by the myeloperoxidase system of neutrophils, *Proceedings of the National Academy of Sciences* 106: 18686–18691.

49. H. Rosen, R. Rakita, A. Waltersdorph, S. Klebanoff, 1987, Myeloperoxidase-mediated damage to the

succinate oxidase system of *Escherichia coli*. Evidence for selective inactivation of the dehydrogenase component, *Journal of Biological Chemistry* 262: 15004–15010.

50. J. Albrich, J. Hurst, 1982, Oxidative inactivation of *Escherichia coli* by hypochlorous acid: rates and differentiation of respiratory from other reaction sites, *FEBS letters* 144: 157–161.

51. S.J. Klebanoff, 1968, Myeloperoxidase-halide-hydrogen peroxide antibacterial system, *Journal of Bacteriology* 95: 2131–2138.

52. A.K. Camper, G.A. McFeters, 1979, Chlorine injury and the enumeration of waterborne coliform bacteria, *Applied and Environmental Microbiology* 37: 633–641.

53. M.J. Blaser, P. Smith, W.-L. Wang, J. Hoff, 1986, Inactivation of Campylobacter jejuni by chlorine and monochloramine, *Applied and Environmental Microbiology* 51: 307–311.

54. P.V. Scarpino, G. Berg, S.L. Chang, D. Dahling, M. Lucas, 1972, A comparative study of the inactivation of viruses in water by chlorine, *Water Research* 6: 959–965.

55. C. Butterfield, E. Wattie, S. Megregian, C. Chambers, 1943, Influence of pH and temperature on the survival of coliforms and enteric pathogens when exposed to free chlorine, *Public Health Reports (1896–1970)*: 1837–1866.

56. R.W. Bonvillain, R.G. Painter, E.M. Ledet, G. Wang, 2011, Comparisons of resistance of CF and non-CF pathogens to hydrogen peroxide and hypochlorous acid oxidants in vitro, *BMC Microbiology* 11: 112.

57. C.C. Winterbourn, A.J. Kettle, 2013, Redox reactions and microbial killing in the neutrophil phagosome, *Antioxidants & Redox Signaling* 18: 642–660.

58. F. Lanza, 1998, Clinical manifestation of myeloperoxidase deficiency, *Journal of Molecular Medicine* 76: 676–681.

59. N. Dickerhof, V. Isles, P. Pattemore, M.B. Hampton, A.J. Kettle, 2019, Exposure of Pseudomonas aeruginosa to bactericidal hypochlorous acid during neutrophil phagocytosis is compromised in cystic fibrosis, *Journal of Biological Chemistry* 294: 13502–13514.

60. J.N. Green, A.J. Kettle, C.C. Winterbourn, 2014, Protein chlorination in neutrophil phagosomes and correlation with bacterial killing, *Free Radical Biology and Medicine* 77: 49–56.

61. M.B. Grisham, M.M. Jefferson, D. Melton, E. Thomas, 1984, Chlorination of endogenous amines by isolated neutrophils. Ammonia-dependent bactericidal, cytotoxic, and cytolytic activities of the chloramines, *Journal of Biological Chemistry* 259: 10404–10413.

62. M.S. Coker, W.-P. Hu, S.T. Senthilmohan, A.J. Kettle, 2008, Pathways for the decay of organic dichloramines and liberation of antimicrobial chloramine gases, *Chemical Research in Toxicology* 21: 2334–2343.

63. M.S. Coker, L.V. Forbes, M. Plowman-Holmes, et al., 2018, Interactions of staphyloxanthin and enterobactin with myeloperoxidase and reactive chlorine species, *Archives of Biochemistry and Biophysics* 646: 80–89.

64. E.L. Thomas, 1979, Myeloperoxidase, hydrogen peroxide, chloride antimicrobial system: nitrogen-chlorine derivatives of bacterial components in bactericidal action against Escherichia coli, *Infection and Immunity* 23: 522–531.

65. D. Pattison, M. Davies, 2006, Reactions of myeloperoxidase-derived oxidants with biological substrates: gaining chemical insight into human inflammatory diseases, *Current Medicinal Chemistry* 13: 3271–3290.

66. C. Storkey, M.J. Davies, D.I. Pattison, 2014, Reevaluation of the rate constants for the reaction of hypochlorous acid (HOCl) with cysteine, methionine, and peptide derivatives using a new competition kinetic approach, *Free Radical Biology and Medicine* 73: 60–66.

67. J.M. Albrich, C.A. McCarthy, J.K. Hurst, 1981, Biological reactivity of hypochlorous acid: implications for microbicidal mechanisms of leukocyte myeloperoxidase, *Proceedings of the National Academy of Sciences* 78: 210–214.

68. D. Maitra, J. Byun, P.R. Andreana, et al., 2011, Reaction of hemoglobin with HOCl: mechanism of heme destruction and free iron release, *Free Radical Biology and Medicine* 51: 374–386.

69. E.L. Thomas, 1979, Myeloperoxidase-hydrogen peroxide-chloride antimicrobial system: effect of exogenous amines on antibacterial action against Escherichia coli, *Infection and Immunity* 25: 110–116.

70. W.C. Barrette Jr., D.M. Hannum, W.D. Wheeler, J.K. Hurst, 1989, General mechanism for the bacterial toxicity of hypochlorous acid: abolition of ATP production, *Biochemistry* 28: 9172–9178.

71. W. Barrette, J. Albrich, J. Hurst, 1987, Hypochlorous acid-promoted loss of metabolic energy in Escherichia coli, *Infection and Immunity* 55: 2518–2525.

72. J.M. Albrich, J.H. Gilbaugh, K.B. Callahan, J.K. Hurst, 1986, Effects of the putative neutrophil-generated toxin, hypochlorous acid, on membrane permeability and transport systems of *Escherichia coli*, *The Journal of Clinical Investigation* 78: 177–184.

73. S.M. McKenna, K. Davies, 1988, The inhibition of bacterial growth by hypochlorous acid. Possible role in the bactericidal activity of phagocytes, *Biochemical Journal* 254: 685–692.

74. H. Rosen, J. Orman, R.M. Rakita, B.R. Michel, D.R. VanDevanter, 1990, Loss of DNA-membrane interactions and cessation of DNA synthesis in myeloperoxidase-treated Escherichia coli, *Proceedings of the National Academy of Sciences* 87: 10048–10052.

75. L.I. Leichert, F. Gehrke, H.V. Gudiseva, et al., 2008, Quantifying changes in the thiol redox proteome upon oxidative stress in vivo, *Proceedings of the National Academy of Sciences* 105: 8197–8202.

76. K. Xie, C. Bunse, K. Marcus, L.I. Leichert, 2019, Quantifying changes in the bacterial thiol redox proteome during host-pathogen interaction, *Redox Biology* 21: 101087.

77. R.M. Rakita, B.R. Michel, H. Rosen, 1989, Myeloperoxidase-mediated inhibition of microbial respiration: damage to Escherichia coli ubiquinol oxidase, *Biochemistry* 28: 3031–3036.

78. H. Rosen, S. Klebanoff, 1982, Oxidation of Escherichia coli iron centers by the myeloperoxidase-mediated microbicidal system, *Journal of Biological Chemistry* 257: 13731–13735.

79. H. Rosen, S.J. Klebanoff, 1985, Oxidation of microbial iron-sulfur centers by the myeloperoxidase-H_2O_2-halide antimicrobial system, *Infection and Immunity* 47: 613–618.

80. J.K. Hurst, W.C. Barrette Jr., B.R. Michel, H. Rosen, 1991, Hypochlorous acid and myeloperoxidase-catalyzed oxidation of iron-sulfur clusters in bacterial respiratory dehydrogenases, *European Journal of Biochemistry* 202: 1275–1282.

81. S. Dukan, D. Touati, 1996, Hypochlorous acid stress in *Escherichia coli*: resistance, DNA damage, and comparison with hydrogen peroxide stress, *Journal of Bacteriology* 178: 6145–6150.

82. J.P. Henderson, J. Byun, J.W. Heinecke, 1999, Molecular chlorine generated by the myeloperoxidase-hydrogen peroxide-chloride system of phagocytes produces 5-chlorocytosine in bacterial RNA, *Journal of Biological Chemistry* 274: 33440–33448.

83. J. Winter, M. Ilbert, P. Graf, D. Özcelik, U. Jakob, 2008, Bleach activates a redox-regulated chaperone by oxidative protein unfolding, *Cell* 135: 691–701.

84. A. Degrossoli, A. Müller, K. Xie, et al., 2018, Neutrophil-generated HOCl leads to non-specific thiol oxidation in phagocytized bacteria, *Elife* 7: e32288.

85. G. Roos, J. Messens, 2011, Protein sulfenic acid formation: from cellular damage to redox regulation, *Free Radical Biology and Medicine* 51: 314–326.

86. M. Hillion, J. Bernhardt, T. Busche, et al., 2017, Monitoring global protein thiol-oxidation and protein S-mycothiolation in *Mycobacterium smegmatis* under hypochlorite stress, *Scientific Reports* 7: 1–20.

87. M. Imber, N.T.T. Huyen, A.J. Pietrzyk-Brzezinska, et al., 2018, Protein S-bacillithiolation functions in thiol protection and redox regulation of the glyceraldehyde-3-phosphate dehydrogenase Gap in Staphylococcus aureus under hypochlorite stress, *Antioxidants & Redox Signaling* 28: 410–430.

88. N. Linzner, L.V. Vu, V.N. Fritsch, et al., 2019, Staphylococcus aureus uses the bacilliredoxin (BrxAB)/bacillithiol disulfide reductase (YpdA) pathway to defend against oxidative stress under infections, *Frontiers in Microbiology* 10: 1355.

89. R.C. Fahey, 2013, Glutathione analogs in prokaryotes, *Biochimica et Biophysica Acta (BBA)-General Subjects* 1830: 3182–3198.

90. A.P. Fernandes, A. Holmgren, 2004, Glutaredoxins: glutathione-dependent redox enzymes with functions far beyond a simple thioredoxin backup system, *Antioxidants & Redox Signaling* 6: 63–74.

91. A. Gaballa, B.K. Chi, A.A. Roberts, et al., 2014, Redox regulation in *Bacillus subtilis*: the bacilliredoxins BrxA (YphP) and BrxB (YqiW) function in de-bacillithiolation of S-bacillithiolated OhrR and MetE, *Antioxidants & Redox Signaling* 21: 357–367.

92. K. Van Laer, L. Buts, N. Foloppe, et al., 2012, Mycoredoxin-1 is one of the missing links in the oxidative stress defence mechanism of Mycobacteria, *Molecular Microbiology* 86: 787–804.

93. H.A. Parker, N. Dickerhof, L. Forrester, et al. 2021, *Mycobacterium smegmatis* resists the bactericidal activity of hypochlorous acid produced in neutrophil phagosomes, *Journal of Immunology*. 206: 1901–1912.

94. N. Dickerhof, L. Paton, A.J. Kettle, 2020, Oxidation of bacillithiol by myeloperoxidase-derived oxidants, *Free Radical Biology and Medicine* 158: 74–83.

95. D.-C. Pöther, P. Gierok, M. Harms, et al., 2013, Distribution and infection-related functions of bacillithiol in Staphylococcus aureus, *International Journal of Medical Microbiology* 303: 114–123.

96. V.V. Loi, M. Harms, M. Müller, et al., 2017, Real-time imaging of the bacillithiol redox potential in the human pathogen Staphylococcus aureus using a genetically encoded bacilliredoxin-fused redox biosensor, *Antioxidants & Redox Signaling* 26: 835–848.

97. B.K. Chi, A.A. Roberts, T.T.T. Huyen, et al., 2013, S-bacillithiolation protects conserved and essential proteins against hypochlorite stress in firmicutes bacteria, *Antioxidants & Redox Signaling* 18: 1273–1295.

98. C. Johansen, P. Falholt, L. Gram, 1997, Enzymatic removal and disinfection of bacterial biofilms, *Applied and Environmental Microbiology* 63: 3724–3728.

99. J. Oram, B. Reiter, 1966, The inhibition of streptococci by lactoperoxidase, thiocyanate and hydrogen peroxide. The oxidation of thiocyanate and the nature of the inhibitory compound, *Biochemical Journal* 100: 382.

100. E.L. Thomas, T.W. Milligan, R.E. Joyner, M.M. Jefferson, 1994, Antibacterial activity of hydrogen peroxide and the lactoperoxidase-hydrogen peroxide-thiocyanate system against oral streptococci, *Infection and Immunity* 62: 529–535.

101. J. Tenovuo, O. Anttila, M. Lumikari, G. Sievers, 1988, Antibacterial effect of myeloperoxidase against *Streptococcus mutans*, *Oral Microbiology and Immunology* 3: 68–71.

102. J. Carlsson, Y. Iwami, T. Yamada, 1983, Hydrogen peroxide excretion by oral streptococci and effect of lactoperoxidase-thiocyanate-hydrogen peroxide, *Infection and Immunity* 40: 70–80.

103. D. McC. Hogg, G. Jago, 1970, The antibacterial action of lactoperidoxase. The nature of the bacterial inhibitor, *Biochemical Journal* 117: 779–790.

104. M. Lumikari, T. Soukka, S. Nurmio, J. Tenovuo, 1991, Inhibition of the growth of *Streptococcus mutans*, *Streptococcus sobrinus* and *Lactobacillus casei* by oral peroxidase systems in human saliva, *Archives of Oral Biology* 36: 155–160.

105. S. Klebanoff, W. Clem, R. Luebke, 1966, The peroxidase-thiocyanate-hydrogen peroxide antimicrobial system, *Biochimica et Biophysica Acta (BBA)-General Subjects* 117: 63–72.

106. J. Oram, B. Reiter, 1966, The inhibition of streptococci by lactoperoxidase, thiocyanate and hydrogen peroxide. The effect of the inhibitory system on susceptible and resistant strains of group N streptococci, *Biochemical Journal* 100: 373.

107. E.L. Thomas, T.M. Aune, 1978, Lactoperoxidase, peroxide, thiocyanate antimicrobial system: correlation of oxidation with antimicrobial action, *Infection and Immunity* 20: 456–463.

108. L. Björck, C. Rosen, V. Marshall, B. Reiter, 1975, Antibacterial activity of the lactoperoxidase system in milk against pseudomonads and other gram-negative bacteria, *Applied and Environmental Microbiology* 30: 199–204.

109. J.D. Chandler, D.P. Nichols, J.A. Nick, R.J. Hondal, B.J. Day, 2013, Selective metabolism of hypothiocyanous acid by mammalian thioredoxin reductase promotes lung innate immunity and antioxidant defense, *Journal of Biological Chemistry* 288: 18421–18428.

110. B. Reiter, V. Marshall, C. Rosén, 1976, Nonspecific bactericidal activity of the lactoperoxidases-thiocyanate-hydrogen peroxide system of milk against *Escherichia coli* and some gram-negative pathogens, *Infection and Immunity* 13: 800–807.

111. K. Shin, K. Yamauchi, S. Teraguchi, H. Hayasawa, I. Imoto, 2002, Susceptibility of Helicobacter pylori and its urease activity to the peroxidase-hydrogen peroxide-thiocyanate antimicrobial system, *Journal of Medical Microbiology* 51: 231–237.

112. E.L. Thomas, 1981, Lactoperoxidase-catalyzed oxidation of thiocyanate: equilibriums between oxidized forms of thiocyanate, *Biochemistry* 20: 3273–3280.

113. C.B. Hamon, S.J. Klebanoff, 1973, A peroxidase-mediated, Streptococcus mitis-dependent antimicrobial system in saliva, *The Journal of Experimental Medicine* 137: 438–450.

114. B.J. Day, P.E. Bratcher, J.D. Chandler, et al., 2019, The thiocyanate analog selenocyanate is a more potent antimicrobial pro-drug that also is selectively detoxified by the host, *Free Radical Biology and Medicine* 146: 324–332.

115. D. Steinmann, T. Nauser, W.H. Koppenol, 2010, Selenium and sulfur in exchange reactions: a comparative study, *The Journal of Organic Chemistry* 75: 6696–6699.

116. K. Caldwell, A. Tappel, 1964, Reactions of seleno- and sulfoamino acids with hydroperoxides, *Biochemistry* 3: 1643–1647.

117. R. Huber, R. Criddle, 1967, Comparison of the chemical properties of selenocysteine and selenocystine with their sulfur analogs, *Archives of Biochemistry and Biophysics* 122: 164–173.

118. M. Adamson, J. Carlsson, 1982, Lactoperoxidase and thiocyanate protect bacteria from hydrogen peroxide, *Infection and Immunity* 35: 20–24.

119. P. Courtois, M. Pourtois, 1996, Purification of NADH: hypothiocyanite oxidoreductase in Streptococcus sanguis, *Biochemical and Molecular Medicine* 57: 134–138.

120. R. Ihalin, V. Loimaranta, M. Lenander-Lumikari, J. Tenovuo, 1998, The effects of different (pseudo) halide substrates on peroxidase-mediated killing of *Actinobacillus actinomycetemcomitans, Journal of Periodontal Research* 33: 421–427.

121. T. van der Poll, S.M. Opal, 2009, Pathogenesis, treatment, and prevention of pneumococcal pneumonia, *The Lancet* 374: 1543–1556.

122. M. Exner, M. Hermann, R. Hofbauer, et al., 2004, Thiocyanate catalyzes myeloperoxidase-initiated lipid oxidation in LDL, *Free Radical Biology and Medicine* 37: 146–155.

123. R. Zhang, Z. Shen, W.M. Nauseef, S.L. Hazen, 2002, Defects in leukocyte-mediated initiation of lipid peroxidation in plasma as studied in myeloperoxidase-deficient subjects: systematic identification of multiple endogenous diffusible substrates for myeloperoxidase in plasma, *Blood, The Journal of the American Society of Hematology* 99: 1802–1810.

124. G.R. Stark, 1972, [53]. Modification of proteins with cyanate, *Methods in Enzymology*, Elsevier, pp. 579–584.

125. Z. Wang, S.J. Nicholls, E.R. Rodriguez, et al., 2007, Protein carbamylation links inflammation, smoking, uremia and atherogenesis, *Nature Medicine* 13: 1176–1184.

126. M.T. Ashby, A.C. Carlson, M.J. Scott, 2004, Redox buffering of hypochlorous acid by thiocyanate in physiologic fluids, *Journal of the American Chemical Society* 126: 15976–15977.

127. M. Mickelson, 1979, Antibacterial action of lactoperoxidase-thiocyanate-hydrogen peroxide on *Streptococcus agalactiae, Applied and Environmental Microbiology* 38: 821–826.

128. M. Mickelson, 1977, Glucose transport in *Streptococcus agalactiae* and its inhibition by lactoperoxidase-thiocyanate-hydrogen peroxide, *Journal of Bacteriology* 132: 541–548.

129. V. Loimaranta, J. Tenovuo, H. Korhonen, 1998, Combined inhibitory effect of bovine immune whey and peroxidase-generated hypothiocyanite against glucose uptake by *Streptococcus mutans, Oral Microbiology and Immunology* 13: 378–381.

130. B.A. Law, P. John, 1981, Effect of the lactoperoxidase bactericidal system on the formation of the electrochemical proton gradient in E. coli, *FEMS Microbiology Letters* 10: 67–70.

131. V.M. Marshall, B. Reiter, 1980, Comparison of the antibacterial activity of the hypothiocyanite anion towards *Streptococcus lactis* and *Escherichia coli, Microbiology* 120: 513–516.

132. K. Shin, H. Hayasawa, B. Lönnerdal, 2001, Inhibition of Escherichia coli respiratory enzymes by the lactoperoxidase-hydrogen peroxide-thiocyanate antimicrobial system, *Journal of Applied Microbiology* 90: 489–493.

133. N.W. De Jong, K.X. Ramyar, F.E. Guerra, et al., 2017, Immune evasion by a staphylococcal inhibitor of myeloperoxidase, *Proceedings of the National Academy of Sciences* 114: 9439–9444.

134. A. Ulfig, L.I. Leichert, 2020, The effects of neutrophil-generated hypochlorous acid and other hypohalous acids on host and pathogens, *Cellular and Molecular Life Sciences*: 1–30.

135. M.J. Gray, W.-Y. Wholey, U. Jakob, 2013, Bacterial responses to reactive chlorine species, *Annual Review of Microbiology* 67: 141–160.

136. B. Groitl, J.U. Dahl, J.W. Schroeder, U. Jakob, 2017, Pseudomonas aeruginosa defense systems against microbicidal oxidants, *Molecular Microbiology* 106: 335–350.

137. A.J. Potter, C. Trappetti, J.C. Paton, 2012, Streptococcus pneumoniae uses glutathione to defend against oxidative stress and metal ion toxicity, *Journal of Bacteriology* 194: 6248–6254.

138. A.C. Posada, S.L. Kolar, R.G. Dusi, et al., 2014, Importance of bacillithiol in the oxidative stress response of *Staphylococcus aureus, Infection and Immunity* 82: 316–332.

139. I.V. Mikheyeva, J.M. Thomas, S.L. Kolar, et al., 2019, YpdA, a putative bacillithiol disulfide reductase, contributes to cellular redox homeostasis and virulence in Staphylococcus aureus, *Molecular Microbiology* 111: 1039–1056.

140. M. Mickelson, 1966, Effect of lactoperoxidase and thiocyanate on the growth of *Streptococcus pyogenes* and *Streptococcus agalactiae* in a chemically defined culture medium, *Microbiology* 43: 31–43.

CHAPTER ELEVEN

Priming the Innate Immune System to Combat Respiratory Disease

Brian J. Day

National Jewish Health

CONTENTS

ABBREVIATIONS

CF:	Cystic fibrosis
CFTR:	Cystic fibrosis transmembrane conductance regulator protein
COPD:	Chronic obstructive pulmonary disease
DAMP:	Damage-associated molecular pattern
DUOX:	Dual NADPH oxidase
β-ENaC:	Beta-epithelium sodium channel
EPO:	Eosinophil peroxidase
GSA:	Glutathione sulfonamide
GSH:	Glutathione
HIV:	Human immunodeficiency virus
HMGB1:	High-mobility group box 1 protein
HOBr:	Hypobromous acid
HOCl:	Hypochlorous acid
HOI:	Hypoiodous acid
HOSCN:	Hypothiocyanous acid
IκB:	Inhibitory kappa B
IL-4:	Interleukin-4
LPO:	Lactoperoxidase
MAPK:	Mitogen-activated protein kinase
MPO:	Myeloperoxidase
MRP:	Multidrug resistance-associated protein
NF-κB:	Nuclear factor kappa B
NOX:	NADPH oxidase
RAGE:	Receptors for advanced glycation end products
$^-$SCN:	Thiocyanate
Sec:	Selenocysteine
Tg:	Transgenic
TLR:	Toll-like receptor
TrxR:	Thioredoxin reductase

INNATE IMMUNITY OXIDANT GENERATING NETWORK IN THE LUNG

The respiratory system contains two separate arms of the innate immune system's oxidant generating network. One arm resides in the mucosal epithelium, and the other arm resides in

DOI: 10.1201/9781003212287-14

circulating leukocytes. Both systems employ halo-peroxidases, NADPH oxidases (NOXs), halides and pseudohalides to generate broad spectrum hypo-halous acids that are effective biocides to prevent infection [1]. Mammals express a large number of haloperoxidases that include myeloperoxidase (MPO), lactoperoxidase (LPO), eosinophil peroxi-dase (EPO) and peroxidasin [2,3]. NOXs gener-ate superoxide that is dismutated into hydrogen peroxide [4,5]. Hydrogen peroxide activates hal-operoxidases in the presence of halides or pseu-dohalides to generate a broad range of oxidants. Haloperoxidases can employ pseudohalides such as thiocyanate ($^-$SCN) or halides such as chloride, bromide or iodide to generate their respective hypohalous acids, hypothiocyanous (HOSCN), hypochlorous (HOCl), hypobromous (HOBr) and hypoiodous (HOI), respectively [1,6]. Hypohalous acids have antimicrobial activities against a broad range of pathogens including bacteria, fungi and virus [6–10]. Many of these oxidants are thought to kill pathogens by oxidizing essential cellular macromolecules [11,12]. Unfortunately, one of the unintended consequences of oxidant generat-ing network activation is damage to the host dur-ing chronic inflammation (Figure 11.1). Oxidant damage in the lung leads to edema and airway constriction that impairs gas exchange. A large number of respiratory diseases are associated with chronic inflammation and oxidative stress due, in large part, to oxidants generated by the innate immune system [13–15].

The lung mucosal epithelium is armed with a secreted haloperoxidase, LPO [16,17]. LPO is an abundant protein in the lung epithelial lining fluid that bathes the airway surface [16,18]. Lung epithelium also express NADPH dual oxidase (DUOX) that sits on the cell membrane surface and generates superoxide, which is dismutated either spontaneously or enzymatically by super-oxide dismutase to hydrogen peroxide [19–21]. DUOXs are activated to generate hydrogen per-oxide through Toll-like receptor (TLR) engage-ment [22,23]. Epithelial cells secrete LPO that is activated in the presence of hydrogen peroxide to turn the pseudohalide thiocyanate ($^-$SCN) or the halides bromide or iodide into their respec-tive hypohalous acids. This system allows the site-specific generation of hypohalous acids in response to pathogen signals.

A subset of leukocytes known as granulocytes contain vesicles loaded with high levels of halo-peroxidase and NOX [4,5]. These vesicles can fuse with phagolysosomes to supply haloperoxi-dase and hydrogen peroxide for the generation of hypohalous acids [1]. These oxidants aid in kill-ing the encapsulated pathogens [24]. MPO is the predominant haloperoxidase in neutrophils and in some tissue resident macrophages [11]. MPO is the only haloperoxidase that can use chloride as a substrate to generate HOCl [2,25]. However, $^-$SCN is the preferred substrate for MPO with a lower K_m than chloride [26]. It has been calcu-lated that MPO produces equal molar amounts of HOCl and HOSCN at physiological levels of chlo-ride and $^-$SCN [26]. This feature enables $^-$SCN to be used pharmacologically to change the balance of HOCl and HOSCN produced during inflam-mation [27–29]. Eosinophil granules contain high levels of EPO that can use $^-$SCN, iodide or bromide to generate their respective hypoha-lous acids [30,31]. Hypohalous acids have broad

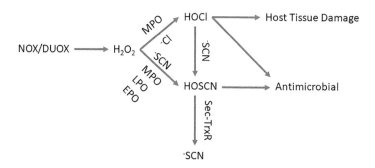

Figure 11.1 Formation of innate immune oxidants by haloperoxidases in the airways. Hydrogen peroxide (H$_2$O$_2$) is gener-ated by neutrophil NADPH oxidase (NOX) or epithelial dual oxidase (DUOX). Haloperoxidases, such as leukocyte myeloper-oxidase (MPO), eosinophil peroxidase (EPO) or epithelial lactoperoxidase (LPO), consume H$_2$O$_2$ and chloride or thiocyanate ($^-$SCN) to generate hypochlorous acid (HOCl) or hypothiocyanous acid (HOSCN). $^-$SCN can also directly react with HOCl to form HOSCN. HOSCN can be detoxified by host selenocysteine (Sec) containing thioredoxin reductase (Sec-TrxR).

antimicrobial activities and defend the body from pathogens. Granulocytes can also secrete this system into the extracellular environment through a process called exocytosis or NETosis [32]. HOCl formation has also been shown to trigger NETosis [33,34]. This process is particularly useful when the pathogen is too large to be phagocytized as is the case for many fungi and helminths [35].

ANTIMICROBIAL ACTIVITY OF THE LUNG'S INNATE IMMUNE OXIDANTS

Common microbes in the environment, under some circumstances, can become pathogens. An excellent example is Pseudomonas aeruginosa that is ubiquitously found in soil and water. This microbe is normally not a pathogen in healthy people, but can become a lethal pathogen in those with a compromised immune system, or those that have the genetic disease cystic fibrosis (CF) [36]. The innate immune system is thought to act as a defense against microbes by utilizing many nonspecific defenses including oxidants to kill trapped microbes. Microbes can be trapped by engulfment in phagolysosomes, mucus or by neutrophil extracellular traps formed during NETosis [37]. Each of these circumstances also contains many of the elements for the generation of hypohalous acids. The source of hydrogen peroxide for hypohalous acid formation during NETosis is still an open question but may be supplied by epithelial DUOX, leukocyte NOX or even the microbes themselves.

Hypohalous acids damage microbial cellular macromolecules by oxidizing functional groups [12]. Some hypohalous acids, such as HOBr, can readily oxidize aromatic rings [38,39], others can readily oxidize amino groups [40], thiol groups [41,42] and unsaturated bonds in fatty acids [43,44]. These disruptive processes can damage cell membrane transporters and adversely affect the microbe's ability to obtain vital nutrients from their environment for growth and replication [45]. Energy generation in microbes occurs close to the cell membrane and can be readily damaged by hypohalous acids [46,47]. Enzymes that are critical for the production of nucleic acids used for energy production and replication are also sensitive to oxidative inactivation [48]. Oxidation of microbe's ribonucleic acid (RNA) and deoxyribonucleic acid (DNA) can disrupt protein synthesis, cell signaling and replication [49].

Microbes have a number of defenses against innate immune oxidants to evade host defense. Microbes have antioxidants and antioxidant enzyme systems that can scavenge innate immune system oxidants. Many of these antioxidants are similar to the host such as glutathione (GSH) [50], but many are unique to the microbe such as bacillthiol [51] and mycothiol [52]. Some of the defenses are used by the microbe for other purposes but can serve to detoxify innate immune oxidants. The generation of polyphosphates is an example that confers resistance to innate immune oxidants [53]. It is interesting to note that many CF-associated pathogens have higher gene expression encoding proteins to adapt to the higher levels of lung oxidative stress [54]. Similarly, the host has also evolved defense systems against innate immune oxidants to limit self-inflicted damage. An example is the incorporation of selenocysteine (Sec) in mammalian thioredoxin reductase (Sec-TrxR) to detoxify HOSCN [55].

INFLAMMATORY CELL SIGNALING BY INNATE IMMUNE SYSTEM OXIDANTS

Hydrogen peroxide is the most studied oxidant in regard to inflammatory cell signaling as a regulator of transcriptional activation [56]. Hydrogen peroxide is a relatively stable oxidant that can readily diffuse across cell membranes [57]. Hydrogen peroxide levels are determined by the rates of formation and consumption by a network of oxidases, antioxidants and antioxidant enzymes [58]. Some oxidant generating enzymes, such as haloperoxidase, can consume hydrogen peroxide at relatively high rate constants that are comparable to those of antioxidant enzymes [59,60]. Hydrogen peroxide can affect the activities of cellular kinases and phosphatases that are critical players in proinflammatory signaling pathways [61,62]. Many cell signaling proteins contain low pK_a cysteine (Cys) residues that are readily oxidized and referred to as redox switches [63]. HOSCN formed from the reaction between hydrogen peroxide, $^-$SCN and a haloperoxidase has similar oxidizing properties to hydrogen peroxide. HOSCN readily and selectively reacts with low pK_a thiol switches but has much faster rates of reaction than hydrogen peroxide [60,64]. The haloperoxidases could effectively facilitate hydrogen peroxide signaling through the generation of more reactive and selective species such as HOSCN.

Hypohalous acids have been reported to activate inflammatory cell signaling pathways. HOSCN has been reported to induce tissue factor and nuclear factor kappa B (NF-κB) expression that play a role in eosinophil-induced thrombosis [65]. HOSCN can increase NF-κB signaling in cultured macrophages resulting in increased inflammatory cytokine expression [66]. HOSCN can also modulate mitogen-activated protein kinase (MAPK) through the inhibition of protein tyrosine phosphatases [67]. HOSCN has been shown to increase the expression of intracellular adhesion molecules and vascular cell adhesion molecules on endothelial cells [68]. Conversely, the innate immune system could use ⁻SCN as a chemical switch to shift oxidant formation away from HOCl to HOSCN as a mechanism to resolve inflammation while maintaining host defense. Proteins oxidized by HOSCN may be easier for the host to repair than those oxidized by HOCl. The anion ⁻SCN passivates through the CF transmembrane conductance regulator protein (CFTR), and its deficit in myeloid cells leads to decreased resolution of bacterial infection and inflammation that are hallmarks of CF lung disease [69].

Oxidation products of cellular macromolecules can also participate in receptor-mediated inflammatory cell signaling. The TLRs and receptors for advanced glycation end products (RAGE) recognize oxidized cellular macromolecules also known as damage-associated molecular patterns (DAMPs) [70]. A well-studied DAMP is the high-mobility group box 1 protein (HMGB1) [71]. HMGB1 is a thiol-containing redox-sensitive protein that normally resides in the cell nucleus [72]. Oxidation of thiols in HMGB1 is thought to regulate its release from the cell nucleus and binding to its receptors [73,74]. Released HMGB1 can engage TLRs and RAGE receptors to mediate cell signaling pathways in response to infection and inflammation [75,76]. Excessive signaling of these types of inflammatory pathways is a common mechanism that drives lung disease.

Oxidants can also trigger excessive inflammation by disrupting negative regulators of the NF-κB system [77]. NF-κB is held in the cytoplasm as an inactive complex by inhibitory kappa B (IκB) and oxidants can modify IκB to release NF-κB to traffic to the nucleus and turn on pro-inflammatory genes [78]. Recent reports suggest that HOSCN may also inhibit mitochondrial respiration in macrophages [79] and may be involved

in the Warburg effect seen in macrophages during infection [80]. HOSCN is a more moderate oxidant than HOCl. Again, the severity and degree of oxidation and the ability of the host to repair or reverse thiol oxidation may act as a gating mechanism for the degree of inflammatory response. Disruption of negative regulation on pro-inflammatory signaling pathways and a loss of inflammation resolution are important features of chronic inflammation associated with many pulmonary diseases.

HARNESSING ENDOGENOUS INNATE IMMUNITY PATHWAYS TO DIMINISH INFLAMMATION IN RESPIRATORY DISEASES

The lung is an organ that has evolved to adapt to continuous exposure to ambient air containing a vast array of pathogens and particulate matter. Pathogens and particulate matter can activate the innate immune system and signal the recruitment and activation of leukocytes that mediate edema and injury. The lung's primary function of gas exchange requires that the alveolar septa maintains close proximity to the blood capillaries for efficient gas exchange. Inflammation disrupts the close proximity of the alveolar septa with the blood capillaries by stimulation of edema. The lung has developed a number of defenses to limit edema and injury responses that are detrimental to lung function.

There are numerous ways oxidants can promote inflammation and disrupt resolution. Endogenous generation of hypohalous acids plays important roles in host defense but not much focus has been given to which of these oxidants drive inflammation and whether some are involved in resolution. There are concerns that developing therapeutics that may increase the production of these oxidants may lead to excessive tissue injury and damage [81]. A key question is whether one can boost endogenous production of hypohalous acids in vivo to achieve beneficial effects on host defense without paradoxically exacerbating lung inflammation and damage.

THIOCYANATE AS AN ANTIOXIDANT AND CLOAKED OXIDANT

⁻SCN is a low-molecular-weight anion ubiquitously found in all extracellular fluids that interface with the external environment [82]. ⁻SCN has paradoxical roles as both an antioxidant and a cloaked oxidant as its redox couple, HOSCN. ⁻SCN originates from the diet as an intact molecule or through sulfur transferase metabolism of cyanide from the breakdown of dietary glucosides and glucosinolate-containing plants [83]. It is interesting that vegans have higher plasma levels of ⁻SCN than the general population [84]. ⁻SCN is secreted and concentrated in extracellular fluids through anion channels, including the CFTR anion channel that is dysfunctional in the genetic disease CF [85]. CF patients have 21% lower levels of ⁻SCN in their saliva compared with controls [86]. CFTR knockout mice have 75% lower levels of ⁻SCN in their bronchoalveolar lavage fluid compared with wild-type mice [87].

⁻SCN is the preferred substrate for all haloperoxidases [2]. This feature allows ⁻SCN to compete with chloride, bromide and iodide as substrates for all haloperoxidases. Another unique property of ⁻SCN is its ability to directly react at high rate constants with all hypohalous acids and secondary by-products to form HOSCN nonenzymatically [27]. These properties allow ⁻SCN to act like a funnel and direct a diverse group of oxidants to HOSCN. HOSCN can then be detoxified by the host Sec-containing TrxR to ⁻SCN and water [55]. Selenium plays two important processes in selenocysteine compared with sulfur in Cys. Selenocysteine has faster rate of reaction with HOSCN than Cys [88]. Secondly, selenocysteine is less likely to form irreversible higher oxidation states than Cys [89]. On the other hand, pathogen TrxR, which lacks selenocysteine due to evolutionary divergence [90], is actually inhibited by HOSCN [55] (Figure 11.2).

The unique properties of ⁻SCN including its ability to directly react with other hypohalous acids, being a preferred substrate by all haloperoxidases, and its oxidation product being a substrate for host Sec-TrxR, allow ⁻SCN to protect the lung from oxidants of the innate immune system [29,55]. Regulation of ⁻SCN levels can act as a master switch of the haloperoxidase system by titrating the ratio of HOSCN/hypohalous acids formed during infection and inflammation [29]. As concentrations of ⁻SCN rise in the extracellular fluids, the levels of hypohalous acids drop and may be one way the immune system switches from a host damaging response to a less damaging response and resolution without the loss of pathogen suppression (Figure 11.3). It could be speculated that the body evolved this system as a mechanism to resolve inflammation, a process defective in many human diseases.

THERAPEUTIC APPLICATIONS FOR THE ⁻SCN/HOSCN REDOX COUPLE

Although endogenous generation of hypohalous acids plays important roles in host defense, too often they are lumped together as a group when they may have very different roles during inflammation and infection. A key question is whether one can boost the endogenous

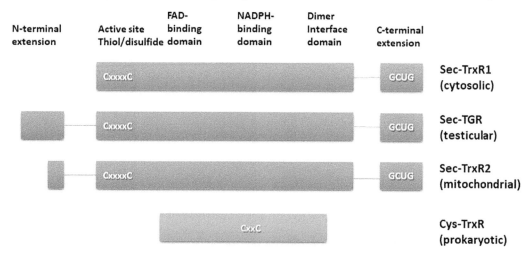

Figure 11.2 Evolutionary diversity of thioredoxin reductases (TrxR) among mammalian isoforms (Sec-TrxR1, Sec-TrxR2 and thioredoxin-glutathione reductase (TGR)) and Cys-TrxR prokaryotic form. Notice the lack of C-terminal selenocysteine motif (GCUG) and different location of the active site thiol/disulfide catalytic centers between mammalian Sec-TrxRs and the prokaryotic Cys-TrxR.

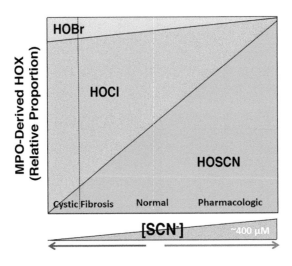

Figure 11.3 Thiocyanate (⁻SCN) can act as a switch to drive innate immune oxidant formation toward hypothiocyanous acid (HOSCN) during inflammation. As the concentration of ⁻SCN rises in the extracellular fluid, a greater proportion of oxidant becomes HOSCN. Under normal concentrations of halides and ⁻SCN, the oxidant output is around equal parts of hypochlorous acid (HOCl) and HOSCN. Modeling estimates that when the ⁻SCN concentration reaches 400 μM, the oxidant output from MPO is mostly HOSCN. As the concentrations of ⁻SCN decrease, there is a shift in the proportion of oxidant formed to the more damaging HOCl.

production of hypohalous acids to achieve beneficial effects on host defense without paradoxically exacerbating tissue inflammation and damage [14,81]. There is some controversy in the field with a number of studies showing adverse effects of HOSCN when applied directly to cells and tissues [79,81,91,92]. HOSCN can efficiently oxidize cellular macromolecules when it overwhelms endogenous antioxidant defenses [41–43]. It is important to note whether ⁻SCN or its oxidant HOSCN is used in these studies and the concentration of HOSCN used to produce the adverse effects. ⁻SCN is actually considered relatively nontoxic with an oral LD_{50} in rats of 764 mg/kg [93]. Most studies that treat with ⁻SCN do not show these adverse effects and paradoxically protect against inflammation and damage [28,29,55,94]. One can view ⁻SCN as a prodrug that activates only at sites of inflammation where it is a substrate of haloperoxidases or reacts directly with hypohalous acids generating HOSCN that can be readily metabolized by the host (Figure 11.4).

The use of ⁻SCN as an antioxidant and a cloaked oxidant may be key to overcoming this dilemma. ⁻SCN can limit inflammation and oxidative damage while preserving host defense and cell signaling processes needed to target pathogens and begin resolving inflammation. ⁻SCN has been given to humans long ago as an antihypertension agent, but fell out of use in the mid-20th century upon the development of better and more potent antihypertensive agents [95]. Some of the literature from ⁻SCN uses as an oral antihypertension agent reported large plasma levels of 1–2 mM, which had only a modest effect on lowering blood pressure [96,97]. Toxicology on ⁻SCN used during this period suggested that most patients tolerated plasma ⁻SCN concentrations that were ten-fold higher than endogenous levels. The plasma levels of ⁻SCN used to treat hypertension were twofold more than the ⁻SCN concentration needed to saturate the oxidative output of haloperoxidases. Potassium and sodium salts of ⁻SCN have high oral bioavailability [98] and are effectively absorbed into the blood after inhalation [28,29].

ANTIMICROBIAL ACTIVITIES OF THE ⁻SCN/HOSCN REDOX COUPLE

The ⁻SCN/HOSCN redox couple is a major component of innate immune response to pathogens [99]. Bacteria are more sensitive to the cytotoxic effects of the ⁻SCN/HOSCN redox couple than mammalian cells [55]. This is not true for the chloride/HOCl redox couple where equal fluxes produced damage to both bacteria and

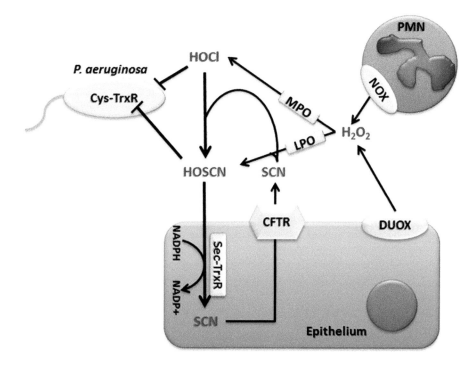

Figure 11.4 Selective detoxification of hypothiocyanous acid (HOSCN) by lung epithelium. Both MPO and LPO can generate HOSCN from H_2O_2 released by neutrophil (PMN) NADPH oxidase (NOX) or epithelial dual oxidase (DUOX). Hypochlorous acid (HOCl) generated from MPO can also be directly converted to HOSCN by reaction with SCN. HOSCN can be readily detoxified and recycled back to $^-$SCN by mammalian epithelial and PMN thioredoxin reductase (Sec-TrxR) but not by prokaryotic Cys-TrxR found in P. *aeruginosa* (PA). Recycled $^-$SCN is transported back through anion channels such as CFTR into the airway fluid.

mammalian cells [55]. HOSCN has been reported to be 10–500-fold more potent than hydrogen peroxide in inhibiting the growth and metabolism of oral streptococci [99–101]. HOSCN has also been shown to be an effective antimicrobial agent against a broad range of Gram-negative and Gram-positive bacteria [102,103]. Some of the reported targets for the antimicrobial action of HOSCN include glycolytic enzymes such as hexokinase, glucose-6-phosphate dehydrogenase and aldolase [99]. HOSCN can target bacterial membrane-bound transport proteins and interferes with nutrient uptake and induces cellular leakage of glucose, amino acids and potassium [102,104]. HOSCN inhibits Helicobacter pylori viability and urease activity required to alkalinize gastric juice for stomach colonization [105]. Bacterial Cys-TrxR is a newly identified target of HOSCN inhibition, which in stark contrast to its counterpart mammalian Sec-TrxR, actually metabolizes HOSCN [55]. The thioredoxin/TrxR system transfers electrons to ribonucleotide reductases that are essential for DNA synthesis and repair and their inhibition

may lead to bacterial growth arrest [106]. HOSCN is very reactive toward low pK_a thiols found in a number of enzymes involved in DNA synthesis including bacterial thioredoxin, thioredoxin reductase, glutaredoxin and ribonucleotide reductase that convert RNA to DNA (Figure 11.5).

In addition to bacteria, HOSCN has been shown to inhibit the growth of fungi, viruses and parasites. HOSCN has been reported to inhibit the viability of Candida albicans [9,107]. HOSCN antiviral activities have been published for a wide range of human viral pathogens including influenza [108]. In this study, HOSCN was found to decrease viral plaque formation in MDCK cells with an IC_{50} that ranged from 57 to 148 μM. Another study tested HOSCN against 12 different influenza A and B strains in vitro and demonstrated viral inactivation [10]. HOSCN has also been shown to suppress poly I:C-induced viral responses by modulating interferon regulatory factor 3 phosphorylation in human airway epithelial cells [109]. Similarly, HOSCN has antiviral activity against respiratory syncytial virus, Herpes, echovirus and

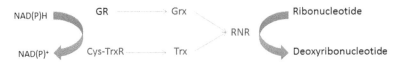

RNR contributes to DNA synthesis in bacteria.
Red: contains thioredoxin fold (CxxC) active sequence

Figure 11.5 Ribonucleotide reductase (RNR) requires either reduced glutaredoxin (Grx) or thioredoxin (Trx) as cofactors for deoxyribonucleotide synthesis. Both Grx and Trx have thioredoxin folds that contain low pK_a thiols that may be sensitive to HOSCN inactivation as has been shown with Cys-TrxR.

human immunodeficiency virus (HIV) [110,111]. HOSCN's ability to inhibit HIV replication also occurred without any cytopathic effects on reporter host cells [112]. This is consistent with the hypothesis of ⁻SCN redirecting oxidants to those that are well tolerated by the host. HOSCN has similar potency in killing parasitic schistosomula as HOBr and HOCl [113].

ANTI-INFLAMMATORY AND ANTIMICROBIOCIDAL ACTIVITIES OF ⁻SCN/HOSCN REDOX COUPLE IN CYSTIC FIBROSIS LUNG DISEASE

CF is a genetic disease caused by mutations in the gene that encodes the CFTR protein [114]. The CFTR protein is an anion transporter responsible for maintaining hydration of secreted mucus into the airway lining fluid [115–117]. However, since the initial discovery of a deficit in chloride transport, a number of other functions for CFTR have been described. The gene that encodes for CFTR is actually most closely associated with the multidrug resistance-associated protein (ABCC gene family) rather than classical chloride transporters [118]. Many of the transporters in the ABCC gene family can also transport an important endogenous antioxidant, GSH [119]. Early studies found decreased levels of GSH in the airway fluids of CF subjects [120]. Later, a number of groups demonstrated the ability of CFTR to also transport GSH apically into the airway lining fluid [87,121–125]. Impaired transport of important anions that regulate airway fluid mucus viscosity [126], pH [127,128] and host defense [85] through the CFTR protein are important contributors to CF lung disease.

The major rationale for the use of ⁻SCN in lung disease came from studies of CF cell culture and animal models. Although it was well known that ⁻SCN was an anion that could be transported through CFTR [129], the connection between ⁻SCN and CF was first noted when Fragoso et al. reported that apical transport of ⁻SCN was blocked in primary airway epithelial cells by CFTR inhibitors and stimulated by cAMP and forskolin [130]. Moskwa et al. later showed that airway epithelial cells containing a ΔF508 mutation were less efficient at exporting ⁻SCN and could be restored by transfection with functional CFTR [131]. Further research went on to show that this CFTR-mediated ⁻SCN efflux to be important in bacterial killing [85,131]. Deficiencies of ⁻SCN in extracellular fluids has also been reported in CF subjects and mutant CFTR model systems [86,87]. However, this may not always be the case, due to the fact that ⁻SCN is not solely dependent upon CFTR for transport [13,132]. A number of apical channels can also transport ⁻SCN, including pendrin [133] and the calcium chloride channel protein [134]. It is interesting to note that infection status and respiratory symptoms may work in tandem to upregulate ⁻SCN efflux in the lung. Pedemonte et al. reported that cytokines like interleukin 4 (IL-4) can stimulate cells to upregulate the expression of pendrin and ⁻SCN efflux [133]. Similarly, others have shown a wide range of cytokines (IL-4, interleukin-13 and interferon-gamma) associated with allergic responses and infection to regulate pendrin expression [135].

The efficacy of inhaled ⁻SCN in animal models of bacterial lung infection has been reported [28,29]. In these studies, the nebulization of an isotonic 0.5% NaSCN solution twice daily 1 day after *Pseudomonas aeruginosa* lung infection improved bacterial lung clearance, decreased neutrophil influx, decreased cytokine production and decreased markers of oxidative stress [28,29]. One of these studies used the beta-epithelial sodium channel (β-ENaC) transgenic (Tg) mouse model that is associated with chronic lung inflammation and mucus obstruction [136]. Nebulization of ⁻SCN in the β-ENaC Tg mouse resulted in anti-inflammatory effects even in the uninfected mice, and these actions were greatly enhanced in the infected mice [29]. This study also demonstrated the ability of exogenously delivered ⁻SCN to change the ratio of HOCl/HOSCN produced in an infected lung. HOCl reacts with GSH producing a selective biomarker, glutathione sulfonamide (GSA) [137]. GSA has been detected in airway lining fluid from CF subjects [138] and infected mice [29]. Infected β-ENaC Tg mice treated with ⁻SCN had lower levels of GSA in their airway lining fluids [29].

Other lung diseases may also be prime candidates for the development of ⁻SCN as a potential therapeutic. Many chronic pulmonary diseases including chronic obstructive pulmonary disease (COPD), asthma and acute respiratory distress syndrome are exacerbated by infections and may benefit from ⁻SCN therapy. Recently it has been reported that COPD subjects have decreased levels of CFTR expression in their lungs and are at increased risk of infections [139]. Current therapeutics target either inflammation or pathogen survival. Maintaining the positive host defense features of inflammation while limiting oxidative injury may provide ⁻SCN a novel therapeutic niche.

CONCLUSION

The bivalent mechanism of ⁻SCN gives more flexible utility on preserving host defense while limiting host damage and inflammation. The ⁻SCN/HOSCN redox couple can act as an antioxidant with the ability to promote host defense. The host ability to readily metabolize HOSCN with Sec-TrxR prevents further amplification of host damage and inflammation and may play a role in resolving inflammation. The ability of ⁻SCN levels to funnel hypohalous acid formation to HOSCN that can be metabolized by host Sec-TrxR and recycled creates a unique self-contained system (Figure 11.6). This system can be leveraged as a pharmacological approach to treat chronic lung diseases associated with infectious exacerbation as seen in CF and COPD where ⁻SCN transport may be impaired.

REFERENCES

1. W.M. Nauseef, 2007, How human neutrophils kill and degrade microbes: an integrated view, *Immunol. Rev.* 219: 88–102.
2. P.G. Furtmuller, M. Zederbauer, W. Jantschko, et al., 2006, Active site structure and catalytic mechanisms of human peroxidases, *Arch. Biochem. Biophys.* 445: 199–213.
3. H. Li, Z. Cao, G. Zhang, V.J. Thannickal, G. Cheng, 2012, Vascular peroxidase 1 catalyzes the formation of hypohalous acids: characterization of its substrate specificity and enzymatic properties, *Free Radic. Biol. Med.* 53: 1954–1959.
4. P. Patriarca, R. Cramer, M. Marussi, F. Rossi, D. Romeo, 1971, Mode of activation of granule-bound NADPH oxidase in leucocytes during phagocytosis, *Biochim. Biophys. Acta* 237: 335–338.
5. M. Hoffman, A.P. Autor, 1980, Production of superoxide anion by an NADPH-oxidase from rat pulmonary macrophages, *FEBS Lett.* 121: 352–354.
6. S.J. Klebanoff, W.H. Clem, R.G. Luebke, 1966, The peroxidase-thiocyanate-hydrogen peroxide antimicrobial system, *Biochim. Biophys. Acta* 117: 63–72.

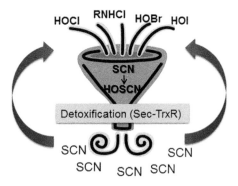

Figure 11.6 Thiocyanate (⁻SCN) can act as a funnel to convert a number of innate immune oxidants to hypothiocyanous acid (HOSCN). This can be metabolized by host selenocysteine (Sec)-containing thioredoxin reductase (Sec-TrxR). ⁻SCN can directly react with a diverse array of innate immune system oxidants including hypochlorous acid (HOCl), hypobromous acid (HOBr), hypoiodous acid (HOI) and secondary oxidants such as chloramines (RNHCl) forming HOSCN. The HOSCN formed is converted back to ⁻SCN and water and recycled back to the airway lining fluid.

7. J. Tenovuo, K.K. Makinen, G. Sievers, 1985, Antibacterial effect of lactoperoxidase and myeloperoxidase against Bacillus cereus, *Antimicrob. Agents Chemother.* 27: 96–101.

8. P. Courtois, P. Majerus, M. Labbe, et al., 1992, Susceptibility of anaerobic microorganisms to hypothiocyanite produced by lactoperoxidase, *Acta Stomatol. Belg.* 89: 155–162.

9. P.M. Majerus, P.A. Courtois, 1992, Susceptibility of *Candida albicans* to peroxidase-catalyzed oxidation products of thiocyanate, iodide and bromide, *J. Biol. Buccale* 20: 241–245.

10. U. Patel, A. Gingerich, L. Widman, et al., 2018, Susceptibility of influenza viruses to hypothiocyanite and hypoiodite produced by lactoperoxidase in a cell-free system, *PLoS One* 13: e0199167.

11. C.C. Winterbourn, A.J. Kettle, 2013, Redox reactions and microbial killing in the neutrophil phagosome, *Antioxid. Redox Signal.* 18: 642–660.

12. M.J. Davies, 2011, Myeloperoxidase-derived oxidation: mechanisms of biological damage and its prevention, *J. Clin. Biochem. Nutr.* 48: 8–19.

13. E. Thomson, S. Brennan, R. Senthilmohan, et al., 2010, Identifying peroxidases and their oxidants in the early pathology of cystic fibrosis, *Free Radic. Biol. Med.* 49: 1354–1360.

14. J.D. Chandler, B.J. Day, 2012, Thiocyanate: a potentially useful therapeutic agent with host defense and antioxidant properties, *Biochem. Pharmacol.* 84: 1381–1387.

15. B.S. Rayner, Y. Zhang, B.E. Brown, et al., 2018, Role of hypochlorous acid (HOCl) and other inflammatory mediators in the induction of macrophage extracellular trap formation, *Free Radic. Biol. Med.* 129: 25–34.

16. M. Salathe, M. Holderby, R. Forteza, et al., 1997, Isolation and characterization of a peroxidase from the airway, *Am. J. Respir. Cell Mol. Biol.* 17: 97–105.

17. C. Wijkstrom-Frei, S. El-Chemaly, R. Ali-Rachedi, et al., 2003, Lactoperoxidase and human airway host defense, *Am. J. Respir. Cell Mol. Biol.* 29: 206–212.

18. S. El-Chemaly, M. Salathe, S. Baier, G.E. Conner, R. Forteza, 2003, Hydrogen peroxide-scavenging properties of normal human airway secretions, *Am. J. Respir. Crit. Care Med.* 167: 425–430.

19. M. Geiszt, J. Witta, J. Baffi, K. Lekstrom, T.L. Leto, 2003, Dual oxidases represent novel hydrogen peroxide sources supporting mucosal surface host defense, *FASEB J.* 17: 1502–1504.

20. H. Fischer, 2009, Mechanisms and function of DUOX in epithelia of the lung, *Antioxid. Redox Signal.* 11: 2453–2465.

21. A. van der Vliet, 2008, NADPH oxidases in lung biology and pathology: host defense enzymes, and more, *Free Radic. Biol. Med.* 44: 938–955.

22. Y. Wu, J. Lu, S. Antony, et al., 2013, Activation of TLR4 is required for the synergistic induction of dual oxidase 2 and dual oxidase A2 by IFN-gamma and lipopolysaccharide in human pancreatic cancer cell lines, *J. Immunol.* 190: 1859–1872.

23. Y. Huang, Y. Yu, S. Zhan, et al., 2020, Dual oxidase Duox and Toll-like receptor 3 TLR3 in the Toll pathway suppress zoonotic pathogens through regulating the intestinal bacterial community homeostasis in Hermetia illucens L, *PLoS One* 15: e0225873.

24. S.J. Klebanoff, 1968, Myeloperoxidase-halide-hydrogen peroxide antibacterial system, *J. Bacteriol.* 95: 2131–2138.

25. J.E. Harrison, J. Schultz, 1976, Studies on the chlorinating activity of myeloperoxidase, *J. Biol. Chem.* 251: 1371–1374.

26. C.J. van Dalen, M.W. Whitehouse, C.C. Winterbourn, A.J. Kettle, 1997, Thiocyanate and chloride as competing substrates for myeloperoxidase, *Biochem. J.* 327: 487–492.

27. M.T. Ashby, A.C. Carlson, M.J. Scott, 2004, Redox buffering of hypochlorous acid by thiocyanate in physiologic fluids, *J. Am. Chem. Soc.* 126: 15976–15977.

28. J.D. Chandler, E. Min, J. Huang, D.P. Nichols, B.J. Day, 2013, Nebulized thiocyanate improves lung infection outcomes in mice, *Br. J. Pharmacol.* 169: 1166–1177.

29. J.D. Chandler, E. Min, J. Huang, et al., 2015, Antiinflammatory and antimicrobial effects of thiocyanate in a cystic fibrosis mouse model, *Am. J. Respir. Cell Mol. Biol.* 53: 193–205.

30. G.T. Archer, 1962, Release of peroxidase from eosinophil granules in vitro, *Nature* 194: 973–974.

31. J. Wang, A. Slungaard, 2006, Role of eosinophil peroxidase in host defense and disease pathology, *Arch. Biochem. Biophys.* 445: 256–260.

32. N.G. Almyroudis, M.J. Grimm, B.A. Davidson, et al., 2013, NETosis and NADPH oxidase: at the intersection of host defense, inflammation, and injury, *Front. Immunol.* 4: 45.

33. Y. Zhang, B.S. Rayner, M. Jensen, C.L. Hawkins, 2019, In vitro stimulation and visualization

of extracellular trap release in differentiated human monocyte-derived macrophages, J. Vis. Exp. 153: e60541.

34. K. Akong-Moore, O.A. Chow, M. von Kockritz-Blickwede, V. Nizet, 2012, Influences of chloride and hypochlorite on neutrophil extracellular trap formation, PLoS One 7: e42984.

35. C. Diaz-Godinez, J.C. Carrero, 2019, The state of art of neutrophil extracellular traps in protozoan and helminthic infections, Biosci. Rep. 39: BSR20180916.

36. C. Winstanley, S. O'Brien, M.A. Brockhurst, 2016, Pseudomonas aeruginosa evolutionary adaptation and diversification in cystic fibrosis chronic lung infections, Trends Microbiol. 24: 327–337.

37. B.G. Yipp, B. Petri, D. Salina, et al., 2012, Infection-induced NETosis is a dynamic process involving neutrophil multitasking in vivo, Nat. Med. 18: 1386–1393.

38. C.L. Hawkins, D.I. Pattison, N.R. Stanley, M.J. Davies, 2008, Tryptophan residues are targets in hypothiocyanous acid-mediated protein oxidation, Biochem. J. 416: 441–452.

39. A.J. Szuchman-Sapir, D.I. Pattison, N.A. Ellis, et al., 2008, Hypochlorous acid oxidizes methionine and tryptophan residues in myoglobin, Free Radic. Biol. Med. 45: 789–798.

40. C.L. Hawkins, D.I. Pattison, M.J. Davies, 2003, Hypochlorite-induced oxidation of amino acids, peptides and proteins, Amino Acids 25: 259–274.

41. T.J. Barrett, D.I. Pattison, S.E. Leonard, et al., 2012, Inactivation of thiol-dependent enzymes by hypothiocyanous acid: role of sulfenyl thiocyanate and sulfenic acid intermediates, Free Radic. Biol. Med. 52: 1075–1085.

42. M.T. Ashby, H. Aneetha, 2004, Reactive sulfur species: aqueous chemistry of sulfenyl thiocyanates, J. Am. Chem. Soc. 126: 10216–10217.

43. J. Arnhold, O.M. Panasenko, J. Schiller, A. Vladimirov Yu, K. Arnold, 1995, The action of hypochlorous acid on phosphatidylcholine liposomes in dependence on the content of double bonds. Stoichiometry and NMR analysis, Chem. Phys. Lipids 78: 55–64.

44. S.M. McKenna, K.J. Davies, 1988, The inhibition of bacterial growth by hypochlorous acid. Possible role in the bactericidal activity of phagocytes, Biochem. J. 254: 685–692.

45. J.M. Albrich, J.H. Gilbaugh, 3rd, K.B. Callahan, J.K. Hurst, 1986, Effects of the putative neutrophil-generated toxin, hypochlorous acid,

on membrane permeability and transport systems of Escherichia coli, J. Clin. Invest. 78: 177–184.

46. H. Rosen, S.J. Klebanoff, 1982, Oxidation of Escherichia coli iron centers by the myeloperoxidase-mediated microbicidal system, J. Biol. Chem. 257: 13731–13735.

47. H. Rosen, S.J. Klebanoff, 1985, Oxidation of microbial iron-sulfur centers by the myeloperoxidase-H_2O_2-halide antimicrobial system, Infect. Immun. 47: 613–618.

48. H. Rosen, J. Orman, R.M. Rakita, B.R. Michel, D.R. VanDevanter, 1990, Loss of DNA-membrane interactions and cessation of DNA synthesis in myeloperoxidase-treated Escherichia coli, Proc. Natl. Acad. Sci. U.S.A. 87: 10048–10052.

49. J.P. Henderson, J. Byun, J.W. Heinecke, 1999, Chlorination of nucleobases, RNA and DNA by myeloperoxidase: a pathway for cytotoxicity and mutagenesis by activated phagocytes, Redox Rep. 4: 319–320.

50. J.A. Chesney, J.W. Eaton, J.R. Mahoney, Jr., 1996, Bacterial glutathione: a sacrificial defense against chlorine compounds, J. Bacteriol. 178: 2131–2135.

51. V.R. Perera, G.L. Newton, K. Pogliano, 2015, Bacillithiol: a key protective thiol in Staphylococcus aureus, Expert Rev. Anti. Infect. Ther. 13: 1089–1107.

52. A.M. Reyes, B. Pedre, M.I. De Armas, et al., 2018, Chemistry and redox biology of mycothiol, Antioxid. Redox Signal. 28: 487–504.

53. M.J. Gray, U. Jakob, 2015, Oxidative stress protection by polyphosphate--new roles for an old player, Curr. Opin. Microbiol. 24: 1–6.

54. X. Shi, Z. Gao, Q. Lin, et al., 2019, Meta-analysis reveals potentialiInfluence of oxidative stress on the airway microbiomes of cystic fibrosis patients, Genomics Proteomics Bioinformatics 17: 590–602.

55. J.D. Chandler, D.P. Nichols, J.A. Nick, R.J. Hondal, B.J. Day, 2013, Selective metabolism of hypothiocyanous acid by mammalian thioredoxin reductase promotes lung innate immunity and antioxidant defense, J. Biol. Chem. 288: 18421–18428.

56. H.S. Marinho, C. Real, L. Cyrne, H. Soares, F. Antunes, 2014, Hydrogen peroxide sensing, signaling and regulation of transcription factors, Redox Biol. 2: 535–562.

57. F. Antunes, E. Cadenas, 2000, Estimation of H_2O_2 gradients across biomembranes, FEBS Lett. 475: 121–126.

58. H.J. Forman, M. Torres, 2002, Reactive oxygen species and cell signaling: respiratory burst in

macrophage signaling, *Am. J. Respir. Crit. Care Med.* 166: S4–8.

59. W. Jantschko, P.G. Furtmuller, M. Zederbauer, et al., 2005, Reaction of ferrous lactoperoxidase with hydrogen peroxide and dioxygen: an anaerobic stopped-flow study, *Arch. Biochem. Biophys.* 434: 51–59.

60. F. Antunes, P.M. Brito, 2017, Quantitative biology of hydrogen peroxide signaling, *Redox Biol.* 13: 1–7.

61. Y.S. Bae, S.W. Kang, M.S. Seo, et al., 1997, Epidermal growth factor (EGF)-induced generation of hydrogen peroxide. Role in EGF receptor-mediated tyrosine phosphorylation, *J. Biol. Chem.* 272: 217–221.

62. T.C. Meng, T. Fukada, N.K. Tonks, 2002, Reversible oxidation and inactivation of protein tyrosine phosphatases in vivo, *Mol. Cell* 9: 387–399.

63. D.P. Jones, H. Sies, 2015, The redox code, *Antioxid. Redox Signal* 23: 734–746.

64. O. Skaff, D.I. Pattison, M.J. Davies, 2009, Hypothiocyanous acid reactivity with low-molecular-mass and protein thiols: absolute rate constants and assessment of biological relevance, *Biochem. J.* 422: 111–117.

65. J.G. Wang, S.A. Mahmud, J.A. Thompson, et al., 2006, The principal eosinophil peroxidase product, HOSCN, is a uniquely potent phagocyte oxidant inducer of endothelial cell tissue factor activity: a potential mechanism for thrombosis in eosinophilic inflammatory states, *Blood* 107: 558–565.

66. G.J. Pan, B.S. Rayner, Y. Zhang, D.M. van Reyk, C.L. Hawkins, 2018, A pivotal role for NF-kappaB in the macrophage inflammatory response to the myeloperoxidase oxidant hypothiocyanous acid, *Arch. Biochem. Biophys.* 642: 23–30.

67. A.E. Lane, J.T. Tan, C.L. Hawkins, A.K. Heather, M.J. Davies, 2010, The myeloperoxidase-derived oxidant HOSCN inhibits protein tyrosine phosphatases and modulates cell signalling via the mitogen-activated protein kinase (MAPK) pathway in macrophages, *Biochem. J.* 430: 161–169.

68. J.G. Wang, S.A. Mahmud, J. Nguyen, A. Slungaard, 2006, Thiocyanate-dependent induction of endothelial cell adhesion molecule expression by phagocyte peroxidases: a novel HOSCN-specific oxidant mechanism to amplify inflammation, *J. Immunol.* 177: 8714–8722.

69. T.L. Bonfield, C.A. Hodges, C.U. Cotton, M.L. Drumm, 2012, Absence of the cystic fibrosis transmembrane regulator (CFTR) from myeloid-derived cells slows resolution of inflammation and infection, *J. Leukoc. Biol.* 92: 1111–1122.

70. M.E. Bianchi, 2007, DAMPs, PAMPs and alarmins: all we need to know about danger, *J. Leukoc. Biol.* 81: 1–5.

71. J.R. Klune, R. Dhupar, J. Cardinal, T.R. Billiar, A. Tsung, 2008, HMGB1: endogenous danger signaling, *Mol. Med.* 14: 476–484.

72. U. Andersson, H. Erlandsson-Harris, H. Yang, K.J. Tracey, 2002, HMGB1 as a DNA-binding cytokine, *J. Leukoc. Biol.* 72: 1084–1091.

73. E. Venereau, M. Casalgrandi, M. Schiraldi, et al., 2012, Mutually exclusive redox forms of HMGB1 promote cell recruitment or proinflammatory cytokine release, *J. Exp. Med.* 209: 1519–1528.

74. H. Yang, P. Lundback, L. Ottosson, et al., 2012, Redox modification of cysteine residues regulates the cytokine activity of high mobility group box-1 (HMGB1), *Mol. Med.* 18: 250–259.

75. Y. Zhang, R. Karki, O.J. Igwe, 2015, Toll-like receptor 4 signaling: a common pathway for interactions between prooxidants and extracellular disulfide high mobility group box 1 (HMGB1) protein-coupled activation, *Biochem. Pharmacol.* 98: 132–143.

76. R. Kokkola, A. Andersson, G. Mullins, et al., 2005, RAGE is the major receptor for the proinflammatory activity of HMGB1 in rodent macrophages, *Scand. J. Immunol.* 61: 1–9.

77. R. Karki, O.J. Igwe, 2013, Toll-like receptor 4-mediated nuclear factor kappa B activation is essential for sensing exogenous oxidants to propagate and maintain oxidative/nitrosative cellular stress, *PLoS One* 8: e73840.

78. Y. Zhang, F. Chen, 2004, Reactive oxygen species (ROS), troublemakers between nuclear factor-kappaB (NF-kappaB) and c-Jun NH(2)-terminal kinase (JNK), *Cancer Res.* 64: 1902–1905.

79. D.T. Love, C. Guo, E.I. Nikelshparg, et al., 2020, The role of the myeloperoxidase-derived oxidant hypothiocyanous acid (HOSCN) in the induction of mitochondrial dysfunction in macrophages, *Redox Biol.* 36: 101602.

80. P. Escoll, C. Buchrieser, 2018, Metabolic reprogramming of host cells upon bacterial infection: why shift to a Warburg-like metabolism? *FEBS J.* 285: 2146–2160.

81. T.J. Barrett, C.L. Hawkins, 2012, Hypothiocyanous acid: benign or deadly? *Chem. Res. Toxicol.* 25: 263–273.

82. J.D. Chandler, B.J. Day, 2015, Biochemical mechanisms and therapeutic potential of pseudohalide thiocyanate in human health, *Free Radic. Res.* 49: 695–710.

83. H. Han, H. Kwon, 2009, Estimated dietary intake of thiocyanate from Brassicaceae family in Korean diet, *J. Toxicol. Environ. Health A* 72: 1380–1387.

84. A.M. Leung, A. Lamar, X. He, L.E. Braverman, E.N. Pearce, 2011, Iodine status and thyroid function of Boston-area vegetarians and vegans, *J. Clin. Endocrinol. Metab.* 96: E1303–1307.

85. G.E. Conner, C. Wijkstrom-Frei, S.H. Randell, V.E. Fernandez, M. Salathe, 2007, The lactoperoxidase system links anion transport to host defense in cystic fibrosis, *FEBS Lett.* 581: 271–278.

86. L. Minarowski, D. Sands, A. Minarowska, et al., 2008, Thiocyanate concentration in saliva of cystic fibrosis patients, *Folia Histochem. Cytobiol.* 46: 245–246.

87. N.S. Gould, S. Gauthier, C.T. Kariya, et al., 2010, Hypertonic saline increases lung epithelial lining fluid glutathione and thiocyanate: two protective CFTR-dependent thiols against oxidative injury, *Respir. Res.* 11: 119–128.

88. L. Carroll, D.I. Pattison, S. Fu, et al., 2015, Reactivity of selenium-containing compounds with myeloperoxidase-derived chlorinating oxidants: second-order rate constants and implications for biological damage, *Free Radic. Biol. Med.* 84: 279–288.

89. G.W. Snider, E. Ruggles, N. Khan, R.J. Hondal, 2013, Selenocysteine confers resistance to inactivation by oxidation in thioredoxin reductase: comparison of selenium and sulfur enzymes, *Biochemistry* 52: 5472–5481.

90. R.P. Hirt, S. Muller, T.M. Embley, G.H. Coombs, 2002, The diversity and evolution of thioredoxin reductase: new perspectives, *Trends Parasitol.* 18: 302–308.

91. S.M. Bozonet, A.P. Scott-Thomas, P. Nagy, M.C. Vissers, 2010, Hypothiocyanous acid is a potent inhibitor of apoptosis and caspase 3 activation in endothelial cells, *Free Radic. Biol. Med.* 49: 1054–1063.

92. M.M. Lloyd, D.M. van Reyk, M.J. Davies, C.L. Hawkins, 2008, Hypothiocyanous acid is a more potent inducer of apoptosis and protein thiol depletion in murine macrophage cells than hypochlorous acid or hypobromous acid, *Biochem. J.* 414: 271–280.

93. ScienceLab, 2011, Sodium thiocyanate, MSDS: 1–5.

94. A. Zietzer, S.T. Niepmann, B. Camara, et al., 2019, Sodium thiocyanate treatment attenuates atherosclerotic plaque formation and improves endothelial regeneration in mice, *PLoS One* 14: e0214476.

95. L.F. Blaney, A.J. Geiger, R.G. Ernst, 1941, Potassium thiocyanate in the treatment of hypertension, *Yale J. Biol. Med.* 13: 493–508.

96. A. Ruskin, K.W. Mc, 1947, Comparative study of potassium thiocyanate and other drugs in the treatment of essential hypertension, *Am. Heart J.* 34: 691–701.

97. K.S. Alstad, 1949, The effects of thiocyanate on basal and supplemental blood pressures, *Br. Heart J.* 11: 249–256.

98. V. Schulz, 1984, Clinical pharmacokinetics of nitroprusside, cyanide, thiosulphate and thiocyanate, *Clin. Pharmacokinet.* 9: 239–251.

99. J.D. Oram, B. Reiter, 1966, The inhibition of streptococci by lactoperoxidase, thiocyanate and hydrogen peroxide. The oxidation of thiocyanate and the nature of the inhibitory compound, *Biochem. J.* 100: 382–388.

100. S.J. Klebanoff, R.G. Luebke, 1965, The antilactobacillus system of saliva. Role of salivary peroxidase, *Proc. Soc. Exp. Biol. Med.* 118: 483–486.

101. E.L. Thomas, T.W. Milligan, R.E. Joyner, M.M. Jefferson, 1994, Antibacterial activity of hydrogen peroxide and the lactoperoxidase-hydrogen peroxide-thiocyanate system against oral streptococci, *Infect. Immun.* 62: 529–535.

102. V.M. Marshall, B. Reiter, 1980, Comparison of the antibacterial activity of the hypothiocyanite anion towards Streptococcus lactis and *Escherichia coli*, *J. Gen. Microbiol.* 120: 513–516.

103. B.J. Day, P.E. Bratcher, J.D. Chandler, et al., 2020, The thiocyanate analog selenocyanate is a more potent antimicrobial pro-drug that also is selectively detoxified by the host, *Free Radic. Biol. Med.* 146: 324–332.

104. M.N. Mickelson, 1977, Glucose transport in *Streptococcus agalactiae* and its inhibition by lactoperoxidase-thiocyanate-hydrogen peroxide, *J. Bacteriol.* 132: 541–548.

105. K. Shin, K. Yamauchi, S. Teraguchi, H. Hayasawa, I. Imoto, 2002, Susceptibility of *Helicobacter pylori*

and its urease activity to the peroxidase-hydrogen peroxide-thiocyanate antimicrobial system, *J. Med. Microbiol.* 51: 231–237.

106. R. Sengupta, A. Holmgren, 2014, Thioredoxin and glutaredoxin-mediated redox regulation of ribonucleotide reductase, *World J. Biol. Chem.* 5: 68–74.

107. M. Lenander-Lumikari, 1992, Inhibition of *Candida albicans* by the peroxidase/SCN-/H$_2$O$_2$ system, *Oral Microbiol. Immunol.* 7: 315–320.

108. C. Sugita, K. Shin, H. Wakabayashi, et al., 2018, Antiviral activity of hypothiocyanite produced by lactoperoxidase against influenza A and B viruses and mode of its antiviral action, *Acta Virol.* 62: 401–408.

109. T.T. Nguyen, S. Suzuki, R. Sugamata, et al., 2018, Hypothiocyanous acid suppresses polyI:C-induced antiviral responses by modulating IRF3 phosphorylation in human airway epithelial cells, *Tohoku J. Exp. Med.* 245: 131–140.

110. H. Mikola, M. Waris, J. Tenovuo, 1995, Inhibition of herpes simplex virus type 1, respiratory syncytial virus and echovirus type 11 by peroxidase-generated hypothiocyanite, *Antiviral Res.* 26: 161–171.

111. M. Pourtois, C. Binet, N. Van Tieghem, et al., 1990, Inhibition of HIV infectivity by lactoperoxidase-produced hypothiocyanite, *J. Biol. Buccale* 18: 251–253.

112. N. Moguilevsky, M. Steens, C. Thiriart, et al., 1992, Lethal oxidative damage to human immunodeficiency virus by human recombinant myeloperoxidase, *FEBS Lett.* 302: 209–212.

113. M. Arlandson, T. Decker, V.A. Roongta, et al., 2001, Eosinophil peroxidase oxidation of thiocyanate. Characterization of major reaction products and a potential sulfhydryl-targeted cytotoxicity system, *J. Biol. Chem.* 276: 215–224.

114. B. Kerem, J.M. Rommens, J.A. Buchanan, et al., 1989, Identification of the cystic fibrosis gene: genetic analysis, *Science* 245: 1073–1080.

115. P.M. Quinton, 1983, Chloride impermeability in cystic fibrosis, *Nature* 301: 421–422.

116. M.R. Knowles, M.J. Stutts, A. Spock, et al., 1983, Abnormal ion permeation through cystic fibrosis respiratory epithelium, *Science* 221: 1067–1070.

117. J.A. Regnis, M. Robinson, D.L. Bailey, et al., 1994, Mucociliary clearance in patients with cystic fibrosis and in normal subjects, *Am. J. Respir. Crit. Care Med.* 150: 66–71.

118. F.S. Collins, 1992, Cystic fibrosis: molecular biology and therapeutic implications, *Science* 256: 774–779.

119. N. Ballatori, C.L. Hammond, J.B. Cunningham, S.M. Krance, R. Marchan, 2005, Molecular mechanisms of reduced glutathione transport: role of the MRP/CFTR/ABCC and OATP/SLC21A families of membrane proteins, *Toxicol. Appl. Pharmacol.* 204: 238–255.

120. J.H. Roum, R. Buhl, N.G. McElvaney, Z. Borok, R.G. Crystal, 1993, Systemic deficiency of glutathione in cystic fibrosis, *J. Appl. Physiol.* 75: 2419–2424.

121. B.J. Day, A.M. van Heeckeren, E. Min, L.W. Velsor, 2004, Role for cystic fibrosis transmembrane conductance regulator protein in a glutathione response to bronchopulmonary pseudomonas infection, *Infect. Immun.* 72: 2045–2051.

122. N.S. Gould, E. Min, R.J. Martin, B.J. Day, 2012, CFTR is the primary known apical glutathione transporter involved in cigarette smoke-induced adaptive responses in the lung, *Free Radic. Biol. Med.* 52: 1201–1206.

123. L.W. Velsor, A. van Heeckeren, B.J. Day, 2001, Antioxidant imbalance in the lungs of cystic fibrosis transmembrane conductance regulator protein mutant mice, *Am. J. Physiol. Lung Cell Mol. Physiol.* 281: L31–38.

124. P. Linsdell, J.W. Hanrahan, 1998, Glutathione permeability of CFTR, *Am. J. Physiol.* 275: C323–326.

125. L. Gao, K.J. Kim, J.R. Yankaskas, H.J. Forman, 1999, Abnormal glutathione transport in cystic fibrosis airway epithelia, *Am. J. Physiol.* 277: L113–118.

126. A.T. Adewale, E. Falk Libby, L. Fu, et al., 2020, Novel therapy of bicarbonate, glutathione and ascorbic acid improves cystic fibrosis mucus transport, *Am. J. Respir. Cell Mol. Biol.* 63: 362–373.

127. J.H. Poulsen, H. Fischer, B. Illek, T.E. Machen, 1994, Bicarbonate conductance and pH regulatory capability of cystic fibrosis transmembrane conductance regulator, *Proc. Natl. Acad. Sci. U.S.A.* 91: 5340–5344.

128. R.D. Coakley, B.R. Grubb, A.M. Paradiso, et al., 2003, Abnormal surface liquid pH regulation by cultured cystic fibrosis bronchial epithelium, *Proc. Natl. Acad. Sci. U.S.A.* 100: 16083–16088.

129. P. Linsdell, 2001, Thiocyanate as a probe of the cystic fibrosis transmembrane conductance regulator chloride channel pore, *Can. J. Physiol. Pharmacol.* 79: 573–579.

130. M.A. Fragoso, V. Fernandez, R. Forteza, et al., 2004, Transcellular thiocyanate transport by human airway epithelia, J. Physiol. 561: 183–194.

131. P. Moskwa, D. Lorentzen, K.J. Excoffon, et al., 2007, A novel host defense system of airways is defective in cystic fibrosis, Am. J. Respir. Crit. Care Med. 175: 174–183.

132. D. Lorentzen, L. Durairaj, A.A. Pezzulo, et al., 2011, Concentration of the antibacterial precursor thiocyanate in cystic fibrosis airway secretions, Free Radic. Biol. Med. 50: 1144–1150.

133. N. Pedemonte, E. Caci, E. Sondo, et al., 2007, Thiocyanate transport in resting and IL-4-stimulated human bronchial epithelial cells: role of pendrin and anion channels, J. Immunol. 178: 5144–5153.

134. L. Ferrera, O. Zegarra-Moran, L.J. Galietta, 2011, Ca^{2+}-activated Cl^- channels, Compr. Physiol. 1: 2155–2174.

135. Y. Nakagami, S. Favoreto, Jr., G. Zhen, et al., 2008, The epithelial anion transporter pendrin is induced by allergy and rhinovirus infection, regulates airway surface liquid, and increases airway reactivity and inflammation in an asthma model, J. Immunol. 181: 2203–2210.

136. M.A. Mall, J.R. Harkema, J.B. Trojanek, et al., 2008, Development of chronic bronchitis and emphysema in beta-epithelial Na^+ channel-overexpressing mice, Am. J. Respir. Crit. Care Med. 177: 730–742.

137. D.T. Harwood, A.J. Kettle, S. Brennan, C.C. Winterbourn, 2009, Simultaneous determination of reduced glutathione, glutathione disulphide and glutathione sulphonamide in cells and physiological fluids by isotope dilution liquid chromatography-tandem mass spectrometry, J. Chromatogr. B. Analyt. Technol. Biomed. Life Sci. 877: 3393–3399.

138. N. Dickerhof, R. Turner, I. Khalilova, et al., 2017, Oxidized glutathione and uric acid as biomarkers of early cystic fibrosis lung disease, J. Cyst. Fibros. 16: 214–221.

139. A. Rab, S.M. Rowe, S.V. Raju, et al., 2013, Cigarette smoke and CFTR: implications in the pathogenesis of COPD, Am. J. Physiol. Lung Cell Mol. Physiol. 305: L530–541.

PART FOUR

Peroxidases in Pathology

CHAPTER TWELVE

Imaging the Reactivity of Myeloperoxidase *In Vivo*

Cuihua Wang, Negin Jalali Motlagh, Enrico G. Kuellenberg, and John W. Chen
Institute for Innovation in Imaging
Massachusetts General Hospital and Harvard Medical School

CONTENTS

INTRODUCTION

Modern molecular imaging uses a variety of imaging technologies such as magnetic resonance imaging (MRI), positron emission tomography (PET), fluorescent imaging, and computed tomography (CT). These technologies provide noninvasive and powerful tools to advance our understanding of pathogenesis and disease progression by observing biological and pathological processes *in vivo* and can track treatment efficacy. Molecular imaging agents for MRI and PET are potential translational candidates. However, bioluminescence and fluorescent imaging agents may also be used in the clinical setting through the use of endoscopes and goggles. Molecular imaging technologies allow us to visualize activities of molecular targets such as myeloperoxidase (MPO) in living organisms to further our understanding of the pathophysiology in the endogenous environment without the need to sacrifice animals or perform procedures that can potentially alter the biology through *ex vivo* and *in vitro* manipulations.

MPO is a highly oxidative enzyme secreted by neutrophils and activated macrophages in response to pathogen and microbial stimulus. Aberrant MPO activity and its oxidative products have been pathologically implicated in many diseases, including

DOI: 10.1201/9781003212287-16

cardiovascular, neurological, and rheumatological diseases, among others. MPO is emerging as an important imaging and therapeutic target. The past two decades have witnessed a rapid development of activatable imaging methods to detect MPO activity utilizing the oxidative property of MPO, including generating reactive oxidative species and oxidizing substrates containing a 5-hydroxyindole (5-HI) moiety. The current imaging strategies to detect MPO activity fall into two major categories (Table 12.1): (i) agents that detect reactive species generated by MPO and (ii) agents based on MPO substrates or inhibitors. In this chapter, we will discuss recent progress in imaging MPO activity with a focus on those with translational potential to report MPO activity in vivo.

AGENTS THAT DETECT MPO-GENERATED REACTIVE SPECIES

Under oxidative stress, MPO released from neutrophils/macrophages uses hydrogen peroxide (H_2O_2) and chloride to produce reactive oxygen/nitrogen species (ROS/RNS), including hypochlorous acid (HOCl), hydroxy radical (OH·), singlet oxygen ($^1O_2$), and nitrogen dioxide radical (NO$_2$·), of which HOCl is recognized as an initial and specific product of MPO [1,2]. These highly reactive species can modify lipids, induce DNA damage, and interrupt protein function, resulting in tissue damage [2]. Imaging agents can be designed to take advantage of the high reactivity of these ROS/RNS to develop "turn-on" optical imaging agents. These agents can turn from an "off" state (non- or weakly fluorescent/luminescent) into an "on" state in the presence of ROS/RNS. The first part of Table 12.1 summarizes the imaging agents that can detect HOCl and other reactive species according to their excitation/emission mechanism and their applications/validation in animal models. Note that in this chapter, we do not cover agents that detect H_2O_2, since while it is a substrate for MPO, H_2O_2 production reflects NADPH oxidase and superoxide dismutase activity rather than MPO activity. We also do not include agents that have only been tested in vitro for which there are already several excellent reviews [3,4].

Fluorescence Imaging

Fluorescence imaging agents are designed to absorb light (excitation) to raise it to a higher excited state. When the agent returns to the ground state, it results in the emission of fluorescent light that can be detected. Photostability, tissue penetration, and quantum yield of the fluorophores are important parameters that affect fluorescence imaging. Near infrared (NIR) emission (650–900 nm) is frequently used in the design of these molecular imaging agents as these wavelengths confer deeper tissue penetration. Major fluorescent imaging agents targeting MPO-generated reactive species are listed in Table 12.1.

As the specific product generated by MPO, multiple "turn-on" imaging agents for detecting HOCl have been developed [3,5], but most have been evaluated only in vitro. Table 12.1 lists agents that have been validated in preclinical animal models. One of the earliest fluorescent imaging agents to target HOCl was developed by Shepherd et al. and called SNAPF (sulfonaphthoaminophenyl fluorescein) [6]. This agent can selectively detect HOCl over other reactive species. SNAPF was designed based on a xanthene dye scaffold linked to a cleavable 4-aminophenylether "mask' that shows weak fluorescence, but upon activation by strong oxidants, the "mask" is removed from SNAPF that can generate a strong fluorescence signal (Figure 12.1a). SNAPF has an emission wavelength of 676 nm, within the NIR range of 650–900 nm, and was able to detect HOCl generation in vivo in a mouse model of peritonitis induced by thioglycolate with a 1.4-fold signal increase compared with that of control mice. It has also been used to detect HOCl in human atherosclerotic plaques [6]. SNAPF was also utilized to detect MPO activity in a rat model of acute lung injury induced by lipopolysaccharide (LPS) using endoscopic confocal microscopy [7]. Another agent targeting HOCl was described by Wei et al. that is a deformylation reaction-based NIR "turn-on" probe called FDOCl-1; its specificity to MPO was shown using live cells stimulated by LPS/PMA (phorbol 12-myristate 13-acetate) with the MPO inhibitor 4-aminobenzoic acid hydrazide (ABAH) [8]. FDOCl-1 was applied in vivo in a mouse model of arthritis induced by λ-carrageenan. HKOCl-3 is another small-molecule fluorescent agent that showed superior specificity to HOCl in vitro over other ROS/RNS and can detect HOCl in a zebrafish model of embryo development [9]. Recently Liu et al. reported an NIR "turn-on" agent FD-301 that is specific to HOCl [10]. The specificity of FD-301 to

TABLE 12.1

Imaging probes that can detect MPO-generated reactive species

Detection modes	Modality/probes	Excitation (nm)	Emission (nm)	Targets	Preclinical models	Signal increase (fold change)
Detection of reactive species generated by MPO[a]				Fluorescence		
	SNAPF	614	676	HOCl	Perionitis; acute lung injury	1.4–1.8
	HKOCl-3	490	527	HOCl	Zebrafish embryo development	–
	FD-301	620	686	HOCl	Arthritis; ulcerative colitis	–
	KDOCl-1	635	720	HOCl	Arthritis	–
	Oxazine NPs	620	672	ONOO$^-$, HOCl	Myocardial infarction (MI)	–
				Bioluminescence (BLI)		
	Luminol	–	425	HOCl, OH, HOBr, ONOO$^-$, O$_2^-$	Acute dermatitis; focal arthritis; cancer	13–30
	L-012	–	425	HOCl, OH, HOBr, ONOO$^-$, O$_2^-$	Inflammation induced by LPS and PMA; arthritis	8–15
	Luminol-QD800	745	800	HOCl, OH, HOBr, ONOO$^-$, O$_2^-$	Pulmonary inflammation; tumor metastasis	–
				Other optical imaging modalities		
	Luminol+DiI-DiD	540	670	HOCl, OH, HOBr, ONOO$^-$, O$_2^-$	LPS-induced inflammation; breast cancer	24
	RSPN	Laser: 700	IR775S: 820	HOCl, ONOO$^-$	Acute edema	2.7
MPO substrates/inhibitors[b]	5HT-DOTA(Gd)	Magnetic resonance imaging (MRI)		MPO	MPO implant	1.7
	MPO-Gd	MRI		MPO	MPO implant; MI; EAE; NASH atherosclerosis; cancer	2

(Continued)

TABLE 12.1 (*Continued*)

Imaging probes that can detect MPO-generated reactive species

Detection modes	Modality/probes	Excitation (nm)	Emission (nm)	Targets	Preclinical models	Signal increase (fold change)
	5HT-DOTAGA-Gd	MRI		MPO	Lung inflammation	2
	heMAMP	MRI		MPO	Subcutaneous inflammation; tandem stenosis	4–10
	[18F]-MAPP	Positron emission tomography (PET)		MPO	Paw inflammation; MI	4
	[18F]-AlF-bis-5HT-NOTA	PET		MPO	Paw inflammation	–
	MABS	Fluorescence	Computed tomography (CT)	MPO	Dermatitis; paw inflammation; brain abscess	2–4
	[11C]AZD3241	PET		MPO	–	–

CAIA, collagen antibody-induced arthritis; EAE, experimental autoimmune encephalomyelitis; LGL, large granular lymphocytic tumor; MI, myocardial infarction; NASH, nonalcoholic steatohepatitis; SNAPF, sulfonaphthoaminophenyl fluorescein; NPs, nanoparticles; RSPN, ratiometric semiconducting polymer nanoparticles.

a Due to the shallow depth of penetration of optical imaging, these agents are best suited for in vitro and small animal studies, as well as catheter-based studies. Because it is impossible to test these agents against all potential oxidative products, specificity to HOCl/MPO for some of these agents may need further investigation.

b These imaging agents for MRI, CT, and PET are suitable for in vivo studies in animals and potentially humans. The 5HT-based agents have been validated against eosinophil peroxidase and lactoperoxidase. However, they are less sensitive than luminol-based imaging agents.

MPO was demonstrated in vitro with ABAH inhibition and in vivo in a mouse model of arthritis (with ABAH as an inhibitor) and ulcerative colitis (with 5-aminosalicylic acid as an inhibitor).

It is possible to conjugate the small-molecule fluorescent dyes to nanoparticles to increase the circulation time and accumulation of the agent. Panizzi et al. developed such a fluorescent sensor by coating quenched oxazine to an Alexa Flour 488-modified magnetic nanoparticle, which increased its blood half-life from ~40 min to > 9 h, compared with the free dye [11]. The oxazine dye is released from the nanoparticles in the presence of HOCl or ONOO$^-$ and becomes fluorescent. This sensor was validated with sorted neutrophils pretreated with the MPO inhibitor ABAH, resulting in 95% reduction in fluorescent signal, and was applied to detecting HOCl and ONOO$^-$ in a mouse model of myocardial infarction (Figure 12.1b).

A potential limitation of some of these fluorescent agents is that they may be activated by reactive species that are not specific to MPO, such as ONOO$^-$. Several of these agents lacked validation against products from other peroxidases, such as eosinophil peroxidase (EPO) and lactoperoxidase (LPO), as well as testing in vivo with MPO inhibitors or in MPO-deficient mice. Therefore, the specificity of these agents for MPO will need further investigation. Nevertheless, these agents are suitable for detecting oxidative stress if specificity to MPO is not important or necessary. In addition, these agents may serve as templates to spur future development of MPO-specific fluorescent imaging agents.

Bioluminescence Imaging (BLI)

Bioluminescent probes comprise another class of noninvasive optical imaging agents to detect MPO activity in vivo. Unlike fluorescence imaging,

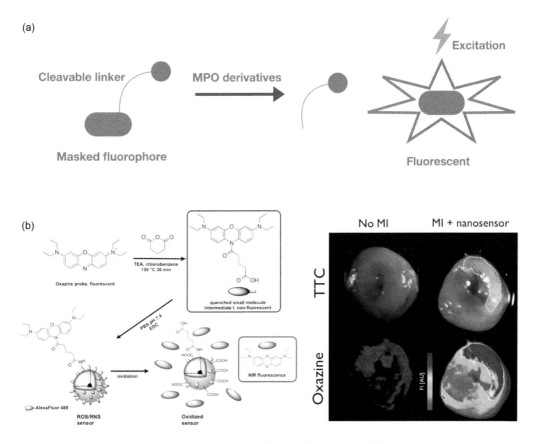

Figure 12.1 Fluorescence and bioluminescence imaging. (a) "Turn-on" mechanism of fluorescent probes activated by MPO-generated reactive species. (b) Left: Synthesis of oxazine-based NPs and its activation by ROS/RNS; Right: ex vivo fluorescence reflectance imaging (FRI) of heart slices with and without myocardial infarction. Infarcted region highlighted by the dashed line throughout. (Reprinted with permission from Panizzi et al., 2009, J. Am. Chem. Soc. 131: 15739–15744.)

bioluminescence imaging (BLI) utilizes light energy emitted through a chemical reaction without needing an external light source. Luminol is the most widely used chemiluminescent probe for BLI due to its stability and low cost. Luminol has been used to detect MPO activity in mouse models of acute dermatitis, focal arthritis [12], and mammary tumors [13]. While specificity of luminol to MPO was demonstrated in vivo using MPO inhibition with ABAH and in MPO-deficient mice [12], it should be noted that luminol is sensitive to multiple ROS/RNS species including HOCl, OH, and ONOO. Interestingly, whereas luminol reacts with products of reactions with EPO in vitro [14], Gross et al., using an allergic inflammation model in MPO-deficient mice and histology to verify that eosinophils infiltrated the site, demonstrated that luminol was not sensitive to EPO in vivo [12]. Since luminol emits blue light with emission maximum at 425 nm, tissue absorption and scatter limit its penetration depth to 0.5 mm. One strategy to enhance the bioluminescent signal is to increase the photon flux of the probe's emission. L-012, an analogue of luminol, was reported to have higher sensitivity to $ONOO^-$ and O_2^- and can produce 10–100 times stronger signal than luminol in vitro. It was used to detect inflammation induced by LPS and PMA as well as collagen antibody-induced arthritis (CAIA) in animals [15]. To improve tissue penetration depth, Zhang and colleagues described coadministering NIR-emitting quantum dot nanoparticles to red shift the blue light emitted by luminol (luminol-QD800) through chemiluminescent resonance energy transfer (CRET) [16]. With this approach, a 37-fold increase in luminescence emission signal over luminol alone was achieved in detecting reactive species in LPS-induced pulmonary inflammation. The specificity of luminol-QD800 was validated in vitro with LPO, in MPO-deficient mice and in mice treated with an NF-kB inhibitor MLN120B, which demonstrated 70% inhibition in the same model. Luminol-QD800 BLI can also effectively detect deep tumor foci in a mouse model of MDA-MB-231-luc2-induced tumor metastases.

Miscellaneous Technologies

Besides the ongoing efforts to develop more specific and optimized NIR probes for detecting MPO-generated ROS/RNS, new technologies

such as photoacoustic (PA) technique are also under development. PA imaging combines the high contrast of fluorescence or bioluminescence with the higher spatial resolution of ultrasound imaging to achieve deeper tissue penetration, greater specificity, and better resolution [17]. Liu et al. [18] reported an agent combining luminol with DiI-DiD nanobubbles (NBs) as a bioluminescence/ultrasound dual-modal imaging agent to detect inflammation (Figure 12.2a and b). Luminol + DiI-DiD NBs imaging through the BRET-FRET process showed a 24-fold luminescence signal increase than that with luminol alone and demonstrated significantly decreased luminescence signal when pretreated with the irreversible MPO inhibitor ABAH in a mouse model of LPS-induced inflammation, supporting its specificity to MPO. This dual-modal imaging agent was also capable of detecting inflammation in a xenograft model of breast cancer induced by 4T1-luc cells (Figure 12.2c). A photoacoustic probe developed by Pu et al. combined semiconducting polymer nanoparticles (SPNs) with a cyanine dye derivative (IR775S) [19]. The resultant probe is called ratiometric SPN (RSPN), which was found to be specific to $ONOO^-$ and ClO^-. RSPN was capable of detecting ROS/RNS in an acute edema model induced by zymosan with a twofold increase in signal.

Optical imaging is sensitive, convenient, and relatively inexpensive. As such, it is widely used in biological studies. However, its inherent disadvantage in tissue penetration limits its in vivo applications, especially in translational uses. Nonetheless, emerging efforts to translate these techniques for the bedside are ongoing. NIR-fluorescence imaging has been evaluated as a guide for intraoperative navigation and is gaining clinical acceptance [20]. NIR-fluorescence catheters and its combinations with other imaging modalities, such as optical coherence tomography–NIR fluorescence (OCT-NIRF) imaging, intravascular ultrasound-NIR fluorescence (IVUS-NIRF) imaging, have been developed in recent years for intravascular imaging that allows in vivo detection of high-risk plaques in atherosclerosis [21–28]. These technologies provide ways to overcome the penetration issue and use optical imaging to obtain high-quality three-dimensional images for clinical use. We envision these technologies could apply to MPO imaging.

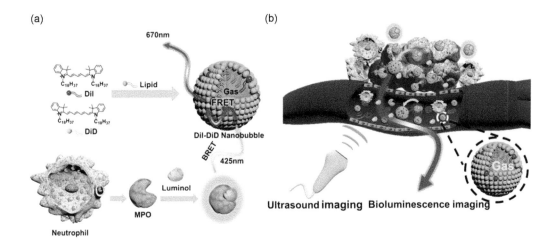

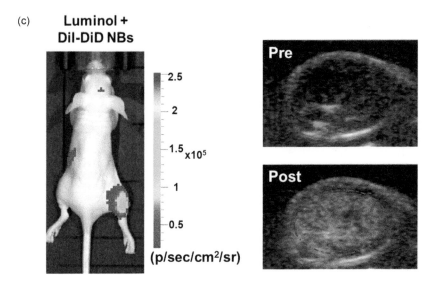

Figure 12.2 Photoacoustic imaging of luminol+DiI-DiD NBs. (a) and (b) Schematic illustration of luminol+DiI-DiD NBs for dual-modal imaging of MPO activity. DiI and DiD were co-incorporated in the lipid layer of the nanobubbles (NBs). The blue light generated by luminol at 425 nm can activate the NBs through the BRET, and the following FRET between DiI and DiD the agent red shifts into red light with a peak at 670 nm (a). Luminol can freely penetrate into inflamed tissues such as tumors, to interact with MPO and activate the DiI-DiD NBs through the BRET-FRET for bioluminescence imaging. The echogenicity of DiI-DiD also detects the tissues by contrast-enhanced ultrasound imaging (b). (c) Bioluminescence imaging of MPO activity (left) and contrast-enhanced ultrasound imaging of the tumor at the same site indicated in BLI with lumoinol+DiI-DiD NBs injection (right) in a mouse model of breast cancer. The red dashed line indicated the area of the tumor. (Reprinted with permission from Liu et al., 2019, *ACS Nano.* 13: 5124–5132.)

AGENTS BASED ON MPO SUBSTRATES/INHIBITORS

Another strategy to detect MPO activity is to target and interact with MPO. The most commonly used method to target enzymes is to introduce moieties that can interact with the enzymes. One approach is to use inhibitors for MPO. However, the low concentration of the enzyme may affect the sensitivity of the agent and saturation of the enzyme may limit its efficacy. Another class of imaging probes is based on MPO substrates, taking advantage of their unique interaction with MPO in the MPO catalytic cycle [29,30]. The

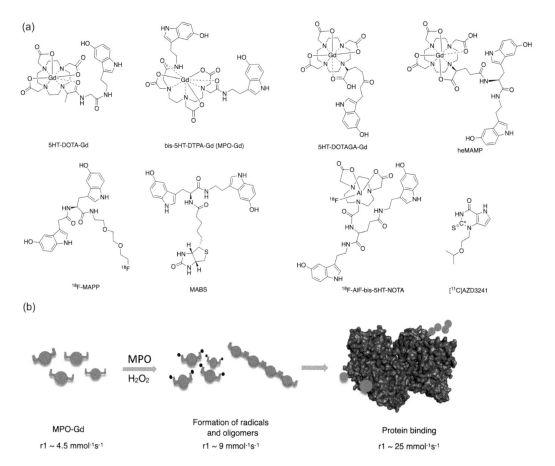

(a)

5HT-DOTA-Gd

bis-5HT-DTPA-Gd (MPO-Gd)

5HT-DOTAGA-Gd

heMAMP

18F-MAPP

MABS

18F-AlF-bis-5HT-NOTA

[11C]AZD3241

(b)

MPO
H2O2

MPO-Gd	Formation of radicals and oligomers	Protein binding
r1 ~ 4.5 mmol⁻¹s⁻¹	r1 ~ 9 mmol⁻¹s⁻¹	r1 ~ 25 mmol⁻¹s⁻¹

Figure 12.3 (a) Structures of imaging probes that interact with MPO (* = 11C). (b) Schematic illustration of the activation of MPO-Gd by MPO. The activated MPO-Gd forms oligomers or binds to proteins, and the relaxivity increases accordingly.

structures of the MPO imaging probes developed using MPO substrates/inhibitors are summarized in Figure 12.3a.

"

ACTIVATABLE IMAGING PROBES TARGETING MPO

5-Hydroxyindol (5-HI)-Based Activatable Imaging Agents

In the catalytic cycle of MPO, phenolic and indolic compounds can interact with MPO-compound I to form radicals through one electron transfer [1]. Our group had tested a variety of MPO substrates and identified 5-hydroxyindoles such as 5-hydroxytryptamine (5-HT) to be the best substrates for imaging applications, as they have favorable kinetics and can outcompete Cl⁻ even in the presence of 5,000 times higher excess of Cl⁻ over 5-HT [29,31]. For MRI agent design, it is important to note that 5-HT does not lose its redox potential once incorporated into a chelating structure [32]. In addition, because 5-HT is a substance already present in the body, no toxicity concern is present over the concentration range used for imaging. These properties make 5-HT an ideal substrate to detect MPO activity in imaging applications. After interaction with MPO-compound I, the 5-HI moiety on the imaging agents forms radicals that then combine into oligomers and bind to proteins and become "activated" [32,33]. The binding of the 5-HI unit to proteins after activation not only increases the retention of the agent in inflammatory sites containing elevated MPO activity but also eliminates nonspecific signal over time – thereby increasing the sensitivity and specificity of the imaging signal. Unlike the mechanism-based inhibitors that chemically bind to the heme group of the active site after activation by MPO and subsequently block the enzymatic activity of MPO [34,35], 5-HI-based imaging agents are substrates of MPO and exit the active site after activation. While it is theoretically possible that the activated agent can bind to sites on MPO that contain tyrosine/tryptophan, there are no tyrosine or tryptophan residues within the binding pocket [36], and thus there are no targets that block the active site and reduce MPO activity. Using this mechanism, our group and other investigators have developed a series of imaging agents based on 5-HI and validated their specificity to MPO and over other peroxidases, including EPO and LPO, and applied them to study multiple diseases and treatment effects in animal models, including MPO-deficient mouse models. TPO has not been tested since it is mainly secreted locally within the thyroid, so reactivity with TPO is not excluded [32,37].

5-HT-Based Imaging Agents

MPO-Gd

Magnetic resonance imaging (MRI) is a noninvasive, widely used imaging modality for disease diagnosis and treatment monitoring in the clinic and provides detailed anatomical images without ionizing radiation or radioactive agents.

The first MPO-activatable MR imaging agent is 5HT-DOTA-Gd (Figure 12.3a), reported in 2004 by Chen et al. [31]. This agent contained a single 5-HT moiety and was replaced by bis-5HT-DTPA-Gd in 2005 that features two 5-HT moieties [33,38]. The latter agent was found to have improved sensitivity over 5HT-DOTA-Gd [33], and bis-5HT-DTPA-Gd was dubbed "MPO-Gd." Note that this does not mean that the agent is composed of MPO conjugated to Gd. After activation, MPO-Gd's longitudinal relaxivity (r1) increases from 4.5 to ~9 and ~25 mmol^{-1}s^{-1} for oligomers and protein binding, respectively (Figure 12.3b). The efficacy of MPO-Gd was validated in vivo in Matrigel implant experiments, which showed more than twofold contrast-to-noise ratio (CNR) increase on the MPO-containing side compared with the side without MPO [32]. MPO-Gd was found to

be only activatable by MPO but not by EPO [32]. The specificity and efficacy of MPO-Gd were further demonstrated in multiple disease models where MPO plays critical roles in the disease pathology and progress. We introduce these studies below.

MYOCARDIAL INFARCTION

Ischemic myocardial infarction (MI) caused by the occlusion of coronary arteries elicits an inflammatory response characterized by influx of neutrophils and monocytes from the blood pool. As part of the immunological function to combat infection, these cells release MPO, which in the injured tissue generates ROS/RNS that are thought to be responsible for reperfusion damage following ischemia. MR imaging with MPO-Gd in a mouse model of MI showed significantly delayed washout kinetics and higher CNRs in the infarcted myocardium compared with wild-type MI mice imaged with the nonspecific Gd-DTPA and to MPO-deficient MI mice imaged with MPO-Gd, thus confirming the in vivo specificity of MPO-Gd (Figure 12.4a) [39]. Furthermore, MPO imaging tracked the changes in MPO activity over time in MI and noninvasively monitored treatment response to the MPO inhibitor PF-1355 (Figure 12.4b) [40] and the anti-inflammatory drug atorvastatin [39].

ATHEROSCLEROSIS

Atherosclerosis is the underlying cause of most cardiovascular diseases, which remain one of the leading causes of morbidity and mortality around the globe. Inflammation plays a pivotal role in atherosclerotic plaque formation, development, and rupture. Vulnerable plaques prone to rupture contain a greater number of infiltrating macrophages that secrete MPO than do stable plaques [41,42]. MPO contributes to the plaque destabilization by modifying LDL and the activation state of matrix metalloproteases (MMPs). Identification of vulnerable, highly inflamed plaque and early prevention could prevent adverse cardiovascular events from occurring. In a rabbit model of atherosclerosis, MR imaging with MPO-Gd displayed a signal increase greater than twofold in diseased vessel walls compared with normal vessel walls or to diseased vessel walls imaged with conventional DTPA-Gd (Figure 12.4c). The increased signal correlated to a threefold increase of MPO concentration by tissue

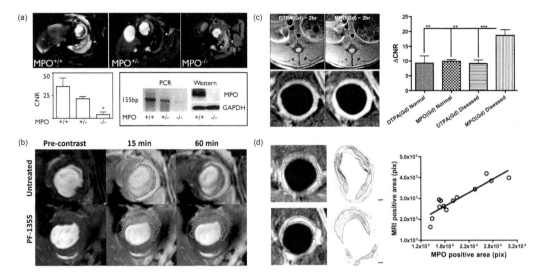

Figure 12.4 MR imaging of MPO in cardiovascular diseases. (a) Myocardial infarction. Imaging of infarcted myocardium in MPO-deficient mice establishes specificity of MPO-Gd for MPO. MR imaging and contrast-to-noise ratio (CNR) analysis showed that the signal of the infarct in wild-type mice 2 h after injection of MPO-Gd is brightly enhanced, intermediate enhanced in heterozygous MPO-deficient mice, and significantly reduced in homozygous MPO-deficient mice. Polymerase chain reaction and western blotting of representative genotypes correspond to the imaging data. (Reprinted with permission from Nahrendorf et al., 2008, *Circulation* 117: 1153–1160.) (b) MPO-Gd imaging on day 2 demonstrated reduced MPO activity in PF-1355-treated mice compared with untreated mice with MI. Dotted areas represent the infarcted areas. (Reprinted with permission from Ali et al., 2016, *JACC: Basic Transl. Sci.* 1: 633–643.) (c) In a rabbit model of atherosclerosis, delayed MPO-Gd images 2 h after MPO-Gd injection showed substantially increased enhancement in diseased vessels compared with DTPA-Gd and in normal vessels. (d) MPO-Gd imaging identified distinct foci of MPO activity in diseased atherosclerotic wall and correlated well with matched immunostained sections rich in MPO. (c and d, Reprinted with permission from Ronald et al., 2009, *Circulation* 120: 592–599.)

analysis, and imaging results correlated well with histological analysis (Figure 12.4d) [43]. Similarly, in a murine model of tandem carotid atherosclerosis, MPO-Gd imaging showed greater than twofold signal increase in vulnerable plaques compared with stable plaques. MPO-deficient mice and mice treated with the MPO inhibitor AZM198 demonstrated significantly attenuated MRI signal in the atherosclerotic plaques, further validating the in vivo specificity of MPO-Gd [44].

DEMYELINATING DISEASE

Multiple sclerosis (MS) is the leading cause of non-traumatic neurological disability in young adults. MS is characterized by inflammatory demyelinating plaques in the CNS caused by an immune-mediated inflammatory response. MPO is found to be highly expressed in active MS plaques and a major contributor to demyelination [45]. Detecting active inflammation in MS patients is a key diagnostic tool in the management of MS patients, as earlier and timely treatment of active inflammation decreases disability. However, current MR

imaging reflects only the breakdown of the blood–brain barrier (BBB) and penetration of the contrast agent instead of active inflammation, which do not always correspond to each other [46]. In mice with experimental autoimmune encephalomyelitis (EAE), a commonly used murine model of MS, Chen and colleagues demonstrated that MPO-Gd imaging is capable of detecting 40%–90% more and smaller inflammatory lesions than does conventional Gd-enhanced MR imaging (Figure 12.5a) and that in vivo MPO activity detected by MPO-Gd imaging correlated with the degree of demyelination, immune cell infiltration, and clinical disease severity [47,48]. Unlike conventional nonspecific MRI agents, MPO-Gd imaging was able to detect the earliest time point at which pro-inflammatory cells are present in the brain and is able to detect preclinical and subclinical active disease even during apparent clinical remission [48]. Furthermore, MPO-Gd imaging can track the changes in the brains of EAE mice treated with the MPO inhibitor ABAH (Figure 12.5b) [49] or ABAH in combination with glatiramer acetate (GA) [50], a first-line

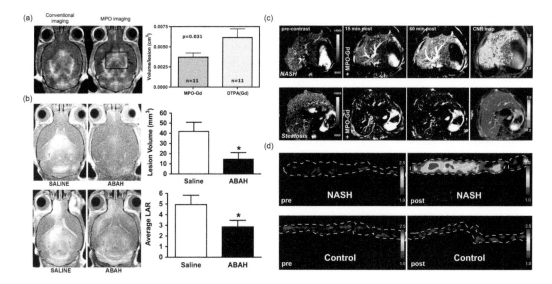

Figure 12.5 MPO-Gd imaging in EAE and NASH. (a) MPO-Gd imaging of experimental autoimmune encephalomyelitis (EAE) model revealed smaller volume lesions than did that with conventional Gd-DTPA. (Reprinted with permission from Chen et al., 2008, *Brain* 131: 1123–1133.) (b) MPO-Gd imaging of EAE mice demonstrated that lesion volume and average lesion activation ratio (LAR) in ABAH-treated mice were significantly decreased compared with that in saline-treated mice. (Reprinted with permission from Forghani et al., 2012, *Radiology* 263: 451–460.) (c) MPO-Gd MR imaging is able to detect inflammatory activity in diet-induced NASH (up) and steatosis (down). (d) MPO-Gd MR imaging showed increased MPO activity in liver biopsy samples of NASH patients compared with controls. (c and d, Reprinted with permission from Pulli et al., 2017, *Radiology* 284: 390–400.)

immunomodulatory drug targeting lymphocytes. These findings showed that MPO imaging may advance the care of MS patients once translated.

NONALCOHOLIC STEATOHEPATITIS

Nonalcoholic fatty liver disease (NAFLD) is the most common liver disease in the world. When NAFLD is associated with inflammation, it is called nonalcoholic steatohepatitis (NASH), which can progress to fibrosis or cirrhosis in 30%–50% of the cases. Currently, there is no imaging technique that can differentiate NASH from steatosis, and diagnosis can only be obtained by performing an invasive transcutaneous liver biopsy. Studies have shown that inflammation and oxidative stress are key features of NASH, and human NASH contains higher amounts of MPO than do steatotic liver specimens [51]. We and others have shown that in experimental NASH, MPO plays important roles in hepatocyte death, activation of hepatic stellate cells, and fibrosis – three hallmarks of progressive disease [52,53]. In both mouse models of NASH induced by LPS or diet, Pulli and coworkers revealed that MPO-Gd imaging detected elevated MPO activity in the livers of NASH mice compared with those of control and MPO-deficient mice

(Figure 12.5c) [54]. This was further validated in human liver biopsy samples where MPO-Gd distinguished between NASH and steatotic control samples (Figure 12.5d), underscoring its translational potential.

5HT-DOTAGA-Gd

Another 5-HT-based MRI probe for *in vivo* imaging is 5HT-DOTAGA-Gd. Similar to 5HT-DOTA-Gd (Figure 12.3a) [31], 5HT-DOTAGA-Gd also has one 5-HT moiety linked to the macrocyclic ligand DOTA [55]. Rodríguez-Rodríguez et al. reported imaging pulmonary inflammation with 5HT-DOTAGA-Gd MR imaging using a mouse model of bleomycin-induced lung injury and demonstrated twofold higher signal increase in diseased mice compared with that in control mice as well as in diseased mice imaged with the non-specific analogue T-DOTAGA-Gd, confirming the sensitivity and specificity of Gd-5HT-DOTAGA [56]. Wadghiri et al. also demonstrated that Gd-5HT-DOTAGA MRI was able to detect MPO activity in human samples of brain aneurysm [55], again demonstrating that this class of agents has high translational potential.

The applications of MPO MR imaging in multiple diseases confirmed the specificity and efficacy of these agents in detecting MPO activity. The activatable mechanism of MPO-Gd and its analogs makes it possible to detect biologically relevant concentration of MPO in vivo. MPO-Gd imaging could provide a useful noninvasive tool to improve diagnosis and prognosis in multiple inflammatory diseases. However, MPO-Gd has limited translational potential due to the use of a linear chelating backbone, which has much lower kinetic stability to maintain chelation to Gd compared with that of macrocyclic chelates. Older macrocyclic versions of MPO-Gd (5HT-DOTA-Gd and 5HT-DOTAGA-Gd) contain only one 5-HT-based moiety and have lower sensitivity compared with that of MPO-Gd with two 5-HT-based moieties [32]. To improve both the safety and efficacy of these agents, Wang et al. recently developed and validated a new generation of highly efficient MPO activatable MRI probe (heMAMP) that uses a DOTA-based macrocyclic backbone as well as containing two 5-HT moieties (Figure 12.3a). Interestingly, heMAMP not only possesses high kinetic stability for Gd, it also has up to 3 times higher efficacy in vivo compared with prior agents – demonstrating a similar signal enhancement at 1/3 the dose compared with MPO-Gd in a mouse model of unstable atherosclerotic plaque [57].

Other 5-HI-Based Imaging Agents

18F-MAPP: Positron Emission Tomography Imaging of MPO Activity

PET is a highly sensitive and quantitative imaging modality using radiotracer as low as picomolar in concentration. PET combined with CT imaging is widely used in detecting tumor/metastasis, infectious diseases, and neurological diseases. Wang et al. developed an ^{18}F-labeled MPO-activatable PET probe (^{18}F-MAPP) that comprises two 5- HI (5-hydroxytryptophan and 5-hydroxyindole acetic acid) moieties and a linker to incorporate the radioactive moiety [58]. Being a small molecule, ^{18}F-MAPP has a short blood half-life (<2 min), and only those agents that are activated by MPO and bound to protein remain in inflamed sites. ^{18}F-MAPP was validated both in vitro using autoradiography demonstrating binding to proteins after activation by MPO and in vivo in Matrigel implant experiment, demonstrating 2.5-fold

higher standard uptake value (SUV) ratio in the MPO-containing side compared with the control side without MPO and linear increase corresponding to the MPO activity.

The efficacy and specificity of ^{18}F-MAPP PET imaging were further validated in two disease models. In a mouse model of complete Freund's adjuvant (CFA)-induced paw inflammation, ^{18}F-MAPP imaging detected a fourfold higher uptake in the CFA-injected forepaw than in the PBS-injected forepaw. ^{18}F-MAPP also accurately tracked the treatment effect of the irreversible MPO inhibitor PF-1355, reporting an average of 57% inhibition, corresponding to ~50% of inhibition detected by biochemical assays (Figure 12.6a) [40]. In a mouse model of myocardial infarction, ^{18}F-MAPP uptake in the infarcted myocardium was more than fourfold higher than in normal myocardium without infarct and in the infarcted myocardium in MPO-deficient mice, further confirming its specificity to MPO in vivo (Figure 12.6b). Importantly, ^{18}F-MAPP can cross the blood–brain barrier, making it a potential candidate for neuroimaging applications.

Recently, Tang et al. reported a theranostic agent based on bis-5HT-linked nanoparticles (NPs) to target neutrophils to enhance cancer treatment [59]. They described a 5-HT-based PET imaging agent ^{18}F-AlF-bis-5HT-NOTA (Figure 12.3a) and performed tests in vitro using plasma for protein binding and in vivo in a mouse model of paw inflammation induced by turpentine. Using the MPO inhibitor PF-1355, the PET agent demonstrated 53% signal decrease after treatment. They then labeled NPs with the PET imaging agent (HZ-5-^{64}Cu) and a leukotriene inhibitor to target neutrophils induced by photodynamic therapy (PDT) to improve cancer treatment in a mouse model of breast cancer.

MABS as a Platform for Fluorescence and CT Imaging of MPO Activity

Employing a pre-targeting approach, Wang et al. developed an MPO-activatable biotinylated sensor (MABS) [37]. Distinct from most imaging probes, MABS itself does not contain either a fluorophore or a modality-specific element but is comprised of two 5-HI moieties (5-hydroxytryptophan and 5-hydroxyindole acetic acid) specific to MPO conjugated to a biotin moiety (Figure 12.3a). MABS can be oxidized by MPO and stays in inflammatory sites through protein binding, then detected by a streptavidin-labeled secondary imaging reporter via the biotin–streptavidin interaction. The specificity and versatility of MABS were demonstrated in multiple models combined with several secondary imaging detectors for a variety of imaging applications at different scales, described below.

MABS with Streptavidin-Alexa-Fluoro647 (SAF-647) for Fluorescence Imaging

The specificity of MABS to MPO over EPO and LPO was validated in vitro by experiments employing coincubation with fibrinogen and subsequent native PAGE [37]. The sensitivity and specificity of MABS were validated in vivo in Matrigel implant experiments, in which the signal increase was linearly proportional to the amount of MPO present (Figure 12.6c). No significant signal was detected when Matrigel did not contain MPO, in MPO-deficient mice or in mice treated with ABAH, or when imaged with a nonspecific analogue of MABS. MABS fluorescence imaging was validated in a mouse model of irritant contact dermatitis induced by PMA and in a mouse model of cerebritis induced by the bacteria salmonella. MABS fluorescence imaging was also applied to tissue sections mounted on slides and identified a short distance away from the cerebritis a distinct population of cells that contains inactive MPO (positive for MPO antibody immunostaining but negative for MABS signal) and may represent cells that are primed but not yet participating in inflammation. This finding suggests that studies that only use MPO antibody to determine the presence

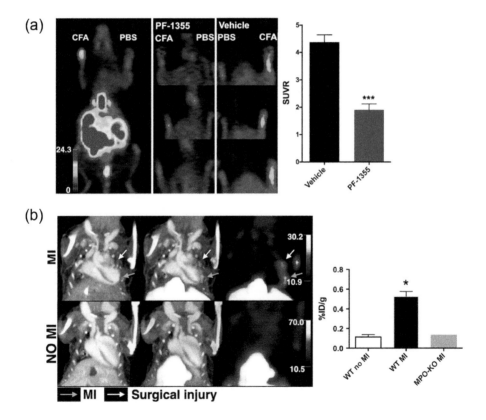

Figure 12.6 ^{18}F-MAPP and MABS imaging. – (a) In a mouse model of inflammation induced by complete Freund's adjuvant (CFA), ^{18}F-MAPP uptake in the CFA-injected side was fourfold higher than that in the PBS-injected control side, and ^{18}F-MAPP uptake in mice treated with the specific MPO inhibitor PF-1355 after CFA injection is markedly decreased (57% of mean inhibition) relative to that of the vehicle-treated control mice. (b) In a mouse model of myocardial infarction (MI), ^{18}F-MAPP uptake is much higher than that in mice without MI or MPO-deficient mice with MI. (a and b, Reprinted with permission from Wang et al., 2019, *Proc. Natl. Acad. Sci. U.S.A.* 116: 11966–11971.)

(*Continued*)

(c)

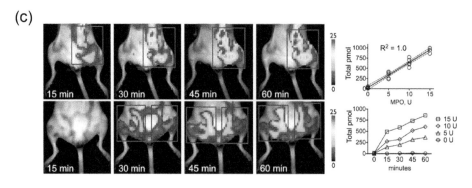

(d)

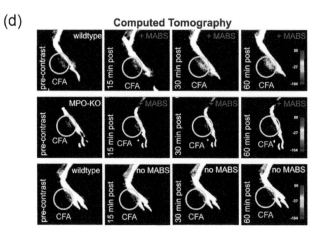

Figure 12.6 (Continued) ^{18}F-MAPP and MABS imaging. – (c) Fluorescence molecular tomography (FMT) imaging after injection of MABS and streptavidin-AlexaFluor-647 (SAF-647) at different concentrations of MPO embedded in Matrigel revealed a linear increase with increasing quantities of MPO and fluorescence signal increase over 60 min and (d) CT imaging after MABS and streptavidin-gold-conjugated nanoparticles injection in CFA-induced paw inflammation showed contrast enhancement on the CFA side over 60 min, but not in MPO-deficient mice or in wild-type mice without MABS. (c and d, Reprinted with permission from Wang et al., 2019, *Theranostics* 9: 7525–7536).

and location of MPO activity may not detect the actual biological response; a strategy that combines detection of MPO protein and MABS fluorescence imaging to detect MPO activity would provide a more complete and biologically relevant picture of the MPO response. Finally, MABS imaging can also detect MPO activity in neutrophil extracellular traps (NETs) induced by *Streptococcus pneumoniae*.

MABS with Streptavidin-Gold Nanoparticles for CT Imaging

When combined with streptavidin-labeled gold nanoparticles, MABS was able to detect MPO activity in a mouse model of inflammation induced by CFA using molecular CT imaging. Approximately twofold higher signal-to-noise ratio (SNR) was observed in the CFA-injected side compared with

the PBS-injected side and in MPO-deficient mice with CFA injection (Figure 12.6d).

In addition to SAF-647 and streptavidin-labeled gold nanoparticles, MABS can be used with streptavidin-labeled fluorophores of different absorptions and emissions for parallel imaging of different targets in the same subjects, with radionuclides for PET imaging or with iron oxide for MR imaging. By choosing different secondary probes, MABS provides a versatile platform for multimodal molecular imaging.

INHIBITOR-BASED IMAGING PROBES TARGETING ENZYMATIC MPO

[11C]AZD3241 is the only MPO inhibitor-based PET imaging probe reported so far, where the MPO inhibitor AZD3241 was labeled with carbon-11 in the thio-carbonyl position (Figure 12.3a) [60]. The biodistribution study of [^{11}C]AZD3241 imaging in cynomolgus monkeys showed that [^{11}C]AZD3241 rapidly entered the brain with a maximum concentration of 1.9%–2.6% of the injected radioactivity within 1.5 min and was homogeneously distributed in the brain. However, this agent has not been tested in a disease model, and thus its sensitivity and applications are yet to be determined.

PERSPECTIVES

MPO imaging is emerging to be a powerful and useful technology to improve our understanding of MPO biology and involvement in diseases. Currently, two different strategies have been used to detect MPO activity, namely by detecting MPO-generated reactive species or by interacting with MPO either via a substrate or an inhibitor. The former strategy employs optical imaging agents that have a somewhat limited translational potential. The latter strategy includes a wider variety of imaging modalities that can be used, including MRI and PET that have higher translational potential. When translated into clinical practice, MPO imaging will provide a diagnostic tool to realize early detection and to improve accuracy in the diagnosis of many inflammatory diseases. MPO imaging could also provide a highly specific and accurate noninvasive means to evaluate emerging novel therapeutics and to monitor treatment effects that target MPO-related inflammatory and immune response.

REFERENCES

1. S.J. Klebanoff, 2005, Myeloperoxidase: friend and foe, J. Leukoc. Biol. 77: 598–625.
2. B.S. van der Veen, M.P. de Winther, P. Heeringa, 2009, Myeloperoxidase: molecular mechanisms of action and their relevance to human health and disease, Antioxid. Redox Signal. 11: 2899–937.
3. T. Yudhistira, S.V. Mulay, Y. Kim, M.B. Halle, D.G. Churchill, 2019, Imaging of hypochlorous acid by fluorescence and applications in biological systems, Chem. Asian J. 14: 3048–3084.
4. J. Huang, A. Milton, R.D. Arnold, et al., 2016, Methods for measuring myeloperoxidase activity toward assessing inhibitor efficacy in living systems, J. Leukoc. Biol. 99: 541–548.
5. C. Ma, G. Zhong, Y. Zhao, et al., 2020, Recent development of synthetic probes for detection of hypochlorous acid/hypochlorite, Spectrochim. Acta A. Mol. Biomol. Spectrosc. 240: 118545.
6. J. Shepherd, S.A. Hilderbrand, P. Waterman, et al., 2007, A fluorescent probe for the detection of myeloperoxidase activity in atherosclerosis-associated macrophages, Chem. Biol. 14: 1221–1231.
7. F. Chagnon, A. Bourgouin, R. Lebel, et al., 2015, Smart imaging of acute lung injury: exploration of myeloperoxidase activity using in vivo endoscopic confocal fluorescence microscopy, Am. J. Physiol. Lung Cell Mol. Physiol. 309: L543–L551.
8. P. Wei, W. Yuan, F. Xue, et al., 2018, Deformylation reaction-based probe for in vivo imaging of HOCl, Chem. Sci. 9: 495–501.
9. J.J. Hu, N.K. Wong, M.Y. Lu, et al., 2016, HKOCl-3: a fluorescent hypochlorous acid probe for live-cell and in vivo imaging and quantitative application in flow cytometry and a 96-well microplate assay, Chem. Sci. 7: 2094–2099.
10. L. Liu, P. Wei, W. Yuan, et al., 2020, Detecting basal myeloperoxidase activity in living systems with a near-infrared emissive "turn-on" probe, Anal. Chem. 92: 10971–10978.
11. P. Panizzi, M. Nahrendorf, M. Wildgruber, et al., 2009, Oxazine conjugated nanoparticle detects in vivo hypochlorous acid and peroxynitrite generation, J. Am. Chem. Soc. 131: 15739–15744.
12. S. Gross, S.T. Gammon, B.L. Moss, et al., 2009, Bioluminescence imaging of myeloperoxidase activity in vivo, Nat. Med. 15: 455–461.
13. H.S. Alshetaiwi, S. Balivada, T.B. Shrestha, et al., 2013, Luminol-based bioluminescence imaging of mouse mammary tumors, J. Photochem. Photobiol. B. 127: 223–228.
14. A.S. Haqqani, J.K. Sandhu, H.C. Birnboim, 1999, A myeloperoxidase-specific assay based upon bromide-dependent chemiluminescence of luminol, Anal. Biochem. 273: 126–132.
15. A. Kielland, T. Blom, K.S. Nandakumar, et al., 2009, In vivo imaging of reactive oxygen and nitrogen species in inflammation using the luminescent probe L-012, Free Radic. Biol. Med. 47: 760–766.
16. N. Zhang, K.P. Francis, A. Prakash, D. Ansaldi, 2013, Enhanced detection of myeloperoxidase activity in deep tissues through luminescent excitation of near-infrared nanoparticles, Nat. Med. 19: 500–505.
17. P. Beard, 2011, Biomedical photoacoustic imaging, Interface Focus 1: 602–631.

18. R. Liu, J. Tang, Y. Xu, Z. Dai, 2019, Bioluminescence imaging of inflammation in vivo based on bioluminescence and fluorescence resonance energy transfer using nanobubble ultrasound contrast agent, *ACS Nano.* 13: 5124–5132.

19. K. Pu, A.J. Shuhendler, J.V. Jokerst, et al., 2014, Semiconducting polymer nanoparticles as photoacoustic molecular imaging probes in living mice, *Nat. Nanotechnol.* 9: 233–239.

20. L. van Manen, H.J.M. Handgraaf, M. Diana, et al., 2018, A practical guide for the use of indocyanine green and methylene blue in fluorescence-guided abdominal surgery, *J. Surg. Oncol.* 118: 283–300.

21. F.A. Jaffer, C. Vinegoni, M.C. John, et al., 2008, Real-time catheter molecular sensing of inflammation in proteolytically active atherosclerosis, *Circulation* 118: 1802–1809.

22. F.A. Jaffer, M.A. Calfon, A. Rosenthal, et al., 2011, Two-dimensional intravascular near-infrared fluorescence molecular imaging of inflammation in atherosclerosis and stent-induced vascular injury, *J. Am. Coll. Cardiol.* 57: 2516–2526.

23. H. Yoo, J.W. Kim, M. Shishkov, et al., 2011, Intra-arterial catheter for simultaneous microstructural and molecular imaging in vivo, *Nat. Med.* 17: 1680–1684.

24. S. Lee, M.W. Lee, H.S. Cho, et al., 2014, Fully integrated high-speed intravascular optical coherence tomography/near-infrared fluorescence structural/molecular imaging in vivo using a clinically available near-infrared fluorescence-emitting indocyanine green to detect inflamed lipid-rich atheromata in coronary-sized vessels, *Circ. Cardiovasc. Interv.* 7: 560–569.

25. S. Kim, M.W. Lee, T.S. Kim, et al., 2016, Intracoronary dual-modal optical coherence tomography-near-infrared fluorescence structural-molecular imaging with a clinical dose of indocyanine green for the assessment of high-risk plaques and stent-associated inflammation in a beating coronary artery, *Eur. Heart J.* 37: 2833–2844.

26. T. Hara, G.J. Ughi, J.R. McCarthy, et al., 2017, Intravascular fibrin molecular imaging improves the detection of unhealed stents assessed by optical coherence tomography in vivo, *Eur. Heart J.* 38: 447–455.

27. A.J. Dixon, J.A. Hossack, 2013, Intravascular near-infrared fluorescence catheter with ultrasound guidance and blood attenuation correction, *J. Biomed. Opt.* 18: 56009.

28. M.J. Bertrand, M. Abran, F. Maafi, et al., 2019, In vivo near-infrared fluorescence imaging of atherosclerosis using local delivery of novel targeted molecular probes, *Sci. Rep.* 9: 2670.

29. H.B. Dunford, Y. Hsuanyu, 1999, Kinetics of oxidation of serotonin by myeloperoxidase compounds I and II, *Biochem. Cell Biol.* 77: 449–457.

30. A. Reimer, G. Heuther, F. Schmidt, P. Schuff-Werner, M.M. Brudny, 1990, Oxidation of the indole nucleus of 5-hydroxytryptamine and formation of dimers in the presence of peroxidase and H_2O_2, *Neural Transm. Suppl.* 32: 249–257.

31. J.W. Chen, W. Pham, R. Weissleder, A. Bogdanov, Jr., 2004, Human myeloperoxidase: a potential target for molecular MR imaging in atherosclerosis, *Magn. Reson. Med.* 52: 1021–1028.

32. E. Rodriguez, M. Nilges, R. Weissleder, J.W. Chen, 2010, Activatable magnetic resonance imaging agents for myeloperoxidase sensing: mechanism of activation, stability, and toxicity, *J. Am. Chem. Soc.* 132: 168–177.

33. J.W. Chen, M. Querol Sans, A. Bogdanov, Jr., R. Weissleder, 2006, Imaging of myeloperoxidase in mice by using novel amplifiable paramagnetic substrates, *Radiology* 240: 473–481.

34. W. Zheng, R. Warner, R. Ruggeri, et al., 2015, PF-1355, a mechanism-based myeloperoxidase inhibitor, prevents immune complex vasculitis and anti-glomerular basement membrane glomerulonephritis, *J. Pharmacol. Exp. Ther.* 353: 288–298.

35. A.K. Tiden, T. Sjogren, M. Svensson, et al., 2011, 2-thioxanthines are mechanism-based inactivators of myeloperoxidase that block oxidative stress during inflammation, *J. Biol. Chem.* 286: 37578–37589.

36. T.J. Fiedler, C.A. Davey, R.E. Fenna, 2000, X-ray crystal structure and characterization of halide-binding sites of human myeloperoxidase at 1.8 A resolution, *J. Biol. Chem.* 275: 11964–11971.

37. C. Wang, B. Pulli, N. Jalali Motlagh, et al., 2019, A versatile imaging platform with fluorescence and CT imaging capabilities that detects myeloperoxidase activity and inflammation at different scales, *Theranostics* 9: 7525–7536.

38. M. Querol, J. Chen, R. Weissleder, A. Bogdanov, 2005, DTPA-bisamide-based MR sensor agents for peroxidase imaging, *Org. Lett.* 7: 1719–1722.

39. M. Nahrendorf, D. Sosnovik, J.W. Chen, et al., 2008, Activatable magnetic resonance imaging agent reports myeloperoxidase activity in

healing infarcts and noninvasively detects the antiinflammatory effects of atorvastatin on ischemia-reperfusion injury, *Circulation* 117: 1153–1160.

40. M. Ali, B. Pulli, G. Courties, et al., 2016, Myeloperoxidase inhibition improves ventricular function and remodeling after experimental myocardial infarction, *JACC: Basic Transl. Sci.* 1: 633–643.

41. A. Daugherty, J.L. Dunn, D.L. Rateri, J.W. Heinecke, 1994, Myeloperoxidase, a catalyst for lipoprotein oxidation, is expressed in human atherosclerotic lesions, *J. Clin. Invest.* 94: 437–444.

42. S.J. Nicholls, S.L. Hazen, 2005, Myeloperoxidase and cardiovascular disease, *Arterioscler. Thromb. Vasc. Biol.* 25: 1102–1111.

43. J.A. Ronald, J.W. Chen, Y. Chen, et al., 2009, Enzyme-sensitive magnetic resonance imaging targeting myeloperoxidase identifies active inflammation in experimental rabbit atherosclerotic plaques, *Circulation* 120: 592–599.

44. I. Rashid, G.J. Maghzal, Y.C. Chen, et al., 2018, Myeloperoxidase is a potential molecular imaging and therapeutic target for the identification and stabilization of high-risk atherosclerotic plaque, *Eur. Heart J.* 39: 3301–3310.

45. R.M. Nagra, B. Becher, W.W. Tourtellotte, et al., 1997, Immunohistochemical and genetic evidence of myeloperoxidase involvement in multiple sclerosis, *J. Neuroimmunol.* 78: 97–107.

46. F. Cotton, H.L. Weiner, F.A. Jolesz, C.R. Guttmann, 2003, MRI contrast uptake in new lesions in relapsing-remitting MS followed at weekly intervals, *Neurology* 60: 640–646.

47. J.W. Chen, M.O. Breckwoldt, E. Aikawa, G. Chiang, R. Weissleder, 2008, Myeloperoxidase-targeted imaging of active inflammatory lesions in murine experimental autoimmune encephalomyelitis, *Brain* 131: 1123–1133.

48. B. Pulli, G.R. Wojtkiewicz, Y. Iwamoto, M. Ali, D. Li, S. Schob, K.L. Hsieh, A.H. Jacobs, J.W. Chen, 2015, Multiple sclerosis: myeloperoxidase immunoradiology improves detection of acute and chronic disease in experimental model, *Radiology* 275: 480–489.

49. R. Forghani, G.R. Wojtkiewicz, Y. Zhang, et al., 2012, Demyelinating diseases: myeloperoxidase as an imaging biomarker and therapeutic target, *Radiology* 263: 451–460.

50. A. Li, Y. Wu, B. Pulli, et al., 2019, Myeloperoxidase molecular MRI reveals synergistic combination therapy in murine experimental autoimmune neuroinflammation, *Radiology* 293: 158–165.

51. S.S. Rensen, Y. Slaats, J. Nijhuis, et al., 2009, Increased hepatic myeloperoxidase activity in obese subjects with nonalcoholic steatohepatitis, *Am. J. Pathol.* 175: 1473–1482.

52. B. Pulli, M. Ali, Y. Iwamoto, et al., 2015, Myeloperoxidase-hepatocyte-stellate cell cross talk promotes hepatocyte injury and fibrosis in experimental nonalcoholic steatohepatitis, *Antioxid. Redox Signal.* 23: 1255–1269.

53. S.S. Rensen, V. Bieghs, S. Xanthoulea, et al., 2012, Neutrophil-derived myeloperoxidase aggravates non-alcoholic steatohepatitis in low-density lipoprotein receptor-deficient mice, *PLoS One* 7: e52411.

54. B. Pulli, G. Wojtkiewicz, Y. Iwamoto, et al., 2017, Molecular MR imaging of myeloperoxidase distinguishes steatosis from steatohepatitis in nonalcoholic fatty liver disease, *Radiology* 284: 390–400.

55. Y.Z. Wadghiri, D.M. Hoang, A. Leporati, et al., 2018, High-resolution imaging of myeloperoxidase activity sensors in human cerebrovascular disease, *Sci. Rep.* 8: 7687.

56. A. Rodriguez-Rodriguez, S. Shuvaev, N. Rotile, et al., 2019, Peroxidase sensitive amplifiable probe for molecular magnetic resonance imaging of pulmonary inflammation, *ACS Sens.* 4: 2412–2419.

57. Wang, D. Cheng, N. Jalali Motlagh, et al., 2021. Highly efficient activatable MRI probe to sense myeloperoxidase activity. *J. Med. Chem.* 64(9), 5874–5885. doi:10.1021/acs.jmedchem.1c00038

58. C. Wang, E. Keliher, M.W.G. Zeller, et al., 2019, An activatable PET imaging radioprobe is a dynamic reporter of myeloperoxidase activity in vivo, *Proc. Natl. Acad. Sci. U.S.A.* 116: 11966–11971.

59. L. Tang, Z. Wang, Q. Mu, et al., 2020, Targeting neutrophils for enhanced cancer theranostics, *Adv. Mater.* 32: e2002739.

60. P. Johnstrom, L. Bergman, K. Varnas, et al., 2015, Development of rapid multistep carbon-11 radiosynthesis of the myeloperoxidase inhibitor AZD3241 to assess brain exposure by PET microdosing, *Nucl. Med. Biol.* 42: 555–560.

CHAPTER THIRTEEN

Role of Myeloperoxidase in Endothelial Dysfunction and Altered Cell Signaling in Atherosclerosis

Benjamin S. Rayner
Heart Research Institute
University of Sydney

CONTENTS

VASOACTIVE MPO EXERTS DETRIMENTAL EFFECTS ON ENDOTHELIAL NITRIC OXIDE SIGNALING

The endothelium lines the inner surface of the circulatory system and comprises a cellular monolayer, which functions as a structural barrier between the blood and vessel wall, producing a range of bioactive molecules that serve to maintain and regulate vascular tone and hemostasis. Furthermore, through production of a variety of signaling molecules, endothelial cells protect against inflammation, oxidative stress, and the coagulation cascade upon injury. As such the endothelium is crucial to and involved in every aspect in the modulation of blood flow in the body [1].

The endothelium regulates blood vessel dilatation through the production and release of nitric oxide (NO), by endothelial nitric oxide synthase (eNOS). NO diffuses and acts on the underlying vascular smooth muscle, causing relaxation through the stimulation of soluble guanylate cyclase (sGC) and cyclic guanosine monophosphate (cGMP) signaling (Figure 13.1), a mechanism that also has antiproliferative and anti-migratory effects on the vascular smooth muscle cells [2,3]. Any disruption, therefore, to the mechanisms of NO production and delivery results in ongoing vasoconstriction, adversely effecting vessel homeostasis. The process of atherosclerosis is characterized by abnormal endothelium-derived NO bioavailability, and as such endothelial dysfunction directly contributes to plaque formation and activation within the setting of atherosclerosis, as well as being inexorably linked to ongoing clinical manifestations, such as myocardial ischemia and resultant heart failure [3].

The production and release of MPO by infiltrating immune cells, such as neutrophils, monocytes, and macrophages, occur at sites of inflammation within the vasculature (Figure 13.2) and have a direct effect on the endothelium through its interaction with the endothelial glycocalyx [4]. Additionally, MPO can further affect NO bioavailability through mechanisms that include altering expression and activity of eNOS, as well as MPO favoring NO as a physiological substrate [5]. MPO-derived reactive intermediates are also able to oxidize this signaling molecule, leading to its reduced bioavailability [6,7].

DOI: 10.1201/9781003212287-17

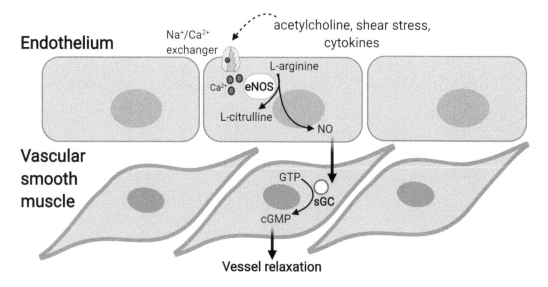

Figure 13.1 Endothelial cell production of nitric oxide (NO) leading to vessel relaxation.

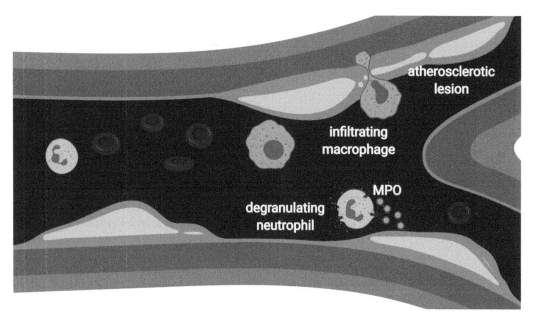

Figure 13.2 The production and release of myeloperoxidase by immune cells within the vasculature.

Both MPO and its reaction products are present and active within human atherosclerotic plaques [8,9]. In addition, MPO is an independent risk factor for the development of coronary artery disease [10], with circulating MPO levels strongly correlating with the risk of endothelial dysfunction in humans [11]. However, somewhat paradoxical to the traditional notion of the involvement of MPO directly in the progression of atherosclerosis, early modeling of atherosclerosis in mice deficient in MPO demonstrated an increase in lesion formation, compared with wild-type controls [12]. In this study, lesions from MPO-deficient mice were found to be 50% larger than those within their control counterparts, concurrent with increased infiltration of monocytes. The authors hypothesized that a potential protective effect of MPO within the setting of atherosclerosis may be due to the ability of the enzyme to oxidatively inhibit the activation of pro-inflammatory molecules, including chemokines, cytokines, and proteases, resulting in reduced phagocyte infiltration and activity.

More recent data obtained in mouse models using a pharmacological MPO inhibitor revealed the crucial role of MPO activity and subsequent oxidation of sGC as the underlying cause of the reduced NO bioavailability that results in endothelial dysfunction within the setting of atherosclerosis [13]. Contrasting with the study by Brennan et al., MPO inhibition in this case did not affect either arterial MPO content or circulating inflammatory cytokines. It is possible, therefore, that any adverse effects shown in the earlier study are derived only from the complete absence of MPO in the setting of atherosclerosis, rather than the inhibition of active circulating MPO. In the latter study, the authors demonstrate a role for MPO activity in endothelial dysfunction through the use of a number of inflammatory-mediated models of endothelial dysfunction relevant to atherosclerosis [13]. Here, mice received a dietary supplement of AZM198 that resulted in 95% inhibition of extracellular MPO. AZM198 is a specific suicide inhibitor of MPO, which has a 2-thioxanthine structure [14]. It irreversibly inactivates the enzyme, through covalent attachment to the heme prosthetic group. As such, the inhibitor can prevent oxidative stress to the surrounding cells and tissue during the inflammatory response [14]. Supplementation with AZM198 significantly decreased the conversion of exogenously added hydroethidine to 2-Cl-E$^+$, a surrogate marker for the chlorinating activity of MPO [15], in the mouse plasma, and improved vessel function [13]. Moreover, the arteries from MPO/ApoE double-knockout mice demonstrated a greater endothelium-dependent relaxation compared with their ApoE knockout mouse counterparts [13]. This was dependent on eNOS activity and was inhibited by prior incubation of the vessel segments with the eNOS inhibitor N-nitroarginine methyl ester (L-NAME) [13]. Lastly, while NO levels were not affected by MPO blockage, inhibition of MPO increased arterial cGMP concentration, consistent with oxidation and subsequent inhibition of sGC as the underlying mechanism of endothelial dysfunction [13].

Hypochlorous acid (HOCl) is one of the major oxidants produced through MPO activity [16]. In addition to the direct role of active MPO (and resultant oxidant generation) on NO bioavailability and endothelial dysfunction, exposure to pathophysiological concentrations of HOCl has also been shown to selectively impair endothelial function in both a time- and concentration-dependent

manner [3]. Here incubation of thoracic aorta, obtained from atherosclerotic rabbits, with HOCl concentrations as low as 100 μM caused impairment of endothelial-dependent acetylcholine-induced relaxation within 5 min of exposure to the oxidant. Furthermore, it was shown that this vessel impairment occurred in the absence of any endothelial morphological changes or loss of cell viability, but with significant increases to the amount of HOCl-modified proteins within the endothelium. Subsequent endothelial cellular studies determined that exposure to HOCl caused a dose-dependent decrease in eNOS activity and resultant NO bioavailability, strikingly similar to the results demonstrated in the inhibition studies of MPO activity mentioned above [13].

In humans, increased eNOS oxidation as evidenced by disruption of the dimer structure is associated with MPO in atherosclerotic plaques isolated from carotid arteries [17]. This was attributed to the production of HOCl, as exposure of recombinant eNOS or human umbilical vein endothelial cells (HUVEC) to this oxidant resulted in the release of zinc and enzyme inactivation via disruption of the eNOS dimers [17]. Interestingly, in HUVECs, the eNOS uncoupling was associated with an increase in superoxide ($O_2^{\bullet-}$) production, translocation of NADPH oxidase subunits p67^{phox} and p47^{phox}, and the phosphorylation protein kinase C [17]. Similarly, treatment of isolated murine aortic tissue with HOCl increased the oxidation of eNOS dimers and promoted $O_2^{\bullet-}$ and peroxynitrite (ONOO$^-$) formation [17]. This led to the conclusion that HOCl could uncouple eNOS by a pathway involving the generation of ONOO$^-$ and activation of NADPH oxidase [17].

It has long been established within the setting of atherosclerosis that overproduction of $O_2^{\bullet-}$ can adversely affect NO bioavailability, resulting in endothelial dysfunction [18]. Indeed, pharmacological inhibition of superoxide production or supplementation of the endogenous antioxidant superoxide dismutase (SOD) is able to, at least partially, restore vessel function within the setting of atherosclerosis [19,20]. Interestingly, $O_2^{\bullet-}$ itself can enhance MPO production of HOCl, with SOD able to inhibit the chlorinating ability of the enzyme [21], providing a link between these two oxidant species. HOCl-mediated impairment of NO bioactivity and eNOS dimer instability are both prevented by the addition of a SOD mimetic, consistent with HOCl-induced endothelial dysfunction being at least in part, dependent on $O_2^{\bullet-}$ production [3,17].

The other major MPO-derived oxidant, hypothiocyanous acid (HOSCN), also exerts detrimental effects on NO signaling by endothelial cells. Exposure of either cultured HCAEC or rat aortic segments to HOSCN decreases l-citrulline formation and the subsequent reduction of cGMP activity [22]. Similarly, exposure of isolated recombinant human eNOS to increasing pathophysiological concentrations of HOSCN results in the dose-dependent inactivation of the enzyme, results mirroring the previous experiments assaying active MPO [5] or HOCl [3,17]. As with HOCl, exposure of eNOS to HOSCN was accompanied by a parallel release of Zn^{2+}, indicating the targeting of the zinc–sulfur cluster of the enzyme [22].

In addition to the ongoing endothelial dysfunction and chronic inflammation, atherosclerosis in its earliest stages is characterized by the accumulation of oxidized low-density lipoprotein (oxLDL) within the vessel wall [23]. The formation of oxLDL can also cause endothelial dysfunction through impairment of NO bioavailability [24,25]. It is well established that low-density lipoprotein is target for MPO and HOCl in vivo (see Chapter 7). Briefly, MPO-LDL complexes are present in the circulation of patients with atherosclerosis [26–28] and the MPO-derived oxidants, HOCl and HOSCN, both react to produce modified LDL, which has numerous pro-atherogenic properties (e.g. [27,29–31]). Thus, modification LDL by HOCl decreases the endothelial synthesis of NO [32]. Similarly, incubation of rat aortic vessel segments with HOCl or HOSCN-modified LDL results in significant impairment of endothelial-dependent relaxation in response to acetylcholine [33]. This was attributed to loss of eNOS activity and subsequent NO production upon exposure to the modified LDL, on the basis of the in vitro experiments with human coronary arterial endothelial cells (HCAECs) [33].

In summary, it is evident that MPO itself, oxidants linked to MPO activity, or MPO-modified LDL are all capable of causing vessel dysfunction within the setting of atherosclerosis, with the in vivo detrimental perturbations largely dependent on the endothelial maintenance of the NO signaling pathway. Not only is endothelial dysfunction one of the major hallmarks of the atherosclerotic process, endothelial cells are recognized as one of the primary targets of MPO-derived oxidant-mediated damage. However, in addition to HOCl being able to cause impairment of endothelium-dependent relaxation and inducing endothelial cell dysfunction [34], an infusion of HOCl into carotid arteries in vivo is sufficient enough to result in neointima formation, which is also relevant to atherosclerosis [35]. Similarly, HOCl modulates endothelium function through decreasing the adhesiveness of extracellular matrix proteins for endothelial cells [36] and by converting matrix metalloproteinases into their active form [37]. This destabilizes the vascular and tissue environment surrounding the endothelial cells [38]. Furthermore, HOCl and HOSCN both cause ongoing endothelial cell damage, dysfunction, and death, potentially contributing to the pathophysiology of atherosclerosis (discussed below).

ENDOTHELIAL INTRACELLULAR SIGNALING MECHANISMS INVOKED BY MPO-DERIVED OXIDANTS

The activation of endothelial cell signaling pathways following exposure to HOCl was first demonstrated in HUVECs [39]. Exposure of HUVECs to between 20 and $40\,\mu M$ HOCl resulted in rapid activation of the extracellular signal-regulated mitogen-activated protein (MAP) kinase (ERK 1/2) pathway within 2 min and activation of the p38 MAP kinase pathway within 15 min, which was sustained for as long as 60 min post-oxidant exposure before returning to basal levels [39]. ERK 1/2 activation plays a pivotal function in cell growth and differentiation and, along with p38 activation, is increasingly being shown to confer a survival advantage to cells as a part of their adaptive response to detrimental environmental conditions such as when exposed to oxidative stress. In confirmation of the pro-survival nature of ERK 1/2 activation in this setting, pharmacological inhibition of the ERK MAP kinase pathway significantly decreased the proportion of viable cells across all concentrations of HOCl tested [39].

In comparison, endothelial cell exposure to HOSCN results in the activation of cellular signaling mechanisms that are associated with the thrombotic events that lead to the development of atherosclerosis [40]. Exposure of HUVEC to up to $100\,\mu M$ HOSCN leads to a significant sevenfold increase in tissue factor (TF) activity, one of the primary initiators of thrombosis. Mirroring the pathway activation shown in these cells upon incubation with HOCl [39], induction of

TF activity by HOSCN was shown to be dependent on the phosphorylation of the extracellular signal-regulated kinases (ERK) 1/2 pathway, here through NFκB activation.

The expression of a variety of adhesion molecules, including E-selectin, intercellular adhesion molecule 1 (ICAM-1), and vascular cell adhesion molecule 1 (VCAM-1), on the endothelial cell surface is also regulated by NFκB activity [41]. Exposure of HUVEC to pathophysiological levels of HOSCN resulted in the increased surface expression of E-selectin, ICAM-1, and VCAM-1, with inhibition of NFκB activity blocking the expression of these adhesion molecules. The subsequent coculturing of HOSCN-activated endothelial cells with isolated human neutrophils resulted in a significant increase in neutrophil adhesion to the endothelial cell surface, demonstrating a functional consequence of upregulation of cell surface marker expression by HOSCN [41]. Antibody blocking of E-selectin on the endothelial cell surface or, similarly, the counter-ligand for ICAM-1 on neutrophils, CD11b/CD18, decreased the HOSCN-induced neutrophil adhesion by approximately 40%. Furthermore, the pivotal role for NFκB in these processes was ascertained using the specific NFκB inhibitor andrographolide, also attenuating these processes.

ENDOTHELIAL GLUTATHIONE IS A MAJOR TARGET OF MPO-DERIVED OXIDANTS

Glutathione (GSH) is the major low-molecular-weight thiol in most cells and is one of the initial cellular targets for HOCl, playing a crucial role against oxidative injury. Perfusion of the lungs with 1 μM HOCl caused a sixfold increase in vascular permeability that was associated with a 60% decrease in tissue concentrations of both GSH and nonprotein thiols [42]. Similarly, in vitro exposure of endothelial cells to increasing concentrations of HOCl results in a dose-dependent decrease in protein thiols, with 50% of cellular protein thiols modified upon exposure to 50 μM HOCl, indicating that at least one in four HOCl molecules were reacting with a protein thiol within the cell at this concentration [43]. Exposure of cultured HCAEC to HOCl concentrations of above 50 μM caused a 50% decrease in cellular GSH levels over controls within 15 min of exposure that was accompanied by significant decreases in overall cellular thiols in endothelial cells exposed to HOCl concentrations

between 100 and 200 μM [44]. Interestingly, despite the propensity of HOSCN for thiol groups, in this study the authors were unable to show loss of GSH upon HOSCN exposure and only significant loss of total thiols within these cells upon exposure to the pathophysiological level of 400 μM HOSCN. Use of thiol-specific, fluorescent, intracellular labeling provided further evidence for protein thiol oxidation in HCAEC following exposure to HOCl, but not HOSCN, suggesting that HOSCN may exert cellular effects through its interaction with membrane receptors, rather than intracellular processes [44].

MPO-DERIVED OXIDANTS PERTURB CALCIUM HANDLING IN ENDOTHELIAL CELLS

HOCl-induced oxidation of protein thiols can lead to irreversible modification of cellular enzymes [45]. A pertinent example of this is found in the activity of sarco/endoplasmic reticulum (SR) control of the flux of Ca^{2+} between intracellular stores and the cytosol, which is controlled by the SR Ca^{2+} ATPases (SERCA). Within the SR, more than 90% of free protein thiols are located on SERCA with each molecule possessing 26 thiol-containing cysteine residues, six of which are in disulfide bonds, leaving 20 free thiol groups susceptible to potential oxidation [46]. Importantly, these free thiol groups are crucial to the activity of SERCA, as indicated by studies showing that oxidation or blocking of these thiol groups with thiol-directed reagents leads to the loss of SERCA activity that is concomitant with cytosolic Ca^{2+} accumulation [47]. Isolated SR vesicles exposed to either HOCl or HOSCN result in the oxidation of thiol residues on SERCA [48]. In this study, the authors exposed SR vesicles to either HOCl for 1 h or HOSCN for 2 h and found that oxidant concentrations as low as 10 μM were able to induce a significant 60% reduction in SERCA activity [48]. This was accompanied by the significant loss of SERCA thiol groups, measurable upon exposure to ≥25 μM of either oxidant [48]. Furthermore, exposure of HCAEC to <20 μM HOCl or HOSCN resulted in a concentration-dependent increase in intracellular Ca^{2+} release from internal stores, which could be abolished by blocking of SERCA activity through the use of thapsigargin [48].

It has become increasingly apparent that disruption to cellular Ca^{2+} handling mechanisms is a critical determinate of endothelial cell survival.

One of the major intracellular outcomes of cytosolic increases in free Ca^{2+} due to the disruption in the Ca^{2+} handling abilities of cells is an increase in the extent of mitochondrial dysfunction. Mitochondria are responsible for cellular respiration and maintenance of cellular energy stores through the production of ATP. While cytosolic Ca^{2+} accumulation can be compensated for by mitochondrial Ca^{2+} uptake to some extent, an increase in mitochondrial Ca^{2+} accelerates the rate of respiration. This results in a reduction of membrane potential ($\Delta\Psi_m$) causing further cellular dysfunction and death through the increased generation of reactive oxygen species and loss of cellular ATP. Exposure of HCAEC to concentrations of $\geq 25\,\mu M$ HOCl resulted in a significant decrease in $\Delta\Psi_m$, reaching 50% of that of control cells within 1 h of treatment [44]. In contrast, exposure of HCAEC to $100\,\mu M$ HOSCN for 2 h was required in order to achieve an equivalent extent of mitochondrial dysfunction (altered $\Delta\Psi_m$). In support of the notion that HOSCN exerts detrimental effects on mitochondrial and cellular function, exposure of HCAEC cells to $100\,\mu M$ HOSCN in this instance also resulted in the significant release of mitochondrial proapoptotic proteins cytochrome c, apoptosis-inducing factor, and endonuclease G within 2 h of exposure [44]. Similarly, the oxidative inactivation of mitochondrial aconitase has been implicated in mitochondrial dysfunction within a number of disease settings, owing to its role in the Krebs citric acid cycle and function as iron response protein-1, binding specific mRNA sequences to regulate cellular iron levels [49]. Exposure of HCAEC to HOSCN resulted in a significant reduction in cellular aconitase activity and increase in iron release from the cells [49]. Interestingly, HCAEC exposure to HOCl required substantially higher concentrations of the oxidant in order to effect a significant decrease in aconitase activity and resultant iron release from the cells [49]. This was attributed to the greater thiol specificity of HOSCN compared with HOCl (see Chapter 4), resulting in direct targeting of Cys residues at or near the iron–sulfur cluster active site of aconitase [49], consistent with the ability of HOSCN to disrupt the zinc–sulfur clusters within eNOS [22]. Together, these data confirm the ability of both MPO-derived oxidants to induce mitochondrial dysfunction within endothelial cells and highlight specific mechanisms involved in potentiating cell death.

EXPOSURE TO MPO-DERIVED OXIDANTS CAUSES ENDOTHELIAL CELL DEATH

Exposure to either HOCl or HOSCN induces endothelial cell death, which is dependent on both the timing and concentrations of the oxidants studied. Within HUVECs, concentrations of $25–40\,\mu M$ HOCl cause hallmarks of an apoptotic cell death mechanism including cell membrane blebbing, nuclear chromatin condensation, increased binding of Annexin V, and caspase activation of up to tenfold compared with controls, which can be blocked by preincubation with the pan-caspase inhibitor Z-VAD-fmk [50]. This apparent initiation of apoptosis at lower concentrations of oxidant has also been obtained through the use of a variety of sources of endothelial cells including cells isolated from human saphenous veins [38] as well as HCAEC [44]. Consistently, lower doses between 5 and $25\,\mu M$ HOCl caused significant increases in the extent of apoptotic cell death with increased binding of Annexin V, DNA fragmentation, caspase activity, and mitochondrial cytochrome c release that was coupled with decreased expression of the antiapoptotic Bcl-2 [38]. In comparison, exposure of endothelial cells to HOCl concentrations of greater than $25\,\mu M$ led to an increasing proportion of necrotic cell death [38,44].

The occurrence of necrotic cell death was evidenced in some of the earliest investigations into the effect of HOCl on the endothelium, performed within HUVEC cultures. Two such studies published simultaneously [50,51] both demonstrate the rapid and dose-dependent release of radiolabeled ^{51}Cr into the cell culture supernatant upon exposure to concentrations of HOCl between 10 and $50\,\mu M$. This release of ^{51}Cr, indicative of cell lysis, occurred within 15–30 min and equated to approximately 50% cell lysis following exposure to $50\,\mu M$ HOCl. Increasing the concentration of HOCl to $100\,\mu M$ resulted in the complete lysis of the cells within 2 h of exposure, confirming the susceptibility of endothelial cells to concentrations of HOCl well within the range that is physiologically achievable within in vivo situations [50]. Similarly, subsequent studies utilizing either HCAEC [44] or porcine brain microvascular endothelial cells (BMVEC) [52] both confirmed the ability of HOCl to cause rapid cell death. Similarly, in HUVEC cultures exposed to concentrations of HOCl greater than $50\,\mu M$, extensive cell necrosis was evident commencing within 15 min of exposure and remaining elevated for up to 6 h.

In comparison, assessment of HCAEC cell death upon exposure to increasing concentrations of HOSCN demonstrated that over a 2 h period, there was no increase over controls of the level of necrosis evident. Concentrations of the oxidant as low as 25 μM were, however, able to induce significant 30% increase in the extent of apoptosis within 1 h of exposure, with apoptotic cell death accountable within 60% of the cell population when measured at 2 h exposure to 100 μM of the oxidant [44]. However, the treatment conditions employed and cell type are important in determining the extent and nature of HOSCN-mediated cell death (reviewed in Refs. [53,54]). Thus, exposure of HUVECs to HOSCN, while resulting in marked morphological changes, did not show any evidence of apoptosis [55]. Moreover, HOSCN treatment actually inhibited apoptosis in this case via inactivation of thiol-dependent caspases [55]. Taken together, the combination of these results confirms the ability of the two major MPO-derived oxidants in the vasculature, HOCl and HOSCN, to invoke endothelial cell death that is mechanistically relevant within the chronic inflammatory setting of atherosclerosis.

CONCLUSION

Endothelial cell exposure to MPO and MPO-derived oxidants causes substantial cell dysfunction and death, involving mechanisms of altered Ca^{2+} handling, leading to mitochondrial dysfunction and, ultimately, both apoptotic and necrotic death. The in vivo manifestation of exposure to active MPO and its products in the circulation is the detrimental alteration to vascular function [56,57], accentuated by the disruption to endothelial NO signaling and the endothelial inflammatory response [11,17]. Together, these effects play a critical role in driving atherosclerotic lesion formation and disease progression. These factors combined highlight MPO activity as a potential therapeutic target for the treatment of cardiovascular diseases.

REFERENCES

1. S. Giannitsi, M. Bougiakli, A. Bechlioulis, K. Naka, 2019, Endothelial dysfunction and heart failure: a review of the existing bibliography with emphasis on flow mediated dilation, JRSM Cardiovasc. Dis. 8: 2048004019843047.

2. S. Moncada, E.A. Higgs, 1991, Endogenous nitric oxide: physiology, pathology and clinical relevance, Eur. J. Clin. Invest. 21: 361–374.

3. R. Stocker, A. Huang, E. Jeranian, et al., 2004, Hypochlorous acid impairs endothelium-derived nitric oxide bioactivity through a superoxide-dependent mechanism, Arterioscler. Thromb. Vasc. Biol. 24: 2028–2033.

4. K. Manchanda, H. Kolarova, C. Kerkenpass, et al., 2018, MPO (myeloperoxidase) reduces endothelial glycocalyx thickness dependent on its cationic charge, Arterioscler. Thromb. Vasc. Biol. 38: 1859–1867.

5. D. Lau, S. Baldus, 2006, Myeloperoxidase and its contributory role in inflammatory vascular disease, Pharmacol. Ther. 111: 16–26.

6. S.L. Maiocchi, J.C. Morris, M.D. Rees, S.R. Thomas, 2017, Regulation of the nitric oxide oxidase activity of myeloperoxidase by pharmacological agents, Biochem. Pharmacol. 135: 90–115.

7. J.P. Eiserich, S. Baldus, M.L. Brennan, et al., 2002, Myeloperoxidase, a leukocyte-derived vascular NO oxidase, Science 296: 2391–2394.

8. A. Daugherty, J.L. Dunn, D.L. Rateri, J.W. Heinecke, 1994, Myeloperoxidase, a catalyst for lipoprotein oxidation, is expressed in human atherosclerotic lesions, J. Clin. Invest. 94: 437–444.

9. S.L. Hazen, J.W. Heinecke, 1997, 3-Chlorotyrosine, a specific marker of myeloperoxidase-catalysed oxidation, is markedly elevated in low density lipoprotein isolated from human atherosclerotic intima, J. Clin. Invest. 99: 2075–2081.

10. R. Zhang, M.L. Brennan, X. Fu, et al., 2001, Association between myeloperoxidase levels and risk of coronary artery disease, J. Am. Med. Assoc. 286: 2136–2142.

11. J.A. Vita, M.L. Brennan, N. Gokce, et al., 2004, Serum myeloperoxidase levels independently predict endothelial dysfunction in humans, Circulation 110: 1134–1139.

12. M.L. Brennan, M.M. Anderson, D.M. Shih, et al., 2001, Increased atherosclerosis in myeloperoxidase-deficient mice, J. Clin. Invest. 107: 419–430.

13. D. Cheng, J. Talib, C.P. Stanley, et al., 2019, Inhibition of MPO (myeloperoxidase) attenuates endothelial dysfunction in mouse models of vascular inflammation and atherosclerosis, Arterioscler. Thromb. Vasc. Biol. 39: 1448–1457.

14. A.K. Tiden, T. Sjogren, M. Svensson, et al., 2011, 2-thioxanthines are mechanism-based inactivators of myeloperoxidase that block oxidative stress during inflammation, *J. Biol. Chem.* 286: 37578–37589.

15. G.J. Maghzal, K.M. Cergol, S.R. Shengule, et al., 2014, Assessment of myeloperoxidase activity by the conversion of hydroethidine to 2-chloroethidium, *J. Biol. Chem.* 289: 5580–5595.

16. J.E. Harrison, J. Schultz, 1976, Studies on the chlorinating activity of myeloperoxidase, *J. Biol. Chem.* 251: 1371–1374.

17. J. Xu, Z. Xie, R. Reece, D. Pimental, M.H. Zou, 2006, Uncoupling of endothelial nitric oxidase synthase by hypochlorous acid: role of NAD(P) H oxidase-derived superoxide and peroxynitrite, *Arterioscler. Thromb. Vasc. Biol.* 26: 2688–2695.

18. J.S. Beckman, T.W. Beckman, J. Chen, P.A. Marshall, B.A. Freeman, 1990, Apparent hydroxyl radical production by peroxynitrite: implications for endothelial injury from nitric oxide and superoxide, *Proc. Natl. Acad. Sci. U.S.A.* 87: 1620–1624.

19. A. Mugge, J.H. Elwell, T.E. Peterson, et al., 1991, Chronic treatment with polyethylene-glycolated superoxide dismutase partially restores endothelium-dependent vascular relaxations in cholesterol-fed rabbits, *Circ. Res.* 69: 1293–1300.

20. Y. Ohara, T.E. Peterson, D.G. Harrison, 1993, Hypercholesterolemia increases endothelial superoxide anion production, *J. Clin. Invest.* 91: 2546–2551.

21. A.J. Kettle, C.C. Winterbourn, 1988, Superoxide modulates the activity of myeloperoxidase and optimizes the production of hypochlorous acid, *Biochem. J.* 252: 529–536.

22. J. Talib, J. Kwan, A. Suryo Rahmanto, P.K. Witting, M.J. Davies, 2014, The smoking-associated oxidant hypothiocyanous acid induces endothelial nitric oxide synthase dysfunction, *Biochem. J.* 457: 89–97.

23. R. Stocker, J.F. Keaney, Jr., 2004, Role of oxidative modifications in atherosclerosis, *Physiol. Rev.* 84: 1381–1478.

24. A. Blair, P.W. Shaul, I.S. Yuhanna, P.A. Conrad, E.J. Smart, 1999, Oxidized low density lipoprotein displaces endothelial nitric-oxide synthase (eNOS) from plasmalemmal caveolae and impairs eNOS activation, *J. Biol. Chem.* 274: 32512–32519.

25. T.W. Hein, J.C. Liao, L. Kuo, 2000, oxLDL specifically impairs endothelium-dependent, NO-mediated dilation of coronary arterioles, *Am. J. Physiol. Heart Circ. Physiol.* 278: H175–H183.

26. A.C. Carr, M.C. Myzak, R. Stocker, M.R. McCall, B. Frei, 2000, Myeloperoxidase binds to low-density lipoprotein: potential implications for atherosclerosis, *FEBS Lett.* 487: 176–180.

27. C. Delporte, K.Z. Boudjeltia, C. Noyon, et al., 2014, Impact of myeloperoxidase-LDL interactions on enzyme activity and subsequent posttranslational oxidative modifications of apoB-100, *J. Lipid Res.* 55: 747–757.

28. A.V. Sokolov, V.A. Kostevich, O.L. Runova, et al., 2014, Proatherogenic modification of LDL by surface-bound myeloperoxidase, *Chem. Phys. Lipids* 180: 72–80.

29. F.O. Ismael, T.J. Barrett, D. Sheipouri, et al., 2016, Role of myeloperoxidase oxidants in the modulation of cellular lysosomal enzyme function: a contributing factor to macrophage Dysfunction in Atherosclerosis? *PLoS One* 11: e0168844.

30. E. Malle, G. Marsche, J. Arnhold, M.J. Davies, 2006, Modification of low-density lipoprotein by myeloperoxidase-derived oxidants and reagent hypochlorous acid, *Biochim. Biophys. Acta* 1761: 392–415.

31. L.J. Hazell, R. Stocker, 1993, Oxidation of low-density lipoprotein with hypochlorite causes transformation of the lipoprotein into a high-uptake form for macrophages, *Biochem. J.* 290: 165–172.

32. A. Nuszkowski, R. Grabner, G. Marsche, et al., 2001, Hypochlorite-modified low density lipoprotein inhibits nitric oxide synthesis in endothelial cells via an intracellular dislocalization of endothelial nitric-oxide synthase, *J. Biol. Chem.* 276: 14212–14221.

33. A.I. Abdo, B.S. Rayner, D.M. van Reyk, C.L. Hawkins, 2017, Low-density lipoprotein modified by myeloperoxidase oxidants induces endothelial dysfunction, *Redox Biol.* 13: 623–632.

34. C. Zhang, R. Patel, J.P. Eiserich, et al., 2001, Endothelial dysfunction is induced by proinflammatory oxidant hypochlorous acid, *Am. J. Physiol. Heart Circ. Physiol.* 281: H1469–H1475.

35. J. Yang, Y. Cheng, R. Ji, C. Zhang, 2006, Novel model of inflammatory neointima formation reveals a potential role of myeloperoxidase in neointimal hyperplasia, *Am. J. Physiol. Heart Circ. Physiol.* 291: H3087–H3093.

36. M.C. Vissers, C. Thomas, 1997, Hypochlorous acid disrupts the adhesive properties of subendothelial matrix, *Free Radic. Biol. Med.* 23: 401–411.

37. X. Fu, S.Y. Kassim, W.C. Parks, J.W. Heinecke, 2001, Hypochlorous acid oxygenates the cysteine switch domain of pro-matrilysin (MMP-7). A mechanism for matrix metalloproteinase activation and atherosclerotic plaque rupture by myeloperoxidase, J. Biol. Chem. 276: 41279–41287.

38. S. Sugiyama, K. Kugiyama, M. Aikawa, et al., 2004, Hypochlorous acid, a macrophage product, induces endothelial apoptosis and tissue factor expression: involvement of myeloperoxidase-mediated oxidant in plaque erosion and thrombogenesis, Arterioscler. Thromb. Vasc. Biol. 24: 1309–1314.

39. R.G. Midwinter, M.C. Vissers, C.C. Winterbourn, 2001, Hypochlorous acid stimulation of the mitogen-activated protein kinase pathway enhances cell survival, Arch. Biochem. Biophys. 394: 13–20.

40. J.G. Wang, S.A. Mahmud, J.A. Thompson, et al., 2006, The principal eosinophil peroxidase product, HOSCN, is a uniquely potent phagocyte oxidant inducer of endothelial cell tissue factor activity: a potential mechanism for thrombosis in eosinophilic inflammatory states, Blood 107: 558–565.

41. J.G. Wang, S.A. Mahmud, J. Nguyen, A. Slungaard, 2006, Thiocyanate-dependent induction of endothelial cell adhesion molecule expression by phagocyte peroxidases: a novel HOSCN-specific oxidant mechanism to amplify inflammation, J. Immunol. 177: 8714–8722.

42. S. Hammerschmidt, H. Wahn, 2004, The oxidants hypochlorite and hydrogen peroxide induce distinct patterns of acute lung injury, Biochim. Biophys. Acta 1690: 258–264.

43. J.M. Pullar, M.C. Vissers, C.C. Winterbourn, 2001, Glutathione oxidation by hypochlorous acid in endothelial cells produces glutathione sulfonamide as a major product but not glutathione disulfide, J. Biol. Chem. 276: 22120–22125.

44. M.M. Lloyd, M.A. Grima, B.S. Rayner, et al., 2013, Comparative reactivity of the myeloperoxidase-derived oxidants hypochlorous acid and hypothiocyanous acid with human coronary artery endothelial cells, Free Radic. Biol. Med. 65: 1352–1362.

45. A.V. Peskin, C.C. Winterbourn, 2006, Taurine chloramine is more selective than hypochlorous acid at targeting critical cysteines and inactivating creatine kinase and glyceraldehyde-3-phosphate dehydrogenase, Free Radic. Biol. Med. 40: 45–53.

46. M. Strosova, M. Skuciova, L. Horakova, 2005, Oxidative damage to Ca^{2+}-ATPase sarcoplasmic reticulum by HOCl and protective effect of some antioxidants, Biofactors 24: 111–116.

47. T.G. Favero, D. Colter, P.F. Hooper, J.J. Abramson, 1998, Hypochlorous acid inhibits $Ca(^{2+})$-ATPase from skeletal muscle sarcoplasmic reticulum, J. Appl. Physiol. 84: 425–430.

48. N.L. Cook, H.M. Viola, V.S. Sharov, et al., 2012, Myeloperoxidase-derived oxidants inhibit sarco/endoplasmic reticulum Ca^{2+}-ATPase activity and perturb Ca^{2+} homeostasis in human coronary artery endothelial cells, Free Radic. Biol. Med. 52: 951–961.

49. J. Talib, M.J. Davies, 2016, Exposure of aconitase to smoking-related oxidants results in iron loss and increased iron response protein-1 activity: potential mechanisms for iron accumulation in human arterial cells, J. Biol. Inorg. Chem. 21: 305–317.

50. M.C. Vissers, J.M. Pullar, M.B. Hampton, 1999, Hypochlorous acid causes caspase activation and apoptosis or growth arrest in human endothelial cells, Biochem. J. 344: 443–449.

51. J.M. Pullar, C.C. Winterbourn, M.C. Vissers, 1999, Loss of GSH and thiol enzymes in endothelial cells exposed to sublethal concentrations of hypochlorous acid, Am. J. Physiol. 277: H1505–H1512.

52. A. Ullen, G. Fauler, E. Bernhart, et al., 2012, Phloretin ameliorates 2-chlorohexadecanal-mediated brain microvascular endothelial cell dysfunction in vitro, Free Radic. Biol. Med. 53: 1770–1781.

53. B.S. Rayner, D.T. Love, C.L. Hawkins, 2014, Comparative reactivity of myeloperoxidase-derived oxidants with mammalian cells, Free Radic. Biol. Med. 71: 240–255.

54. M.J. Davies, C.L. Hawkins, 2020, The role of myeloperoxidase in biomolecule modification, chronic inflammation, and disease, Antioxid. Redox Signal. 32: 957–981.

55. S.M. Bozonet, A.P. Scott-Thomas, P. Nagy, M.C. Vissers, 2010, Hypothiocyanous acid is a potent inhibitor of apoptosis and caspase 3 activation in endothelial cells, Free Radic. Biol. Med. 49: 1054–1063.

56. T.K. Rudolph, S. Wipper, B. Reiter, et al., 2012, Myeloperoxidase deficiency preserves vasomotor function in humans, Eur. Heart J. 33: 1625–1634.

57. A. Klinke, E. Berghausen, K. Friedrichs, et al., 2018, Myeloperoxidase aggravates pulmonary arterial hypertension by activation of vascular Rho-kinase, JCI Insight 3: e97530.

CHAPTER FOURTEEN

Myeloperoxidase in Ischemic Heart Disease

Dennis Mehrkens, Simon Geißen, and Stephan Baldus
University Hospital Cologne
University of Cologne

Volker Rudolph
University Hospital of the Ruhr-University Bochum

CONTENTS

ABBREVIATIONS

ACS:	Acute coronary syndrome
Apo A-I:	Apolipoprotein A-I
Apo B-100:	Apolipoprotein B-100
CAD:	Coronary artery disease
ECM:	Extracellular matrix
ECs:	Endothelial cells
FMD:	Flow-mediated dilatation
HDL:	High-density lipoproteins
HOCl:	Hypochlorous acid
LDL:	Low-density lipoproteins
MI:	Myocardial infarction
MMP:	Matrix metalloproteinase
MPO:	Myeloperoxidase
NO$^\bullet$:	Nitric oxide
PMNs:	Polymorphonuclear neutrophils
ROS:	Reactive oxygen species
SMCs:	Smooth muscle cells

INTRODUCTION

The term ischemic heart disease refers to the consequences of reduced blood flow to the myocardium, which is typically caused by coronary artery disease (CAD) and its most serious complication, myocardial infarction (MI). CAD is the coronary manifestation of the systemic disease atherosclerosis, a pathological transition of the large and medium-sized arteries, which is one of the most common diseases in the world and the primary cause of death in industrialized nations [1]. Atherosclerosis is considered a chronic inflammatory disease underlying the pathologies of coronary heart disease, peripheral arterial disease and cerebrovascular disease [2]. The CANTOS study has shown for the first time a clinical benefit for Canakinumab as the first anti-inflammatory drug that is able to lower cardiovascular endpoints independent of lipid

DOI: 10.1201/9781003212287-18

reduction [3]. More recently, the LoDoCo2 trial in a similar manner demonstrated that colchicine, an inhibitor of cell proliferation that exhibits anti-inflammatory effects, significantly reduces the risk of adverse events in CAD patients [4]. The initial stages of the disease are driven by the dysfunction of endothelial cells (ECs), abnormal deposition of lipids in the intima and increased oxidative stress, followed by stimulation of the immune system. The first indication for a pivotal role of myeloperoxidase (MPO) in the development of atherosclerosis was the discovery that the enzyme is enriched within human atheroma [5]. This is further corroborated by chlorination of proteins within atheroma by the MPO-specific product hypochlorous acid (HOCl) [6]. Over the ensuing years, further biochemical and immuno-histochemical analyses confirmed the presence of MPO and its products within human atherosclerotic lesions [5,7–11]. Clinical studies have shown that MPO plasma levels identify risk patients with acute coronary syndromes, correlate with subsequent cardiovascular events and act as a strong predictor of mortality following MI [12,13]. This chapter focuses in particular on the role of MPO in the pathogenesis of ischemic heart disease and provides an overview of past and current experimental and clinical studies.

MPO PROMOTES ENDOTHELIAL DYSFUNCTION

Every major risk factor for atherosclerosis has been shown to promote a subclinical pathologic vascular phenotype called endothelial dysfunction. It constitutes one of the earliest changes of vessels undergoing atherosclerotic transformation [14]. Apart from classical risk factors, which certainly play the major part in its development (hypercholesterolemia, high blood pressure, smoking and diabetes mellitus), nonclassical risk factors such as air pollution, psychological stress or chronic inflammatory diseases (e.g. rheumatoid arthritis, psoriasis) are also involved in the development of endothelial dysfunction [15]. This condition is characterized by abnormal endothelial reactivity, releasing pro-fibrotic and pro-inflammatory factors that interfere with the vasoprotective mechanisms of the endothelium and disrupt nitric oxide (NO$^{\bullet}$)-dependent signal transduction [16]. The release of inflammatory cytokines initiates leukocyte recruitment to the

vascular wall. Among other leukocyte species, predominantly macrophages, polymorphonuclear neutrophils (PMNs) are also recruited to the site of endothelial dysfunction and upon activation secrete MPO from azurophilic granules [17]. As a cationic protein, MPO binds to the endothelial surface via electrostatic interactions [18]. Mechanistically, the study of Manchanda et al. showed that MPO leads to a collapse of the endothelial glycocalyx (EG) via physical interaction with heparan sulfate glycosaminoglycan residues of the endothelium, promoting leukocyte adhesion and potentially disrupting mechanosensing of the EG [19] (Figure 14.1, Table 14.1).

MPO then undergoes transcytosis into the sub-endothelial space and accumulates in proximity of NO$^{\bullet}$-producing ECs and the NO$^{\bullet}$ target, i.e. smooth muscle cells (SMC) [20,21]. A hallmark of endothelial dysfunction is the reduction of NO$^{\bullet}$ bioavailability, impairing vasodilation [22]. In this context, MPO-derived oxidants can disrupt endothelial function. NO$^{\bullet}$ is oxidized to nitrite and nitrogen dioxide either directly or by small radical intermediates that are formed when MPO enters the peroxidase cycle. In addition, HOCl derived from MPO can lead to chlorination of L-arginine, the substrate of endothelial nitric oxide synthase (eNOS), thereby inducing not only substrate depletion but also direct inhibition of eNOS [23]. Ex vivo studies in explanted rabbit aortic rings exposed to HOCl demonstrated an impaired endothelium-dependent relaxation [24,25] (Table 14.1). Various reactive oxygen species (ROS) produced by MPO uncouple eNOS, leading to reduced NO$^{\bullet}$ production and release of superoxide ($O_2^{\bullet-}$) [26]. The reaction of ROS with high-density lipoproteins (HDL) leads to delocalization of eNOS within the plasma membrane [27]. HOCl also compromises the activity of dimethylarginine dimethylaminohydrolase 1 (DDAH-1), which under inflammatory conditions leads to increased accumulation of the eNOS inhibitor asymmetric dimethylarginine (ADMA) and consequently to a reduction in NO$^{\bullet}$ production [28] (Figure 14.1).

These effects are reflected by functional consequences in animal models. The vasorelaxation of explanted aortas of MPO-deficient mice was less impaired when mice were treated with lipopolysaccharide compared with wild-type (WT) animals [29]. Furthermore, infusion of MPO-loaded red blood cells in mice provoked increased peripheral vasoconstriction [30]. In a large animal model, left atrial injection of MPO resulted

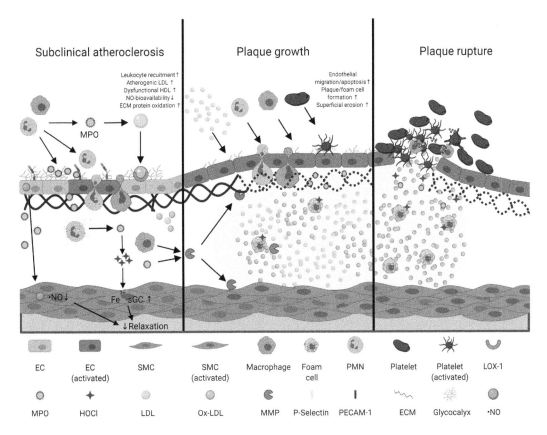

Figure 14.1 MPO promotes the development and progression of atherosclerosis. Abbreviations used: EC, endothelial cell; SMC, smooth muscle cell; PMN, polymorphonuclear neutrophil; LOX-1, lectin-like oxidized low-density lipoprotein 1; MPO, myeloperoxidase; HOCl, hypochlorous acid; LDL, low-density lipoprotein; Ox-LDL, oxidized low-density lipoprotein; MMP, matrix metalloproteinase; PECAM-1, platelet endothelial cell adhesion molecule 1; ECM, extracellular matrix; ·NO, nitric oxide.

TABLE 14.1
Effect of MPO and MPO-derived molecules on endothelial function

Authors	Year	Journal	Mechanistic claim	Experimental model	Key finding
Zhang et al.	2001	J. Biol. Chem.	L-Arginine chlorination	In vitro/ex vivo (rat aorta)	HOCl chlorinates L-arginine, compromising NO· synthase
Eiserich et al.	2002	Science	NO oxidation	In vitro/ex vivo (rat aorta)	MPO reduces NO bioavailability in the subendothelial space
Stocker et al.	2004	Arterioscler. Thromb.Vasc. Biol.	Superoxide formation	In vitro/ex vivo (rabbit aorta)	HOCl affects endothelial NO production due to a superoxide-dependent reduction of eNOS stability
Baldus et al.	2006	Circulation	MPO immobilized at EC layer	In vivo (human)	CAD patients exhibit increased amounts of immobilized MPO at the endothelium, impairing endothelial function

(Continued)

TABLE 14.1 (*Continued*)
Effect of MPO and MPO-derived molecules on endothelial function

Authors	Year	Journal	Mechanistic claim	Experimental model	Key finding
Rudolph et al.	2010	*Eur. Heart J.*	Vasomotor properties	In vivo (porcine and human)	PMN activation causes FMD reduction in humans that is alleviated in individuals with low MPO activity
Liu et al.	2012	*PLoS One*	Favorable effect of small molecule inhibitor	In vivo (ApoE$^{-/-}$ mice)	Small molecule inhibition of MPO alleviates endothelial dysfunction
Manchanda et al.	2018	*Arterioscler. Thromb.Vasc. Biol.*	Electrostatic interaction	In vitro/in vivo (mouse)	MPO leads to a collapse of the endothelial glycocalyx
Etwebi et al.	2018	*Hypertension*	Calpain activation, eNOS inhibition	In vitro/ex vivo (mouse aorta)	MPO increases the protease calpain and decreases Ser^{1177} phosphorylation of eNOS, thereby inflicting endothelial dysfunction
Cheng et al.	2019	*Arterioscler. Thromb.Vasc. Biol.*	Oxidation of sGC	In vivo (mouse)	MPO inhibition attenuates endothelial dysfunction by reduced oxidation of soluble guanylatecyclase

in reduced myocardial and peripheral blood flow [31]. Recently, MPO inhibition could attenuate endothelial dysfunction in multiple murine models of vascular injury and atherosclerosis, coinciding with reduced oxidation of soluble guanylate cyclase (sGC) [32,33] (Figure 14.1, Table 14.1**)**.

Clinical data support these experimental findings. MPO plasma levels were a strong and independent predictor of endothelial dysfunction in a cohort of 298 patients and volunteers without clinical evidence of congestive heart failure, CAD or high blood pressure. Even after adjustment for traditional risk factors, widespread cardiovascular disease (CVD) and medication, MPO remains a strong predictor of endothelial dysfunction [34]. Furthermore, plasma levels of MPO in patients with symptomatic CAD correlated inversely with endothelial vascular function [35]. In patients undergoing coronary angiography due to symptoms indicative of CAD, administration of heparin liberated vessel bound MPO and thereby unmasked a correlation of coronary lesions and intravascular MPO content. Additionally, removing the enzyme from the endothelial cell surface in this manner improved flow-mediated dilatation (FMD) of the brachial artery, which reflects

NO$^\bullet$-dependent vasodilation [21]. Even healthy individuals showed an inverse correlation of vascular endothelial function with the number of circulating neutrophils and MPO plasma levels due to the decreased NO$^\bullet$ response [36]. In persons with hereditary MPO deficiency, FMD was not affected by the activation of neutrophils, in contrast to MPO-competent subjects [31].

Overall, there is substantial experimental and clinical evidence that MPO impairs endothelial function in inflamed vessels. This effect is mediated by several catalytic and non-catalytic activities that altogether result in a reduction of NO$^\bullet$ bioavailability.

LIPIDS AND LIPOPROTEINS AND HOW THEY ARE AFFECTED BY THE RELEASE OF MPO

Apart from endothelial dysfunction, perhaps the most decisive factor in the pathogenesis of atherosclerosis is an imbalance in lipid metabolism. Of importance is the level of circulating cholesterol, which is present in the forms of lipoproteins in various density – high-density lipoprotein (HDL), low-density lipoprotein (LDL) and very low-density lipoprotein (VLDL) – conglomerates of phospholipids and apolipoproteins containing a core of cholesterol and cholesteryl esters. Specifically, increased LDL concentration is strongly associated with an increased risk of atherosclerosis and its coronary consequence, CAD [37]. Its abundance in the circulation impacts the probability of cholesterols infiltrating the vessel intima of arteries, most impressively apparent in the case of familial hypercholesteremia, where mutations in the LDL receptor, apolipoprotein B-100 (Apo B-100) or proprotein convertase subtilisin/kexin type 9 (PSCK9) reduce cellular uptake of LDL. Patients suffering from any of these conditions have an up to fivefold increase in risk of atherosclerotic CVD independent of other risk factors [38] and reduction of LDL serum levels is a pillar stone of CAD therapy.

But it is not only the abundancy of LDL in the circulation that is a risk factor for atherosclerosis. The pathogenic character of LDL apparently depends on its oxidation: Highly oxidized LDL, so-called ox-LDL, is not capable of binding to the LDL receptor and therefore is unable to leave the circulation in a physiological manner [39]. Additionally, it is more prone to uptake by monocytes and macrophages, which detect it via scavenger receptors such as cluster of differentiation 36/platelet glycoprotein 4 (CD36) or lectin-type oxidized LDL receptor 1 (LOX-1) [40,41]. Continuous intracellular accumulation of cholesterol then leads to the much described transition of beneficial, scavenging phagocytes to pathogenic foam cells [42]. Early in vitro studies suggested that MPO-generated nitrating intermediates lead to the formation of NO_2-LDL, which in turn represents a high-uptake form for intimal macrophages [43,44] (Table 14.2). More recently, it has been shown that foam cells originate from immune cells and smooth muscle cells alike, although the exact composition in humans remains unclear [45]. However, macrophages at different stages of transformation to foam cells express MPO [9], which in turn is highly abundant in atheroma, potentially causing modifications of lipoproteins that further enhance atherosclerotic pathology [8].

TABLE 14.2

Atherogenic lipid-modifying processes of MPO and MPO-derived molecules

Authors	Year	Journal	Mechanistic claim	Experimental model	Key finding
Daugherty et al.	1994	Clin. Invest.	Potential oxidative modification in the vascular wall	Human ex vivo	MPO is found in atherosclerotic lesions of human patients
Hazen et al.	1997	Clin. Invest.	Oxidative modification of LDL	In vitro/human ex vivo	3-Chlorotyrosine was increased in LDL isolated from human atheroma
Podrez et al.	1999	Clin. Invest.	Nitrogen species convert LDL	In vitro/human ex vivo	LDL of the human atherosclerotic aorta is enriched in nitrotyrosine
Bergt et al.	2004	PNAS	Oxidative modification of HDL	In vitro/human ex vivo	Cholesterol efflux from lipip-laden macrophages is impaired by MPO in vitro
Zheng et al.	2004	J. Clin. Invest.	Nitration of human Apo A-I	In vitro/human ex vivo	Nitration and chlorythyrosination of Apo A-I in human atheroma
Shao et al.	2006	J. Biol. Chem.	Mutant forms of Apo A-I protein	In vitro	Lysin residue mediated modification of Apo A-I
Delporte et al.	2014	J. Lipid Res.	LC-MS/MS derived posttranslational modifications	In vitro/human	Mapping several posttranslational modifications on apoB-100 in humans

MPO has been shown to strongly modify Apo B-100, creating an MPO-dependent highly oxidized LDL commonly called Mox-LDL (see also Chapter 7). Its formation appears to be the product of a specific interaction of MPO with the protein moiety of LDL in addition to an indirect and unspecific effect of the oxidative burst created by the formation of HOCl [46]. Thereby, circulating MPO as well as MPO in the subendothelial space promotes atherosclerosis by modification of LDL and specifically Apo B-100 (Figure 14.1, Table 14.2).

On the other hand, levels of HDL, commonly branded as the "benign cholesterol," are inversely correlated with CAD [47]. Several mechanisms for a protective effect in atherosclerosis have been proposed, the most intensely studied one being reverse cholesterol transport, a process that can remove and scavenge cholesterol from foam cells [48]. Despite the strong correlation between HDL levels and cardiovascular health, there is an ongoing debate about whether it has a causal protective function or whether decreased HDL levels constitute more of an epiphenomenon of disturbed LDL metabolism [49]. Two groups independently found evidence for the MPO-dependent tyrosination and chlorination of HDL residues in plasma and atheroma of subjects suffering from ischemic heart disease, reducing the cholesterol reverse transport capacity of HDL granules [50,51]. Specifically for its component apolipoprotein A-I (Apo A-I), in vitro studies demonstrated site-specific effects for tyrosine modifications on Apo A-I exposed to MPO in vitro, disrupting its lipid exchange capacity [52,53]. Similar functional impairment of HDL and reverse cholesterol transport upon inflammation has also been described in human cohorts and may add to the atherogenic properties of MPO [54,55]. For the interested reader, Chapter 7 contains a detailed description of the interaction of MPO and lipoproteins across disease models.

ADVANCED ATHEROSCLEROTIC LESIONS – HOW MPO AFFECTS PLAQUE STABILITY

Postmortem studies have established atherosclerotic plaque rupture to be responsible for up to 75% of episodes of acute coronary syndrome (ACS), the result of a sudden total or subtotal occlusion of a coronary artery [56]. Several key mechanisms underlying the molecular and cellular processes leading to plaque rupture have been identified. These can be distinguished into fibrous cap thinning, inflammation of plaque content and necrotic core proliferation. This process, among others, involves matrix metalloproteinase (MMPs) activation, apoptosis and dysfunction of endothelial and smooth muscle cells, continuous thrombogenesis and cytokine signaling [57] (Figure 14.1). MMPs are proteolytic enzymes that, when activated, facilitate the breakdown of extracellular matrix (ECM) during tissue transformation. They fulfill complex roles in atherosclerotic plaques, but are mainly considered to destabilize the plaque, ultimately promoting rupture [58]. MPO and its oxidative products have been found to activate MMPs in vitro [59], an effect that might be further amplified by inhibition of the endogenous tissue inhibitors of MMPs (TIMPs) [60].

Furthermore, direct interactions with, and cleavage of, components of the ECM of SMCs such as laminins, fibronectins and perlecan have been described [61–64]. HOCl-derived protein modifications are present in the ECM of human atheroma [65]. These interactions, coinciding with the presence of PMNs [66], abundancy of active MPO in coronary atherosclerotic plaques and its colocalization with MMP-7 [59], suggest that the enzyme promotes the degradation of the ECM. Additionally, direct oxidation and chlorination of ECM components by MPO and HOCl may come into play, as they have recently been shown for laminin-111 and fibronectin in vitro [20,63,67] (Table 14.3). The chlorination and oxidation activities of MPO further appear to be potentiated by the glycosaminoglycan-dependent binding to ECM proteins due to the cationic charge of the enzyme [68]. MPO-mediated modifications of ECM further induce a phenotypical switch of human coronary artery SMCs toward reduced adhesion, increased proliferation and pro-inflammatory changes in gene expression [69].

Although ECM degradation is a plausible and potentially necessary function in tissue reorganization after local infection or injury, it is disadvantageous in atherosclerosis since it causes plaque instability. The translational relevance of these findings is supported by a study identifying macrophage-derived MPO in postmortem analysis of human coronary plaques [9]. Special care must be taken when investigating the role of MPO in the development and stability of atherosclerotic plaques in mouse models, as the publication history shows partly contradictory results. The study in which MPO-deficient animals were

TABLE 14.3

MPO and MPO-derived molecules mediated effects on plaque stability

Authors	Year	Journal	Interaction partner(s)	Experimental approach	Key finding
Fu et al.	2001	J. Biol. Chem.	MMP-7	In vitro/human biopsies	MMP-7 is activated via chlorination by HOCl, driving plaque rupture
Baldus et al.	2001	J. Clin. Invest.	Fibronectin	In vitro (BAECs)/ex vivo (rat aorta)	Transcytosed MPO facilitates nitration of tyrosine residues of fibronectin
Woods/Davies	2003	Biochem. J.	ECM proteins and polysaccharides	In vitro (VSMC)	HOCl induces fragmentation of ECM proteins and polysaccharides
Woods et al.	2003	Biochem. J.	ECM proteins	Ex vivo analysis of human plaques	HOCl derived oxidations are present in the ECM of human aortic plaques
Wang et al.	2007	J. Biol. Chem.	TIMP-1	In vitro/human BAL samples	MPO inactivates TIMP-1 via oxidation by HOCl resulting in higher proteolytic activity
Sugiyama et al.	2004	Arterioscler. Thromb. Vasc. Biol.	HOCl induces caspase-3 activation	In vitro	HOCl provokes apoptosis in ECs
Rees et al.	2010	Matrix. Biol.	Perlecan	In vitro	MPO and HOCl oxidize the protein core of perlecan, potentially increasing permeability of the subendothelial space
Kubala et al.	2013	Biochim. Biophys. Acta.	Glycosaminoglycans	In vitro	Chlorination and oxidation activity of MPO is elevated due to statically induced binding to glycosaminoglycans
Rashid et al.	2018	Eur. Heart J.	Reduced fibrin and hemosidirin deposition	In vitro/in vivo	Pharmacological Inhibition of MPO increases plaque stability
Nybo et al.	2018	Redox. Biol.	Fibronectin	In vitro	MPO and HOCl induce chlorination and oxidation of human fibronectin, compromising SMC function
Nybo et al.	2019	Redox. Biol.	Laminin-111	In vitro	HOCl oxidizes and chlorinates numerous sites of laminin
Cai et al.	2019	Free. Radic. Biol. Med.	Various ECM components	In vitro (HCASMC)	MPO and HOCl derived oxidation of ECM changes SMC phenotype
Cai et al.	2020	Sci. Rep.	Fibronectin and type IV collagen	In vitro (HCASMC)	MPO/HOCl/H_2O_2 modifies collagen and fibronectin in SCM derived ECM

first described reported an increase in lesion size in the absence of MPO in an Ldlr$^{-/-}$ model, but could not detect MPO or 3-chloro-tyrosine in the disease model used [70]. Thus, the applicability to human disease, in which both are reliably detected, was questioned by the authors. In contrast, later studies showed a therapeutic effect of MPO deficiency or inhibition in the Apoe$^{-/-}$ and Ldlr$^{-/-}$ model, in which the enzyme is also found in atherosclerotic plaques [71–73]. However, specifically Rashid et al. discuss that MPO influences phenotype, i.e. stability, rather than size of atherosclerotic lesions [71].

There is evidence that MPO may also render the antithrombotic endothelial surface thrombogenic, since MPO-dependent NO$^{\bullet}$ consumption and oxidative stress increase platelet activation, adhesion and aggregation and thereby enhance the expression of pro-thrombotic factor plasminogen activator inhibitor-1 (PAI-1) [74]. In addition, the surface expression of Pselectin in ECs, which promotes platelet adhesion, is enhanced by MPO-derived lipid oxidation products accumulated in atheroma [11]. More recently, MPO activity within atherosclerotic plaques was measured in vivo using an MRI probe, in a model facilitating the tandem-stenosis model in Apoe$^{-/-}$ mice [71]; future research may therefore see the use of MPO activity within plaques as a radiological biomarker of plaque instability.

In patients with acute coronary syndromes and MI, recent findings suggest a significant role of MPO, as PMN accumulation in culprit lesions is a strong and independent predictor of mortality [75]. MPO plasma levels are associated with the transition of stable to vulnerable plaques and serve as a biomarker for the risk of cardiac events and adverse cardiac outcome [76,77]. Additionally, high levels of plasma MPO are associated with coronary plaque erosion in patients with acute coronary syndromes [12,78].

MPO PROMOTES NEOINTIMA FORMATION

Coronary atherosclerosis and coronary artery occlusion can be provoked by extensive hyperplasia of the innermost arterial layer (intima) [79–81]. This so-called neointima formation is of utmost relevance since established and new therapies of atherosclerosis, e.g. coronary angioplasty, drug eluting stent implantation or bioresorbable vascular scaffold, still lead to restenosis to a significant percentage [82,83]. During intimal growth, SMCs migrate from the media into the inner vascular

wall, which leads to vascular remodeling often followed by atherosclerosis [80]. In a model of vascular injury, MPO-deficient mice showed significantly reduced neointima formation compared with WT control animals. This effect could also be induced by treating WT mice with the MPO inhibitor 4-aminobenzoic acid hydrazide (4-ABAH). Transplantation of MPO-competent neutrophils in MPO-deficient animals resulted in increased intima proliferation after vascular injury [72]. The fact that HOCl has been shown to induce EC apoptosis followed by hyperproliferation in rat vessels confirms that MPO can induce intima proliferation via its enzymatic activity [84,85] (Table 14.3). However, MPO has also been reported to inhibit the proliferation and migration of SMCs via the oxidative modification of HDL in atherosclerotic lesions, thereby destabilizing plaques at risk (Figure 14.1). ROS can induce SMC apoptosis and inhibit proliferation [86]. It is known that hydrogen peroxide (H_2O_2) stimulates the proliferation of SMCs, while other ROS induce proliferation to a lesser degree [87]. In contrast, other studies report a more stimulatory effect on SMC proliferation that depends on the level and origin of ROS, growth factors, transcription factors and other mediators such as the modified lipoproteins involved [88,89]. Taken together, the role of MPO in SMC proliferation and intimal hyperplasia is sometimes controversial, and further research is needed to decipher the role of MPO in this pathology.

MPO IN MYOCARDIAL INFARCTION

Coronary plaque rupture frequently results in the obliteration of vessels, causing MI, the most severe consequence of coronary atherosclerosis. Upon cardiac ischemia, immune cells infiltrate the myocardium to facilitate resorption of apoptotic cells and to initiate wound healing. As canonical first responders to tissue injury, PMNs play an important part during the early stages of MI [90–92]. It is therefore reasonable to assume that MPO, as an abundant and highly reactive component of the cytotoxic armamentarium of PMNs, plays a significant role in the lysis of the destroyed infarct tissue. Whereas inflammatory response, subsequent fibrotic remodeling and scar tissue formation are vital in preventing cardiac rupture, the presence of immune cells has been shown to be indispensable for the orchestration of tissue repair, the activity of innate immune cells also undoubtedly damages healthy tissue [93–96].

Importantly, modern interventional therapy usually achieves reperfusion of the occluded artery within 2 h after the onset of symptoms. Using catheter-based restoration of coronary blood flow, mortality from MI could be substantially reduced, but the reperfusion of ischemic tissue causes reperfusion injury that is to a large extent regulated by immune cells infiltrating myocardial tissue [97]. Although the inhibition of central junctions of pro-inflammatory signaling pathways in animal models has led to therapeutic success, no anti-inflammatory therapy has yet been established for infarction patients. Therefore, it is crucial for translational research to better understand the role and balance of individual elements of local leukocyte activation in MI. Regarding MPO, epidemiological studies clearly associate diminished enzyme activity with reduced burden of CVD; however, to which extent this is due to reduced atherosclerotic remodeling in the first place or modulation of on-site activity of PMNs after infarction is not clear; although most cardiovascular research on the enzyme focused on its role in NO• homeostasis, endothelial dysfunction and plaque formation, several individual studies suggest that it also has a direct role in post-infarct remodeling.

Like endogenous cardiac infarction in human patients, PMN infiltration is seen within hours after coronary artery ligation in animal models. MPO-deficient mice exhibit less total immune cell content in the infarct zone – further suggesting its role as a chemotactic factor, but also a reduction of adverse hypertrophic left ventricular remodeling and improved systolic ventricular function as compared with WT mice; consecutively, are less prone to the development of ventricular arrhythmia [98,99]. However, MPO deficiency does not impact infarct size, although it delays fibrotic scar formation [98]. These overall protective effects are in clear contrast to an adverse outcome after MI that is observed when PMNs are depleted in total [96,100]. An important role of MPO in MI was confirmed by an additional study facilitating MPO inhibition by a suicide substrate, where strong attenuation of consecutive cardiac failure after infarction specifically revealed an effect of the enzyme and its catalytic activity on post-infarct remodeling [101]. Of note, an impact of MPO on tissue remodeling after ischemic injury is not specific for the heart: Both MPO deficiency and inhibition protect from cell death and tissue inflammation in a murine model of ischemic stroke, whereas MPO deficiency attenuated loss of glomerular filtration rate after ischemic renal injury in mice [102,103].

ASSOCIATION OF MPO AND CARDIOVASCULAR OUTCOME

The majority of clinical studies have shown a prognostic value of MPO levels, but most of them include only few patients and were therefore not adequately powered [12,13,104–108]. However, in 2003, the authors of this chapter and others successfully conducted a prospective clinical trial, assessing the occurrence of recurrent infarction or death from MI in patients with ACS [12]. We could identify a cutoff value for MPO >350 µg/L based on which patients had a significantly increased risk of death or nonfatal infarction within 6 months (18.1% vs. 8.8%, P=0.002 [12]). Interestingly, we could identify a subgroup of patients with low Troponin T levels at baseline but elevated MPO levels, who have an increased risk of acute myocardial ischemia. Almost in parallel, Brennan et al. showed in a similar trial enrolling 604 patients, presenting with acute chest pain, that the MPO plasma level predicted an increased early risk of myocardial infarction, independently of other markers of inflammation or myocardial damage [77].

In contrast, Apple et al., in one of the few studies with a negative outcome, investigated the association between several biomarkers including MPO and adverse events (MI, need for revascularization or death) and found no increased risk for patients with MPO levels >125.6 versus <125.6 µg/L in patients with ACS. In total, 457 patients with ACS were observed over a period of 4 months. More recently, similar results were obtained in an analysis of CVD and death in a subgroup of the Chronic Renal Insufficiency Cohort (CRIC). The study group included 3,872 patients with chronic kidney disease who had measured MPO at baseline. The study results displayed an increased risk for cardiovascular events and death in patients with higher MPO levels, but the association lost significance after adjustment for cardiac biomarkers [109]. Because of the divergent results and limited power of previous studies, Abdel-Latif et al. combined 13 studies with a total 9,090 subjects in a meta-analysis to address the question whether high MPO level predicts major adverse cardiac events (MACE) and mortality in patients presenting with ACS.

Subjects with high MPO levels demonstrated a significantly increased mortality (odds ratio 2.03 confidence interval (CI): 1.40–2.94; P<0.001), whereas the risk of MACE or recurrent MI was not increased. The effect on mortality was not influenced by other cardiovascular risk factors, such as hypertension or diabetes mellitus [110]. Although the analysis demonstrated a trend toward a correlation of high MPO level with MACE, it failed to reach statistical significance. The authors discuss again the heterogeneous study population in most of the studies and a lack of statistical power in individual studies, which also influences the result of the meta-analysis. However, the prognostic value of MPO was highest for the subgroup of studies that included a higher proportion of acute MI patients compared with studies that mainly included unstable angina pectoris patients [13,111]. The authors conclude that integrating MPO in risk stratification models could have an additional value in identifying patients at higher risk of developing heart failure, recurrent ischemia and clinical events specially mortality. Still, further studies are warranted and could help to reduce the variability.

CONCLUSION

Taken together, MPO promotes atherosclerotic plaque formation and rupture in animal models of vascular disease. Low MPO activity is associated with a reduced incidence of CAD in humans, consolidating the translational relevance of these observations. Furthermore, the enzyme appears to be one of the main agents responsible for the adverse effects of neutrophils in ischemic injury and subsequent scar formation. MPO inhibition might therefore be an attractive therapeutic strategy for individuals at high risk of atherosclerosis and patients immediately after cardiac infarction.

REFERENCES

1. Roth G.A., Abate D., Abate K.H., et al. 2018, Global, regional, and national age-sex-specific mortality for 282 causes of death in 195 countries and territories, 1980–2017: A systematic analysis for the Global Burden of Disease Study 2017. *Lancet* 392: 1736–1788.
2. Libby P. 2012, Inflammation in atherosclerosis. *Arterioscler. Thromb. Vasc. Biol.* 32: 2045–2051.
3. Ridker P.M., Everett B.M., Thuren T., et al. 2017, Anti-inflammatory therapy with Canakinumab for atherosclerotic disease. *N. Engl. J. Med.* 377: 1119–1131.
4. Nidorf S.M., Fiolet A.T.L., Mosterd A., et al. 2020, Colchicine in patients with chronic coronary disease. *N. Engl. J. Med.* 383: 1838–1847
5. Daugherty A., Dunn J.L., Rateri D.L., Heinecke J.W. 1994, Myeloperoxidase, a catalyst for lipoprotein oxidation, is expressed in human atherosclerotic lesions. *J. Clin. Invest.* 94: 437–444.
6. Hazell L.J., Arnold L., Flowers D., Waeg G., Malle E., Stocker R. 1996, Presence of hypochlorite-modified proteins in human atherosclerotic lesions. *J. Clin. Invest.* 97: 1535–1447.
7. Beckmann J.S., Ye Y.Z., Anderson P.G., et al. 1994, Extensive nitration of protein tyrosines in human atherosclerosis detected by immunohistochemistry. *Biol. Chem. Hoppe Seyler* 375: 81–88.
8. Hazen S.L., Heinecke J.W. 1997, 3-Chlorotyrosine, a specific marker of myeloperoxidase-catalyzed oxidation, is markedly elevated in low density lipoprotein isolated from human atherosclerotic intima. *J. Clin. Invest.* 99: 2075–2081.
9. Sugiyama S., Okada Y., Sukhova G.K., Virmani R., Heinecke J.W., Libby P. 2001, Macrophage myeloperoxidase regulation by granulocyte macrophage colony-stimulating factor in human atherosclerosis and implications in acute coronary syndromes. *Am. J. Pathol.* 158: 879–891.
10. Hazell L.J., Baernthaler G., Stocker R. 2001, Correlation between intima-to-media ratio, apolipoprotein B-100, myeloperoxidase, and hypochlorite-oxidized proteins in human atherosclerosis. *Free Radic. Biol. Med.* 31: 1254–1262.
11. Thukkani A.K., McHowat J., Hsu F.F., Brennan M.L., Hazen S.L., Ford D.A. 2003, Identification of α-chloro fatty aldehydes and unsaturated lysophosphatidylcholine molecular species in human atherosclerotic lesions. *Circulation* 108: 3128–3133.
12. Baldus S., Heeschen C., Meinertz T., et al. 2003, Myeloperoxidase serum levels predict risk in patients with acute coronary syndromes. *Circulation* 108: 1440–1513.
13. Mocatta T.J., Pilbrow A.P., Cameron V.A., et al. 2007, Plasma concentrations of myeloperoxidase predict mortality after myocardial infarction. *J. Am. Coll. Cardiol.* 49: 1993–2000.
14. Perticone F., Ceravolo R., Pujia A., et al. 2001, Prognostic significance of endothelial dysfunction in hypertensive patients. *Circulation* 104: 191–196.

15. Daiber A., Chlopicki S. 2020, Revisiting pharmacology of oxidative stress and endothelial dysfunction in cardiovascular disease: Evidence for redox-based therapies. *Free Radic. Biol. Med.* 157: 15–37.

16. Della Rocca D.G., Pepine C.J. 2010, Endothelium as a predictor of adverse outcomes. *Clin. Cardiol.* 33: 730–732

17. Lacy P. 2006, Mechanisms of degranulation in neutrophils. *Allergy, Asthma Clin. Immunol.* 2: 98–108.

18. Klinke A., Nussbaum C., Kubala L., et al. 2011, Myeloperoxidase attracts neutrophils by physical forces. *Blood* 117: 1350–1358.

19. Manchanda K., Kolarova H., Kerkenpaß C., et al. 2018, MPO (Myeloperoxidase) reduces endothelial glycocalyx thickness dependent on its cationic charge. *Arterioscler. Thromb. Vasc. Biol.* 38: 1859–1867.

20. Baldus S., Eiserich J.P., Mani A., et al. 2001, Endothelial transcytosis of myeloperoxidase confers specificity to vascular ECM proteins as targets of tyrosine nitration. *J. Clin. Invest.* 108: 1759–1770.

21. Baldus S., Rudolph V., Roiss M., et al. 2006, Heparins increase endothelial nitric oxide bioavailability by liberating vessel-immobilized myeloperoxidase. *Circulation* 113: 1871–1878.

22. Harrison D.G. 1997, Cellular and molecular mechanisms of endothelial cell dysfunction. *J. Clin. Invest.* 100: 2153–2157.

23. Zhang C., Reiter C., Eiserich J.P., et al. 2001, L-Arginine chlorination products inhibit endothelial nitric oxide production. *J. Biol. Chem.* 276: 27159–27165.

24. Stocker R., Huang A., Jeranian E., et al. 20014, Hypochlorous acid impairs endothelium-derived nitric oxide bioactivity through a superoxide-dependent mechanism. *Arterioscler. Thromb. Vasc. Biol.* 24: 2028–2033.

25. Storkey C., Davies M.J., Pattison D.I. 2014, Reevaluation of the rate constants for the reaction of hypochlorous acid (HOCl) with cysteine, methionine, and peptide derivatives using a new competition kinetic approach. *Free Radic. Biol. Med.* 73: 60–66.

26. Elahi M.M., Kong Y.X., Matata B.M. 2009, Oxidative stress as a mediator of cardiovascular disease. *Oxid. Med. Cell Longev.* 2: 920580.

27. Nuszkowski A., Gräbner R., Marsche G., Unbehaun A., Malle E., Heller R. 2001, Hypochlorite-modified low density lipoprotein inhibits nitric oxide synthesis in endothelial cells via an intracellular dislocalization of endothelial nitric-oxide synthase. *J. Biol. Chem.* 276: 14212–14221.

28. Von Leitner E.C., Klinke A., Atzler D., et al. 2011, Pathogenic cycle between the endogenous nitric oxide synthase inhibitor asymmetrical dimethylarginine and the leukocyte-derived hemoprotein myeloperoxidase. *Circulation* 124: 2735–2745.

29. Eiserich J.P., Baldus S., Brennan M.-L.L., et al. 2002, Myeloperoxidase, a leukocyte-derived vascular NO oxidase. *Science* 296: 2391–2394.

30. Adam M., Gajdova S., Kolarova H., et al. 2014, Red blood cells serve as intravascular carriers of myeloperoxidase. *J. Mol. Cell. Cardiol.* 74: 353–363.

31. Rudolph T.K.K., Wipper S., Reiter B., et al. 2012, Myeloperoxidase deficiency preserves vasomotor function in humans. *Eur. Heart J.* 33: 1625–1634

32. Cheng D., Talib J., Stanley C.P., et al. 2019, Inhibition of MPO (myeloperoxidase) attenuates endothelial dysfunction in mouse models of vascular inflammation and atherosclerosis. *Arterioscler. Thromb. Vasc. Biol.* 39: 1448–1457.

33. Liu C., Desikan R., Ying Z., et al. 2012, Effects of a novel pharmacologic inhibitor of myeloperoxidase in a mouse atherosclerosis model. *PLoS One* 7: e50767.

34. Vita J.A., Brennan M.L., Gokce N., et al. 2004, Serum myeloperoxidase levels independently predict endothelial dysfunction in humans. *Circulation* 110: 1134–1139.

35. Baldus S., Heitzer T., Eiserich J.P., et al. 2004, Myeloperoxidase enhances nitric oxide catabolism during myocardial ischemia and reperfusion. *Free Radic. Biol. Med.* 37: 902–911.

36. Walker A.E., Seibert S.M., Donato A.J., Pierce G.L., Seals D.R. 2010, Vascular endothelial function is related to white blood cell count and myeloperoxidase among healthy middle-aged and older adults. *Hypertension* 55: 363–369.

37. Borén J., John Chapman M., Krauss R.M., et al. 2020, Low-density lipoproteins cause atherosclerotic cardiovascular disease: Pathophysiological, genetic, and therapeutic insights: A consensus statement from the European Atherosclerosis Society Consensus Panel. *Eur. Heart J.* 41: 2313–2330.

38. Perak A.M., Ning H., De Ferranti S.D., Gooding H.C., Wilkins J.T., Lloyd-Jones D.M. 2016, Long-term risk of atherosclerotic cardiovascular disease in US adults with the familial hypercholesterolemia phenotype. *Circulation* 134: 9–19.

39. Li D., Mehta J.L. 2005, Oxidized LDL, a critical factor in atherogenesis. *Cardiovasc. Res.* 68: 353–440.

40. Ganesan R., Henkels K.M., Wrenshall L.E., et al. 2018, Oxidized LDL phagocytosis during foam cell formation in atherosclerotic plaques relies on a PLD2–CD36 functional interdependence. *J. Leukoc. Biol.* 103: 867–883.

41. Pirillo A., Norata G.D., Catapano A.L. 2013, LOX-1, OxLDL, and atherosclerosis. *Mediators Inflamm.* 2013: 152786.

42. Tall A.R., Yvan-Charvet L. 2015, Cholesterol, inflammation and innate immunity. *Nat. Rev. Immunol.* 15: 104–116.

43. Podrez E.A., Schmitt D., Hoff H.F., Hazen S.L. 1999, Myeloperoxidase-generated reactive nitrogen species convert LDL into an atherogenic form in vitro. *J. Clin. Invest.* 103: 1547–1560.

44. Hazen S.L., Zhang R., Shen Z., et al. 1999, Formation of nitric oxide–derived oxidants by myeloperoxidase in monocytes. *Circ. Res.* 85: 950–958.

45. Wang Y., Dubland J.A., Allahverdian S., et al. 2019, Smooth muscle cells contribute the majority of foam cells in ApoE (Apolipoprotein E)-deficient mouse atherosclerosis. *Arterioscler. Thromb. Vasc. Biol.* 39: 876–887.

46. Delporte C., Van Antwerpen P., Vanhamme L., Roumeguère T., Zouaoui Boudjeltia K. 2013, Low-density lipoprotein modified by myeloperoxidase in inflammatory pathways and clinical studies. *Mediators Inflamm.* 2013: 971579.

47. Gordon D.J., Probstfield J.L., Garrison R.J., et al. 1989, High-density lipoprotein cholesterol and cardiovascular disease. Four prospective American studies. *Circulation* 79: 8–15.

48. Ouimet M., Barrett T.J., Fisher E.A. 2019, HDL and reverse cholesterol transport: Basic mechanisms and their roles in vascular health and disease. *Circ. Res.* 124: 1505–1518.

49. Barter P., Genest J. HDL cholesterol and ASCVD risk stratification: A debate. *Atherosclerosis* 283: 7–12.

50. Zheng L., Nukuna B., Brennan M.L., et al. 2004, Apolipoprotein A-I is a selective target for myeloperoxidase-catalyzed oxidation and function impairment in subjects with cardiovascular disease. *J. Clin. Invest.* 114: 529–541.

51. Bergt C., Pennathur S., Fu X., et al. 2004, The myeloperoxidase product hypochlorous acid oxidizes HDL in the human artery wall and impairs ABCA1-dependent cholesterol transport. *Proc. Natl. Acad. Sci. U.S.A.* 101: 13032–13037.

52. Smith J.D. 2010, Myeloperoxidase, inflammation, and dysfunctional high-density lipoprotein. *J. Clin. Lipidol.* 4: 382–388.

53. Shao B., Oda M.N., Bergt C., et al. 2006, Myeloperoxidase impairs ABCA1-dependent cholesterol efflux through methionine oxidation and site-specific tyrosine chlorination of apolipoprotein A-I. *J. Biol. Chem.* 281: 9001–9004.

54. Reilly M.P., McGillicuddy F.C., De La Moya M.L., et al. 2009, Inflammation impairs reverse cholesterol transport in vivo. *Circulation* 119: 1135–1145.

55. Sorrentino S.A., Besler C., Rohrer L., et al. 2010, Endothelial-vasoprotective effects of high-density lipoprotein are impaired in patients with type 2 diabetes mellitus but are improved after extended-release niacin therapy. *Circulation* 121: 110–122.

56. Narula J., Nakano M., Virmani R., et al. 2013, Histopathologic characteristics of atherosclerotic coronary disease and implications of the findings for the invasive and noninvasive detection of vulnerable plaques. *J. Am. Coll. Cardiol.* 61: 1041–1051.

57. Aikawa M., Libby P. 2004, The vulnerable atherosclerotic plaque: Pathogenesis and therapeutic approach. *Cardiovasc. Pathol.* 13: 125–138.

58. Johnson J.L. 2017, Metalloproteinases in atherosclerosis. *Eur. J. Pharmacol.* 816: 93–106.

59. Fu X., Kassimm S.Y., Parks W.C., Heinecke J.W. 2001, Hypochlorous acid oxygenates the cysteine switch domain of pro-matrilysin (MMP-7): A mechanism for matrix metalloproteinase activation and atherosclerotic plaque rupture by myeloperoxidase. *J. Biol. Chem.* 276: 41279–41287.

60. Wang Y., Rosen H., Madtes D.K., et al. 2007, Myeloperoxidase inactivates TIMP-1 by oxidizing its N-terminal cysteine residue: An oxidative mechanism for regulating proteolysis during inflammation. *J. Biol. Chem.* 282: 31826–31834.

61. Nybo T., Cai H., Chuang C.Y., Gamon L.F., Rogowska-Wrzesinska A., Davies M.J. 2018, Chlorination and oxidation of human plasma fibronectin by myeloperoxidase-derived oxidants, and its consequences for smooth muscle cell function. *Redox Biol.* 19: 388–400.

62. Rees M.D., Whitelock J.M., Malle E., et al. 2010, Myeloperoxidase-derived oxidants selectively disrupt the protein core of the heparan sulfate proteoglycan perlecan. *Matrix Biol.* 29: 63–73.

63. Nybo T., Dieterich S., Gamon L.F., et al. 2019, Chlorination and oxidation of the extracellular matrix protein laminin and basement membrane extracts by hypochlorous acid and myeloperoxidase. *Redox Biol.* 20: 496–513.

64. Woods A.A., Davies M.J. 2003, Fragmentation of extracellular matrix by hypochlorous acid. *Biochem. J.* 376: 219–227.

65. Woods A.A., Linton S.M., Davies M.J. 2003, Detection of HOCl-mediated protein oxidation products in the extracellular matrix of human atherosclerotic plaques. *Biochem. J.* 370: 729–735.

66. Naruko T., Ueda M., Haze K., et al. 2002, Neutrophil infiltration of culprit lesions in acute coronary syndromes. *Circulation* 106: 2894–2900.

67. Cai H., Chuang C.Y., Hawkins C.L., Davies M.J. 2020, Binding of myeloperoxidase to the extracellular matrix of smooth muscle cells and subsequent matrix modification. *Sci. Rep.* 10: 666.

68. Kubala L., Kolářová H., Víteček J., et al. 2013, The potentiation of myeloperoxidase activity by the glycosaminoglycan- dependent binding of myeloperoxidase to proteins of the extracellular matrix. *Biochim. Biophys. Acta* 1830: 4524–4536.

69. Cai H., Chuang C.Y., Vanichkitrungruang S., Hawkins C.L., Davies M.J. 2019, Hypochlorous acid-modified extracellular matrix contributes to the behavioral switching of human coronary artery smooth muscle cells. *Free Radic. Biol. Med.* 134: 516–526.

70. Brennan M.L., Anderson M.M., Shih D.M., et al. 2001, Increased atherosclerosis in myeloperoxidase-deficient mice. *J. Clin. Invest.* 107: 419–430.

71. Rashid I., Maghzal G.J., Chen Y.-C.C., et al. 2018, Myeloperoxidase is a potential molecular imaging and therapeutic target for the identification and stabilization of high-risk atherosclerotic plaque. *Eur. Heart J.* 39: 3301–3310.

72. Tiyerili V., Camara B., Becher M.U., et al. 2016, Neutrophil-derived myeloperoxidase promotes atherogenesis and neointima formation in mice. *Int. J. Cardiol.* 204: 29–36.

73. Roth Flach R.J., Su C., Bollinger E., et al. 2019, Myeloperoxidase inhibition in mice alters atherosclerotic lesion composition. *PLoS One* 14: e0214150.

74. Bouchie J.L., Hansen H., Feener E.P. 1998, Natriuretic factors and nitric oxide suppress plasminogen activator inhibitor-1 expression in vascular smooth muscle cells: Role of cGMP in the regulation of the plasminogen system. *Arterioscler. Thromb. Vasc. Biol.* 18: 1771–1779.

75. Distelmaier K., Winter M.P., Dragschitz F., et al. 2014, Prognostic value of culprit site neutrophils in acute coronary syndrome. *Eur. J. Clin. Invest.* 44: 257–265.

76. Baldus S., Heeschen C., Meinertz T., et al. 2003, Myeloperoxidase serum levels predict risk in patients with acute coronary syndromes. *Circulation* 108: 1440–1445.

77. Brennan M.L., Penn M.S., Van Lente F., et al. 2003, Prognostic value of myeloperoxidase in patients with chest pain. *N. Engl. J. Med.* 349: 1595–1604.

78. Ferrante G., Nakano M., Prati F., et al. 2010, High levels of systemic myeloperoxidase are associated with coronary plaque erosion in patients with acute coronary syndromes: A clinicopathological study. *Circulation* 122: 2505–2513.

79. Subbotin V.M. 2016, Excessive intimal hyperplasia in human coronary arteries before intimal lipid depositions is the initiation of coronary atherosclerosis and constitutes a therapeutic target. *Drug Discov. Today* 21: 1578–1595.

80. Hoglund V.J., Rong Dong X., Majesky M.W. 2010, Neointima formation: A local affair. *Arterioscler. Thromb. Vasc. Biol.* 30: 1877–1879.

81. Milutinović A., Šuput D., Zorc-Pleskovič R. 2020, Pathogenesis of atherosclerosis in the tunica intima, media, and adventitia of coronary arteries: An updated review. *Bosn. J. Basic Med. Sci.* 20: 21–30.

82. De Meyer G.R., Bult H. 1997, Mechanisms of neointima formation – Lessons from experimental models. *Vasc. Med.* 2: 179–189.

83. Torrado J., Buckley L., Durán A., et al. 2018, Restenosis, stent thrombosis, and bleeding complications. *J. Am. Coll. Cardiol.* 71: 1676–1695.

84. Yang J., Cheng Y., Ji R., Zhang C. 2006, Novel model of inflammatory neointima formation reveals a potential role of myeloperoxidase in neointimal hyperplasia. *Am. J. Physiol. Heart Circ. Physiol.* 291: H3087–3093.

85. Sugiyama S., Kugiyama K., Aikawa M., Nakamura S., Ogawa H., Libby P. 2004, Hypochlorous acid, a macrophage product, induces endothelial apoptosis and tissue factor expression: Involvement of myeloperoxidase-mediated oxidant in plaque erosion and thrombogenesis. *Arterioscler. Thromb. Vasc. Biol.* 24: 1309–1314.

86. Li P.F., Dietz R., von Harsdorf R. 1997, Reactive oxygen species induce apoptosis of vascular smooth muscle cell. *FEBS Lett.* 404: 249–252.

87. Rao G.N., Berk B.C. 1992, Active oxygen species stimulate vascular smooth muscle cell growth and proto-oncogene expression. *Circ. Res.* 70: 593–599.

88. Taniyama Y., Griendling K.K. 2003, Reactive oxygen species in the vasculature: Molecular and cellular mechanisms. *Hypertension* 42: 1075–1081.

89. Burtenshaw D., Kitching M., Redmond E.M., Megson I.L., Cahill P.A. 2019, Reactive oxygen species (ROS), intimal thickening, and subclinical atherosclerotic disease. *Front. Cardiovasc. Med.* 26: 89.

90. Prabhu S.D., Frangogiannis N.G. 2016, The biological basis for cardiac repair after myocardial infarction. *Circ. Res.* 119: 91–112.

91. Puhl S.L., Steffens S. 2019, Neutrophils in post-myocardial infarction inflammation: Damage vs. resolution? *Front. Cardiovasc. Med.* 6: 25.

92. Ma Y., Yabluchanskiy A., Lindsey M.L. 2013, Neutrophil roles in left ventricular remodeling following myocardial infarction. *Fibrogenes. Tissue Repair* 6: 11.

93. Nahrendorf M., Pittet M.J., Swirski F.K. 2010, Monocytes: Protagonists of infarct inflammation and repair after myocardial infarction. *Circulation* 121: 2437–2445.

94. Schloss M.J., Horckmans M., Nitz K., et al. 2016, The time-of-day of myocardial infarction onset affects healing through oscillations in cardiac neutrophil recruitment. *EMBO Mol. Med.* 8: 937–948.

95. Dittrich A., Lauridsen H. 2019, Myocardial infarction and the immune response - Scarring or regeneration? A comparative look at mammals and popular regenerating animal models. *J. Immunol. Regen. Med.* 4: 100016.

96. Horckmans M., Ring L., Duchene J., et al. 2017, Neutrophils orchestrate post-myocardial infarction healing by polarizing macrophages towards a reparative phenotype. *Eur. Heart J.* 38: 187–197.

97. Hausenloy D.J., Yellon D.M. 2013, Myocardial ischemia-reperfusion injury: A neglected therapeutic target. *J. Clin. Invest.* 123: 92–100.

98. Askari A.T., Brennan M.-L.L., Zhou X., et al. 2003, Myeloperoxidase and plasminogen activator inhibitor 1 play a central role in ventricular remodeling after myocardial infarction. *J. Exp. Med.* 197: 615–624.

99. Mollenhauer M., Friedrichs K., Lange M., et al. 2017, Myeloperoxidase mediates postischemic arrhythmogenic ventricular remodeling. *Circ. Res.* 121: 56–70.

100. Clements-Jewery H., Hearse D.J., Curtis M.J. 2007, Neutrophil ablation with anti-serum does not protect against phase 2 ventricular arrhythmias in anaesthetised rats with myocardial infarction. *Cardiovasc. Res.* 73: 761–769.

101. Ali M., Pulli B., Courties G., et al. 2016, Myeloperoxidase inhibition improves ventricular function and remodeling after experimental myocardial infarction. *JACC Basic Transl. Sci.* 1: 633–643.

102. Kim H.J., Wei Y., Lee J.Y., et al. 2016, Myeloperoxidase inhibition increases neurogenesis after ischemic stroke. *J. Pharmacol. Exp. Ther.* 359: 262–272.

103. Matthijsen R.A., Huugen D., Hoebers N.T., et al. 2007, Myeloperoxidase is critically involved in the induction of organ damage after renal ischemia reperfusion. *Am. J. Pathol.* 171: 1743–1752.

104. Koch C., Henrich M., Heidt M.C. 2014, Sequential analysis of myeloperoxidase for prediction of adverse events after suspected acute coronary ischemia. *Clin. Cardiol.* 37: 744–749.

105. Chang L-T., Chua S., Sheu J-J., et al. 2009, Level and prognostic value of serum myeloperoxidase in patients with acute myocardial infarction undergoing primary percutaneous coronary intervention. *Circ. J.* 73: 726–731.

106. Scirica B.M., Sabatine M.S., Jarolim P., et al. 2011, Assessment of multiple cardiac biomarkers in non-ST-segment elevation acute coronary syndromes: Observations from the MERLIN-TIMI 36 Trial. *Eur. Heart J.* 32: 697–705.

107. Meuwese M.C., Stroes E.S.G., Hazen S.L., et al. 2007, Serum myeloperoxidase levels are associated with the future risk of coronary artery disease in apparently healthy individuals. The EPIC-Norfolk prospective population study. *J. Am. Coll. Cardiol.* 50: 159–165.

108. Zhang R., Brennan M.L., Fu X., et al. 2001, Association between myeloperoxidase levels and risk of coronary artery disease. *J. Am. Med. Assoc.* 286: 2136–2142.

109. Correa S., Pena-Esparragoza J.K., Scovner K.M., Waikar S.S., Mc Causland F.R. 2020, Myeloperoxidase and the risk of CKD progression, cardiovascular disease, and death in the chronic renal insufficiency cohort (CRIC) study. *Am. J. Kidney Dis.* 76: 32–41.

110. Kolodziej A.R., Abo-Aly M., Elsawalhy E., Campbell C., Ziada K.M., Abdel-Latif A. 2019, Prognostic role of elevated myeloperoxidase in patients with acute coronary syndrome: A systemic review and meta-analysis. *Mediators Inflamm.* 2019: 2872607.

111. Kaya M.G., Yalcin R., Okyay K., et al. 2012, Potential role of plasma myeloperoxidase level: In predicting long-term outcome of acute myocardial infarction. *Texas Heart Inst. J.* 39: 500–506.

CHAPTER FIFTEEN

The Role of Myeloperoxidase in Neurodegenerative Disease

Wanda F. Reynolds and Richard A. Maki
Sanford Burnham Prebys Medical Discovery Institute

CONTENTS

DOI: 10.1201/9781003212287-19

INTRODUCTION

MPO Is a Double-Edged Sword

Myeloperoxidase (MPO) is a component of the innate immune system, present at high levels in neutrophils and monocytes [1,2] where it generates oxidants that kill phagocytosed microbes but can also damage normal cells. MPO is conventionally considered a myeloid-specific gene expressed in bone marrow myeloid precursor cells, but the human MPO (hMPO) gene has been found to escape this restriction in stress situations and can be expressed in other cells, such as astrocytes, neurons, or microglia in Alzheimer's disease (AD) [3–5], Parkinson's disease (PD), [6–8] and multiple sclerosis (MS) [9,10]. To enable investigation into the effects of hMPO expression in neurodegenerative disease, a humanized mouse model was created that is transgenic for a single copy of the intact hMPO gene injected as a 32 kb DNA restriction fragment from a bacterial artificial chromosome (Jackson# 035208 C57BL-Tg (MPO* -463G) 1Wfr/J) [11]. The inserted MPO gene has several kb of 5' and 3' flanking sequences and is located on the X chromosome. When the hMPO transgenic mice were crossed to mouse models of AD or PD, the hMPO transgene was expressed robustly in subsets of astrocytes, neurons, or microglia [4,8]. MPO expression led to increased lipid peroxidation, carbamylation, chlorination, nitration, and greater memory impairment in a model of AD [4] and motor impairment and earlier death in a model of PD [8]. The atypical expression of hMPO involves an upstream Alu element encoding binding sites for members of the nuclear receptor superfamily of transcription factors such as PPARγ as well as SP1 [12–15]. The murine MPO gene, lacking the primate-specific Alu, is not expressed in the brain in these mouse disease models. A polymorphism in this Alu, −463G, RS2333227, increases hMPO expression and has been linked to risk for AD [3,16–20] cardiovascular disease [21–26], and epithelial cancers [27,28]. This chapter discusses the evidence of aberrant MPO expression in AD, PD, and MS and the resultant oxidative damage associated with memory impairment in AD or motor impairment in PD through analysis of post-mortem human brain and mouse disease models expressing the human MPO gene.

MPO EXPRESSION IN BRAIN PROMOTES ALZHEIMER'S DISEASE

AD is the most common neurodegenerative disease in humans and the leading cause of dementia. The hallmarks of AD are extracellular deposits of amyloid-β (Aβ) in diffuse or neuritic plaques and the presence in neurons of neurofibrillary tangles (NFTs) containing hyperphosphorylated Tau (reviewed in Refs. [29,30]). The brain's innate immune cells, astrocytes and microglia, play a role in AD, promoting neurotoxicity through generation of reactive oxygen species (ROS) and inflammatory cytokines (reviewed in Refs. [31,32]).

Amyloid Plaques Are a Defining Feature of AD

Amyloid plaques are insoluble deposits consisting primarily of amyloid beta (Aβ) [33,34], a 39–42 residue peptide derived from proteolysis of amyloid precursor protein (APP) [35]. Amyloid deposits are typically associated with clusters of activated microglia, along with astrocytes and degenerating neurites [36]. Considerable evidence supports a causative role for Aβ in AD, including the ubiquitous occurrence of Aβ in plaques, the toxicity of Aβ (1–42) for neuronal cells [37–39], and the linkage of familial AD to mutations in APP and the presenilin genes, which promote secretion of the toxic Aβ peptide [40,41]. Deposition of Aβ is known to increase under oxidative conditions and oxidizing radicals are implicated in AD [42–45], possibly due to radical-induced cross-linking of Aβ into insoluble beta sheet structures or fibrils [45,46]. Activated microglia, the resident brain macrophages, are a major source of oxidizing radicals [47]. These myeloid cells exist in a quiescent state in normal brain tissue but can become activated in response to neuronal damage or various other stimuli, including aggregated Aβ [37,48], thereupon phagocytizing the Aβ particles [49] and releasing oxidizing species such as superoxide anion and reactive nitrogen intermediates [48,50].

MPO Generates Oxidants in AD

Several studies support a role for MPO in the pathophysiology of AD [3–5,7,51]. While MPO is a potential source of reactive radicals in microglia, this myeloid enzyme is not expressed in quiescent microglia in normal brain tissue. MPO catalyzes a reaction between hydrogen peroxide, produced by NADPH oxidase, and chloride to generate hypochlorous acid (HOCl), a toxic oxidizing agent, which further reacts with other biological molecules to generate other reactive products [52].

MPO-generated reactive oxidizing and nitrating species serve as weapons against invading bacteria and fungi but can also damage normal cells such that expression is generally restricted to bone marrow myeloid precursor cells, then packaged in granules in circulating neutrophils and monocytes. While MPO is not expressed in normal aged brain, there is evidence that the human MPO gene may be induced in stressed neurons, astrocytes, or microglia in AD [3–5] or other neurodegenerative diseases such as PD [6–8], where this enzyme can lead to nitration, chlorination, and carbamylation of proteins as well as lipid peroxidation.

MPO Is Abundant in AD Brain Co-localizing with Aβ in Amyloid Plaques

Immunohistochemical analysis of normal aged brain compared with AD cases revealed that most AD cases exhibited an abundance of MPO-positive plaques in the cerebral cortex (Figure 15.1b) while MPO was not detected outside of vessels in normal aged brain tissue (Figure 15.1a) [3]. In addition to the amorphous deposition of MPO in amyloid plaques, MPO was often detected in cells at the periphery of plaques (Figure 15.1c–g), while there were relatively few MPO-positive cells observed distant from the immediate plaque areas. The observation that MPO-positive cells tend to be restricted to the immediate areas around plaques suggested that Aβ or other plaque components induce MPO expression. Higher magnification revealed short processes on the MPO positive cells (Figure 15.1c and e), and in some cases, MPO staining could be seen to be vesicular (Figure 15.1e), consistent with the typical lysosomal localization of MPO in monocytes or other myeloid cells [53,54].

MPO Is Expressed in Microglia Associated with Amyloid Plaques

To determine if the MPO-positive cells were microglia, the macrophages of the brain, the sections were costained with monoclonal antibodies to CD68, a lysosomal glycoprotein specific for monocytes macrophages and often used to identify microglia at AD plaques [37,55]. CD68-positive microglia (arrows) were detected by immunofluorescence at the periphery of a plaque (Figure 15.1f), and these cells costained with MPO antibodies detected with peroxidase substrate (Figure 15.1g), indicating these MPO-positive cells at plaques were microglia macrophages.

MPO Co-localizes with Aβ on the Walls of Blood Vessels in AD

Confocal microscopy demonstrated colocalization of MPO (Figure 15.1h, green) and Aβ (Figure 15.1i, red) in plaques and along the periphery of a blood vessel (Figure 15.1j, merged). MPO was also detected within the vessel lumen (arrow), consistent with MPO released from circulating neutrophils and monocytes, while Aβ was restricted to the vessel periphery (Figure 15.1i, arrow). These results are consistent with prior reports of perivascular Aβ deposition in AD known as cerebral amyloid angiopathy [56]. This observation raises the possibility that MPO oxidants enhance formation of insoluble Aβ aggregates along vessel walls in AD or that Aβ induces MPO expression.

The −463G Promoter Polymorphism Is Associated with Increased Incidence of AD in Females

The question arises as to whether MPO presence in plaques is a causative agent in AD or is it a secondary effect in reactive macrophages at the site. One means to address this question involves a functional polymorphism, −463G/A (rs2333227), in the human MPO promoter. The −463G site creates an SP1-binding site and is a more potent activator of a reporter gene in transfection assays [13]. Moreover, the homozygous GG genotype is associated with higher MPO expression in primary myeloid leukemia cells [57]. This GG homozygous genotype is predominant in the general population (61%) and was found in early studies to be overrepresented in females with early onset

Human brain

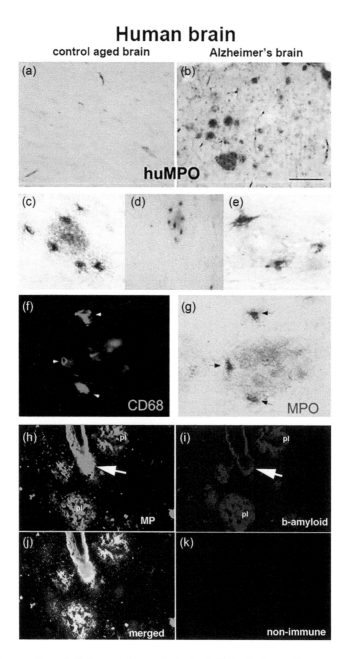

Figure 15.1 MPO is present in amyloid plaques in human AD brain. (a, b) Cerebral cortex from normal aged human brain (a) and human AD brain (b) were immunostained with antibodies against human MPO. There was virtually no MPO immunostaining in normal aged brain parenchyma, yet MPO was abundant in plaques in AD brain. MPO-positive cells are often found at the periphery of plaques (c–e), some with processes (c, e), some with MPO in vesicles (e). CD68 immunostaining (f) co-localizing in cells expressing MPO (g) identifies cells as microglia. (h–j) Co-localization of MPO with Aβ in plaques and walls of blood vessel. Sections were double-stained with rabbit antibodies to MPO (h) and monoclonal antibodies to Aβ (i) and imaged with confocal microscopy (j, merged). (h) MPO is detected in plaques and within the lumen of a blood vessel. (i) Aβ is detected in plaques and along the periphery of the vessel. (j) Co-localization is seen in plaques and at the vessel periphery. (k) The no primary control. (Panels a and b are reprinted from Maki et al., 2009 [4], Aberrant expression of myeloperoxidase in astrocytes promotes phospholipid oxidation and memory deficits in a mouse model of Alzheimer's disease, J. Biol. Chem. 284: 3158–3169, (Figure 1a, b) with permission from Elsevier. Panels c–k are reprinted from Reynolds et al., 1999, Myeloperoxidase polymorphism is associated with gender-specific risk for Alzheimer's disease, Exp. Neurol. 155: 31–41, (Figures 1a, b and 2b–d) with permission from Elsevier.)

MS (86%), suggesting that higher MPO expression accelerates damage to the myelin sheath by macrophages/microglia [9]. To determine if the polymorphism was associated with AD incidence, the MPO genotypes of 69 AD cases were determined and found to be 73% GG homozygotes [3]. These findings suggested that the −463G allele may enhance MPO gene expression in microglia or other cells in AD or other neurodegenerative states. The −463G/A site is within a primate-specific Alu element and thus is absent from the murine MPO gene. The site is within the first of four hexamer half-sites recognized by members of the nuclear receptor superfamily of transcription factors, including PPARγ, estrogen receptor, thyroid hormone receptor, and LXR [12,13]. This raised the possibility that these nuclear receptor transcription factors could modulate or induce abnormal MPO expression in various cell types and disease states.

Other case-control studies have examined the role of the rs2333227 polymorphism in AD. A study of 127 Finnish patients found the −463A allele increased risk of AD in males by 3.8-fold when in association with the ApoE4 allele [19]. A study of 148 Italian AD patients found that the association of −463G along with an A2M polymorphism synergistically increased the risk of AD by 25-fold [20]. A study of 315 Spanish AD patients found no association of the −463G/A with AD risk [58]. These varied findings suggest that the effects of the MPO polymorphism are influenced by gender and by interactions with other polymorphisms.

The −463GA/rs2333227 polymorphism has been associated with risk for various cancers, including lung, gastric, prostate, breast, colorectal, and cervical, as well as inflammatory diseases including lupus (SNPedia, NIH dbSNP site lists 161 publications). The greatest number of association studies have focused on rs2333227 effects in lung cancer and coronary heart disease, and again the results can vary depending on ethnicity and gender as well as interactions with other polymorphisms. As one example, a meta-analysis [59] compiled data from 19 case-control studies of coronary heart disease, amassing 4,008 cases and 3,460 controls, and found that the lower expressing −463A polymorphism was associated with reduced risk of coronary heart disease in Asians but not in Caucasians. Another meta-analysis examined the effect of the −463G/A polymorphism on lung

cancer risk in smokers [60]. Data were pooled from ten lung cancer studies including 3,688 cases and 3,874 controls. The higher expressing GG genotype was found to increase risk for lung cancer in smokers in Caucasians and possibly in Asians. Interestingly, there are ethnic differences in the frequencies of the −463G or A alleles. Africans have the lowest percentage (50%) of GG genotype, Caucasians have higher levels (60%), and Asians have the highest levels (71%), raising the possibility that selective pressures, such as infectious diseases, increased the frequency of the −463G allele during the migration of humans from Africa to Europe and Asia.

ApoE4 Allele Correlates with Greater Deposition of MPO in Plaques in AD

The ApoE4 allele is the major genetic link to AD, being associated with earlier onset and higher incidence of disease [61–63]. Individuals with one or two E4 alleles have increased amounts of Aβ deposition in plaques [61]. To investigate the possible correlation of APOE genotype and MPO deposition, the amounts of MPO in plaques in 17 AD cases were determined by densitometer scan of immunostained sections. Analyses indicated a correlation between the presence of the ApoE4 allele and the amount of MPO in plaques [3]. Highest average MPO deposits were found in ApoE4-E4 homozygotes, intermediate levels were seen in E4-E2 or E4-E3 heterozygotes, and lowest amounts were seen in cases lacking the E4 allele (P = 0.01). This finding suggested that the ApoE4 variant is linked to increased expression or deposition of MPO in AD brain.

MPO-Generated Oxidants May Promote Aβ Aggregation Thereby Contributing to AD

The most likely mechanism by which MPO contributes to AD is through the generation of reactive oxidizing species. Lipid peroxidation and other oxidative damage are among the earliest pathological changes associated with senile plaques [64,65]. ApoE is highly susceptible to oxidation by MPO-HOCl [66], and oxidation of ApoE, especially ApoE4, enhances complex formation with Aβ [62,67]. These observations suggested that MPO-generated oxidants may contribute to AD pathology by promoting the precipitation of Aβ or the coaggregation of ApoE and Aβ.

MPO Is Deposited in Plaques along with Aβ in a Transgenic Mouse Model Expressing the −463G MPO Allele

The hMPO transgenic mouse was crossed to the APP23 mouse model that overexpresses the human APP751 transgene with familial mutations linked to AD [4]. Immunohistochemical analysis of sections revealed abundant amyloid plaques in hippocampus and cortex (Figure 15.2b) with dense MPO deposition in plaques in the cortex, especially the frontal cortex (Figure 15.2a). MPO was also detected to a lesser degree in cells in the hippocampus, striatum, cerebellum, and brain stem, as well as in cells bound along the blood vessels or meningeal lymphatic vessels [4]. In

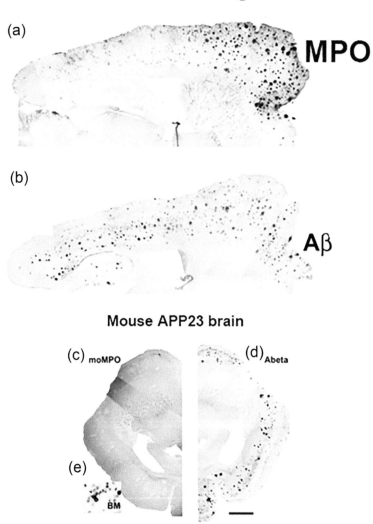

Figure 15.2 The huMPO transgene is expressed at plaques in the APP23 model, unlike mouse MPO. (a) Immunostaining of sagittal brain sections from MPO-APP23 with antibodies to MPO detected robust staining of plaques especially in the frontal cortex. (b) Antibodies to Aβ (6E10) detected abundant plaques throughout the cortex and hippocampus. (d) Immunostaining of coronal sections of the APP23 mouse brain with antibodies to Aβ detected plaques in the cortex, while antibodies to mouse MPO failed to detect plaques (c) but did detect mouse MPO in bone marrow myeloid cells (e). (Panels are reprinted from Maki et al., 2009 [4], Aberrant expression of myeloperoxidase in astrocytes promotes phospholipid oxidation and memory deficits in a mouse model of Alzheimer disease, J. Biol. Chem. 284: 3158–3169, (Figure 1c, e, f, g) with permission from Elsevier.)

contrast, the mouse MPO gene was not expressed at amyloid plaques or in associated cells in APP23 brain (Figure 15.2c and d) but was detected in bone marrow (Figure 15.2e). Thus, the human MPO gene, but not murine MPO, is expressed in the APP overexpressing model of AD.

MPO Co-localizes with Aβ in Plaques and on Vessel Walls in hMPO-APP23 as in AD Brain

Confocal studies were performed to determine the types of cells expressing MPO around plaques in the hMPO-APP23 mouse model as compared with human AD. The example shows human AD in which MPO colocalized with Aβ in the dense core of a plaque (merge) and was present in cytoplasmic vesicles in two cells embedded in a halo of Aβ surrounding the core (Figure 15.3a). In the MPOG-APP23 model (Figure 15.3d),

MPO similarly co-localized with Aβ in plaques (merge) and was also detected in the walls of blood vessels traversing the plaques as was noted in human AD (Figure 15.1j). These findings show that MPO is deposited along with Aβ in plaques and on blood vessel walls in huMPO-APP23 brain as in human AD.

hMPO Is Expressed in Astrocytes in APP23 Mouse Brain

Confocal immunofluorescence microscopy was used to identify cells expressing human MPO in APP23 brain. Confocal images showed MPO to be present in astrocytes, co-localizing with glial fibrillary-associated protein (GFAP), an astrocyte marker (Figure 15.3e). GFAP was predominantly localized to thick processes off the cell body, whereas punctate MPO immunostaining

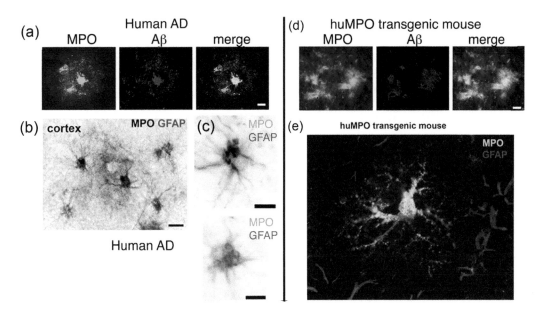

Figure 15.3 MPO is expressed in astrocytes in human AD and in MPOG-APP23 brain. Co-localization of MPO and Aβ in plaques in human AD brain. (a) Confocal fluorescence microscopy detected MPO (green) in the dense core of a plaque in human AD brain and in cytoplasmic vesicles within two associated cells (left panel). Aβ (red) was detected in the dense core and in a halo of particulate material (middle panel). The merged image (right panel) shows co-localization of MPO and Aβ in the plaque core. (b) MPO is expressed in astrocytes in human AD. Immunostaining detects human MPO (Vector SG, blue-black) in large vesicles in GFAP-positive (AEC, red) astrocytes around a plaque in AD tissue. (c) GFAP-positive astrocytes (red) with a cluster of MPO-positive vesicles (SG, blue-black). Scale bars = 20 μm. (d) In the transgenic MPOG-APP23 mice, MPO (left panel, green) and Aβ (middle, red) were detected in plaques, co-localizing in the merged image. MPO and Aβ are also co-localized in the walls of blood vessels traversing the plaques (right and left panels). Scale bars = 20 μm. (e) MPO is expressed in astrocytes in MPOG-APP23. Confocal image shows punctate MPO immunofluorescent staining (Alexa Fluor 488, green) in vesicles throughout a GFAP-positive (Alexa Fluor 594, red) astrocyte. (Panels are reprinted from Maki et ai., 2009 [4], Aberrant expression of myeloperoxidase in astrocytes promotes phospholipid oxidation and memory deficits in a mouse model of Alzheimer disease, J. Biol. Chem. 284: 3158–3169, (Figure 2a, b, d) with permission from Elsevier.)

was present throughout the cell body and in finer ramifications. Although the great majority (~95%) of MPO-positive cells clearly costained for GFAP, only a fraction (~5%) of GFAP-positive astrocytes costained for MPO, as illustrated by the GFAP-positive astrocyte projections in the background of Figure 15.3e, which lack MPO staining. In situ hybridization confirmed the presence of hMPO mRNA in astrocytes that costained for GFAP [4].

MPO Is Expressed in GFAP-Positive Astrocytes in Human AD Brain

While earlier studies detected MPO in CD68-positive microglia [3] and neuronal-appearing cells in human AD [5], later analysis of human AD cortical sections also detected MPO in clustered vesicles in GFAP-positive astrocytes (Figure 15.3b and c) [4]. As in the MPOG-APP23 mouse model, MPO was present in only a subset (~5%) of GFAP-positive astrocytes in plaque-laden regions or associated white matter tracts. These findings demonstrate that MPO is expressed in a subset of astrocytes in human AD as in the MPOG-APP23 model, consistent with findings of MPO in GFAP-positive astrocytes in PD brain [6]. Another study did not find MPO in GFAP-positive astrocytes in human AD brain [7], instead finding MPO only in cells associated with blood vessels and plaques.

MPO-APP23 Mice Exhibit Greater Memory Impairment Than APP23

To investigate the possible effects of MPO-generated oxidants on neural function in the mouse model of AD, spatial memory was tested by Morris water maze comparing MPO-APP23 and APP23 mice over 7 days (Figure 15.4a). In this experiment, the mice are first trained over several days to go to the visible escape platform in a 5-foot-wide pool of water. The platform is then hidden below the surface of the water made opaque by nontoxic white paint and the mice are introduced to the pool and given 1 min to find the hidden platform. Within 3 days, wild-type (WT) mice learn the position of the platform and find it within 10 s [4]. The APP23 mice require 7 days to reach the 10 s latency criteria, while the MPO-APP mice were significantly slower to find the hidden platform with mean latency of 20 s at day 7. This

indicated that MPO expression in APP23 brain leads to greater memory impairment.

Increased Lipid Peroxidation in MPOG-APP23 Brain

Lipid peroxides decompose to generate aldehydes such as 4-hydroxynonenal (4-HNE), a neurotoxic product that is increased in serum of AD patients [68]. 4-HNE forms stable adducts with proteins that provide an assay for lipid peroxidation by ELISA. There was a striking increase in 4-HNE levels in MPO-APP23 as compared with APP23 (Figure 15.4b). There was no increase in 4-HNE in hMPO brain lacking the APP transgene, indicating that Aβ toxicity is required to promote MPO-dependent lipid peroxidation.

Unsaturated phospholipids in neuronal tissue are vulnerable to free radical attack leading to lipid peroxidation. An oxidative lipidomics approach was undertaken to identify and characterize peroxidized phospholipids in brain. Mass spectrometry and fluorescence HPLC detected higher levels of oxidized anionic phospholipids phosphatidylserine hydroperoxides (PS-OOH) and phosphatidylinositol hydroperoxides (PS-OOH), particularly PS-OOH (Figure 15.4c) in MPO-APP23 brain, correlating with increased levels of peroxidized PS and PI products in postmortem brain samples from AD patients (Figure 15.4d). Strikingly, accumulation of the same individual molecular species of PS-OOH and PI-OOH was characteristic of brain samples from AD patients and MPOG-APP23 mice, providing evidence that the hMPO-APP23 mouse is a valid model for investigation of lipid peroxidation in AD.

Another subclass of phospholipids are plasmalogens, which contain a cis-vinyl ether linkage at the sn-1 position of the glycerol backbone (reviewed in Ref. [69]). Plasmalogens are major structural components of cell membranes and are predominant in the brain but also present in the kidney, lung, and skeletal muscle [69]. One variety of plasmalogens, ethanolamine plasmalogens (PlsEtns), has been found to decrease in AD patients, and this change correlated with cognition and severity of disease [70–72]. The cause of reduced PlsEtns in AD is not clear. One possible mechanism is oxidative stress, particularly from MPO-generated HOCl [73]. One consequence of HOCl-modified plasmalogens is endothelial dysfunction and the breakdown of the blood–brain

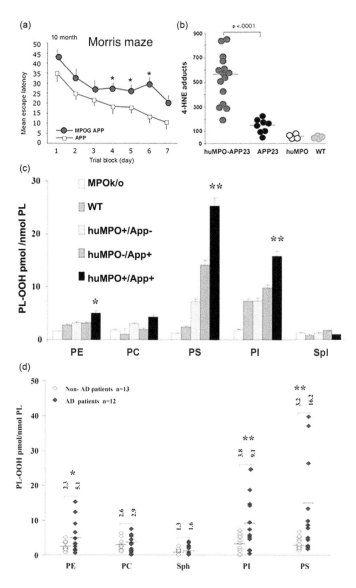

Figure 15.4 Increased lipid peroxidation in MPOG-APP23 brain correlating with greater spatial memory impairment. (a) Greater spatial memory impairment in MPO-APP23 mice. Morris water maze experiments were carried out with MPOG-APP23 (n = 8) and APP23 (n = 7) mice. Each data point represents mean escape latency (seconds) ±S.E. for the combined latency of four daily trials. Asterisks indicate significant differences (*, P < 0.05) between control APP23 and MPOG-APP23 values as determined by analysis of variance (Fisher's post-hoc least significant difference). The MPOG-APP23 exhibited significantly greater escape latency than APP23 controls on days 4–7. (b) ELISA assays were performed to measure 4-HNE-histidine adducts in frontal cortical extracts from 15 huMPO-APP, 8 APP23, 4 huMPO, and four wild-type (WT) mice. There was a significant increase in mean levels of 4-HNE-histidine between MPOG-APP23 and APP23 (P < 0.0001). (c) Increased peroxidation of anionic phospholipids in MPO-APP brain. Profiles of hydroperoxide content in major classes of phospholipids in samples of frontal cortex from wild-type, MPO-knockout, and MPO-APP23 mice. Selective and robust accumulation of PL-OOH in PS and PI from MPOG-APP23 versus WT animals was observed (**, P < 0.01 versus WT brain samples). PE of MPO-APP23 animals contained slightly but significantly elevated levels of hydroperoxides (*, P < 0.05 versus WT brain samples). (d) Increased peroxidation of anionic phospholipids in human AD. Profiles of hydroperoxides content in major classes of phospholipids in brain samples from non-AD and AD patients. Note that 3–5 times higher levels of hydroperoxides were found in PS and PI from AD brain tissue than non-demented controls (*, P < 0.05 and **, P < 0.01). A twofold increase of hydroperoxides was detected in PE from AD brain versus controls. (Panels are reprinted from Maki et al., 2009 [4], Aberrant expression of myeloperoxidase in astrocytes promotes phospholipid oxidation and memory deficits in a mouse model of Alzheimer disease, J. Biol. Chem. 284: 3158–3169, (Figures 5a, 6a, b, 7a) with permission from Elsevier.)

barrier [74,75]. As discussed below, this could lead to an influx of neutrophils and the release of MPO. The evidence linking phospholipids and MPO in neurodegenerative diseases such as AD is now well established and provides an important avenue for further research as well as possible therapeutic options in the future.

The Role of Neutrophils in AD

In addition to MPO expression in the brain resident cell types described above, there is evidence that MPO in neutrophils plays an important role in the development of AD [51]. Neutrophils contain the highest levels of MPO, comprising 5% of the total cellular protein [2]. While neutrophils are primarily localized to the bloodstream, reactive neutrophils can attach along blood vessel walls (see Figure 15.1) and extravasate into the brain parenchyma, producing HOCl and other oxidants that contribute to AD pathology. Release of MPO from neutrophils attached along veins in AD brain could also compromise the blood–brain barrier and impair the clearance of Aβ from the brain. Analysis of whole blood from AD patients and controls showed that there were higher numbers of hyperactivated neutrophils in AD patients, correlating with increased ROS as well as neutrophil extracellular traps [76]. Moreover, the ratio of harmful hyperreactive CXCR4-high senescent neutrophils versus immunosuppressive neutrophils rose in the later stages of AD in fast declining patients.

In mouse models of AD, neutrophils were found to extravasate from vessels and traffick to areas with amyloid deposits where they released neutrophil traps [77]. Another method by which neutrophils can promote neuropathology is by binding to cortical capillary walls, thus blocking blood flow. To look at the effects of stalled neutrophils in mouse AD models, antibodies against the neutrophil marker Ly6G were used to deplete neutrophils, resulting in increased blood flow and improved spatial memory performance [78]. While these studies show that neutrophils can promote AD pathology, MPO is not necessarily implicated. To directly examine the effects of elimination of neutrophil MPO in AD mouse models, the 5XFAD mice were irradiated, and the mice transplanted with bone marrow from MPO-deficient mice. Results showed improved spatial memory in the water maze and reduced levels of inflammatory mediators [51].

This study provides evidence that neutrophil-derived MPO can promote AD-related pathology in the 5XFAD mouse model.

Histology, performed by our lab, clearly shows much higher MPO protein levels in neutrophils in vessels as compared with resident astrocytes, neurons, or microglia, yet there are higher numbers of MPO-positive neurons, astrocytes, and microglia in the parenchyma. Further studies are warranted to understand the relative effects of brain resident cells, as compared with circulatory neutrophils in AD pathology.

Conclusions from Studies of Human MPO Expression in AD and Mouse Models of AD

These studies show that the human MPO gene is normally quiescent in brain tissue but can be induced in AD brain in microglia, astrocytes, or neurons by signals generated by Aβ release or deposition in plaques or along the walls of blood vessels. MPO expression in AD brain was associated with greater Aβ deposition in plaques in carriers of ApoE, the major genetic risk factor for AD. In the MPO-APP23 mouse model, hMPO expression is associated with greater memory impairment in water maze tests. In both human AD and the MPO-APP23 mouse model, hMPO expression leads to increased phospholipid peroxidation, particularly PS-OOH and PI-OOH.

THE ROLE OF MPO IN PARKINSON'S DISEASE

PD, the second most common neurodegenerative human disease, is associated with the selective loss of dopaminergic neurons in the substantia nigra pars compacta (SNpc) leading to tremor, bradykinesia, rigidity, and postural instability (reviewed in Refs. [79,80]). Compelling evidence, both histopathological and epidemiological, implicates α-synuclein (αSyn) oligomers and aggregates as the primary cause of PD. While the mechanisms leading to αSyn aggregation are not fully understood, evidence points to a role for oxidative stress [81–85]. MPO, as a component of the innate immune system and a source of reactive oxygen and nitrogen species, is likely to contribute to the oxidation and aggregation of αSyn [8]. As shown above, the MPO gene can be aberrantly induced in microglia, astrocytes, and neurons in AD [3–5] and, as shown below, also in astrocytes and neurons in PD [6–8].

MPO Is Expressed in PD Substantia Nigra Neurons But Not in Normal Aged Brain

Immunohistological analysis of sections from PD SNpc revealed the presence of MPO in melanized neurons as shown at low magnification (Figure 15.5a–c) and at higher magnification (Figure 15.5d, h, i and k) in contrast to little to no MPO detected in melanized neurons in control aged SNpc (Figure 15.5f and g), providing the first evidence of MPO expression in PD SNpc neurons [8]. Neuromelanin, a degradation product of dopamine, appears as light brown pigment in vesicles (Figure 15.5e–g), while MPO immunostaining is black and granular (Figure 15.5d, h, i and k). Quantitation revealed that ~ 20% of melanized PD SNpc neurons stained for MPO compared with 3% in normal aged brain (Figure 15.5j).

MPO Is Detected in Vesicles in PD SN Neurons That Also Contain αSyn Aggregates, Nitrated αSyn, and HOCl-Modified Epitopes

Confocal fluorescence microscopy revealed the robust presence of MPO in vesicles (red) surrounding intracellular αSyn aggregates (green) in PD SNpc neurons (Figure 15.6a and b). As evidence of MPO-generated oxidative damage, MPO was detected in neurons containing nitrated αSyn (Figure 15.6c). More than 30% of PD SNpc neurons were positive for nitrated αSyn as compared with 6% of neurons in aged control brain (Figure 15.6d). MPO-dependent HOCl-modified epitopes were present in more than 40% of neuromelanin positive dopaminergic neurons in PD SNpc (Figure 15.6e and f). MPO was immunodetected in neurons along with HOCl-modified epitopes in more than half of SNpc neurons, as compared with 10% of age-matched controls (Figure 15.6g and h). As evidence that the MPO expressing cells were neurons, MPO-positive cells costained for the dopaminergic neuron marker tyrosine hydroxylase [8]. In summary, the results showed that the expression of MPO in PD SNpc neurons correlates with the presence of nitrated αSyn and HOCl-modified epitopes.

MPO Expressed in hMPO-A53T Brain Is the Secreted 90 kDa Pro-MPO Form

To enable further study of the effects of hMPO expression in PD, the hMPO mouse model was crossed to a model expressing human αSyn-A53T mutant (hMPO-A53T). The A53T transgene contains the αSyn gene with the familial mutation A53T, which promotes fibril formation and aggregation of αSyn, thereby promoting PD [86].

In humans as well as mice, the MPO protein is expressed in bone marrow myeloid precursor cells as a 90 kDa precursor that is proteolytically cleaved in a post-endoplasmic reticulum (ER) compartment to generate the 59 kDa heavy chain and 15 kDa light chain. In a series of events the protomers are covalently bound through a heme group, and two heavy–light protomers are subsequently linked via a disulfide bond between the two heavy chains (reviewed in Ref. [87]). In promyelocytes MPO is trafficked to azurophilic granules, and when neutrophils phagocytose microbes, the MPO-containing vesicles fuse with the phagosome to release MPO to the interior, whereupon MPO reacts with Cl$^-$ to generate HOCl and other microbicidal oxidants. In some cell lines, the 90 kDa MPO precursor can also enter the secretory pathway leading to extracellular release of active MPO (reviewed in Ref. [87]). MPO cDNA transfected into breast cancer cell lines can be processed as the 90 kDa active monomer, which enters the secretory pathway or is processed as the heavy and light chains and trafficked to the granules [88]. To investigate which form of hMPO is produced by cells in the brain, extracts were made from cortex, midbrain, or cerebellum/spinal base from MPO-A53T and A53T brains. MPO was immunoprecipitated and analyzed by western blot, revealing that the 90 kDa proMPO was the predominant form of MPO in the hMPO-A53T brain with little to no 59 kDa MPO heavy chain detected. Interestingly, the highest concentration of MPO 90 kDa proMPO was in the cortex, with approximately half as much in midbrain, and little to no MPO in cerebellum (Figure 15.7a, lanes 1–3), indicating spatial differences in MPO inducers in the brains. Extracts of the A53T brains lacking the hMPO transgene showed no proMPO and no 59 kDa MPO heavy chain (Figure 15.7, lanes 5–7), indicating that the mouse MPO gene is not induced in A53T brain. The 90 kDa MPO precursor was similarly the predominant form in hMPO-Syn61, expressing the native human αSyn gene (Figure 15.7b, lane 4), and hMPO-APP23 (Figure 15.7b, lane 2), while only the 59 kDa heavy chain was seen in mouse bone marrow cells (Figure 15.7b, lane 3). When immunoprecipitation was performed on human

Human PD substantia nigra

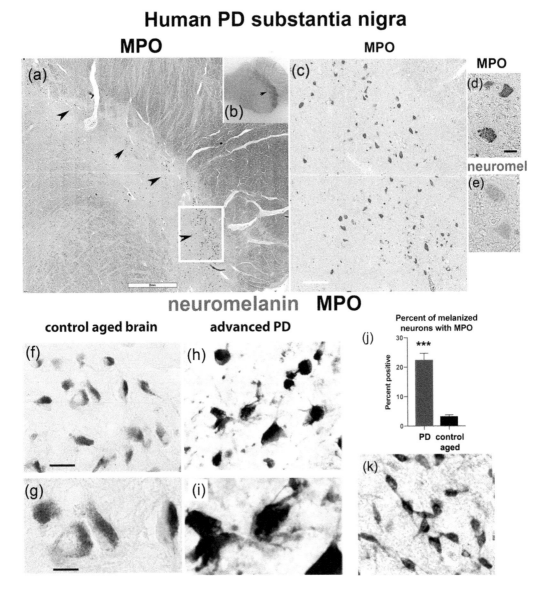

Figure 15.5 MPO is expressed in neurons in PD substantia nigra. Sections of PD SNpc were immunostained with rabbit anti-MPO antibodies followed by biotinylated secondary antibodies and developed with Vector SG peroxidase substrate (black). Arrowheads denote the tract of melanized neurons (a). Boxed area is enlarged in panel c. (b) Paraffin block containing control human SNpc with arrow indicating the melanized tract. (c) MPO immunostaining of melanized neurons in PD SNpc at higher magnification. (d) Magnification of MPO immunostained neurons (black) from the melanized tract. (e) Melanized neurons lacking MPO immunostaining showing brown neuromelanin. (f, g) No MPO immunostaining (black) of melanized neurons (brown) in control aged brain tissue (f) with higher magnification in g. (h, i) MPO immunostaining (black) in dystrophic SNpc neurons exhibiting fibrous dystrophic morphology in advanced stage PD (h), with higher magnification in (i). (j) Percent of melanized neurons expressing MPO. A minimum of three sections from eight PD and eight normal control SN were analyzed. (k) Image of a region adjacent to the melanized tract showing MPO immunostaining in a different type of neurons. Scale bar a 2 mm, c 200 μm, d, e 5 μm, f 20 μm, g 10 μm. (Panels are reprinted from, Maki et al., 2019 [8], Human myeloperoxidase (hMPO) is expressed in neurons in the substantia nigra in Parkinson's disease and in the hMPO-alpha-synuclein-A53T mouse model, correlating with increased nitration and aggregation of alpha-synuclein and exacerbation of motor impairment, *Free. Radic. Biol. Med.* 141: 115–140, (Figure 11a–e, j, k, m, n) with permission from Elsevier.)

Human PD substantia nigra

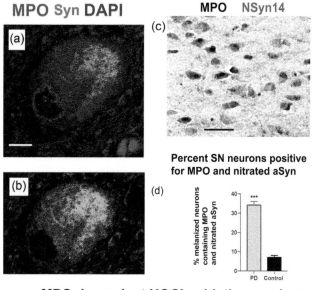

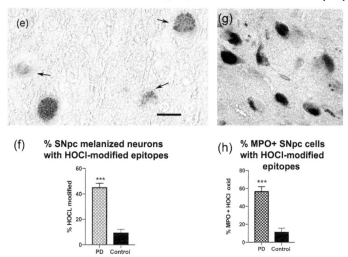

Figure 15.6 MPO-specific HOCl-modification products and nitrated αSyn detected in neurons in PD SNpc. (a) Confocal immunofluorescence staining of a neuron from PD SNpc showing MPO (rabbit anti-hMPO, red), αSyn (mouse Syn505, green), and DAPI (blue) (63×). (b) Single channel immunofluorescence of αSyn alone from a. (c) Immunoperoxidase staining of MPO (rabbit, black) and nitrated αSyn (nSyn14, red) in melanized neurons in human PD SNpc. (d) Percent of melanized neurons costaining for both MPO and nitrated αSyn in human PD SNpc versus aged control SN. (e) Monoclonal antibody 2D10G9 detects HOCl-modified epitopes (black) in vesicles in melanized SN neurons (arrows). (f) Quantitation of neurons positive for HOCl-modified epitopes in PD SNpc versus control SNpc. (g) Immunostaining for MPO (red) in neurons that also stain for HOCl-modified epitopes using 2D10G9 (black). (h) Quantitation of MPO positive neurons with HOCl epitopes in PD SNpc versus control aged SNpc. Statistical significance in d, f, and h was determined by Student's t test. (Panels are reprinted from, Maki et al., 2019 [8]). Human myeloperoxidase (hMPO) is expressed in neurons in the substantia nigra in Parkinson's disease and in the hMPO-alpha-synuclein-A53T mouse model, correlating with increased nitration and aggregation of alpha-synuclein and exacerbation of motor impairment, *Free. Radic. Biol. Med.* 141: 115–140. (Figure 12a, b, e, f, g, i, h, k) with permission from Elsevier.)

PD SNpc extracts, the proMPO 90 kDa protein was present at higher levels than was the 55–59 kDa MPO heavy chain, along with a 70 kDa processing intermediate [8]. These findings indicate that neurons are less able than myeloid precursor cells to process the MPO precursor to the heavy and light chains. This finding raises the important possibility that MPO can be secreted from neurons in PD or AD, resulting in oxidative damage to neighboring cells and potentially propagating PD or AD pathology through the brain. ELISA assays showed that in the humanized MPO mouse and the MPO-A53T mouse brains, there is between about 2,000 and 1,700 pg/mg protein, respectively (Figure

15.7c). Human PD SNpc was found to contain similar levels of MPO protein (between 1,000 and 1,500 pg/mg protein). In contrast, the A53T or C57Bl/6 mouse brains had sixfold lower levels of MPO protein (250 pg/mg), possibly coming from monocytes and neutrophils.

Human MPO Transgene Is Expressed in Neurons in the A53T Model of PD

Sections of hMPO-A53T cortex showed the presence of MPO in neurons costaining for the neuronal marker NeuN (Figure 15.7d and e). Quantitation showed approximately 30% of cortical neurons

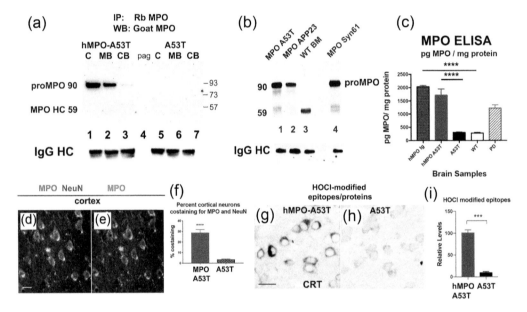

Figure 15.7 MPO is expressed as the secretory 90 kDa precursor in hMPO-A53T brain and leads to increased carbamylation and HOCl-modified epitopes, resulting in greater motor impairment. – (a) Immunoprecipitation of MPO from different regions of hMPO-A53T brain. Antibodies to MPO (rabbit) were added to extracts of isolated regions of mouse brains and bound proteins pulled down with magnetic protein A/G beads. Bound proteins were eluted and fractionated by SDS-PAGE (4%–12%). Western blots were probed with HRP-conjugated goat anti-MPO antibodies (R&D) to reveal immunoprecipitated proteins from hMPO-A53T cortex (C) (lane 1), midbrain (MB) (lane 2), or cerebellum (CB) (lane 3). The control pull-down with Protein A/G beads in the absence of antibodies is in lane 4 (pag). Immunoprecipitation of MPO from extracts of A53T cortex (lane 5), midbrain (MB) (lane 6), and cerebellum/brainstem (CB) (lane 7) showed no detectable MPO (n=4 MPO-A53T brains and 4 A53T brains). Rabbit IgG heavy chain was probed as a loading control (IgG HC). Results show that the 90 kDa proMPO precursor is the predominant form of MPO in hMPO-A53T cortex, with less in midbrain, and little to no MPO in cerebellum. (b) The 90 kDa proMPO is also predominantly expressed in hMPO-APP23 (lane 2) and MPO-Syn61 PD model (lane 4), as in MPO-A53T (lane 1). Mouse WT bone marrow (WT BM) (lane 3) expresses the mature MPO 59 kDa heavy chain. (c) MPO was quantified by ELISA in brain extracts prepared from hMPO tg, hMPO-A53T, A53T, C57Bl/6 WT, and human PD SN. The asterisks indicate a significant difference (P < 0.0001) between the hMPO tg and hMPO-A53T as compared with A53T or C57Bl/6 WT mice. (d–f) Immunofluorescent costaining of MPO (green) and the neuronal marker NeuN (red) in the cortex (d) or only MPO (e). (f) Image analysis determined ~ 30% of cortical cells co-localized for MPO and NeuN in MPO A53T as compared with few cells in A53T. (g, h, i) Immunoperoxidase staining shows MPO-generated HOCl modified epitopes detected in cortical neurons from MPO-A53T (g) of A53T (h) with monoclonal antibody 2D10G9. Quantification of levels of 2D10G9 immunoreactivity in hMPO-A53T versus A53T by ImageJ software (i).

(Continued)

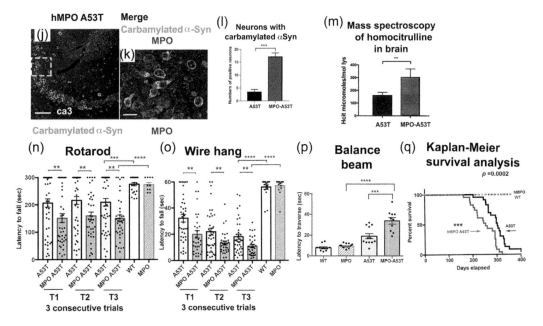

Figure 15.7 (Continued) MPO is expressed as the secretory 90 kDa precursor in hMPO-A53T brain and leads to increased carbamylation and HOCl-modified epitopes, resulting in greater motor impairment. – (j) Confocal immunofluorescence staining of MPO (red) and carbamylated αSyn (green) in MPO-A53T mouse hippocampus CA3 region. (k) Boxed area in j is enlarged. (l) Quantitation of numbers of CA3 neurons positive for carbamylated αSyn in MPO-A53T and A53T hippocampus. (m) Mass spectrometry quantitation of levels of carbamylated lysine (homocitrulline) in the A53T mouse brain as compared with the hMPO-A53T mouse brain (**P<0.005). (n–p) Impaired motor abilities in hMPO-A53T mice compared with A53T. (n) Rotarod analysis was performed with the indicated genotypes A53T, hMPO-A53T, hMPO transgenics (MPO), and wild-type (WT, C57Bl/6). Three consecutive trials (T1–T3) were performed. (o) The wire hang (three trials) was performed with the same genotypes. (p) Balance beam was performed with the genotypes indicated. Behavior data were analyzed using a one-way analysis of variance (ANOVA) followed by Dunnet's post-hoc test and represented as mean±S.E.M. (**P<0.005, ***P<0.001, ****P<0.0001). (q) hMPO-A53T mice reach end-stage paralysis earlier than A53T mice. Statistical significance determined by the Kaplan–Meier survival analysis (Mantel–Cox) for hMPO-A53T and A53T (***P=0.0002). (Panels are reprinted from, Maki et al., 2019 [8]). Human myeloperoxidase (hMPO) is expressed in neurons in the substantia nigra in Parkinson's disease and in the hMPO-a-synuclein mouse model, correlating with increased nitration and aggregation of alpha-synuclein and exacerbation of motor impairment, *Free Radic. Biol. Med.* (Figures 1m–o, 2a–c, 6f–h, 7a, b, g, h, 9a–d), with permission from Elsevier.)

expressing both NeuN and MPO in hMPO-A53T, while there was no significant staining of mouse MPO in A53T (Figure 15.7f). Thus, human MPO, but not mouse MPO, was expressed in neurons in the PD models. RNAscope *in situ* hybridization further confirmed hMPO mRNA expression in cultured embryonic neurons from hMPO-A53T mice [8].

HOCl-Modified Epitopes in MPO-A53T Brain

Chlorination is a specific oxidation product of MPO (reviewed in Refs. [89,90]). When MPO-A53T and A53T cortical brain sections were stained using antibody 2D10G9 that recognizes HOCl-modified epitopes [91,92], higher levels of HOCl-modified epitopes were seen in MPO-A53T as compared with A53T cortex (Figure 15.7g and h),

as quantified in Figure 15.7i. Thus, MPO expression in neurons leads to HOCl-modified epitopes.

Carbamylation of αSyn by MPO in A53T Mouse Brain

Carbamylation (also called carbamoylation) is a reaction between isocyanic acid and the nucleophilic functional groups on proteins [93]. Isocyanic acid can be produced by two reactions: urea deamination and thiocyanate oxidation by myeloperoxidase. MPO is an enzymatic catalyst of protein carbamylation *in vivo*. Confocal images of mouse hippocampus provided evidence of increased carbamylated αSyn in hMPO-A53T compared with A53T brain (Figure 15.7j and k). In order to detect carbamylated lysine, antibodies against carbamylated peptides of αSyn were generated. A low-magnification (20×) image shows immunostaining of carbamylated αSyn (green) and MPO (red) in pyramidal neurons of the hippocampal CA3 region (Figure 15.7j). The boxed area is further enlarged to show colocalization (yellow) of MPO (red) and carbamylated αSyn (green) in a subset of neurons (63×) (Figure 15.7k). To quantitate the level of carbamylation, immunopositive neurons from each genotype were counted, revealing a significant increase of carbamylated lysine-positive neurons in the CA3 region of hMPO-A53T brain versus A53T brain (Figure 15.7l). To further quantitate the amounts of Hcit, extracts were prepared from hMPO-A53T and A53T brains and analyzed by mass spectrometry to confirm significantly higher levels of HCit in the hMPO-A53T brains as compared with A53T brains (Figure 15.7m).

MPO Expression Exacerbates Motor Impairment in the hMPO-A53T Mice

To determine if hMPO expression affects motor abilities in the hMPO-A53T model, several standard motor behavior tests were carried out. The accelerating Rotarod tests balance, coordination, muscle strength, and stamina, as the mice are required to maintain balance on a rotating bar in three consecutive tests of 5 min duration with 5 min rest intervals (Figure 15.7n). Most WT or hMPO mice were able to remain on the rotarod for the entire 300 s time interval. The A53T mice were less able to maintain balance, resulting in a mean latency to fall of 206 s, while the hMPO-A53T mice were the least able to maintain hold, with a mean latency of 151 s. These findings show that the hMPO transgene exacerbates the motor impairment of the A53T mice. Importantly, the hMPO transgene had no effect on motor abilities in the absence of the A53T gene, indicating that hMPO functionally synergizes with αSyn to exacerbate αSyn-mediated motor impairment, possibly due to MPO nitration/carbamylation of αSyn leading to neurotoxic aggregates.

The wire hang is a method to test grip strength, stamina, and neuromuscular dysfunction (Figure 15.7o). The mice are required to support their weight inverted on a cage top for up to 60 s for three consecutive tests with 5 min rest intervals. In most cases, WT mice or hMPO (MPO) mice easily maintained grip through the three 60 s trials (mean latency to fall of 56 s). The A53T mice (gray) fell at a mean of 37 s on the first trial and earlier on succeeding trials. The hMPO-A53T (red) fell even earlier at a mean of 19 s on trial 1 and earlier on successive trials. Again, the hMPO transgene had no effect on grip strength in the absence of the A53T transgene, demonstrating that hMPO and αSyn synergize to exacerbate motor impairment.

The balance beam is another test of balance and motor impairment (Figure 15.7p). Mice are required to traverse a dowel (1 m) with diameter of 1 cm. WT or hMPO mice traverse the beam in less than 10 s, while the A53T mice required a mean of 18 s and the hMPO-A53T mice crossed in mean 34 s. Again, there was no effect of the hMPO transgene alone, indicating a functional interaction between hMPO and αSyn to increase motor impairment at these early stages of αSyn-mediated damage. As further indication of the negative impact of MPO oxidants in association with αSyn, Kaplan–Meier survival analysis showed that hMPO expression in the A53T model leads to earlier onset of end-stage paralysis (Figure 15.7q). Based on these findings, we conclude that hMPO expression in neurons results in greater oxidative damage to neurons that leads to impairment of motor abilities in the A53T model.

The results confirm and extend previous work studying MPO in a different model of PD [6]. In the MPTP model of PD, 1-methyl-4-phenyl-1,2,3,6-tetrahydropyrine is metabolized into the toxic cation 1-methyl-4-phenylpyridinium (MPP+) by the enzyme monoamine oxidase B. MPP+ primarily kills dopamine-producing neurons. The results showed that the intraperitoneal injection of MPTP resulted in reduced numbers of tyrosine hydroxylase-positive neurons and increased MPO expression in astrocytes [6]. In addition, the MPTP-induced neuropathology was reduced in MPO-deficient mice [6]. Taken together these results point to the significant participation of MPO in the oxidative damage and resulting cell death in the MPTP mouse model of PD.

A neurodegenerative disease related to PD is multiple system atrophy (MSA) (reviewed in Ref. [94]). The disease is rare and fatal. It is characterized by a variable combination of parkinsonism, cerebellar impairment, and autonomic dysfunction [94]. MPO expression was shown in microglia in the degenerating areas of human

MSA brains [95]. A mouse model of MSA was developed in which mice overexpressing oligodendroglial αSyn are placed under conditions of oxidative stress induced by 3-nitropropionic acid (3-NP) [96]. In this model, MPO was found to be upregulated in microglia. Interestingly, when an MPO inhibitor, AZD3241, was given to the MSA mice, there was reduced motor impairment and a rescue of vulnerable neurons [95]. Recently, this inhibitor was tested in MSA patients in a Phase 2 study with encouraging results [97]. These studies point to the possible use of an MPO inhibitor for the treatment of MSA as well as other neurodegenerative diseases where MPO is involved.

Conclusions from Studies of MPO in Parkinson's Disease

The findings showed that in PD substantia nigra, the hMPO gene is expressed in neurons containing aggregates of nitrated αSyn and MPO-specific HOCl-modified epitopes. In the hMPO-A53T mouse model, hMPO expression was seen also in neurons while mouse MPO was not expressed. In the A53T model, hMPO was expressed in neurons co-localizing with nitrated αSyn, carbamylated lysine, nitrotyrosine, as well as HOCl-modified epitopes/proteins. RNAscope in situ hybridization confirmed hMPO mRNA expression in cultured MPO-A53T embryonic neurons [8]. Interestingly, as in the APP model, the hMPO protein expressed in hMPO-A53T brain is primarily the precursor proMPO, which enters the secretory pathway potentially resulting in interneuronal transmission of MPO and oxidative species. As evidence of the deleterious impact of MPO oxidants, the hMPO-A53T model exhibited significant exacerbation of motor impairment on the rotating rod, balance beam, and wire hang tests, as compared with A53T lacking hMPO. hMPO expression in the A53T model further resulted in earlier onset of end-stage paralysis. Importantly, hMPO expression in the absence of the αSyn transgene had no effect on motor impairment, indicating a synergistic interaction between MPO and αSyn, likely involving MPO oxidation of αSyn promoting fibrillation and aggregation. Together these findings suggest that MPO plays an important role in nitrative and oxidative damage that contributes to αSyn pathology in PD.

Why Is MPO Expressed in Astrocytes or Neurons in AD or PD Brain?

One likely mechanism involves the upstream Alu element with the −463 G polymorphism creating an SP1 site in the first of four hexamer half-sites recognized by members of the nuclear receptor family of ligand-binding sites including RAR, PPARγ/α, LXR, and ER [12,13]. These four sites, and the G at position 5 in the first hexamer element, are present in all members of the major Alu superfamily, as was first reported for the MPO promoter [13,15]. Alu elements are transposable and derived from a corrupted 7SL gene. During the past 65 million years, more than 1 million Alu elements have inserted throughout primate genomes, and this infiltration of regulatory sites is thought to have enhanced primate evolution by altering gene expression patterns [15] (reviewed in Ref. [98]). The Alu insertion upstream of MPO may have been beneficial, allowing induced expression of MPO in the brains of early primates in the event of microbial infection due to head injury or gum disease. However, in the present epoch, MPO expression in neurons or astrocytes in aging brain can be pathologic, leading to oxidized fibrillar Aβ promoting AD. Because selective pressures work only on people of reproductive age, and AD occurs in people post reproductive age, selective pressures would not disable the Alu sites to prevent MPO expression.

THE ROLE OF MPO IN MULTIPLE SCLEROSIS

MS was the first neurodegenerative disease state in which MPO was implicated by association studies of the −463G/A promoter polymorphism as well as immunohistochemical data [9]. MS is an inflammatory disease of the central nervous system, characterized by multifocal lesions corresponding to sites of demyelination of axons (reviewed in Refs. [99,100]). The autoimmune condition is thought to be initiated by T cells recognizing myelin-associated antigens, such as myelin basic protein [101]. The myelin reactive T cells are thought to secrete cytokines and chemokines, which enhance the infiltration and activation of macrophages and microglia. These activated phagocytes attack and degrade the myelin sheath, a process that is likely to be exacerbated by the release of compounds that generate

ROS [102,103]. There is increasing evidence that MPO is actively involved in the disease process.

As described above, the −463G/A polymorphism in the upstream promoter of the human MPO gene likely contributes to the regulation of MPO gene expression [13] through the creation of an SP1 site associated with several nuclear receptor-binding sites. The −463 GG (originally called SpSp) genotype was first found to be associated with the incidence of myeloid leukemia [57]. Because ROS generated by macrophages and microglia are implicated in neurodegenerative diseases such as MS, an investigation of the possible involvement of MPO in this disease state was subsequently undertaken. An analysis of the MPO polymorphism was examined in 59 MS cases [9]. Of these MS cases, 43 (73%) were females, consistent with the known prevalence of females in MS. The percent of the GG genotype among the

female MS cases was 74%, which is higher than the 61% GG observed in the general population, suggesting that MPO plays a role in MS pathology.

While another study supported the idea that there is an association between the −463GG genotype leading to higher disability and secondary progressive disease in MS [104], other case-control studies did not find this association [105–108]. Various reasons have been proposed for these differences, including ethnic diversity among the participants [108].

To determine if MPO-expressing cells exist in the vicinity of MS lesions, immunohistochemical analysis was performed with brain sections containing MS lesions. MPO-positive cells were detected in and around MS lesions (Figure 15.8), some of which had morphology suggestive of ramified microglia (Figure 15.8a and b). To determine if MPO-positive cells were present at active

MPO expressed in microglia in MS brain

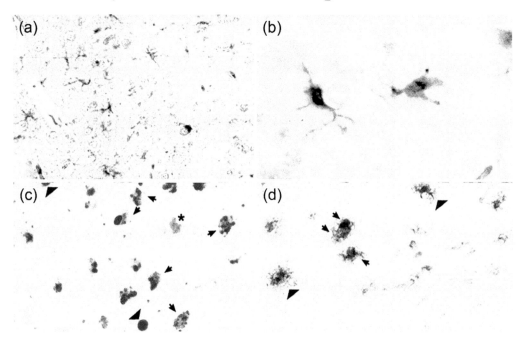

Figure 15.8 Immunohistochemical detection of MPO in MS brain sections. (a) Anti-human MPO immunohistochemical staining of an active MS lesion showing widely distributed brown stained cells (×400). (b) At higher magnification, the MPO-expressing dark brown cells exhibit typical morphology of microglia (×800). (c) Active lesion stained for MPO (brown-yellow) and neutral lipids by Oil Red orange (red) shows co-localization of phagocytosed Oil Red O stained cells expressing MPO (arrows). A few MPO-expressing cells are noted without red staining (*). Oil Red O stained cells with no expression of MPO are also visible (arrowheads) (×800). (d) Double immunostaining for HLA-DR (black), a marker for macrophages, and MPO (red) identifies cells as microglia macrophages (arrows). (Panels are reprinted from Nagra et al., 1997 [9]). Immunohistochemical and genetic evidence of myeloperoxidase involvement in multiple sclerosis, J. Neuroimmunol. 78: 97–107 with permission from Elsevier.)

lesions, sections were costained with Oil Red O, which stains neutral lipids from partially degraded myelin within phagocytic vesicles in macrophages. A cluster of macrophages with multiple Oil Red O stained vesicles was observed to costain for MPO (Figure 15.8c). As evidence that these are macrophages microglia, these cells costained with MPO and HLA-DR a macrophage marker (Figure 15.8d). This places MPO within phagocytic macrophages at MS lesions. A total of 332 lesions were examined from five different donors. MPO-positive cells were detected in approximately 70% of the active lesions in all five donors. Significantly more MPO-positive cells were detected within active lesions than in parenchyma outside lesions or in normal non-MS brain sections. The presence of MPO in microglia/macrophages in MS patients was also demonstrated in the cerebral cortex and was shown to be active [10].

Do microglia express MPO mRNA? Microglia are the macrophages of the brain and like blood borne monocyte macrophages were generally thought to lack MPO mRNA. A PCR approach was used to test for the presence of MPO mRNA in microglia isolated from human brain tissue. Microglia-derived cDNA was tested by PCR with primers spanning two introns to allow the mRNA-derived product to be readily distinguished by size from genomic DNA. A product of the correct size was obtained from the microglial samples from two donors and the DNA sequenced to confirm the presence of MPO cDNA [9]. We conclude that microglia express MPO mRNA.

The Role of MPO in the EAE Model of Multiple Sclerosis

A common animal model of MS is experimental autoimmune encephalomyelitis (EAE). To further delineate the role of MPO in MS, the MPO knockout mouse was used in the EAE model [109]. The MPO knockout on the C57Bl/6 background was treated with MOG 35–55 peptide to induce EAE. There were two primary findings. First, MPO was detected in invading macrophages in the CNS of MOG-treated wild-type mice, and second, unexpectedly, the MPO knockout mice had significantly increased incidence of EAE: 90% of MPO-KO mice developed complete hind limb paralysis as compared with 33% of WT littermates. This paradoxical result suggested that MPO may play a protective role in EAE, possibly linked to later findings of increased iNOS expression and

nitration products in MPO KO monocyte/macrophages [110–112]. Similarly, in a related study, the MPO KO model was unexpectedly found to increase atherosclerosis in the LDL receptor-deficient model [113], in contrast to the human MPO transgenic mouse crossed to the LDL receptor-deficient model, which resulted in increased atherosclerosis, as expected [11].

Recent papers may offer some explanation for the paradoxical effects in MPO KO models. Generalized pustular psoriasis (GPP) is a severe inflammatory disease characterized by increased numbers of neutrophils in pustules in the skin due to impaired clearance of neutrophils by monocytes (efferocytosis). Whole exome sequencing of GPP patients showed the disease is due to various mutations in MPO resulting in loss of MPO activity [114,115] and associated with alterations in protease activity and reduced NET formation [114,115]. Phagocytosis assays in MPO-deficient mice similarly revealed impaired clearance of neutrophils by monocytes.

More recently, in another study of EAE using the MPO knockout mice, it was shown that the MPO knockout mice had less disease [116]. This group also used MOG 35–55 peptide to induce EAE in the MPO knockout on the C57Bl/6 background [116]. The authors point out that the differences between the studies could be due to induction protocols, genetics, and the host microbiota [116]. There is considerable interest in the role of the microbiome in neurodegenerative disease, and this factor probably deserves more study.

The link between MPO and MS has been further strengthened by testing inhibitors of MPO in the EAE model. An irreversible inhibitor of MPO, ABAH, was injected i.p., in the SJL mice treated with proteolipid protein (PLP) in the EAE model [117]. MPO inhibition was accompanied by a decrease in demyelination and lower inflammatory cell recruitment in the brain suggesting a central role for MPO in inflammatory demyelination (see article by Chen in this issue).

A novel tripeptide inhibitor of MPO has also been developed, N-acetyllysyltrosylcysteine amide (KYC) [118]. This inhibitor was developed based on the idea that Tyr* formed by MPO activity is scavenged by the thiol of the adjacent Cys. This prevents Tyr* from leaving the active site of MPO and oxidizing other cellular targets [118]. The authors found that therapeutic administration of KYC for 5 days starting at the peak of disease attenuated

EAE disease severity, resulting in a significant reduction in the level of MPO and reduced myeloid cell numbers and permeability of the blood–brain barrier [116]. A similar result was seen in a progressive model of EAE using NOD mice [119].

There have been some differences in the results in animal models using the MPO knockout mice, likely attributed to protocol design and genetic background of the mice. However, the results as a whole strongly support the idea that MPO inhibition should be considered as a treatment for MS as well as other neurodegenerative diseases, such as PD and AD.

As described in another chapter in this book (see article by Chen in this issue), imaging of MPO in the EAE model has proven to be a valuable indicator of disease progression as well as a measure of the benefits of using MPO inhibitor to treat disease. The role of MPO is now well established in MS and the EAE model. Future efforts will need to explore the value of MPO inhibitors and imaging agents as therapeutics to treat this disease.

CONCLUSIONS

There is convincing evidence of aberrant or atypical MPO expression in astrocytes, neurons, or microglia in neurodegenerative diseases, including AD, PD, and MS. In human AD or PD, MPO expression has been linked to oxidative damage, including nitration, carbamylation, chlorination, and phospholipid peroxidation. Studies using the humanized MPO mouse model crossed to AD and PD models provide evidence that MPO enhances the deleterious effects of Aβ or αSyn in neurodegenerative disease, as the hMPO transgene in the absence of A53T-αSyn or APP23 transgenes has no deleterious effect on memory or motor abilities. This demonstrates that MPO acts in concert with Aβ or αSyn to promote neurodegeneration, likely due to MPO oxidation of Aβ or αSyn that leads to more neurotoxic fibrils or aggregates. Another interesting recent finding is that MPO is produced in the brain as the 90 kD precursor that trafficks through the secretory pathway to be released from neurons or astrocytes, potentially propagating oxidative damage and AD pathology throughout the brain. Future studies should examine the effects of available MPO inhibitors on the course of AD, PD, and MS in mouse models and in humans (reviewed in Refs. [120,121]).

ACKNOWLEDGMENTS

This work was supported in part by the National Institutes of Health (United States) ROI NS074303, ROI AG017879, and ROI AG040623 to WFR. Additional funding to support these studies has been generously provided by Sanford Burnham Prebys Medical Discovery Institute (La Jolla, CA) to WFR.

REFERENCES

1. S.J. Klebanoff, A.J. Kettle, H. Rosen, C.C. Winterbourn, W.M. Nauseef, 2013, Myeloperoxidase: a front-line defender against phagocytosed microorganisms, J. Leukoc. Biol. 93: 185–198.
2. C.C. Winterbourn, A.J. Kettle, M.B. Hampton, 2016, Reactive oxygen species and neutrophil function, Annu. Rev. Biochem. 85: 765–792.
3. W.F. Reynolds, J. Rhees, D. Maciejewski, et al., 1999, Myeloperoxidase polymorphism is associated with gender specific risk for Alzheimer's disease, Exp. Neurol. 155: 31–41.
4. R.A. Maki, V.A. Tyurin, R.C. Lyon, et al., 2009, Aberrant expression of myeloperoxidase in astrocytes promotes phospholipid oxidation and memory deficits in a mouse model of Alzheimer disease, J. Biol. Chem. 284: 3158–3169.
5. P.S. Green, A.J. Mendez, J.S. Jacob, et al., 2004, Neuronal expression of myeloperoxidase is increased in Alzheimer's disease, J. Neurochem. 90: 724–733.
6. D.K. Choi, S. Pennathur, C. Perier, et al., 2005, Ablation of the inflammatory enzyme myeloperoxidase mitigates features of Parkinson's disease in mice, J. Neurosci. 25: 6594–6600.
7. S. Gellhaar, D. Sunnemark, H. Eriksson, L. Olson, D. Galter, 2017, Myeloperoxidase-immunoreactive cells are significantly increased in brain areas affected by neurodegeneration in Parkinson's and Alzheimer's disease, Cell Tissue Res. 369: 445–454.
8. R.A. Maki, M. Holzer, K. Motamedchaboki, et al., 2019, Human myeloperoxidase (hMPO) is expressed in neurons in the substantia nigra in Parkinson's disease and in the hMPO-alpha-synuclein-A53T mouse model, correlating with increased nitration and aggregation of alpha-synuclein and exacerbation of motor impairment, Free Radic. Biol. Med. 141: 115–140.
9. R.M. Nagra, B. Becher, W.W. Tourtellotte, et al., 1997, Immunohistochemical and genetic evidence of myeloperoxidase involvement in multiple sclerosis, J. Neuroimmunol. 78: 97–107.

10. E. Gray, T.L. Thomas, S. Betmouni, N. Scolding, S. Love, 2008, Elevated activity and microglial expression of myeloperoxidase in demyelinated cerebral cortex in multiple sclerosis, *Brain Pathol.* 18: 86–95.

11. L.W. Castellani, J.J. Chang, X. Wang, A.J. Lusis, W.F. Reynolds, 2006, Transgenic mice express human MPO −463G/A alleles at atherosclerotic lesions, developing hyperlipidemia and obesity in −463G males, *J. Lipid Res.* 47: 1366–1377.

12. A.P. Kumar, F.J. Piedrafita, W.F. Reynolds, 2004, Peroxisome proliferator-activated receptor gamma ligands regulate myeloperoxidase expression in macrophages by an estrogen-dependent mechanism involving the −463GA promoter polymorphism, *J. Biol. Chem.* 279: 8300–8315.

13. F.J. Piedrafita, R.B. Molander, G. Vansant, et al., 1996, An Alu element in the myeloperoxidase promoter contains a composite SP1-thyroid hormone-retinoic acid response element, *J. Biol. Chem.* 271: 14412–14420.

14. W.F. Reynolds, A.P. Kumar, F.J. Piedrafita, 2006, The human myeloperoxidase gene is regulated by LXR and PPARalpha ligands, *Biochem. Biophys. Res. Commun.* 349: 846–854.

15. G. Vansant, W.F. Reynolds, 1995, The consensus sequence of a major Alu subfamily contains a functional retinoic acid response element, *Proc. Natl. Acad. Sci. U.S.A.* 92: 8229–8233.

16. F.C. Crawford, M.J. Freeman, J.A. Schinka, et al., 2001, Association between Alzheimer's disease and a functional polymorphism in the Myeloperoxidase gene, *Exp. Neurol.* 167: 456–459.

17. B. Leininger-Muller, A. Hoy, B. Herbeth, et al., 2003, Myeloperoxidase G-463A polymorphism and Alzheimer's disease in the ApoEurope study, *Neurosci. Lett.* 349: 95–98.

18. S.K. Pope, S.B. Kritchevsky, C. Ambrosone, et al., 2006, Myeloperoxidase polymorphism and cognitive decline in older adults in the Health, Aging, and Body Composition Study, *Am. J. Epidemiol.* 163: 1084–1090.

19. W.F. Reynolds, M. Hiltunen, M. Pirskanen, et al., 2000, MPO and APOEepsilon4 polymorphisms interact to increase risk for AD in Finnish males, *Neurology* 55: 1284–1290.

20. M. Zappia, I. Manna, P. Serra, et al., 2004, Increased risk for Alzheimer disease with the interaction of MPO and A2M polymorphisms, *Arch. Neurol.* 61: 341–344.

21. A. Hoy, D. Tregouet, B. Leininger-Muller, et al., 2001, Serum myeloperoxidase concentration in a healthy population: biological variations, familial resemblance and new genetic polymorphisms, *Eur. J. Hum. Genet.* 9: 780–786.

22. R. Pecoits-Filho, L. Nordfors, B. Lindholm, et al., 2003, Genetic approaches in the clinical investigation of complex disorders: malnutrition, inflammation, and atherosclerosis (MIA) as a prototype, *Kidney Int. Suppl.*: S162–167.

23. R. Makela, P.J. Karhunen, T.A. Kunnas, et al., 2003, Myeloperoxidase gene variation as a determinant of atherosclerosis progression in the abdominal and thoracic aorta: an autopsy study, *Lab. Invest.* 83: 919–925.

24. R. Makela, R. Laaksonen, T. Janatuinen, et al., 2004, Myeloperoxidase gene variation and coronary flow reserve in young healthy men, *J. Biomed. Sci.* 11: 59–64.

25. F.W. Asselbergs, W.F. Reynolds, J.W. Cohen-Tervaert, G.A. Jessurun, R.A. Tio, 2004, Myeloperoxidase polymorphism related to cardiovascular events in coronary artery disease, *Am. J. Med.* 116: 429–430.

26. V. Rudolph, T.K. Rudolph, L. Kubala, et al., 2009, A myeloperoxidase promoter polymorphism is independently associated with mortality in patients with impaired left ventricular function, *Free Radic. Biol. Med.* 47: 1584–1590.

27. M.B. Schabath, M.R. Spitz, W.K. Hong, et al., 2002, A myeloperoxidase polymorphism associated with reduced risk of lung cancer, *Lung Cancer* 37: 35–40.

28. J.P. Yang, W.B. Wang, X.X. Yang, et al., 2013, The MPO-463G>A polymorphism and lung cancer risk: a meta-analysis based on 22 case-control studies, *PLoS One* 8: e65778.

29. D.J. Selkoe, J. Hardy, 2016, The amyloid hypothesis of Alzheimer's disease at 25 years, *EMBO Mol. Med.* 8: 595–608.

30. S. Saez-Atienzar, E. Masliah, 2020, Cellular senescence and Alzheimer disease: the egg and the chicken scenario, *Nat. Rev. Neurosci.* 21: 433–444.

31. G.R. Frost, L.A. Jonas, Y.M. Li, 2019, Friend, foe or both? Immune activity in alzheimer's disease, *Front. Aging Neurosci.* 11: 337.

32. R.S. Ray, A. Katyal, 2016, Myeloperoxidase: bridging the gap in neurodegeneration, *Neurosci. Biobehav. Rev.* 68: 611–620.

33. G.G. Glenner, C.W. Wong, 1984, Alzheimer's disease and Down's syndrome: sharing of a unique cerebrovascular amyloid fibril protein, *Biochem. Biophys. Res. Commun.* 122: 1131–1135.

34. D.J. Selkoe, 1994, Cell biology of the amyloid beta-protein precursor and the mechanism of Alzheimer's disease, *Annu. Rev. Cell Biol.* 10: 373–403.

35. C. Haass, D.J. Selkoe, 1993, Cellular processing of beta-amyloid precursor protein and the genesis of amyloid beta-peptide, *Cell* 75: 1039–1042.

36. D.W. Dickson, 1997, The pathogenesis of senile plaques, *J. Neuropathol. Exp. Neurol.* 56: 321–339.

37. C. Geula, C.K. Wu, D. Saroff, et al., 1998, Aging renders the brain vulnerable to amyloid beta-protein neurotoxicity, *Nat. Med.* 4: 827–831.

38. D. Giulian, L.J. Haverkamp, J.H. Yu, et al., 1996, Specific domains of beta-amyloid from Alzheimer plaque elicit neuron killing in human microglia, *J. Neurosci.* 16: 6021–6037.

39. M.P. Lambert, A.K. Barlow, B.A. Chromy, et al., 1998, Diffusible, nonfibrillar ligands derived from Abeta1–42 are potent central nervous system neurotoxins, *Proc. Natl. Acad. Sci. U.S.A.* 95: 6448–6453.

40. M. Citron, D. Westaway, W. Xia, et al., 1997, Mutant presenilins of Alzheimer's disease increase production of 42-residue amyloid beta-protein in both transfected cells and transgenic mice, *Nat. Med.* 3: 67–72.

41. D. Scheuner, C. Eckman, M. Jensen, et al., 1996, Secreted amyloid beta-protein similar to that in the senile plaques of Alzheimer's disease is increased in vivo by the presenilin 1 and 2 and APP mutations linked to familial Alzheimer's disease, *Nat. Med.* 2: 864–870.

42. M.A. Smith, K. Hirai, K. Hsiao, et al., 1998, Amyloid-beta deposition in Alzheimer transgenic mice is associated with oxidative stress, *J. Neurochem.* 70: 2212–2215.

43. S.D. Yan, S.F. Yan, X. Chen, et al., 1995, Nonenzymatically glycated tau in Alzheimer's disease induces neuronal oxidant stress resulting in cytokine gene expression and release of amyloid beta-peptide, *Nat. Med.* 1: 693–699.

44. C.E. Cross, B. Halliwell, E.T. Borish, et al., 1987, Oxygen radicals and human disease, *Ann. Intern. Med.* 107: 526–545.

45. G. Multhaup, T. Ruppert, A. Schlicksupp, et al., 1997, Reactive oxygen species and Alzheimer's disease, *Biochem. Pharmacol.* 54: 533–539.

46. M.A. Smith, 1998, Alzheimer disease, *Int. Rev. Neurobiol.* 42: 1–54.

47. C.A. Colton, D.L. Gilbert, 1993, Microglia, an in vivo source of reactive oxygen species in the brain, *Adv. Neurol.* 59: 321–326.

48. L. Meda, M.A. Cassatella, G.I. Szendrei, et al., 1995, Activation of microglial cells by beta-amyloid protein and interferon-gamma, *Nature* 374: 647–650.

49. D.M. Paresce, H. Chung, F.R. Maxfield, 1997, Slow degradation of aggregates of the Alzheimer's disease amyloid beta-protein by microglial cells, *J. Biol. Chem.* 272: 29390–29397.

50. A. Klegeris, P.L. McGeer, 1997, Beta-amyloid protein enhances macrophage production of oxygen free radicals and glutamate, *J. Neurosci. Res.* 49: 229–235.

51. R. Volkman, T. Ben-Zur, A. Kahana, B.Z. Garty, D. Offen, 2019, Myeloperoxidase deficiency inhibits cognitive decline in the 5XFAD mouse model of Alzheimer's disease, *Front. Neurosci.* 13: 990.

52. M.J. Davies, C.L. Hawkins, 2020, The role of myeloperoxidase in biomolecule modification, chronic inflammation, and disease, *Antioxid. Redox Signal.* 32: 957–981.

53. T. Sagoh, M. Yamada, 1988, Transcriptional regulation of myeloperoxidase gene expression in myeloid leukemia HL-60 cells during differentiation into granulocytes and macrophages, *Arch. Biochem. Biophys.* 262: 599–604.

54. A. Tobler, C.W. Miller, K.R. Johnson, et al., 1988, Regulation of gene expression of myeloperoxidase during myeloid differentiation, *J. Cell. Physiol.* 136: 215–225.

55. H. Li, J. Newcombe, N.P. Groome, M.L. Cuzner, 1993, Characterization and distribution of phagocytic macrophages in multiple sclerosis plaques, *Neuropathol. Appl. Neurobiol.* 19: 214–223.

56. T. Uchihara, H. Akiyama, H. Kondo, K. Ikeda, 1997, Activated microglial cells are colocalized with perivascular deposits of amyloid-beta protein in Alzheimer's disease brain, *Stroke* 28: 1948–1950.

57. W.F. Reynolds, E. Chang, D. Douer, E.D. Ball, V. Kanda, 1997, An allelic association implicates myeloperoxidase in the etiology of acute promyelocytic leukemia, *Blood* 90: 2730–2737.

58. O. Combarros, J. Infante, J. Llorca, et al., 2002, The myeloperoxidase gene in Alzheimer's disease: a case-control study and meta-analysis, *Neurosci. Lett.* 326: 33–36.

59. Y.Q. Zhang, Y.F. Jiang, M. Chen, N.N. Zhang, Y.F. Zhou, 2020, Association between myeloperoxidase rs2333227 polymorphism and susceptibility to coronary heart disease, *Arch. Med. Sci.* 16: 1231–1238.

60. E. Taioli, S. Benhamou, C. Bouchardy, et al., 2007, Myeloperoxidase G-463A polymorphism and lung cancer: a HuGE genetic susceptibility to environmental carcinogens pooled analysis, *Genet. Med.* 9: 67–73.

61. D.E. Schmechel, A.M. Saunders, W.J. Strittmatter, et al., 1993, Increased amyloid beta-peptide deposition in cerebral cortex as a consequence of apolipoprotein E genotype in late-onset Alzheimer disease, *Proc. Natl. Acad. Sci. U.S.A.* 90: 9649–9653.

62. W.J. Strittmatter, A.D. Roses, 1996, Apolipoprotein E and Alzheimer's disease, *Annu. Rev. Neurosci.* 19: 53–77.

63. A.M. Saunders, O. Hulette, K.A. Welsh-Bohmer, et al., 1996, Specificity, sensitivity, and predictive value of apolipoprotein-E genotyping for sporadic Alzheimer's disease, *Lancet* 348: 90–93.

64. L.M. Sayre, D.A. Zelasko, P.L. Harris, et al., 1997, 4-Hydroxynonenal-derived advanced lipid peroxidation end products are increased in Alzheimer's disease, *J. Neurochem.* 68: 2092–2097.

65. S.D. Yan, X. Chen, A.M. Schmidt, et al., 1994, Glycated tau protein in Alzheimer disease: a mechanism for induction of oxidant stress, *Proc. Natl. Acad. Sci. U.S.A.* 91: 7787–7791.

66. C. Jolivalt, B. Leininger-Muller, R. Drozdz, J.W. Naskalski, G. Siest, 1996, Apolipoprotein E is highly susceptible to oxidation by myeloperoxidase, an enzyme present in the brain, *Neurosci. Lett.* 210: 61–64.

67. W.J. Strittmatter, K.H. Weisgraber, D.Y. Huang, et al., 1993, Binding of human apolipoprotein E to synthetic amyloid beta peptide: isoform-specific effects and implications for late-onset Alzheimer disease, *Proc. Natl. Acad. Sci. U.S.A.* 90: 8098–8102.

68. L.T. McGrath, B.M. McGleenon, S. Brennan, et al., 2001, Increased oxidative stress in Alzheimer's disease as assessed with 4-hydroxynonenal but not malondialdehyde, *QJM* 94: 485–490.

69. N.E. Braverman, A.B. Moser, 2012, Functions of plasmalogen lipids in health and disease, *Biochim. Biophys. Acta* 1822: 1442–1452.

70. X. Han, D.M. Holtzman, D.W. McKeel, Jr., 2001, Plasmalogen deficiency in early Alzheimer's disease subjects and in animal models: molecular characterization using electrospray ionization mass spectrometry, *J. Neurochem.* 77: 1168–1180.

71. V. Senanayake, D.B. Goodenowe, 2019, Plasmalogen deficiency and neuropathology in Alzheimer's disease: causation or coincidence? *Alzheimers Dement. (N Y)* 5: 524–532.

72. X.Q. Su, J. Wang, A.J. Sinclair, 2019, Plasmalogens and Alzheimer's disease: a review, *Lipids Health Dis.* 18: 100.

73. E.N.D. Palladino, C.L. Hartman, C.J. Albert, D.A. Ford, 2018, The chlorinated lipidome originating from myeloperoxidase-derived HOCl targeting plasmalogens: metabolism, clearance, and biological properties, *Arch. Biochem. Biophys.* 641: 31–38.

74. A. Ullen, G. Fauler, H. Kofeler, et al., 2010, Mouse brain plasmalogens are targets for hypochlorous acid-mediated modification in vitro and in vivo, *Free Radic. Biol. Med.* 49: 1655–1665.

75. A. Ullen, E. Singewald, V. Konya, et al., 2013, Myeloperoxidase-derived oxidants induce blood-brain barrier dysfunction in vitro and in vivo, *PLoS One* 8: e64034.

76. Y. Dong, J. Lagarde, L. Xicota, et al., 2018, Neutrophil hyperactivation correlates with Alzheimer's disease progression, *Ann. Neurol.* 83: 387–405.

77. E. Zenaro, E. Pietronigro, V. Della Bianca, et al., 2015, Neutrophils promote Alzheimer's disease-like pathology and cognitive decline via LFA-1 integrin, *Nat. Med.* 21: 880–886.

78. J.C. Cruz Hernandez, O. Bracko, C.J. Kersbergen, et al., 2019, Neutrophil adhesion in brain capillaries reduces cortical blood flow and impairs memory function in Alzheimer's disease mouse models, *Nat. Neurosci.* 22: 413–420.

79. C.G. Goetz, A. McGhiey, 2011, The movement disorder society and movement disorders: a modern history, *Mov. Disord.* 26: 939–946.

80. W. Poewe, K. Seppi, C.M. Tanner, et al., 2017, Parkinson disease, *Nat. Rev. Dis. Primers* 3: 17013.

81. T.L. Perry, V.W. Yong, 1986, Idiopathic Parkinson's disease, progressive supranuclear palsy and glutathione metabolism in the substantia nigra of patients, *Neurosci. Lett.* 67: 269–274.

82. P. Jenner, D.T. Dexter, J. Sian, A.H. Schapira, C.D. Marsden, 1992, Oxidative stress as a cause of nigral cell death in Parkinson's disease and incidental Lewy body disease. The Royal Kings and Queens Parkinson's Disease Research Group, *Ann. Neurol.* 32 Suppl: S82–87.

83. A. Yoritaka, N. Hattori, K. Uchida, et al., 1996, Immunohistochemical detection of 4-hydroxynonenal protein adducts in Parkinson disease, *Proc. Natl. Acad. Sci. U.S.A.* 93: 2696–2701.

84. J.E. Duda, B.I. Giasson, Q. Chen, et al., 2000, Widespread nitration of pathological inclusions in neurodegenerative synucleinopathies, *Am. J. Pathol.* 157: 1439–1445.

85. A. Nunomura, P.I. Moreira, H.G. Lee, et al., 2007, Neuronal death and survival under oxidative stress in Alzheimer and Parkinson diseases, *CNS Neurol. Disord. Drug Targets* 6: 411–423.

86. S. Chandra, G. Gallardo, R. Fernandez-Chacon, O.M. Schluter, T.C. Sudhof, 2005, Alpha-synuclein cooperates with CSPalpha in preventing neurodegeneration, *Cell* 123: 383–396.

87. W.M. Nauseef, 2018, Biosynthesis of human myeloperoxidase, *Arch. Biochem. Biophys.* 642: 1–9.

88. R.P. Laura, D. Dong, W.F. Reynolds, R.A. Maki, 2016, T47D Cells expressing myeloperoxidase are able to process, traffic and store the mature protein in lysosomes: studies in T47D cells reveal a role for Cys319 in MPO biosynthesis that precedes its known role in inter-molecular disulfide bond formation, *PLoS One* 11: e0149391.

89. Y.W. Yap, M. Whiteman, N.S. Cheung, 2007, Chlorinative stress: an under appreciated mediator of neurodegeneration? *Cell Signal.* 19: 219–228.

90. O.M. Panasenko, I.V. Gorudko, A.V. Sokolov, 2013, Hypochlorous acid as a precursor of free radicals in living systems, *Biochemistry (Mosc)* 78: 1466–1489.

91. E. Malle, C. Woenckhaus, G. Waeg, et al., 1997, Immunological evidence for hypochlorite-modified proteins in human kidney, *Am. J. Pathol.* 150: 603–615.

92. E. Malle, L. Hazell, R. Stocker, et al., 1995, Immunologic detection and measurement of hypochlorite-modified LDL with specific monoclonal antibodies, *Arterioscler. Thromb. Vasc. Biol.* 15: 982–989.

93. S. Delanghe, J.R. Delanghe, R. Speeckaert, W. Van Biesen, M.M. Speeckaert, 2017, Mechanisms and consequences of carbamoylation, *Nat. Rev. Nephrol.* 13: 580–593.

94. B. Laurens, S. Vergnet, M.C. Lopez, et al., 2017, Multiple system atrophy – state of the art, *Curr. Neurol. Neurosci. Rep.* 17: 41.

95. N. Stefanova, B. Georgievska, H. Eriksson, W. Poewe, G.K. Wenning, 2012, Myeloperoxidase inhibition ameliorates multiple system atrophy-like degeneration in a transgenic mouse model, *Neurotox. Res.* 21: 393–404.

96. N. Stefanova, M. Reindl, M. Neumann, et al., 2005, Oxidative stress in transgenic mice with oligodendroglial alpha-synuclein overexpression replicates the characteristic neuropathology of multiple system atrophy, *Am. J. Pathol.* 166: 869–876.

97. X. Tong, D. Zhou, A. Savage, et al., 2018, Population pharmacokinetic modeling with enterohepatic circulation for AZD3241 in Healthy subjects and patients with multiple system atrophy, *J. Clin. Pharmacol.* 58: 1452–1460.

98. C. Daniel, M. Behm, M. Ohman, 2015, The role of Alu elements in the cis-regulation of RNA processing, *Cell Mol. Life Sci.* 72: 4063–4076.

99. L. Steinman, 2014, Immunology of relapse and remission in multiple sclerosis, *Annu. Rev. Immunol.* 32: 257–281.

100. R. Dobson, G. Giovannoni, 2019, Multiple sclerosis – a review, *Eur. J. Neurol.* 26: 27–40.

101. L. Steinman, A. Waisman, D. Altmann, 1995, Major T-cell responses in multiple sclerosis, *Mol. Med.Today* 1: 79–83.

102. B. Halliwell, 1992, Oxygen radicals as key mediators in neurological disease: fact or fiction? *Ann. Neurol.* 32 Suppl: S10–15.

103. S.J. Klebanoff, 1980, Oxygen metabolism and the toxic properties of phagocytes, *Ann. Intern. Med.* 93: 480–489.

104. B. Zakrzewska-Pniewska, M. Styczynska, A. Podlecka, et al., 2004, Association of apolipoprotein E and myeloperoxidase genotypes to clinical course of familial and sporadic multiple sclerosis, *Mult. Scler.* 10: 266–271.

105. F. Lundmark, H. Salter, J. Hillert, 2007, An association study of two functional promotor polymorphisms in the myeloperoxidase (MPO) gene in multiple sclerosis, *Mult. Scler.* 13: 697–700.

106. I. Nelissen, P. Fiten, K. Vandenbroeck, et al., 2000, PECAM1, MPO and PRKAR1A at chromosome 17q21-q24 and susceptibility for multiple sclerosis in Sweden and Sardinia, *J. Neuroimmunol.* 108: 153–159.

107. O.H. Kantarci, E.J. Atkinson, D.D. Hebrink, C.T. McMurray, B.G. Weinshenker, 2000, Association of two variants in IL-1beta and IL-1 receptor antagonist genes with multiple sclerosis, *J. Neuroimmunol.* 106: 220–227.

108. O.H. Kantarci, E.J. Atkinson, D.D. Hebrink, C.T. McMurray, B.G. Weinshenker, 2000, Association of a myeloperoxidase promoter polymorphism with multiple sclerosis, *J. Neuroimmunol.* 105: 189–194.

109. M. Brennan, A. Gaur, A. Pahuja, A.J. Lusis, W.F. Reynolds, 2001, Mice lacking myeloperoxidase are more susceptible to experimental autoimmune encephalomyelitis, *J. Neuroimmunol.* 112: 97–105.

110. A.P. Kumar, C. Ryan, V. Cordy, W.F. Reynolds, 2005, Inducible nitric oxide synthase expression is inhibited by myeloperoxidase, *Nitric Oxide* 13: 42–53.

111. V. Brovkovych, X.P. Gao, E. Ong, et al., 2008, Augmented inducible nitric oxide synthase expression and increased NO production reduce sepsis-induced lung injury and mortality in myeloperoxidase-null mice, *Am. J. Physiol. Lung Cell Mol. Physiol.* 295: L96–103.

112. K. Ichimori, N. Fukuyama, H. Nakazawa, et al., 2003, Myeloperoxidase has directly-opposed effects on nitration reaction - study on myeloperoxidase-deficient patient and myeloperoxidase-knockout mice, *Free Radic. Res.* 37: 481–489.

113. M.L. Brennan, M.M. Anderson, D.M. Shih, et al., 2001, Increased atherosclerosis in myeloperoxidase-deficient mice, *J. Clin. Invest.* 107: 419–430.

114. S. Haskamp, H. Bruns, M. Hahn, et al., 2020, Myeloperoxidase modulates inflammation in generalized pustular psoriasis and additional rare pustular skin diseases, *Am. J. Hum. Genet.* 107: 527–538.

115. M. Vergnano, M. Mockenhaupt, N. Benzian-Olsson, et al., 2020, Loss-of-function myeloperoxidase mutations are associated with increased neutrophil counts and pustular skin disease, *Am. J. Hum. Genet.* 107: 539–543.

116. H. Zhang, A. Ray, N.M. Miller, et al., 2016, Inhibition of myeloperoxidase at the peak of experimental autoimmune encephalomyelitis restores blood-brain barrier integrity and ameliorates disease severity, *J. Neurochem.* 136: 826–836.

117. R. Forghani, G.R. Wojtkiewicz, Y. Zhang, et al., 2012, Demyelinating diseases: myeloperoxidase as an imaging biomarker and therapeutic target, *Radiology* 263: 451–460.

118. H. Zhang, X. Jing, Y. Shi, et al., 2013, N-acetyl lysyltyrosylcysteine amide inhibits myeloperoxidase, a novel tripeptide inhibitor, *J. Lipid Res.* 54: 3016–3029.

119. G. Yu, S. Zheng, H. Zhang, 2018, Inhibition of myeloperoxidase by N-acetyl lysyltyrosylcysteine amide reduces experimental autoimmune encephalomyelitis-induced injury and promotes oligodendrocyte regeneration and neurogenesis in a murine model of progressive multiple sclerosis, *Neuroreport* 29: 208–213.

120. J. Soubhye, I. Aldib, C. Delporte, et al., 2016, Myeloperoxidase as a target for the treatment of inflammatory syndromes: mechanisms and structure activity relationships of inhibitors, *Curr. Med. Chem.* 23: 3975–4008.

121. S. Galijasevic, 2019, The development of myeloperoxidase inhibitors, *Bioorg. Med. Chem. Lett.* 29: 1–7.

CHAPTER SIXTEEN

The Pathogenesis and Consequences of Myeloperoxidase-Dependent ANCA Vasculitis and Glomerulonephritis

Meghan E. Free, Dominic J. Ciavatta, J. Charles Jennette, and Ronald J. Falk
UNC Chapel Hill

CONTENTS

ABBREVIATIONS

ANCA:	Anti-neutrophil cytoplasmic autoantibody
DNMT1:	DNA (cytosine-5)-methyltransferase 1
GBM:	Glomerular basement membrane
GWA:	Genome-wide association studies
HLA:	Human leukocyte antigen
MPO:	Myeloperoxidase
PR3/PRTN3:	Proteinase 3
TCR:	T cell receptor

INTRODUCTION TO MPO-ANCA VASCULITIS

Anti-neutrophil cytoplasmic autoantibody (ANCA) vasculitis, a small vessel vasculitis with a myriad of symptoms and organ involvement, is characterized by circulating autoantibodies targeting PR3 or MPO. Patients with MPO-ANCA can have a spectrum of clinicopathologic features, including glomerulonephritis without systemic vasculitis, systemic small vessel vasculitis without granulomatous inflammation (microscopic polyangiitis, MPA), systemic vasculitis with granulomatous inflammation but no asthma and blood eosinophilia (granulomatosis with polyangiitis GPA) or systemic vasculitis with granulomatous inflammation, asthma and blood eosinophilia (eosinophilic granulomatosis with polyangiitis, EGPA). Most patients enter remission with immunosuppressive therapy although many will have subsequent relapses requiring adjustments in therapy. Disease activity varies over time and must be monitored, for example, using the Birmingham Vasculitis Activity Score (BVAS).

DOI: 10.1201/9781003212287-20

ANCA VASCULITIS CLINICAL AND PATHOLOGIC FEATURES

The pathologic hallmark of acute ANCA vasculitis is segmental necrotizing inflammation in small vessels that can affect any organ of the body. Small vessels in the skin, kidneys, peripheral nerves, lungs and upper respiratory tract are frequently affected. The acute phase of ANCA vasculitis is characterized by influx of predominantly neutrophils that release destructive inflammatory mediators. This leads to necrosis of vessel walls with hemorrhage and perivascular extravasation of plasma constituents including coagulation factors that are activated to cause fibrinolysis, which results in a characteristic but not specific form of necrosis called fibrinoid necrosis. Segmental fibrinoid necrosis is the initial lesion in kidney glomeruli resulting in necrotizing glomerulonephritis with adjacent cellular responses in Bowman's space called crescents. ANCA crescentic glomerulonephritis differs from immune complex-mediated glomerulonephritis and anti-glomerular basement membrane glomerulonephritis by having little or no glomerular accumulation of immunoglobulin and complement. ANCA glomerulonephritis causes hematuria, proteinuria and kidney failure. Vasculitis in other organs causes many different signs and symptoms, for example, dermal venulitis causing a hemorrhagic rash (purpura), pulmonary capillaritis causing pulmonary hemorrhage, upper respiratory tract vasculitis causing necrotizing sinusitis and inflammation in small arteries (arteritis) causing dysfunction in many organs such as peripheral neuropathy and abdominal pain.

GENETIC PERTURBATIONS OF MPO IN ANCA VASCULITIS

Classic genome-wide association studies (GWAS) from European and North American patient cohorts demonstrated key genetic associations in ANCA vasculitis [1,2]. These studies identified specific HLA as highly associated with ANCA vasculitis, which is not surprising considering that most GWAS with autoimmune diseases reveal HLA associations [3]. In addition, a certain PRTN3 polymorphism was found to be associated with PR3-ANCA disease [1,2]. To date, no associations with MPO polymorphisms have emerged from GWAS, with the caveat that most of these studies have been underpowered to detect differences within the MPO-ANCA vasculitis patient population.

Studies have demonstrated epigenetic and transcriptional perturbations of MPO in patients with ANCA vasculitis [4–7]. Studies examining the expression of DNMT1 in ANCA vasculitis first pointed to potential epigenetic changes in disease [5]. Patients with ANCA vasculitis exhibited lower expression of DNMT1 compared with healthy controls indicating that certain genes could be differentially methylated in patients [5]. Relative DNMT1 was lowest in patients with active disease and rebounded to levels closer to those in healthy controls when patients achieved remission. Methylation at CpG sites essentially silences genes and is one method of epigenetic regulation. The MPO gene has several candidate CpG islands (CGIs) that could be methylated/demethylated for gene regulation. One region within MPO covers exons 5 and 6 and a second region contains exon 7 [5]. Patients with active disease are hypomethylated at these CGIs compared with remission and healthy controls [5]. Providing additional evidence that this hypomethylation contributes to disease is the key finding that mRNA expression of the autoantigen inversely correlates with the degree of DNA methylation [5].

DNA methylation studies focusing on the CGI/exon 5–6 within MPO revealed changes in methylation between periods of active disease and remitting disease with methylation during remission more closely resembling that of healthy controls [5]. Of both clinical and biological interest, the change in methylation at these loci between an individual's disease state could predict probability of time to next flare. While this finding was not statistically significant, there are likely additional MPO epigenetic modifications that have yet to be discerned. To provide insight into disease pathogenesis, the question is whether these changes in methylation correspond to changes in transcription and translation of the autoantigen, MPO (Figure 16.1).

A large cohort of patients with ANCA vasculitis was monitored every 3 months for multiple years to measure changes of MPO expression in total circulating leukocytes [8]. Overall, patients with ANCA vasculitis have significantly increased mRNA expression of MPO compared with healthy controls [8]. Interestingly, patients tend to have

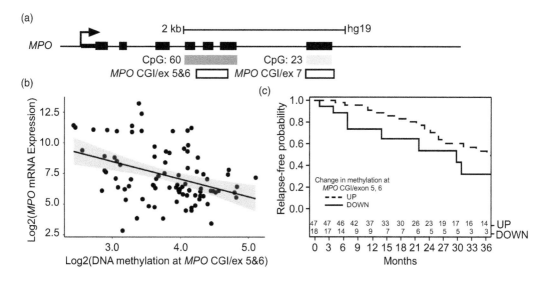

Figure 16.1 DNA methylation of MPO CGI. (a) MPO gene with annotated CGIs. (b) Methylation of MPO CGI/exon 5, 6 inversely correlates with MPO mRNA expression. P<0.0001, r=0.316. (c) Changes in MPO methylation at CGI/exon 5, 6, predict risk of relapse. Log rank=0.41.

either dynamic or static changes of MPO expression between disease relapse and remission. One category of patients (dynamic) exhibited high levels of MPO expression during active disease that decreases during remission while a separate cohort of patients (static) had low MPO expression, with little change between disease states [5].

Through retrospective analysis, the static pattern of autoantigen expression is seen in about 20% of patients who more frequently have disease limited to ear, nose and throat (ENT), while the dynamic pattern of autoantigen gene expression is seen in about 70% of patients who more frequently have disease with extensive renal involvement. This clinical finding has been replicated in additional studies examining specific peripheral cell types [9]. Patients classified as static had disease limited to ENT or cutaneous involvement of the extremities, while patients classified as dynamic had additional organ involvement.

Numerous studies have demonstrated the increased autoantigen expression in leukocytes from patients with ANCA vasculitis, but does this correlate into a functional consequence? By isolating peripheral neutrophils from healthy controls and patients with ANCA vasculitis, this was tested by cellular activation by IgG from either healthy controls or ANCA vasculitis patients. This study demonstrated that there was a positive correlation between expression of MPO autoantigen

and the degree of neutrophil activation by MPO-ANCA IgG [9].

With increased expression of MPO and the finding that expression of MPO correlates with neutrophil activation by MPO-ANCA, the question becomes: is there also increased translation of the autoantigen in ANCA vasculitis? The general consensus has been that granule proteins are formed and stored in cytoplasmic granules while granulocytes are produced in the bone marrow, and upon release from the bone marrow, these cells are terminally differentiated and do not produce additional granule proteins. Because peripheral neutrophils do not live long ex vivo, studies to examine new protein synthesis in human neutrophils have been technically difficult.

However, one study determined not only if new protein synthesis occurs in peripheral neutrophils, but also if MPO is newly synthesized [6]. By culturing neutrophils in vitro first in methionine-free media and then supplementing with a methionine analog, L-aziodohomoalanine, only newly synthesized proteins will incorporate the methionine analog. This analog can be detected through Click-It chemistry by biotinylation of the analog and eventual binding to streptavidin conjugates. This method determined that new protein synthesis occurs in peripheral neutrophils, and importantly — new synthesis of MPO occurs [6]. These studies underscore the relationship of epigenetic and genetic perturbations of MPO in ANCA vasculitis, leading to transcription of the targeted autoantigen.

MPO-ANCAS ARE PATHOGENIC

With the discovery that ANCAs target MPO or PR3, the question that followed was whether ANCAs were merely biomarkers of disease or actually pathogenic. Many autoimmune diseases exhibit hallmark autoantibodies; however, the role of these autoantibodies in the disease process is not clear. Are autoantibodies a by-product of the disease process, or do they initiate and propagate disease?

Multiple animal models provide convincing evidence that MPO-ANCAs are pathogenic [10]. For example, the mouse model utilized by Xiao et al. demonstrates that MPO-ANCA IgG causes glomerulonephritis and systemic vasculitis pathologically identical to lesions on patients with MPO-ANCA disease [11]. To create this model, MPO-deficient mice are immunized with native mouse MPO to generate anti-MPO antibodies. Purified anti-MPO IgG is transferred to wild-type (MPO-sufficient) mice resulting in circulating antibodies that react with mouse MPO (i.e. MPO-ANCA). Within 6 days, mice with circulating MPO-ANCA develop hematuria, proteinuria and leukocyturia, and pathologic examination after 6 days reveals necrotizing and crescentic glomerulonephritis and vasculitis indistinguishable from human MPO-ANCA glomerulonephritis [11].

In this mouse model caused by injection of MPO-ANCA IgG, MPO-ANCA IgG alone causes glomerulonephritis and vasculitis in the absence of functional T cells [11], neutrophils are required for induction of vascular inflammation [12], genetic factors modulate disease severity primarily by modifying the functional status of neutrophils [13], the kinin system modulates pathogenesis [14] and alternative complement pathway activation is required and mediated by C5a engagement of C5a receptor [15]. The elucidation of pathogenic mechanisms provided by this mouse model was translated into novel therapy for patients with ANCA vasculitis in a clinical trial that demonstrated the therapeutic efficacy of the same C5a receptor inhibitor that blocked disease induction in this mouse model [16].

The initial mouse model of MPO-ANCA generated by Xiao et al. relied on the recipient mice

of C57BL/6 in which 100% of mice demonstrate necrotizing crescentic glomerulonephritis; however, only 5%–10% of glomeruli had crescent formation [11]. Additional studies examined the susceptibility of disease within several different mouse strains. The same dose of anti-MPO IgG was injected into 13 genetically different strains of mice to assess induction of glomerulonephritis and the degree of glomerular crescent development [13]. Injection of the 129S6/SvEv strain of mice also resulted in 100% of mice having necrotizing and crescentic glomerulonephritis, but unlike the C57BL/6 mice (average 9.5% glomerular crescents), the 129S6 mice had on average 63.7% crescents [13]. Additionally, some mouse strains had no induction of glomerulonephritis and were protected from disease (NOD, DBA2, AJ). The stark differences in crescent formation between these two strains underscore the contribution of genetics to the severity of ANCA disease.

With further investigation using bone marrow chimeras derived from C57BL/6 and 126S6 mice, the severity of disease was transferred with the bone marrow and not dependent on the host body [13]. Therefore, the genetic determinant of disease severity stemmed from bone-marrow-derived cells, likely neutrophils and/or monocytes. These mouse model studies not only demonstrated that MPO-ANCA are pathogenic, but also revealed that disease severity is modulated by genetics, environment and immune disturbance.

ANCAS INDUCE MYELOID CELL ACTIVATION AND DEGRANULATION TO INJURE VESSEL ENDOTHELIUM

A critical link between ANCA and disease pathogenesis centers on how ANCA binding to autoantigen causes neutrophil or monocyte activation and how this activation results in endothelial damage. ANCAs bind to and interact with target cells through ANCAs binding to cognate antigen (either MPO or PR3) on the surface of neutrophils and monocytes or by Fc receptor engagement to Fc regions of ANCA that is bound to autoantigen (e.g. MPO) on the surface of cells or in the microenvironment [17–19]. This, in turn, initiates neutrophil and monocyte activation. In the case of neutrophil activation, degranulation occurs with the release of proteases and enzymes into the microenvironment. ANCA-induced activation of neutrophils passing through a small blood vessel results in neutrophil adhesion to endothelium; release of inflammatory mediators, destructive enzymes and oxygen radicals; and resultant necrotizing inflammation of the vessel wall.

Another consequence of ANCA activation of neutrophils is the release of neutrophil extracellular traps (NETS) that are DNA extrusions decorated with various cellular proteins including PR3 and MPO. Neutrophils from patients with ANCA vasculitis are more prone to NETosis compared with neutrophils from healthy controls [20]. NETosis may contribute to either the immunogenesis of the ANCA autoimmune response by presenting MPO and PR3 autoantigens in a way that enhances the autoimmune response or may contribute to pathogenesis by mediating some of the inflammatory injury or both. The combination of these findings and factors presents the conundrum as to whether NETosis itself can perpetuate the generation of MPO-ANCA.

ALTERED GLYCOSYLATION OF MPO-ANCA

Because ANCAs are pathogenic, studies of the biology of ANCA immunoglobulin may help understand pathogenic mechanisms and how to target them for therapy. For example, studies of ANCA IgG glycosylation have yielded insight into ANCA pathogenicity [21]. Altered glycosylation of either the Fc or Fab portions of IgGs has been shown to change the function of antibodies with vastly different downstream effects [22–29]. Concerning glycosylation of the Fc portion, N-glycans are attached to the Asn297 residue and alterations of either terminal galactose or sialic acid tend to be at this position [22,23,25,28]. Generally, IgGs without the terminal galactose have an increased pro-inflammatory capacity, and the addition of sialic acid can alter IgGs from pro-inflammatory to anti-inflammatory [22,23,25,28]. These glycosylation changes alter how IgGs interact with immune cells that express Fc receptors.

Additionally, changes in glycosylation in the variable region of IgGs have downstream implications. However, the precise role of different glycans within the Fab has yet to be fully delineated although it is proposed that these alterations can affect the avidity and affinity for the cognate antigen [27,29]. Through mass spectrometry approaches, Lardinois et al. demonstrated altered glycosylation of the Fc and Fab portions of ANCA from patients. By comparing the degree of glycosylation at both the Fc and Fab portions of MPO-ANCA from patients during active disease and remission, this comprehensive analysis provides insight into the relevance of IgG glycosylation and disease [21].

It was determined that ANCA glycosylation differs greatly between PR3-ANCA and MPO-ANCA in the context of disease activity [21]. IgG Fc galactosylation and sialylation correlated with disease activity in PR3-ANCA, with IgG from patients in remission resembling that from healthy controls. However, MPO-ANCAs exhibited a lack of terminal sialic acid and galactosylation, irrespective of patient disease activity [21]. Glycosylation of the Fab portion of IgG changed in MPO-ANCA over the course of disease activity [21]. By separating MPO-ANCA from the pool of other IgGs, the study demonstrated that MPO-ANCA Fabs had higher galactosylation and sialylation compared with non-ANCA IgGs [21]. Collectively, these alterations in glycosylation of both the Fc and Fab portions of MPO-ANCA alter the mechanisms of cellular activation, complement activation and downstream factors leading to disease pathogenesis and severity.

In addition to altered glycosylation patterns of the MPO-ANCA themselves, altered glycosylation of the MPO molecule could play a role in disease pathogenesis including antibody generation to neo-epitopes [30–32]. The heavy chain of MPO contains five sites for glycosylation (therefore ten total sites per dimer), and changes in the degree of glycosylation have the potential to affect the function, folding and antigenicity of MPO [30]. Through mass spectrometry profiling of healthy control MPO, Reiding et al. noted heterogeneity of the degree of MPO glycosylation, which underscores the possibility of altered glycosylation in disease [30]. Changes in glycosylation can also alter protein functionality and how MPO interacts with its natural inhibitor, ceruloplasmin. Using a series of glycosidases to differentially alter the glycosylation of MPO, Wang et al. demonstrated that with sequential deglycosylation, the degree of chlorination decreased as well as the ability of ceruloplasmin to bind [32]. These functional alterations, particularly the decreased binding to the inhibitor ceruloplasmin, can lead to severe infections and inappropriate duration of inflammation [32]. Furthermore, the study by Yu et al. utilized both exoglycosidases and endoglycosidases to treat MPO to alter the degree of glycosylation [31].

With decreased MPO glycosylation, the authors noted more than 50% of serum from anti-glomerular basement membrane (GBM) patients had reactivity to the altered MPO [31]. These studies bring into focus that altered glycosylation of the MPO antigen itself could play a role in increased antigenicity and the development of pathogenic autoantibodies.

THE POLYCLONAL MPO-ANCA RESPONSE DEFINES DISEASE STATUS

While the passive transfer mouse model studies demonstrated the pathogenic potential of polyclonal MPO-ANCA, attempts to cause disease in mice with monoclonal MPO-ANCA have failed. Human MPO-ANCAs are polyclonal and have specificity for multiple different epitopes on the MPO molecule. Clinically, MPO-ANCA titers do not always correlate with disease activity. For example, some patients can be in remission for months or years despite having high MPO-ANCA titers by ELISA. This raises the question as to which autoantibodies within the polyclonal response are pathogenic autoantibodies and which are nonpathogenic (natural or asymptomatic) autoantibodies.

Several studies have performed epitope mapping of the polyclonal ANCA response in patients with MPO-ANCA vasculitis. The study by Fujii et al. utilized recombinant deletion mutants of MPO to screen ANCA reactivity [33]. ANCA had no reactivity to the light chain of MPO, but the majority of patients had reactivity to regions near both MPO N-terminal and C-terminal regions [33]. The authors categorized patients based on clinical features and noted that patients with more restricted reactivity had more alveolar hemorrhage and more relapses compared with patients with broader epitope reactivity.

A caveat of the recombinant deletion mutants is the structural changes of the proteins, especially truncated proteins; therefore, conformational epitopes are likely to be missed. A step strategy to detect antibody epitopes that are dependent on molecular structure is to use mouse/human MPO chimeric molecules [34]. Five different chimeric MPO molecules were generated with large portions of the protein interchanged between mouse and human homologous regions. Patient sera were screened against these chimeric molecules for reactivity. Patient MPO-ANCA had no reactivity to the light chain of MPO. Most patients had

reactivity to the C-terminal region of MPO and pinpointed the regions of amino acids 517–667 and 668–745 [34]. Of interest, the data suggested that while subtle changes in antibody epitope reactivity occurred over time, the majority of patients' antibody reactivity remained stable, suggesting an absence of large-scale antigenic (epitope) drift.

The studies by Fujii et al. and Erdbrugger et al. provided some information on MPO-ANCA epitope specificity, these techniques could only identify large sections of the molecule instead of small amino acid stretches as the epitope. A study by Roth et al. utilized an epitope-excision mass spectrometry–based approach to define MPO-ANCA specificity during active disease, remission and in healthy controls [35]. By including healthy controls, this allows for the detection of natural, asymptomatic autoantibodies. In the epitope-excision method, antibodies are permitted to bind their cognate epitope, trypsin then digests away unbound protein leaving the bound epitope protected. This protected epitope is eluted with strong acid and analyzed by mass spectrometry. These studies elucidated epitopes of MPO that were targeted during active disease, disease in remission and in healthy individuals (natural epitopes) (Figure 16.2).

One of the epitopes (aa447–459) associated with active disease was linear, which permits the generation of peptide-based ELISAs that can be used to study large populations of patients for epitope-specific ANCA reactivity in a longitudinal manner. Initial ELISA studies demonstrated that antibody reactivity to this epitope occurred primarily during disease activity and was undetectable during disease remission [35]. Confirmatory studies utilizing a slightly longer peptide (aa447–461) for solubility issues confirmed that ANCA reactivity not only occurred during disease activity but also could be detected frequently at onset of disease [35,36]. This finding provides insight into the potential immunopathogenesis of disease, i.e. initiation of the MPO-ANCA response.

While this antibody-epitope was associated with active disease and onset of disease, the question became whether this is only a biomarker of disease status or is pathogenic. Isolated epitope-specific ANCAs were tested on neutrophils to determine their ability to induce cellular activation. ANCA reactive to MPO$_{447–459}$ activated neutrophils to the same extent as polyclonal MPO-ANCA from active disease patients. However, ANCA purified with reactivity

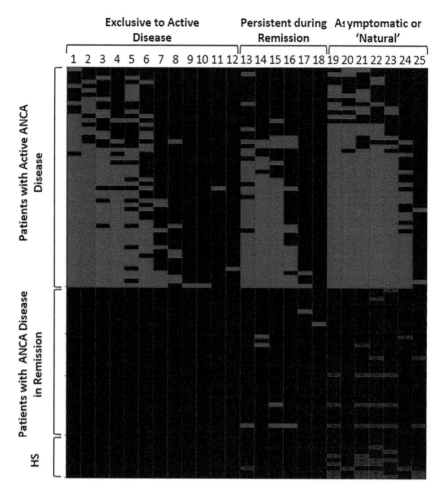

Figure 16.2 MPO-ANCA epitopes differ between disease state. Epitope-excision mass spectrometry revealed ANCA-MPO epitope pairs that are exclusive to active disease, exclusive to disease (irrespective of disease status) and natural/asymptomatic epitopes that are also detected in healthy controls. (This figure is used with permission from Ref. [35].)

to epitopes not associated with active disease did not elicit the same cellular activation exhibited by anti-MPO$_{447-459}$ [35], thus further underscoring the importance of understanding the epitope specificity of ANCA as it relates to disease immunopathogenesis, pathogenesis and progression.

T-CELL RESPONSES ARE MPO EPITOPE-SPECIFIC IN HUMAN AND MURINE DISEASE

While ANCAs are pathogenic and a clinical biomarker of disease, ANCA and the plasma cells producing them only represent half of the adaptive immune system. Moreover, MPO-ANCAs are high-affinity, class-switched IgGs, which indicate that T cell help was necessary to instruct ANCA

formation. Therefore, the T cell repertoire's (both CD4+ and CD8+) response to the autoantigen MPO is also critical to understanding the immunopathogenesis of ANCA vasculitis.

Classically, CD4+ T cells recognize peptides in the context of MHC class II, and CD8+ T cells recognize peptides in the context of MHC class I. These MHCs are found on antigen-presenting cells such as monocytes, macrophages and dendritic cells that activate T cells in an antigen-specific manner. As only peptides can be presented within the binding cleft of MHCs, T cell receptors (TCRs) are genetically encoded to recognize short amino acid sequences as opposed to entire proteins. Certain peptides are known to be more immunogenic than others; therefore epitope mapping of T cell responses to autoantigens provides key insight into how an autoimmune response began and is perpetuated over the course of disease.

Through predictive algorithms, potential peptide–MHC pairings can be imputed [37]. Utilizing this method, several MPO peptides have been predicted to bind several different HLA, and some of these HLA are enriched in the MPO ANCA patient population [36]. To confirm predicted peptide–HLA binding pairs, in vitro binding studies confirm or rule out biologically relevant pairings [36]. These peptides of interest can then be loaded into HLA-appropriate tetramers to test T cell reactivity on ex vivo patient cells. Fluorescently tagged tetramer studies provide the prevalence on a patient-by-patient basis of autoreactive T cells in circulation at a given time and during active disease and remission.

The combination of these lines of investigation led to discovery that the CD4+ T cell response in MPO-ANCA patients is restricted to region of MPO that overlaps with the same region implicated through antibody-epitope mapping studies previously discussed. Patient CD4+ T cells reactive to $MPO_{435-454}$ or $MPO_{447-461}$ were more likely to be antigen-experienced and secrete the pro-inflammatory cytokine IL-17A compared with nonreactive T cells. Additionally, the use of TCR sequencing on autoreactive versus non-autoreactive cells revealed that those MPO-reactive T cells have restricted TCRs indicative of clonal expansion over time [36]. Collectively, the studies examining MPO-reactive CD4+ T cells in patients with ANCA vasculitis determined that autoreactive cells were detectable directly ex vivo without artificial expansion indicating that continuous exposure to MPO could hasten the clonal production of specific autoreactive T cells (Table 16.1).

Similar MPO epitope mapping studies for both CD4+ and CD8+ T cells have emerged from another mouse model of MPO-ANCA disease. This model relies on the injection of native mouse MPO in Freund's complete adjuvant into wild-type mice, followed by a second injection in Freund's incomplete adjuvant a week later to generate an anti-MPO autoimmune response. Analogous to the polyclonal ANCA response, the T cell specificity to MPO is varied by epitope. To decipher which regions of MPO were immunogenic to CD4+ T cells, mice were injected with pools of peptides that spanned sequential regions of the entire MPO molecule [38]. Post-immunization, CD4+ T cells were harvested from mice and stimulated with

TABLE 16.1
CD4+ T cell MPO epitopes

Epitope	In silico score[a]	In vitro affinity (DPB1*04:01)	CD4+ reactivity
$MPO_{105-119}$	10.88	Low/none	ND
$MPO_{245-259}$	1.84	Moderate	ND
$MPO_{409-423}$	3.05	Moderate	Minimal
$MPO_{413-427}$	12.19	Low/none	ND
$MPO_{435-454}$	ND	Moderate	Yes
$MPO_{447-461}$	2.83	High	Yes
$MPO_{488-502}$	7.82	Low/none	ND
$MPO_{545-559}$	2.48	Low/none	Minimal

[a] Lower values indicate higher probability of binding.

either smaller pools of peptides or singular peptides to further define the exact MPO sequences that generated the most robust T cell response. The T cell response was quantified by both cellular proliferation and cytokine production. There were several epitopes that generated robust CD4+ T cell responses; however, one particular epitope elicited a strong T cell response with IL-17A production (peptide 52, $MPO_{409-428}$). Intriguingly, this is the murine homologue of the same peptide ($MPO_{435-454}$) that CD4+ T cells from patients also have reactivity.

To further underscore the pathogenic potential of this region of MPO, injection of $MPO_{409-428}$ into the same mouse model induced disease analogous to the model in which whole native mouse MPO is used as the immunogen. Additionally, immunization with the singular peptide generated a B cell response as evidenced by the detection of circulating MPO-ANCA in those same mice. Mice immunized with $MPO_{409-428}$ exhibited increased albuminuria, increased blood urea nitrogen (BUN) and glomerular necrosis and fibrin deposition almost to the same extent as those mice immunized with whole native mouse MPO [38].

While the role of CD4+ T cells in the generation of the ANCA response is generally accepted and understood for the purposes of directing B cell activation and class switching, the role of CD8+ T cells in the pathogenesis of ANCA vasculitis is less clear. A microarray study has implicated CD8+ T cells in the progression of ANCA vasculitis through the identification of a CD8+ T cell signature that was predictive of relapse [39].

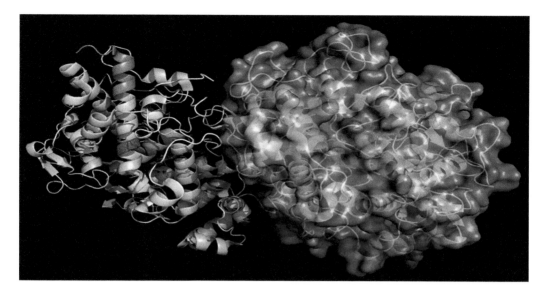

Figure 16.3 The adaptive immune response targets a core region of MPO in ANCA vasculitis. Purple-gold: CD4+ T cell epitope. Gold-fuscia-gold: antibody epitope. Gold-teal: CD8+ T cell epitope. (This figure is used with permission from Ref. [36].)

Combined with evidence that depletion of CD8+ T cells from the mouse model of ANCA glomerulonephritis leads to protection from disease, investigating the MPO specificity of CD8+ T cells has come into focus [40]. Through peptide libraries and dextramer studies, the MPO epitope specificity of CD8+ T cells in the mouse model of anti-MPO immunopathogenesis was determined [40].

Utilizing the same Immune Epitope Database that was used for the human CD4+ epitope predictions, a number of mouse MPO peptides were predicted to bind mouse MHC class I. These peptides were then used to generate CD8+ T cell clones with MPO specificity to determine their cytotoxicity as a measure of functionality. Through a series of studies examining in vitro cytotoxicity, in vivo immunization and identification of epitope-specific CD8+ T cells with dextramers, the mouse MPO$_{431-439}$ epitope triggered a significant CD8+ T cell response. Transfer of MPO$_{431-439}$-specific CD8+ T cells was able to induce disease demonstrated by albuminuria, segmental necrosis and infiltrating CD8+ T cells into the glomerulus [40].

The cumulative data from both human and murine studies examining the epitope specificity of antibodies, CD4+ and CD8+ T cells has pointed to a region of MPO that is targeted by all arms of the adaptive immune response [35,36,38,40]. This region is an alpha helical stretch of amino acids that is buried within the MPO molecule. With the exception of a few amino acids, the majority of this portion of MPO is not exposed to the environment under normal conditions. How this region of MPO is targeted by all arms of the adaptive immune system remains under investigation, although the theory of conformeropathy is valid considering this is the case in anti-GBM disease [41]. Anti-GBM antibodies target the alpha-3 chain of type IV collagen and the precise epitope to which antibodies bind is hidden under homeostatic conditions. While the precise events that lead to the unveiling of the buried epitope is unknown, this is yet another documented example of epitope conformeropathy in autoimmune disease (Figure 16.3).

TARGETING MPO IN ANTIGEN-SPECIFIC IMMUNOTHERAPY

Previous studies determined that MPO is under the control of autoimmune regulator (AIRE) in medullary thymic epithelial cells (mTECs) within the thymus [42]. AIRE promotes the transcription and translation of self-proteins in the thymus for the purpose of T cell education and prevention of autoimmunity. Therefore, the maintenance of self-tolerance to MPO is crucial in the healthy population and preventing the formation of MPO-ANCA. In patients with already established ANCA vasculitis, reestablishment of tolerance to MPO or development of an antigen-specific immunotherapy could be novel therapies that would be more effective and less toxic than current therapies.

With numerous studies, both in humans and in mouse models, demonstrating how the adaptive immune system targets the combined region of $MPO_{435-465}$, this stretch of MPO is a likely candidate for immunotherapy [35,38,40,43]. Because the model of MPO-ANCA disease developed by Holdsworth and Kitching determined the immunodominant CD4+ and CD8+ T cells epitopes, this model could be used to investigate the potential for antigen-specific immunomodulation as proof of principle. Prevention of MPO-ANCA GN was tested by nasal insufflation of $MPO_{409-428}$ prior to initiation of disease. Pretreatment of mice with this singular peptide was able to prevent disease as evidenced by preservation of renal architecture, decreased interferon gamma and IL-17A secretion, decreased total MPO-ANCA titers and decreased segmental glomerular necrosis [44]. However, in current clinical practice, it is unknown which patients will eventually go on to develop ANCA vasculitis. Therefore, interventions within established disease are more clinically relevant. This possibility was tested by initiating experimental disease in mice and then introducing $MPO_{409-428}$ by nasal insufflation on days 10–12 with assessment of disease on day 20 [44]. These experiments demonstrated the partial amelioration of disease as evidenced by a 50% decrease in segmental glomerular necrosis, decreased renal infiltration of CD4+ T cells and macrophages and decreased proteinuria [44].

Through these in-depth profiling studies to delineate the anti-MPO response from all arms of the adaptive immune response, the field is poised to formulate antigen-specific immunotherapies. These studies utilizing a mouse model of immunopathogenesis of the MPO-ANCA response were the first proof-of-concept studies to demonstrate that not only could an MPO peptide elicit a protective immune response, but that this same MPO peptide has the capacity to instruct an anti-inflammatory response in previously established disease. This latter study is key for any future studies and interventions in the human MPO-ANCA vasculitis population.

SUMMARY

The collection of studies of MPO-ANCA vasculitis that have coalesced over the past several decades have not only furthered the fundamental understanding of disease but also have informed new treatment strategies both in practice and in future development. MPO-ANCAs are far more than a biomarker of disease as these autoantibodies play a direct role in binding to MPO on neutrophil and monocytes, thereby causing their activation and downstream pro-inflammatory effects on the microenvironment of the vascular endothelium. This is made possible through genetic and epigenetic dysregulation of MPO in neutrophils and monocytes found circulating in patients with disease. MPO-ANCAs have been shown to have altered glycosylation of both the Fc and Fab portions of the IgGs, which alters their ability to interact with immune cells. These alterations in glycosylation shift these autoantibodies to a more pro-inflammatory capacity and likely alter their affinity and avidity for cognate MPO. Furthermore, intensive studies have mapped the epitope specificity to MPO for the entire adaptive immune response (autoantibodies from plasma cells, CD4+ and CD8+ T cells). Through these studies, a core region of MPO has been repeatedly targeted by all arms of the adaptive immune system and provides key insight into the immunopathogenesis of MPO-ANCA vasculitis. Collectively, this information is the foundation for understanding the immunopathogenesis and pathogenesis of disease while informing the development of future therapies.

REFERENCES

1. Merkel PA, Xie G, Monach PA, et al., 2017, Identification of functional and expression polymorphisms associated with risk for anti-neutrophil cytoplasmic autoantibody-associated vasculitis. Arthritis. Rheumatol. 69: 1054–1066.
2. Lyons PA, Rayner TF, Trivedi S, et al., 2012, Genetically distinct subsets within ANCA-associated vasculitis. N. Engl. J. Med. 367: 214–223.
3. Seldin MF, 2015, The genetics of human autoimmune disease: A perspective on progress in the field and future directions. J. Autoimmun. 64: 1–12.
4. Ciavatta DJ, Yang J, Preston GA, et al., 2010, Epigenetic basis for aberrant upregulation of autoantigen genes in humans with ANCA vasculitis. J. Clin. Invest. 120: 3209–3219.
5. Jones BE, Yang J, Muthigi A, et al., 2017, Gene-specific DNA methylation changes predict remission in patients with ANCA-associated vasculitis. J. Am. Soc. Nephrol. 28: 1175–1187.

6. McInnis EA, Badhwar AK, Muthigi A, et al., 2015, Dysregulation of autoantigen genes in ANCA-associated vasculitis involves alternative transcripts and new protein synthesis. *J. Am. Soc. Nephrol.* 26: 390–399.

7. Yang J, Ge H, Poulton CJ, et al., 2016, Histone modification signature at myeloperoxidase and proteinase 3 in patients with anti-neutrophil cytoplasmic autoantibody-associated vasculitis. *Clin. Epigenetics.* 8: 85.

8. Yang JJ, Pendergraft WF, Alcorta DA, et al., 2004, Circumvention of normal constraints on granule protein gene expression in peripheral blood neutrophils and monocytes of patients with antineutrophil cytoplasmic autoantibody-associated glomerulonephritis. *J. Am. Soc. Nephrol.* 15: 2103–2114.

9. Jones BE, Herrera CA, Agosto-Burgos C, et al., 2020, ANCA autoantigen gene expression highlights neutrophil heterogeneity where expression in normal-density neutrophils correlates with ANCA-induced activation. *Kidney. Int.* 98: 744–757.

10. Jennette JC, Xiao H, Falk R, et al., 2011, Experimental models of vasculitis and glomerulonephritis induced by antineutrophil cytoplasmic autoantibodies. *Contrib. Nephrol.* 169: 211–220.

11. Xiao H, Heeringa P, Hu P, et al., 2002, Antineutrophil cytoplasmic autoantibodies specific for myeloperoxidase cause glomerulonephritis and vasculitis in mice. *J. Clin. Invest.* 110: 955–963.

12. Xiao H, Heeringa P, Liu Z, et al., 2005, The role of neutrophils in the induction of glomerulonephritis by anti-myeloperoxidase antibodies. *Am. J. Pathol.* 167: 39–45.

13. Xiao H, Ciavatta D, Aylor DL, et al., 2013, Genetically determined severity of anti-myeloperoxidase glomerulonephritis. *Am. J. Pathol.* 182: 1219–1226.

14. Hu P, Su H, Xiao H, et al., 2020, Kinin B1 Receptor is important in the pathogenesis of myeloperoxidase-specific ANCA GN. *J. Am. Soc. Nephrol.* 31: 297–307.

15. Xiao H, Dairaghi DJ, Powers JP, et al., 2014, C5a receptor (CD88) blockade protects against MPO-ANCA GN. *J. Am. Soc. Nephrol.* 25: 225–231.

16. Jayne DRW, Bruchfeld AN, Harper L, et al., 2017, Randomized trial of C5a receptor inhibitor Avacopan in ANCA-associated vasculitis. *J. Am. Soc. Nephrol.* 28: 2756–2767.

17. Kettritz R, Jennette JC, Falk RJ, 1997, Cross-linking of ANCA-antigens stimulates superoxide release by human neutrophils. *J. Am. Soc. Nephrol.* 8: 386–394.

18. Porges AJ, Redecha PB, Kimberly WT, et al., 1994, Anti-neutrophil cytoplasmic antibodies engage and activate human neutrophils via Fc gamma RIIa. *J. Immunol.* 153: 1271–1280.

19. Williams JM, Ben-Smith A, Hewins P, et al., 2003, Activation of the G(i) heterotrimeric G protein by ANCA IgG F(ab′)2 fragments is necessary but not sufficient to stimulate the recruitment of those downstream mediators used by intact ANCA IgG. *J. Am. Soc. Nephrol.* 14: 661–669.

20. Kraaij T, Kamerling SWA, van Dam LS, et al., 2018, Excessive neutrophil extracellular trap formation in ANCA-associated vasculitis is independent of ANCA. *Kidney Int.* 94: 139–149.

21. Lardinois OM, Deterding LJ, Hess JJ, et al., 2019, Immunoglobulins G from patients with ANCA-associated vasculitis are atypically glycosylated in both the Fc and Fab regions and the relation to disease activity. *PLoS One* 14: e0213215.

22. Ferrara C, Grau S, Jager C, et al., 2011, Unique carbohydrate-carbohydrate interactions are required for high affinity binding between FcgammaRIII and antibodies lacking core fucose. *Proc. Natl. Acad. Sci. U.S.A.* 108: 12669–12674.

23. Kaneko Y, Nimmerjahn F, Ravetch JV, 2006, Anti-inflammatory activity of immunoglobulin G resulting from Fc sialylation. *Science* 313: 670–673.

24. Malhotra R, Wormald MR, Rudd PM, et al., 1995, Glycosylation changes of IgG associated with rheumatoid arthritis can activate complement via the mannose-binding protein. *Nat. Med.* 1: 237–243.

25. Ohmi Y, Ise W, Harazono A, et al., 2016, Sialylation converts arthritogenic IgG into inhibitors of collagen-induced arthritis. *Nat. Commun.* 7: 11205.

26. Rademacher TW, Williams P, Dwek RA, 1994, Agalactosyl glycoforms of IgG autoantibodies are pathogenic. *Proc. Natl. Acad. Sci. U.S.A.* 91: 6123–6127.

27. Tachibana H, Kim JY, Shirahata S, 1997, Building high affinity human antibodies by altering the glycosylation on the light chain variable region in N-acetylglucosamine-supplemented hybridoma cultures. *Cytotechnology* 23: 151–159.

28. van Timmeren MM, van der Veen BS, Stegeman CA, et al., 2010, IgG glycan hydrolysis attenuates ANCA-mediated glomerulonephritis. *J. Am. Soc. Nephrol.* 21: 1103–1114.

29. Wallick SC, Kabat EA, Morrison SL, 1988, Glycosylation of a VH residue of a monoclonal antibody against alpha (1----6) dextran increases its affinity for antigen. *J. Exp. Med.* 168: 1099–1109.

30. Reiding KR, Franc V, Huitema MG, et al., 2019, Neutrophil myeloperoxidase harbors distinct site-specific peculiarities in its glycosylation. *J. Biol. Chem.* 294: 20233–20245.

31. Yu JT, Li JN, Wang J, et al., 2017, Deglycosylation of myeloperoxidase uncovers its novel antigenicity. *Kidney Int.* 91: 1410–1419.

32. Wang J, Li JN, Cui Z, et al., 2018, Deglycosylation influences the oxidation activity and antigenicity of myeloperoxidase. *Nephrology (Carlton)* 23: 46–52.

33. Fujii A, Tomizawa K, Arimura Y, et al., 2000, Epitope analysis of myeloperoxidase (MPO) specific anti-neutrophil cytoplasmic autoantibodies (ANCA) in MPO-ANCA-associated glomerulonephritis. *Clin. Nephrol.* 53: 242–252.

34. Erdbrugger U, Hellmark T, Bunch DO, et al., 2006, Mapping of myeloperoxidase epitopes recognized by MPO-ANCA using human-mouse MPO chimers. *Kidney Int.* 69: 1799–1805.

35. Roth AJ, Ooi JD, Hess JJ, et al., 2013, Epitope specificity determines pathogenicity and detectability in ANCA-associated vasculitis. *J. Clin. Invest.* 123: 1773–1783.

36. Free ME, Stember KG, Hess JJ, et al., 2020, Restricted myeloperoxidase epitopes drive the adaptive immune response in MPO-ANCA vasculitis. *J. Autoimmun.* 106: 102306.

37. Sette A, Paul S, Vaughan K, et al., 2015, The use of the immune epitope database to study autoimmune epitope data related to Alopecia Areata. *J. Investig. Dermatol. Symp. Proc.* 17: 36–41.

38. Ooi JD, Chang J, Hickey MJ, et al., 2012, The immunodominant myeloperoxidase T-cell epitope induces local cell-mediated injury in anti-myeloperoxidase glomerulonephritis. *Proc. Natl. Acad. Sci. U.S.A.* 109: E2615–2624.

39. McKinney EF, Lyons PA, Carr EJ, et al., 2010, A CD8+ T cell transcription signature predicts prognosis in autoimmune disease. *Nat. Med.* 16: 586–591, 581p following 591.

40. Chang J, Eggenhuizen P, O'Sullivan KM, et al., 2017, CD8+ T cells effect glomerular injury in experimental anti-myeloperoxidase GN. *J. Am. Soc. Nephrol.* 28: 47–55.

41. Pedchenko V, Bondar O, Fogo AB, et al., 2010, Molecular architecture of the Goodpasture autoantigen in anti-GBM nephritis. *N. Engl. J. Med.* 363: 343–354.

42. Tan DS, Gan PY, O'Sullivan KM, et al., 2013, Thymic deletion and regulatory T cells prevent anti-myeloperoxidase GN. *J. Am. Soc. Nephrol.* 24: 573–585.

43. Free ME, Bunch DO, McGregor JA, et al., 2013, Patients with antineutrophil cytoplasmic antibody-associated vasculitis have defective Treg cell function exacerbated by the presence of a suppression-resistant effector cell population. *Arthritis Rheum.* 65: 1922–1933.

44. Gan PY, Tan DS, Ooi JD, et al., 2016, Myeloperoxidase peptide-based nasal tolerance in experimental ANCA-associated GN. *J. Am. Soc. Nephrol.* 27: 385–391.

CHAPTER SEVENTEEN

Role of Peroxidasin in Disease

Gautam Bhave
Vanderbilt University Medical Center

CONTENTS

INTRODUCTION

In 1994, Fessler and colleagues first reported peroxidasin as a basement membrane (BM) protein in *Drosophila*. They purified peroxidasin from a hemocyte cell line secreting BM proteins, cloned its cDNA, and immuno-localized it to BM in developing fly larvae. After the cDNA revealed a prominent peroxidase domain, the authors named the protein peroxidasin [1]. Unique among peroxidases, peroxidasin is a large homo-trimer (~150–180 kDa subunits or ~500 kDa total) with several non-catalytic protein–protein interaction domains, such as leucine-rich repeats (LRRs), immunoglobulin (Ig) domains, and a C-terminal von Willebrand factor type C (wVFc) domain commonly found in extracellular matrix (ECM) proteins.

For much of the decade after the discovery of peroxidasin in *Drosophila*, little was reported except for detection of its cDNA in various contexts but most prominently cancer, such as an upregulated transcript in metastatic melanoma and a p53 inducible gene in a colon cancer cell line [2,3].

Thereafter, the mammalian homologue of peroxidasin was cloned, and based on immunohistochemical localization to vascular BM, the gene was named vascular peroxidase or VPO, presumably to draw analogy to the expression-based nomenclature of classic peroxidases such as myeloperoxidase (MPO), eosinophil peroxidase, and lactoperoxidase (LPO) or salivary gland peroxidase [4]. While the name VPO has historical rationale, it overlooked seminal work in *Drosophila*. Thus, as with nearly all genes first discovered in *Drosophila*, the mammalian homologue is now officially recognized as peroxidasin (human gene PXDN). The name peroxidasin will be used throughout this chapter, even when referring to literature using the VPO rubric. Cloning and genomic sequencing efforts have revealed that most organisms possess a single peroxidasin gene, but some animals, including humans and *C. elegans*, possess two peroxidasin genes [5]. The second gene known as peroxidasin-like in humans (PXDNL) is predicted to be catalytically inactive, but little is known about its function except that PXDNL may inhibit PXDN function [6,7]. This chapter will focus

DOI: 10.1201/9781003212287-21

on peroxidasin (PXDN) function, which remained obscure for at least 15 years after its discovery.

PEROXIDASIN AND BASEMENT MEMBRANE HOMEOSTASIS

Insight into peroxidasin function came from seminal work on the assembly of the collagen IV network of BMs. BMs are specialized forms of ECM classically defined on electron microscopy as an electron dense planar layer found directly underneath epithelial, endothelial, and muscle cells [8]. Indeed, BMs are the primordial form of ECM, arising in evolution with the earliest multicellular animal organisms [9,10]. Interstitial matrix, which primarily surrounds mesenchymal cells, arose later in evolution with tissue complexity and specialization [11]. While ECM clearly provides structural support, this is not its only function. ECM proteins interact with cell surface receptors such as integrins and control growth factor availability to cue cells into their surrounding environment, which in turn modulates nearly all aspects of cell behavior including proliferation, differentiation, and energy metabolism [12].

Four major structural proteins account for most of BM mass: laminins, collagen IV, nidogen, and proteoglycans such as perlecan, agrin, and collagen XVIII. Along with differences in these core constituents, BMs also contain ca. 100–200 ancillary proteins that presumably control cell surface receptor interactions, growth factor binding, post-translational modifications, and turnover and degradation of BM core components [8,13]. Laminins and collagen IV uniquely form sheet-like structures through the oligomerization of trimeric subunits. Laminin heterotrimeric subunits consist of one each of 5 α, 4 β, and 3 γ chains with 16 recognized combinations [14]. Collagen IV trimeric subunits, also known as protomers, are composed of 6 α chains (α1–6), with only three known combinations, denoted as α112, α345, and α556 [15].

Laminin assembly and deposition are considered to define a BM and act as the initiating events in its formation during development. Subsequent collagen IV network formation is thought to structurally reinforce the BM through its triple-helical collagenous structure and the presence of covalent cross-links between protomers [8]. Loss of the γ1 laminin chain, which eliminates nearly all laminin heterotrimers, leads to poor BM formation and early embryonic lethality [16]. Conversely, mice lacking the predominant collagen α112 network demonstrate reasonable BM formation but later embryonic lethality due to mechanical instability and BM rupture [17]. Similarly, lack of the renal glomerular α345 network in Alport Syndrome leads to breaks in the glomerular BM, resulting in hematuria and eventually progressive renal failure [18]. In *Drosophila* egg development, collagen IV acts as a "molecular corset" tightening around the egg and mechanically driving egg elongation via interactions with cell surface integrins [19].

Oligomerization of the collagen IV network occurs at several locations. Four protomer N-termini come together to form the 7S dodecamer, while two C-termini assemble to form the NC1 hexamer (Figure 17.1). The intervening "collagenous" domains also interact through poorly characterized lateral associations. Covalent cross-links between protomers reinforce these non-covalent interactions. Disulfide bonds and lysine–lysine cross-links reinforce the 7S dodecamer, the latter formed by the lysyl oxidase family of enzymes [20]. Disulfide bonds also occur in the collagenous domain [15]. Finally, a sulfilimine (S=N) cross-link between a methionine sulfur on one collagen protomer and (hydroxy)lysine nitrogen on the opposite protomer cross-links the NC1 hexamer [21]. Discovery in collagen IV of the sulfilimine bond, never observed before in a protein, focused significant attention to its mechanism of formation.

Investigation into the formation of the collagen IV sulfilimine cross-link identified peroxidasin as the enzyme responsible for its formation and thus defined a function for peroxidasin [22]. Since collagen IV imparts mechanical stability to BMs, which, in part, is related to covalent cross-links between protomers, one would predict that peroxidasin contributes to BM mechanical strength, since it forms sulfilimine cross-links in collagen IV. Indeed, loss of peroxidasin in *Drosophila* leads to larval lethality due to gut perforation. Examination of the midgut in these animals demonstrated ruptured and torn collagen IV networks, suggesting that sulfilimine cross-links structurally reinforce collagen IV and BMs [22]. In *Drosophila* egg development, loss of peroxidasin subtly reduces egg elongation and represents a milder phenocopy of collagen IV deficiency [23]. In *C. elegans*, lack of peroxidasin results in ultrastructural BM defects similar to collagen IV mutants with early lethality because of body wall muscle rupture. Pharmacologic blockade of body

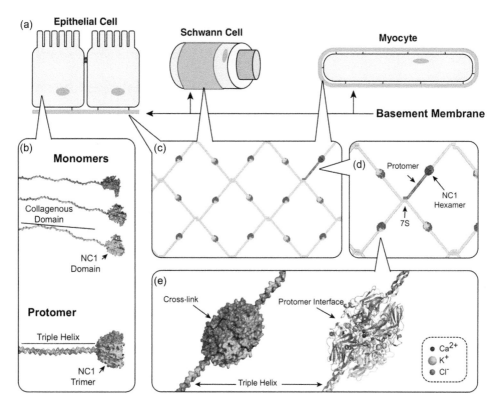

Figure 17.1 Assembly of the collagen IV network of basement membranes (BMs). (a) BMs are specialized layers of extracellular matrix (ECM) that underlie epithelial and endothelial cells and envelop muscle cells and Schwann cells. (b) Collagen IV biosynthesis begins intracellularly as monomeric alpha chains ($\alpha1$–$\alpha6$) that trimerize to form protomers consisting of a C-terminal non-collagenous 1 (NC1) domain and triple helical collagenous region. $\alpha112$, $\alpha345$, and $\alpha556$ are the only known protomer combinations known to exist. (c & d) Trimeric collagen IV protomers are secreted extracellularly and polymerize into a "fence-like" network through two protomers assembling at the NC1 domain to form the NC1 hexamer and four protomers associating to form the 7S dodecamer. Not shown are lateral associations that occur between the intervening collagenous region and yield a more complex meshwork than stylized here. (e) The NC1 hexamer is thought to initially assemble via electrostatic interactions involving chloride ions and then is reinforced by sulfilimine covalent cross-links. (Reproduced with permission from Ref. [99].)

muscle activity ameliorates the phenotype, suggesting that it occurs as a result of tissue instability in response to muscle-contraction-induced mechanical strain [24]. Taken together, peroxidasin forms sulfilimine cross-links in collagen IV, which provides mechanical stability to BMs and tissues. As predicted, loss of function in peroxidasin in invertebrate model systems compromises integrity of tissues under significant mechanical strain during growth and development.

Peroxidases use hydrogen peroxide (H_2O_2) and either directly oxidize substrates (peroxidase cycle) or produce hypohalous acids (halogenation cycle), which in turn modify targets [25]. Mechanistic studies demonstrated that peroxidasin uses H_2O_2 and bromide ion (Br^-) to generate hypobromous acid (HOBr) as a reactive intermediate to form sulfimine cross-links in collagen IV (Figure 17.2). Absence of Br^- prevents formation of collagen IV sulfilimine cross-links in vitro and in cell culture. Furthermore, bromine deprivation of *Drosophila* leads to larval gut perforation, thus phenocopying the loss of peroxidasin. Bromine can thus be envisioned as an essential trace element required to form sulfilimine cross-links in collagen IV and buttress tissue resilience [23]. These mechanistic studies also raise the question of how peroxidasin-generated HOBr is regulated and targeted with the possibility of dysregulation in disease. Dysregulated peroxidasin expression or generation of H_2O_2 substrate in disease might lead to excessive HOBr, which could cause collateral oxidative damage to nearby matrix components and cell surface receptors.

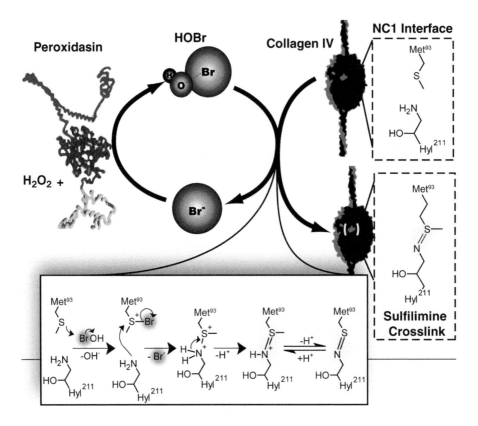

Figure 17.2 Peroxidasin generates hypobromous acid (HOBr) as a reactive intermediate to form sulfilimine (S=N) cross-links in collagen IV. Peroxidasin uses ambient extracellular Br$^-$ and H$_2$O$_2$ from an unknown source to generate HOBr. According to this model, HOBr targets a methionine sulfur on an NC1 subunit to form a bromosulfonium intermediate, which is then attacked by a closely apposed hydroxylysine amine to form a sulfilimine (S=N) cross-link bridging the subunit interface. (Reproduced with permission from Ref. [23].)

PEROXIDASIN EXPRESSION AND FUNCTION IN MAMMALS

Biochemical studies with collagen IV and genetic studies in model invertebrate organisms established that peroxidasin generates HOBr to form sulfilimine cross-links in collagen IV that stabilize tissues under mechanical strain. However, to examine the role peroxidasin might play in human disease, its function in mammals and humans needed further study. mRNA expression by northern blotting and RT-PCR suggested ubiquitous expression at variable levels in nearly all tissues except peripheral blood lymphocytes [2,4,26]. This expression pattern is consistent with a role in collagen IV assembly, since all tissues except peripheral blood cells contain basement membranes. However, data on peroxidasin protein expression are meager. As alluded to in the **Introduction**, initial cloning of the peroxidasin gene in humans (PXDN) suggested ubiquitous

mRNA expression, but with protein expression limited to the heart and vasculature with immunostaining suggestive of BM localization [4]. In a study focused on fibrosis, low-level peroxidasin protein expression appeared to localize to the tubular BM in normal mouse kidney [26]. During development, immunofluorescence of mouse eye found peroxidasin expression in the lens epithelium [27]. Lastly, ECM shot-gun proteomics studies from several tissues have found tryptic peptides corresponding to peroxidasin, leading to its designation as a core matrisome protein [28–30]. A unifying hypothesis is that peroxidasin is expressed at lower levels in many tissues but with higher expression in the cardiovascular system. An intriguing hypothesis for tissue differences in normal expression of peroxidasin may be differential turnover in collagen IV, which may be related to differences in BM mechanical strain. Regardless, definitive data on peroxidasin protein expression await the development of a high-affinity antibody that is validated in the murine knockout.

Prior to the discovery of the role of peroxidasin in stabilizing collagen IV, ophthalmologic geneticists found that rare autosomal recessive PXDN mutations caused anterior segment dysgenesis that often presented with microphthalmia and congenital cataracts [31]. Though extensive phenotypic characterization was not conducted, the affected patients appeared otherwise healthy. Subsequent studies have confirmed that biallelic PXDN mutations primarily cause eye defects, with a minority of patients also exhibiting neurologic impairments in cognition and motor function, brain cortical dysplasia on imaging without apparent clinical consequence, and mild craniofacial and skeletal defects [32,33]. Similar to humans, Pxdn mutant and knockout mice have also demonstrated severe anterior eye defects with microphthalmia or even anophthalmia as well as a white spot on the abdominal wall but without any other significant abnormality [27,34].

In mice, loss of the α112 collagen IV network, the major isoform of collagen IV in most mammalian tissues, leads to embryonic lethality at ca. embryonic day 11 due to rupture of Reichert's membrane, a thickened BM of the parietal yolk sac separating uterine trophoblasts and embryonic parietal endoderm cells. Prominent defects in capillaries with bleeding particularly of the pericardium and pial membrane along with irregular BM ultrastructure were also observed [17]. Autosomal dominant point mutations in the collagen IV α1 and α2 chains in mice and humans affect multiple organs and result in one or more manifestations, including brain small vessel defects resulting in premature intracerebral hemorrhage, porencephaly, ocular abnormalities, including anterior segment dysgenesis with microphthalmia or congenital cataracts, myopathy presenting with severe cramps, and glomerulocystic nephropathy [35–39]. In this context, complete loss of peroxidasin might represent an extremely mild collagen IV phenotype primarily affecting the anterior eye, only one of the manifestations seen in point mutations of a single allele of a collagen IV chain.

The phenotypic difference between peroxidasin and collagen IV loss of function appears much wider in mammals than in invertebrate model systems. For instance, C. elegans null mutants of collagen IV (α1 gene emb-9 and α2 gene let-2) exhibit arrest in late embryogenesis at the three or fourfold stage of elongation with very few hatching as small larvae due to rupture and separation of body wall muscle from the epidermis [40–42]. Severe mutants of C. elegans peroxidasin (pxn-2) also arrest at late embryogenesis due to body wall muscle dysfunction, but unlike collagen IV mutants ca. 70% hatch, eventually arresting as L1 larvae [24]. Thus, the phenotype of peroxidasin null worms is easily identifiable as a milder phenocopy of collagen IV mutants with a prominent defect in BM structural integrity under the mechanical strain of muscle contraction. Conversely, the isolated eye defect in peroxidasin knockout mice is significantly milder than the embryonic lethality and vascular defects observed in collagen IV α112 knockouts. Two main reasons may explain the invertebrate–mammalian discrepancy in phenotype: (i) differences in invertebrate and mammalian development and biology with the lack of significant interstitial matrix as another form of structural support in invertebrates as a conspicuous factor [11], and (ii) intrinsic differences in collagen IV with a greater reliance on the sulfilimine cross-link versus lysyl cross-links or disulfides for mechanical reinforcement in invertebrate collagen IV possibly suggested by the greater chemical solubility of collagen IV in invertebrates [43].

PEROXIDASIN IN EYE DEVELOPMENT

The prominent eye phenotype of peroxidasin loss of function in mice and humans suggests a significant role in the development of the anterior segment of the eye. The anterior segment of the eye refers to the structures in front of the vitreous surface, mainly the cornea, iris, ciliary body and processes, and lens [44]. In terms of ECM, the anterior segment has BMs (from anterior to posterior) underlying the corneal epithelium, corneal endothelium, iris epithelium, and most conspicuously the lens capsule, a specialized thickened BM surrounding the lens [30,45]. Interstitial matrix forms the corneal and iris stroma. The iris further subdivides the anterior segment into a posterior chamber behind and an anterior chamber in front of the iris. Ciliary processes in the posterior chamber secrete aqueous humor, which circulates into the anterior chamber and is reabsorbed at the angle between the iris and cornea via a trabecular meshwork and Schlemm's canal (Figure 17.3). Disruption of this process can lead

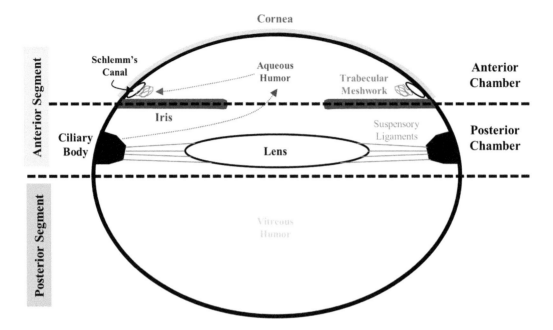

Figure 17.3 Basic anatomy of the eye with an emphasis on the anterior segment. The anterior aspect of the vitreous humor separates the eye into anterior and posterior segments. The iris bisects the anterior segment into an anterior and posterior chamber. The ciliary epithelium secretes aqueous humor, which circulates into the anterior chamber and is absorbed via trabecular meshwork and Schlemm's canal. The cornea covers the anterior surface of the eye.

to accumulation of aqueous humor raising intraocular pressure and resulting in glaucoma [44].

Anterior segment dysgenesis denotes a developmental abnormality of the structures of the anterior segment, with manifestations such as iris hypoplasia (underdevelopment), microcornea, corneal opacity, inappropriate adhesions between the cornea and the iris or lens, malformations of the aqueous humor drainage structures, and congenital cataracts of the lens. In addition to these abnormalities, anterior segment dysgenesis is often accompanied by microphthalmia (small eyes) and glaucoma, due to disruption of aqueous humor drainage [44,46,47].

Anterior segment development is complex, and a detailed description is beyond the scope of this chapter. Briefly, the optic cup derived from neural ectoderm induces the lens to invaginate from the surface ectoderm. Thereafter, periocular mesenchymal cells, mostly of neural crest but also mesodermal origin, migrate in between the lens and surface ectoderm to form the corneal stroma, corneal endothelium, ciliary body, trabecular meshwork and Schlemm's canal, and iris stroma. The surface ectoderm differentiates into corneal epithelium, while migrating neural crest cells simultaneously give rise to ciliary

processes and iris epithelium [47]. Given the complex patterns of cell migration and differentiation, it is not surprising that many patients with anterior segment dysgenesis harbor mutations in transcription factors, most prominently FOXC1 and PITX2 [44]. However, recent work has also focused attention on mutations in structural proteins as causes of anterior segment dysgenesis, particularly BM protein genes, such as PXDN, COL4A1 (collagen IV α1), and LAMB2 (laminin β2 chain) [46].

Many anterior segment abnormalities in patients with PXDN mutations have been described, with congenital cataracts, corneal opacification, and microcornea along with microphthalmia as most prominent [31–33]. In humans with COL4A1 (collagen IV α1 gene) autosomal dominant mutations, similar findings have been described, possibly with broader involvement of anterior segment structures as well as optic nerve hypoplasia in the posterior segment not described in patients with PXDN mutations [48]. These data suggest that, at least in the eye, peroxidasin loss of function appears to be a slightly milder phenocopy of autosomal dominant mutations in collagen IV. However, as noted earlier, autosomal dominant collagen IV mutations also lead to several non-ocular manifestations not found in loss of peroxidasin function.

Detailed characterization during embryonic development of a mouse with a C-terminal truncating mutation in the Pxdn gene suggests that the primary defect is in lens development and growth. The lens forms but then fails to grow, with disorganized lens fibers and eventual lens disruption with lens fibers in the anterior chamber and mesenchymal cells inappropriately present in the posterior segment. Lens epithelial cells in Pxdn mutants proliferate less and fail to differentiate, with decreased expression of Foxe3, a critical transcription factor for lens development. Pax6, the master regulator of eye development, is upregulated in Pxdn mutants, with inappropriate expression in lens fibers and enhanced expression in lens epithelium and retina. Lens disruption also drives ocular inflammation with enhanced TNFα and IL-1 expression. About 3 weeks postnatally, Pxdn mutant mice exhibit adhesions between iris and cornea or lens and cornea, iris hypoplasia, and retinal tract abnormalities. Consistent with a primary role in lens development, peroxidasin expression was primarily found in the lens epithelium and lens fibers, with lesser expression in the inner neuroblastic layer (retina) [27]. Interestingly, spatial expression of an autosomal dominant deletion mutation of the COL4A1 gene restricted to the lens recapitulated anterior segment dysgenesis observed with ubiquitous expression. Expression in the neural crest-derived periocular mesenchymal cells did not produce anterior segment dysgenesis, while vascular endothelial cell expression only generated anterior segment dysgenesis in a sensitized background [48]. Taken together, peroxidasin and collagen IV are critical for lens development and presumably reside in the primordial lens capsule BM to provide mechanical support and interactions with lens epithelial cell surface receptors. With peroxidasin and collagen IV loss of function, disruption of lens development then secondarily derails development of other anterior segment structures, due to absence of lens-derived molecular cues and/or downstream ocular inflammation.

PEROXIDASIN IN CARDIOVASCULAR DISEASE

Early work suggesting prominent peroxidasin expression in subendothelial, cardiomyocyte, and vascular smooth muscle BM pointed to a potential role in cardiovascular homeostasis and disease [4]. This body of work has implicated peroxidasin in nearly every cardiovascular pathology, including hypertension-associated endothelial dysfunction, vascular remodeling, cardiac hypertrophy, atherosclerosis and vascular calcification, aortic aneurysms, ischemic cardiac injury and fibrosis, and pulmonary arterial hypertension.

In spontaneously hypertensive rats, peroxidasin mRNA and protein expression are upregulated in the endothelium and subendothelial BM and in the vascular smooth muscle medial layer ECM, which are also thought to be where peroxidasin is expressed normally [4,49,50]. Angiotensin II (AngII) stimulation of cultured human umbilical vein endothelial cells (HUVEC) and aortic vascular smooth muscle cells were used as in vitro models of hypertension to gain mechanistic insight. In endothelial cells, AngII stimulation increased peroxidasin expression along with H_2O_2 generation thought to be secondary to enhanced NADPH oxidase (NOX) activity. AngII expectedly decreased endothelial nitric oxide synthase (eNOS) expression and activity along with increasing arginine dimethylarginine (ADMA), an endogenous eNOS inhibitor. Pharmacologic blockade of NOX enzymes using nonspecific inhibitors (apocynin and diphenyliodonium) and degradation of H_2O_2 by catalase reversed the effects of AngII on eNOS activity, ADMA levels, and peroxidasin upregulation [49,51]. In unrelated work, H_2O_2 was found to act via Nrf2 to increase peroxidasin transcription [52]. Peroxidasin knockdown using small interfering RNA (siRNA) had similar effects to those seen after NOX inhibition. Peroxidasin is therefore thought to lie downstream of NOX and H_2O_2 and contribute to pathology.

The exact oxidative signaling events however remain unclear. Two reports suggest that peroxidasin produces HOCl as a driver of pathology [49,51], but detailed investigation of peroxidasin catalytic activity demonstrates conclusively that it is incapable of generating HOCl [53]. An alternative hypothesis would be that peroxidasin generates HOBr to promote disease pathology, just as it does in the formation of cross-links in collagen IV. However, disease may not follow normal physiology; peroxidasin may directly oxidize substrates, may generate HOBr that in turn creates other intermediates such as bromamines, or may produce other hypohalous acids such as hypothiocyanous acid (HOSCN) to drive pathology. Given the lack of understanding of the mechanism of peroxidasin activity, we will for now use the term "HOX" as a generic oxidative effector mechanism in the work on peroxidasin and cardiovascular disease until further study clarifies this issue.

A similar picture to endothelial cells has been proposed for peroxidasin action in vascular smooth muscle cells and cardiac myocytes treated with AngII. In this case, excessive proliferation in vascular smooth muscle cells and hypertrophy in cardiac myocytes were proposed as in vitro correlates of hypertension-induced vascular and cardiac remodeling, respectively. AngII drives smooth muscle cell proliferation and increases NOX activity and H_2O_2 production, which in turn upregulate peroxidasin to amplify oxidative signaling via HOX generation. H_2O_2 and HOX activate extracellular regulated kinase (ERK) 1/2, which promotes smooth muscle cell proliferation. However, ERK 1/2 has little effect on NOX activity, peroxidasin expression, or H_2O_2 and HOX generation [50]. Similar events were found to occur in the case of AngII-mediated cardiac myocyte hypertrophy [54].

Peroxidasin may contribute to multiple pathogenic drivers of atherosclerosis. In a mouse model of atherosclerosis, peroxidasin localized to atherosclerotic plaques [55]. Peroxidasin expression also increased in the aorta after administration of proatherogenic oxidized LDL, TNF-alpha, and IL-1, suggesting that upregulated peroxidasin may contribute to generation and/or progression of atherosclerosis [56]. In vitro peroxidasin binds to LDL and can oxidize LDL and apolipoprotein E (ApoE), which in turn promote LDL accumulation in cultured macrophages to form foam cells within atherosclerotic plaques [55,56].

Oxidized LDL (ox-LDL) can influence endothelial cells and vascular smooth muscle cells to promote vascular damage. Similar to AngII, ox-LDL treatment of HUVECs increases NOX activity, H_2O_2 generation, peroxidasin expression and HOX, and activates p38 kinase and receptor interacting protein kinase (RIPK) 1 and 3 to promote apoptosis and necroptosis [57,58]. Pharmacologic inhibition of NOX, knockdown of NOX1, knockdown of peroxidasin, and inhibition of p38 all ameliorate ox-LDL-induced HUVEC apoptosis. While antagonism of NOX and peroxidasin reduces p38 activation, inhibition of p38 has little effect on NOX activity, peroxidasin expression, or generation of H_2O_2 and HOX. Peroxidasin knockdown reduces

ox-LDL-mediated RIPK 1/3 activation as well as upstream modulation of glycogen synthase kinase (GSK-3beta) and beta-catenin [57,58]. Unlike p38 activation and apoptosis, the effects of NOX inhibition on RIPK 1/3 activation and necroptosis were not formally tested but presumably would reduce RIPK activity directly or indirectly by preventing peroxidasin upregulation.

Ox-LDL treatment of vascular smooth muscle cells promotes calcification via activation of ERK 1/2, p38 kinase, and Akt kinases (Ak strain transforming, also known as protein kinase B) and the osteogenic transcription factor Runx2, along with upregulation of NOX1 (but not NOX4) and peroxidasin. A model is proposed wherein NOX generates H_2O_2 and upregulates peroxidasin, which increases HOX. HOX then activates ERK, p38, Akt, and downstream Runx2 to drive ox-LDL-mediated vascular calcification [59]. Taken together, peroxidasin promotes ox-LDL formation in vitro and promotes ox-LDL-mediated dysfunction of endothelial and vascular smooth muscle cells in culture.

In human aortic aneurysm samples and in a mouse model of aortic aneurysms, peroxidasin expression is increased in the medial smooth muscle layer, suggesting a potential pathogenic role. A phenotypic switch in vascular smooth muscle cells from a "contractile" to a "synthetic" phenotype is thought to play a role in weakening of the smooth muscle layer and aneurysm formation. H_2O_2 is thought to promote this phenotypic switch, which is detected by downregulation of contractile smooth muscle proteins and upregulation of matrix metalloproteases such as MMP2 and the transcription factor KLF4 (Kruppel-like Factor). An in vitro correlate of this disease process was modeled using H_2O_2 treatment of cultured vascular smooth muscle cells. Again, H_2O_2 led to peroxidasin upregulation that in turn increased HOX. H_2O_2 and HOX were found to activate ERK 1/2 and drive KLF4-mediated transcription to transform smooth muscle cell phenotype [60].

In heart samples from patients with ischemic cardiomyopathy and in mouse models of post–myocardial infarction (MI) cardiac fibrosis, peroxidasin expression is increased particularly in vimentin-positive fibroblasts in zones of fibrosis [61]. This expression is distinct from that observed normally in cardiac vascular endothelial and vascular smooth muscle cells and cardiomyocytes. Cardiac ischemia-reperfusion injury and subsequent fibrosis are thought to result from ischemic injury to cardiomyocytes resulting in apoptosis. Through cytokines and pro-fibrotic messengers such as TGFβ (transforming growth factor beta), injured cardiomyocytes attract inflammatory cells and activate fibroblasts to eventually resolve the injury by promoting fibrosis. Thus, the role of peroxidasin was investigated in culture using hypoxic injury to cardiomyocytes and TGFβ stimulation of cardiac fibroblasts. Cardiomyocytes upregulated NOX2 and peroxidasin, resulting in elevated H_2O_2 and HOX levels with significant apoptosis in response to hypoxia. Knockdown of NOX2 and peroxidasin attenuated hypoxia-induced cardiomyocyte apoptosis. Direct application of H_2O_2 activated p38 and JNK (c-Jun N-terminal kinase) and increased peroxidasin expression. Kinase inhibitors blocked peroxidasin upregulation, which is a slight departure from other studies where downstream kinase activation did not participate in modifying peroxidasin expression [62]. Stimulation of cultured cardiac fibroblasts with TGFβ led to increased proliferation and production of collagen I along with peroxidasin upregulation. TGFβ activated downstream Smad 2/3 and ERK 1/2, which promoted collagen I production and proliferation, respectively. Peroxidasin knockdown reduced Smad 2/3 and ERK 1/2 activation and attenuated fibroblast proliferation and collagen I production. HOX also activated Smad 2/3 and ERK 1/2 suggesting that peroxidasin drives signaling via generation of HOX, although the role of H_2O_2 and the mechanism of peroxidasin upregulation were not investigated. Uniquely, this work was able to examine the role of peroxidasin in vivo through siRNA tail vein injection to achieve cardiac peroxidasin knockdown after mouse myocardial ischemia. Knockdown ameliorated post-MI fibrosis and loss of function and even reduced mortality [61].

Rats developing pulmonary arterial hypertension in response to hypoxia demonstrated increased pulmonary artery smooth muscle expression of NOX4 and peroxidasin. These findings were recapitulated in an in vitro model where pulmonary artery smooth muscle cells were exposed to hypoxia. In response to hypoxia, these cells exhibit increased proliferation and migration. Peroxidasin knockdown reduced post-hypoxia HOX levels (but not H_2O_2), NFκB (nuclear factor kappa-light-chain-enhancer of activated B cells) activation, and cell proliferation and migration

suggesting a possible role in the pathogenesis of pulmonary arterial hypertension [63].

Taken together, a large body of work suggests a role for peroxidasin in the pathogenesis of a host of cardiovascular diseases. A recurring mechanistic model points to pathologic stimuli, such as AngII, ox-LDL, or hypoxia, increasing peroxidasin expression often via upregulation of NOX enzymes and H_2O_2 generation. H_2O_2, possibly via Nrf2, enhances peroxidasin expression that in turn increases HOX generation. H_2O_2 and HOX collectively drive oxidative signaling to activate downstream kinase networks and transcription factors to promote maladaptive cellular responses.

Given that cardiovascular disease is the leading cause of death in the developed world, these data raise the exciting possibility of therapeutically targeting peroxidasin. However, further work is required to validate these results. First, as discussed earlier, much of the protein expression work used antibodies that have not been clearly validated using Pxdn knockout animals. Second, all of this work assumed that peroxidasin generates HOCl as an oxidative effector molecule, but peroxidasin is unable to produce HOCl [53]. Third, much of the work suggests that peroxidasin uses NOX-generated H_2O_2 to generate HOX. However, peroxidasin does not couple with NOX to generate HOBr in the formation of sulfilimine cross-links [64]. Thus, one would have to hypothesize that NOX provides H_2O_2 for peroxidasin in the setting of disease but not in normal development. Fourth, except in the case of MI [61], little in vivo intervention data exist to determine whether peroxidasin loss of function ameliorates disease. Fifth, multiple groups need to replicate these findings. Regardless, the data so far raise cautious optimism that peroxidasin may be a fruitful target for treating several cardiovascular diseases.

PEROXIDASIN IN TISSUE FIBROSIS

Geiszt and colleagues were the first to suggest a possible role for peroxidasin in tissue fibrosis. Human dermal and pulmonary fibroblasts expressed peroxidasin with significant upregulation and secretion in response to TGFβ stimulation and transformation into myofibroblasts. In addition, supplementation with a heme precursor, delta-aminolevulinic acid, led to deposition of peroxidasin into fibrillar structures co-localizing with fibronectin in fibroblast ECM. More importantly, peroxidasin was upregulated and co-localized with fibronectin in regions of renal interstitial fibrosis after unilateral ureteral obstruction (UUO) in mice, pointing to a role in fibrosis in vivo [26]. Colon and colleagues followed up on these findings by demonstrating that Pxdn knockout mice had reduced fibroblast alpha-smooth muscle actin (SMA) expression, a marker for fibroblast activation, and diminished renal interstitial fibrosis and collagen I deposition in the UUO model of kidney fibrosis [65]. In conjunction with the work discussed earlier on cardiac fibrosis [61], these data suggest that peroxidasin is expressed in fibroblasts, upregulated in fibrosis, and deposited into interstitial ECM rather than BM, as in normal development. However, as in cardiovascular disease, exact mechanisms remain unclear. Peroxidasin generation of HOBr, as in the formation of cross-links in collagen IV to oxidatively amplify pro-fibrotic signaling cascades, is a reasonable hypothesis but with limited supporting data.

In normal development and physiology, peroxidasin generates HOBr as a diffusible intermediate to cross-link collagen IV. HOBr is an extremely reactive oxidant and would require a highly regulated system to target the specific methionine residue in collagen IV to produce sulfilimine cross-links without oxidatively modifying nearby "off-target" residues in collagen IV or other BM proteins. Recent work suggests that the system is slightly inaccurate even in normal development. Nano-SIMS (nanoscale secondary ion mass spectrometry) imaging found that bromine, reflecting brominated amino acids particularly bromotyrosine, is enriched in BM of normal kidney. BM enrichment of bromine is nearly abrogated in Pxdn knockout mice, suggesting that peroxidasin-generated HOBr modifies BM proteins [66]. Moreover, it is not surprising, given its high reactivity, that peroxidasin-generated HOBr acts locally to modify predominantly, though not exclusively, BM proteins [67]. In addition, using conventional mass spectrometry of purified collagen IV, ca. 1.5% of Tyr-1485 in the NC1 domain of the mouse $\alpha2$ chain of collagen IV was found to exist as bromotyrosine, which was nearly absent in Pxdn knockout mice [66]. Similarly, Bathish and colleagues found 3-bromotyrosine (at 1.1 mmol/mol tyrosine) predominantly in ECM of cultured cells that was abolished with loss of peroxidasin function [68]. These data suggest that in normal mice, peroxidasin generates HOBr, which oxidizes collagen IV and probably other BM proteins at "off-target" sites. The efficiency of off-target oxidation seems quite low, but bromotyrosine may not accurately reflect efficiency, as it is a specific, but minor, product of HOBr oxidation [67,69].

Extrapolating from normal physiology to disease to generate a working hypothesis, peroxidasin upregulation in BM or interstitial ECM of fibrosis increases its generation of HOBr, which in turn primarily targets ECM proteins, possibly cell surface receptors and rarely intracellular proteins, to drive maladaptive signaling. Nano-SIMS imaging of bromine in human diabetic kidney disease demonstrated increased bromine accumulation in glomerular and tubular BM. This increase persisted even after accounting for the BM and ECM expansion found in diabetic nephropathy. Interestingly, regions of interstitial fibrosis, where peroxidasin upregulation has been documented in mouse UUO, demonstrated only modest, if any, bromine enrichment [66]. Admittedly, UUO is a tubulointerstitial disease while diabetic kidney disease is predominantly glomerular, so that the compartmental difference may explain this discrepancy. Regardless, increased HOBr-mediated oxidation associates with fibrosis, but the direct molecular targets remain obscure. However, a tentative model based on the work in cardiovascular disease and the work in renal fibrosis may be entertained. Various insults (e.g. hypoxia, ox-LDL, AngII, ureteral obstruction with mechanical stretch) upon epithelial, endothelial, and vascular smooth muscle cells lead to upregulation of peroxidasin in these cells possibly due to increased H_2O_2 and downstream Nrf2 activation. Peroxidasin generates excessive HOBr that targets BM proteins and cell surface receptors in the immediate vicinity and less so intracellular proteins to alter interactions between BM-interacting integrins and their ligands as well as growth factor and other receptor signaling. These alterations, possibly along with H_2O_2, activate downstream kinase and transcription factor signaling and lead to maladaptive responses. In fibrosis, TGFβ among many other signals leads to activation of fibroblasts with increased peroxidasin expression, which through HOBr-mediated oxidation of extracellular targets potentiates fibroblast ECM production (Figure 17.4). Significant work is needed to validate this model; peroxidasin generation of HOBr may not be the only mechanism involved in fibrosis, with other oxidative mechanisms (e.g. direct

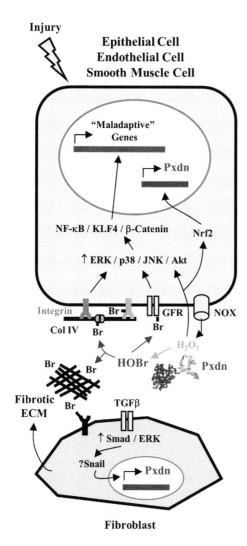

Injury

Epithelial Cell
Endothelial Cell
Smooth Muscle Cell

"Maladaptive" Genes

Pxdn

NF-κB / KLF4 / β-Catenin

Nrf2

↑ ERK / p38 / JNK / Akt

Integrin   Br   GFR   NOX

Col IV   Br   Br

Br   Br   HOBr   H₂O₂   Pxdn

Fibrotic ECM   Br

TGFβ

↑ Smad / ERK

?Snail   Pxdn

Fibroblast

Figure 17.4 Model for peroxidasin involvement in cardiovascular disease and fibrosis. Insults to endothelial, epithelial, or vascular smooth muscle cells, such as AngII, ox-LDL, hypoxia, or mechanical stretch due to urinary tract obstruction, lead to enhanced H_2O_2 generation in these cells through NOX. H_2O_2 in turn activates Nrf2 and upregulates peroxidasin. Peroxidasin generates excessive HOBr, which primarily targets ECM proteins such as collagen IV (col IV) and cell surface receptors such as integrins and modifies cell–matrix interactions and growth factor receptor (GFR) signaling to then drive the activation of kinases (ERK, p38, JNK, Akt) and maladaptive transcription factors (NFκB, β-catenin, KLF4). In fibrosis, TGFβ signaling via Smad 2/3, ERK 1/2, and possibly the transcription factor Snail increases peroxidasin expression, which in turn promotes TGFβ or other signaling to enhance fibroblast activation and deposition of fibrotic ECM. This only represents a hypothetical model that requires further investigation. For instance, peroxidasin may use other mechanisms, such as direct oxidation of substrates or generation of HOSCN to promote fibrosis.

substrate oxidation, generation of bromamines via HOBr, production of other hypohalous acids such as HOSCN) as alternatives, exact molecular targets for HOBr remain unknown, and oxidative modifications that drive pathology are not identified.

PEROXIDASIN IN CANCER

Cancer biology is an enormous field that includes studies of the initiation, growth, invasion, and metastasis of tumors along with their interactions with surrounding stroma and vasculature and immune cells, a detailed description of which is well beyond the scope of this chapter. Interest in the role of peroxidasin in cancer primarily resulted from transcriptomic data pointing to peroxidasin upregulation in many tumors, with the initial identification in melanoma [3]. In some cases, such as basal cell breast cancer and ovarian cancer, enhanced expression of peroxidasin has been shown to associate with poorer patient survival [70,71]. The exact mechanistic role of peroxidasin probably varies depending on tumor and stage.

In some cancers, such as glioblastoma, metastatic brain cancer, and renal cancer, peroxidasin is upregulated along with collagen IV and seems to localize to tumor microvasculature and nearby stroma, suggesting a role in assembly of the collagen IV network in subendothelial BM of tumor capillaries and possibly a broader role in angiogenesis [72,73]. Using normal immortalized aortic endothelial cells, Medfai and colleagues demonstrated that exogenous treatment with recombinant peroxidasin increased endothelial tube formation and vessel density in chicken chorioallantoic membrane, both models of angiogenesis. Exogenous peroxidasin activated ERK 1/2, Akt, and FAK (focal adhesion kinase), findings reminiscent of the studies on endothelial cells focused on cardiovascular disease. Knockdown of peroxidasin decreased endothelial tube formation but only reduced kinase activation resulting from exogenous peroxidase application. Exogenous peroxidasin also upregulated proangiogenic genes and enhanced endogenous peroxidasin transcription, as suggested by the knockdown experiments [74]. Taken together, these data suggest that peroxidasin may not only reinforce collagen IV in BM during the growth of tumor capillaries but also might signal in a paracrine or autocrine fashion to drive angiogenesis.

In breast cancer, peroxidasin may signal in a paracrine fashion to promote cell proliferation. In the MCF10a cell line, expression of an activating mutation in PI3K (phosphoinositide 3-kinase) seen in some forms of breast cancer allows for cell proliferation in the absence of growth factors such as EGF (epidermal growth factor). Mutant cells upregulated peroxidasin, and knockdown of peroxidasin reduced growth-factor-independent cell proliferation. Interestingly, conditioned media from PI3K mutant cells conferred growth-factor-independent growth upon the parental MCF10a cell line. PI3K mutant cells secreted significantly more exosomes, which contained peroxidasin among its cargo, suggesting that peroxidasin acts in a paracrine fashion, possibly even as a soluble messenger rather than an ECM-embedded protein [70].

The role of peroxidasin in tumor epithelial–mesenchymal transition (EMT) has garnered attention. EMT is a complex process with multiple intermediate stages between epithelial and mesenchymal phenotypes, but in general, transition to the mesenchymal phenotype is thought to endow greater invasion and metastatic potential to tumor cells [75]. Melanoma cells with a mesenchymal phenotype overexpress peroxidasin, and knockdown reduces invasion in vitro [76]. The D432 breast cancer cell line can be induced to undergo mesenchymal transition to yield the isogenic D432M cell line. During transition, the microRNA (miRNA) 203a is downregulated with subsequent upregulation of peroxidasin as one of its targets. Knockdown of peroxidasin in D432M cells reduces proliferation, increases sensitivity to chemotherapy-induced apoptosis, but does not alter invasion or migration, thus explaining only part of the mesenchymal phenotype [77]. Interestingly, these studies suggest that peroxidasin contributes to a mesenchymal phenotype, but clearly peroxidasin function in collagen IV assembly is epithelial, as BMs are the canonical ECM of epithelia. While tissues of mesenchymal origin such as muscle are also enveloped in a BM, the increased invasive and metastatic potential of mesenchymal tumor cells seems antithetical to the functions of collagen IV and BMs, which tend to promote cell adhesion and differentiation. Thus, as seen in fibrosis, peroxidasin may promote mesenchymal transition in cancer through a non-collagen IV-related function.

Peroxidasin as a target for miRNAs altered during cancer development has been a focus of studies of hematologic malignancies. In chronic lymphocytic leukemia (CLL), miRNA expression is enhanced, which in turn downregulates peroxidasin, a target of miRNA [78]. Thus, in CLL, peroxidasin uniquely antagonizes malignant transformation. Conversely, in T cell acute lymphoblastic leukemia (ALL), miRNA expression is decreased, leading to peroxidasin upregulation and pointing to a pro-oncogenic role, as suggested in solid tumors [79].

Given its ability to generate HOX from H_2O_2, peroxidasin may participate in redox mechanisms involved in carcinogenesis. Peroxidasin expression is increased in prostate cancer, particularly in advanced stages, and in several prostate cancer cell lines. Knockdown of peroxidasin in these lines decreased cell viability and enhanced fluorescent signals from nonspecific oxidation-sensitive fluorescent probes and increased the ratio of $NADP^+$/ NADPH and GSSG/GSH, suggesting a shift toward an oxidative environment. Peroxidasin knockdown was also accompanied by increased Nrf2, catalase, superoxide dismutase, and peroxiredoxins, presumably in response to the shift toward oxidation. The authors suggest that increased peroxidasin reduces intracellular oxidative potential and thus promotes tumor cell viability [80]. However, earlier work by the same group also suggests an increase in intracellular oxidative potential and Snail overexpression in prostate cancer cells, which in turn leads to a 350-fold increase in peroxidasin mRNA and would thus suggest peroxidasin drives oxidation [81]. This would be more consistent with peroxidasin-mediated conversion of H_2O_2 to HOBr.

Taken together, peroxidasin promotes malignancy, except in CLL. In some tumors, peroxidasin may simply be co-regulated with and cross-link collagen IV, particularly in the assembly of tumor microvasculature BM. In others, peroxidasin may act as an autocrine or paracrine signal to promote tumor cell proliferation or angiogenesis or might act as a miRNA target. Lastly, peroxidasin could regulate tumor redox hemeostasis and signaling and promote cancer progression. However, exact mechanisms remain obscure, and except in the case of endothelial tube formation, it is not clear whether peroxidasin generation of HOBr is involved, as has been implicated in the studies on cardiovascular disease and fibrosis discussed earlier.

PEROXIDASIN IN IMMUNITY

Classic chordata peroxidases in Family 1 of the peroxidase-cyclooxygenase superfamily are notably involved in host defense, with MPO in neutrophils and eosinophil peroxidase in eosinophils serving to generate hypohalous acids to destroy pathogens upon granulocyte activation [82,83]. Epithelia secrete LPO luminally to control pathogens as a form of innate immunity and environmental barrier defense [84]. Can peroxidasin play an analogous role in immune defense? Peroxidasins are the ancestral animal heme peroxidase uniquely conserved along with collagen IV from Cnidaria to man [10]. The conservation might suggest a role in innate immunity particularly in invertebrates lacking chordata peroxidases and specialized leukocytes [83]. Consistent with this hypothesis, mosquito peroxidasin is heavily upregulated in the gut after bacterial infection, and its knockdown reduces bacterial clearance and mosquito survival [85]. Whether peroxidasin universally participates in barrier defense in invertebrates is unknown. A potential difference between peroxidasin and classic chordata peroxidases is the catalytic efficiency of hypohalous acid generation. Peroxidasin is inefficient, which suits its anabolic role in collagen IV assembly where oxidation of bystander ECM proteins might be detrimental [22,86]. Thus, unless there is significant upregulation of expression or posttranslational mechanisms to alter catalytic efficiency, peroxidasin would not be well suited for pathogen destruction, where a large burst of hypohalous production is required. Peroxinectin peroxidases (Family 3 of the peroxidase-cyclooxygenase superfamily) are primarily found in invertebrates and may be an alternative mechanism for pathogen killing in these organisms, but detailed characterization of peroxinectins has not been conducted thus far [83].

Some work has suggested that endothelial cells secrete peroxidasin into the circulation, leading to low micromolar concentrations in mammalian plasma. Peroxidasin was found to generate HOCl at ca. 5%–10% of the efficiency of MPO. Compared with MPO, peroxidasin accounted for an equal or greater fraction of plasma HOCl generation and bacterial killing capacity, suggesting that its catalytic inefficiency was counterbalanced by its 2–3 orders of magnitude greater concentration [87]. Although these data placing peroxidasin as a part of the innate immune defense of circulating plasma are intriguing, other groups have yet to report the presence of peroxidasin in mammalian plasma, and more problematic, strong experimental evidence demonstrates that peroxidasin lacks the capacity to generate HOCl

[53], as described earlier in the discussion of peroxidasin and cardiovascular disease.

Peroxidasin can act as an antigen for antibodies targeting *self* in autoimmune disease particularly involving collagen IV. Goodpasture (GP) disease is characterized by autoantibodies against the α3 and less so α5 NC1 domain. Since the α345 collagen IV network is mainly found in renal glomerular and pulmonary alveolar BM, the primary manifestations of the disease are rapidly progressive glomerulonephritis and renal failure, with or without diffuse alveolar hemorrhage [18,88]. Interestingly, GP antibodies bind poorly to sulfilimine cross-linked collagen IV but avidly interact with uncrosslinked NC1 subunits (Figure 17.5) [88,89]. GP disease is rare and presumably involves a multi-hit process of genetic susceptibility and environmental triggers leading not just to loss of central immune tolerance with anti-collagen IV autoantibody production but also to loss of peripheral tolerance with binding of autoantibodies to their target and activation of downstream immune effector mechanisms [90]. An acquired loss of peroxidasin activity would tip the balance of collagen IV toward uncrosslinked subunits, which in turn would allow for engagement of otherwise inert autoantibodies and thus promote GP disease pathogenesis.

Environmental exposures or inhibitory autoantibodies may block the ability of peroxidasin to generate sulfilimine cross-links in collagen IV. Thiocyanate (SCN$^-$) reduces sulfilimine cross-links in collagen IV, presumably by competing against Br$^-$ for compound I of peroxidasin and forming HOSCN [23,53]. HOSCN, in turn, is incapable of sulfilimine bond formation [91]. Cigarette smokers have significantly higher SCN$^-$ levels, which have the potential to block peroxidasin function [92]. Interestingly, smoking has been associated with an increased incidence or severity of GP disease in some cohorts [93]. Whether exposures to organic solvents also associated with GP disease can similarly antagonize peroxidasin function is unknown [94,95].

A peculiar clinical aspect of GP disease raised the possibility of inhibitory anti-peroxidasin autoantibodies. In ca. 1/3rd of GP cases, anti-MPO (also known as perinuclear anti-neutrophil cytoplasmic or p-ANCA) antibody-mediated vasculitis occurs in combination with GP disease [96]. In these cases, anti-MPO antibodies nearly always predate GP antibodies [97], which would be consistent with a hypothesis of anti-MPO antibodies

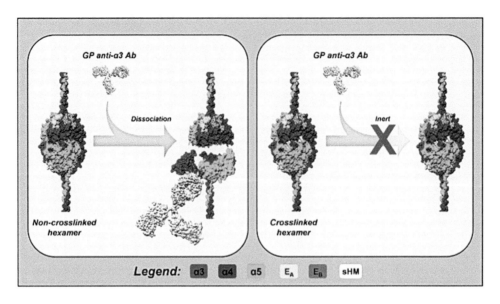

Figure 17.5 Goodpasture (GP) antibodies bind to non-cross-linked NC1 subunits. GP antibodies against the α3 NC1 sub-units can only access their target epitopes known as E_A and E_B in non-cross-linked subunits, which are induced to partially dissociate to allow for antibody engagement (left panel). Sulfilimine cross-linked subunits remain inert, as their epitopes remain protected from GP antibody dissociation and epitope binding. (Reproduced with permission from Ref. [90].)

cross-reacting with and blocking peroxidasin function and increasing susceptibility to subsequent GP disease. McCall and colleagues tested this hypothesis and found that sera from 46% of GP patients had anti-peroxidasin antibodies by ELISA. These patients nearly all exhibited reactivity to plate-adsorbed peroxidasin and MPO, but surprisingly, only soluble peroxidasin, not MPO, blocked immunoreactivity to both adsorbed peroxidasin and MPO, suggesting that these were true anti-peroxidasin antibodies. These antibodies in turn were found to inhibit peroxidasin HOBr generation in vitro. Another set of GP patients exhibited antibodies only recognizing adsorbed MPO that was competed out by soluble MPO but not by soluble peroxidasin, as expected for genuine MPO antibodies. The study also examined whether anti-MPO antibodies in primary ANCA vasculitis might cross-react with peroxidasin. The sera of ca. 13.5% of anti-MPO vasculitis patients reacted with adsorbed peroxidasin but, unlike the patients in primary GP disease, the sera reactivity was abolished by both soluble peroxidasin and MPO, suggesting the presence of cross-reactive antibodies [98]. Taken together, these data suggest that a portion of GP patients possess inhibitory anti-peroxidasin antibodies that predate GP antibodies and might contribute to disease pathogenesis.

CONCLUSION

Peroxidasin is an evolutionarily conserved peroxidase residing in BM that generates HOBr to form sulfilimine cross-links in collagen IV. In invertebrate model systems, loss of peroxidasin nearly phenocopies loss of collagen IV, with muscle rupture during development due to loss of tissue strength. Unlike loss of collagen IV, peroxidasin loss in mammals is dispensable in nearly all tissues except the lens and anterior segment of the eye. While the reason for the discrepancy in mammals is unclear, it raises the exciting possibility that peroxidasin may be therapeutically targeted without adverse consequences to patients. In this regard, peroxidasin is upregulated and might contribute to nearly every cardiovascular disease, renal fibrosis, and several cancers. While a precise mechanism remains unknown, the current hypothesis for peroxidasin action in disease centers around dysregulated generation of HOBr, which, instead of forming sulfimine cross-links in collagen IV, targets other ECM proteins and possibly cell surface receptors and intracellular signaling molecules to promote maladaptive cell signaling. However, in many cases, it is not firmly established that events depend on the catalytic activity of peroxidasin or whether peroxidasin is acting as a soluble messenger or as an ECM-embedded protein. Moreover, precise identification of HOBr oxidation targets and how these oxidation events alter cell behavior are lacking and will hopefully be the focus of future investigation to better understand the role of peroxidasin in disease pathogenesis and gain insight into therapeutic potential.

ACKNOWLEDGMENTS

The author is supported by a grant from the NIH/NIDDK (R01DK116964) and a Burroughs Wellcome Fund Career Award for Medical Scientists (13030995).

REFERENCES

1. R.E. Nelson, L.I. Fessler, Y. Takagi, et al., 1994. Peroxidasin: a novel enzyme-matrix protein of Drosophila development. EMBO J. 13: 3438–3447.

2. N. Horikoshi, J. Cong, N. Kley, T. Shenk, 1999. Isolation of differentially expressed cDNAs from p53-dependent apoptotic cells: activation of the human homologue of the Drosophila peroxidasin gene. Biochem. Biophys. Res. Commun. 261: 864–869.

3. S.R. Weiler, S.M. Taylor, R.J. Deans, et al., 1994. Assignment of a human melanoma associated gene MG50 (D2S448) to chromosome 2p25.3 by fluorescence in situ hybridization. Genomics 22: 243–244.

4. G. Cheng, J.C. Salerno, Z. Cao, P.J. Pagano, J.D. Lambeth, 2008. Identification and characterization of VPO1, a new animal heme-containing peroxidase. Free Radic. Biol. Med. 45: 1682–1694.

5. M. Soudi, M. Zamocky, C. Jakopitsch, P.G. Furtmuller, C. Obinger, 2012. Molecular evolution, structure, and function of peroxidasins. Chem. Biodivers. 9: 1776–1793.

6. I. Cho, G.J. Hwang, J.H. Cho, 2015. Pxn-1 and Pxn-2 may interact negatively during neuronal development and aging in C. elegans. Mol. Cells 38: 729–733.

7. Z. Peterfi, Z.E. Toth, H.A. Kovacs, et al., 2014. Peroxidasin-like protein: a novel peroxidase homologue in the human heart. Cardiovasc. Res. 101: 393–399.

8. P.D. Yurchenco, 2011. Basement membranes: cell scaffoldings and signaling platforms. Cold Spring Harb. Perspect. Biol. 3: a004911.

9. A.L. Fidler, C.E. Darris, S.V. Chetyrkin, et al., 2017. Collagen IV and basement membrane at the evolutionary dawn of metazoan tissues. Elife 6: e24176.

10. A.L. Fidler, R.M. Vanacore, S.V. Chetyrkin, et al., 2014. A unique covalent bond in basement membrane is a primordial innovation for tissue evolution. Proc. Natl. Acad. Sci. U.S.A. 111: 331–336.

11. R.O. Hynes, 2012. The evolution of metazoan extracellular matrix. J. Cell. Biol. 196: 671–679.

12. R.O. Hynes, 2009. The extracellular matrix: not just pretty fibrils. Science 326: 1216–1219.

13. M.J. Randles, M.J. Humphries, R. Lennon, 2017. Proteomic definitions of basement membrane composition in health and disease. Matrix Biol. 57–58: 12–28.

14. J.H. Miner, 2008. Laminins and their roles in mammals. Microsc. Res. Tech. 71: 349–356.

15. J. Khoshnoodi, V. Pedchenko, B.G. Hudson, 2008. Mammalian collagen IV. Microsc. Res. Tech. 71: 357–370.

16. N. Smyth, H.S. Vatansever, P. Murray, et al., 1999. Absence of basement membranes after targeting the LAMC1 gene results in embryonic lethality due to failure of endoderm differentiation. J. Cell. Biol. 144: 151–160.

17. E. Poschl, U. Schlotzer-Schrehardt, B. Brachvogel, et al., 2004. Collagen IV is essential for basement membrane stability but dispensable for initiation of its assembly during early development. Development 131: 1619–1628.

18. B.G. Hudson, K. Tryggvason, M. Sundaramoorthy, E.G. Neilson, 2003. Alport's syndrome, Goodpasture's syndrome, and type IV collagen. N. Engl. J. Med. 348: 2543–2556.

19. S.L. Haigo, D. Bilder, 2011. Global tissue revolutions in a morphogenetic movement controlling elongation. Science 331: 1071–1074.

20. C. Anazco, A.J. Lopez-Jimenez, M. Rafi, et al., 2016. Lysyl oxidase-like-2 cross-links collagen IV of glomerular basement membrane. J. Biol. Chem. 291: 25999–26012.

21. R. Vanacore, A.J. Ham, M. Voehler, et al., 2009. A sulfilimine bond identified in collagen IV. Science 325: 1230–1234.

22. G. Bhave, C.F. Cummings, R.M. Vanacore, et al., 2012. Peroxidasin forms sulfilimine chemical bonds using hypohalous acids in tissue genesis. Nat. Chem. Biol. 8: 784–790.

23. A.S. McCall, C.F. Cummings, G. Bhave, et al., 2014. Bromine is an essential trace element for assembly of collagen IV scaffolds in tissue development and architecture. Cell 157: 1380–1392.

24. J.R. Gotenstein, R.E. Swale, T. Fukuda, et al., 2010. The C. elegans peroxidasin PXN-2 is essential for embryonic morphogenesis and inhibits adult axon regeneration. *Development* 137: 3603–3613.

25. C. Obinger, 2006. Chemistry and biology of human peroxidases. *Arch. Biochem. Biophys.* 445: 197–198.

26. Z. Peterfi, A. Donko, A. Orient, et al., 2009. Peroxidasin is secreted and incorporated into the extracellular matrix of myofibroblasts and fibrotic kidney. *Am. J. Pathol.* 175: 725–735.

27. X. Yan, S. Sabrautzki, M. Horsch, et al., 2014. Peroxidasin is essential for eye development in the mouse. *Hum. Mol. Genet.* 23: 5597–5614.

28. R. Lennon, A. Byron, J.D. Humphries, et al., 2014. Global analysis reveals the complexity of the human glomerular extracellular matrix. *J. Am. Soc. Nephrol.* 25: 939–951.

29. A. Naba, K.R. Clauser, H. Ding, et al., 2016. The extracellular matrix: tools and insights for the "omics" era. *Matrix Biol.* 49: 10–24.

30. G. Uechi, Z. Sun, E.M. Schreiber, W. Halfter, M. Balasubramani, 2014. Proteomic view of basement membranes from human retinal blood vessels, inner limiting membranes, and lens capsules. *J. Proteome Res.* 13: 3693–3705.

31. K. Khan, A. Rudkin, D.A. Parry, et al., 2011. Homozygous mutations in PXDN cause congenital cataract, corneal opacity, and developmental glaucoma. *Am. J. Hum. Genet.* 89: 464–473.

32. A. Choi, R. Lao, P. Ling-Fung Tang, et al., 2015. Novel mutations in PXDN cause microphthalmia and anterior segment dysgenesis. *Eur. J. Hum. Genet.* 23: 337–341.

33. C. Zazo-Seco, J. Plaisancie, P. Bitoun, et al., 2020. Novel PXDN biallelic variants in patients with microphthalmia and anterior segment dysgenesis. *J. Hum. Genet.* 65: 487–491.

34. H.K. Kim, K.A. Ham, S.W. Lee, et al., 2019. Biallelic deletion of pxdn in mice leads to anophthalmia and severe eye malformation. *Int. J. Mol. Sci.* 20: 6144.

35. M. Jeanne, D.B. Gould, 2017. Genotype-phenotype correlations in pathology caused by collagen type IV alpha 1 and 2 mutations. *Matrix Biol.* 57–58: 29–44.

36. S. Zagaglia, C. Selch, J.R. Nisevic, et al., 2018. Neurologic phenotypes associated with col4a1/2 mutations: expanding the spectrum of disease. *Neurology* 91: e2078–e2088.

37. E. Plaisier, O. Gribouval, S. Alamowitch, et al., 2007. COL4A1 mutations and hereditary angiopathy, nephropathy, aneurysms, and muscle cramps. *N. Engl. J. Med.* 357: 2687–2695.

38. K. Vahedi, S. Alamowitch, 2011. Clinical spectrum of type IV collagen (COL4A1) mutations: a novel genetic multisystem disease. *Curr. Opin. Neurol.* 24: 63–68.

39. Z. Chen, T. Migeon, M.C. Verpont, et al., 2016. HANAC Syndrome Col4a1 mutation causes neonate glomerular hyperpermeability and adult glomerulocystic kidney disease. *J. Am. Soc. Nephrol.* 27: 1042–1054.

40. X.D. Guo, J.J. Johnson, J.M. Kramer, 1991. Embryonic lethality caused by mutations in basement membrane collagen of C. elegans. *Nature* 349: 707–709.

41. M.C. Gupta, P.L. Graham, J.M. Kramer, 1997. Characterization of alpha1(IV) collagen mutations in Caenorhabditis elegans and the effects of alpha1 and alpha2(IV) mutations on type IV collagen distribution. *J. Cell Biol.* 137: 1185–1196.

42. M.H. Sibley, P.L. Graham, N. von Mende, J.M. Kramer, 1994. Mutations in the alpha 2(IV) basement membrane collagen gene of Caenorhabditis elegans produce phenotypes of differing severities. *EMBO J.* 13: 3278–3285.

43. M.E. Noelken, B.J. Wisdom, Jr., D.C. Dean, C.H. Hung, B.G. Hudson, 1986. Intestinal basement membrane of Ascaris suum. Molecular organization and properties of the collagen molecules. *J. Biol. Chem.* 261: 4706–4714.

44. Y.A. Ito, M.A. Walter, 2014. Genomics and anterior segment dysgenesis: a review. *Clin. Exp. Ophthalmol.* 42: 13–24.

45. B.P. Danysh, M.K. Duncan, 2009. The lens capsule. *Exp. Eye Res.* 88: 151–164.

46. A.S. Ma, J.R. Grigg, R.V. Jamieson, 2019. Phenotype-genotype correlations and emerging pathways in ocular anterior segment dysgenesis. *Hum. Genet.* 138: 899–915.

47. J.C. Sowden, 2007. Molecular and developmental mechanisms of anterior segment dysgenesis. *Eye (Lond)* 21: 1310–1318.

48. M. Mao, M. Kiss, Y. Ou, D.B. Gould, 2017. Genetic dissection of anterior segment dysgenesis caused by a Col4a1 mutation in mouse. *Dis. Model Mech.* 10: 475–485.

49. Z. Liu, Y. Liu, Q. Xu, et al., 2017. Critical role of vascular peroxidase 1 in regulating endothelial nitric oxide synthase. *Redox Biol.* 12: 226–232.

50. R. Shi, C. Hu, Q. Yuan, et al., 2011. Involvement of vascular peroxidase 1 in angiotensin II-induced

vascular smooth muscle cell proliferation. *Cardio-vasc. Res.* 91: 27–36.

51. H. Peng, L. Chen, X. Huang, et al., 2016. Vascular peroxidase 1 up regulation by angiotensin II attenuates nitric oxide production through increasing asymmetrical dimethylarginine in HUVECs. *J. Am. Soc. Hypertens.* 10: 741–751.

52. K.L. Hanmer, D. Mavri-Damelin, 2018. Peroxidasin is a novel target of the redox-sensitive transcription factor Nrf2. *Gene* 674: 104–114.

53. M. Paumann-Page, R.S. Katz, M. Bellei, et al., 2017. Pre-steady-state kinetics reveal the substrate specificity and mechanism of halide oxidation of truncated human Peroxidasin 1. *J. Biol. Chem.* 292: 4583–4592.

54. W. Yang, Z. Liu, Q. Xu, et al., 2017. Involvement of vascular peroxidase 1 in angiotensin II-induced hypertrophy of H9c2 cells. *J. Am. Soc. Hypertens.* 11: 519–529.

55. Y. Yang, Z. Cao, L. Tian, W.T. Garvey, G. Cheng, 2013. VPO1 mediates ApoE oxidation and impairs the clearance of plasma lipids. *PLoS One* 8: e57571.

56. Y. Yang, R. Shi, Z. Cao, G. Zhang, G. Cheng, 2016. VPO1 mediates oxidation of LDL and formation of foam cells. *Oncotarget* 7: 35500–35511.

57. Y.P. Bai, C.P. Hu, Q. Yuan, et al., 2011. Role of VPO1, a newly identified heme-containing peroxidase, in ox-LDL induced endothelial cell apoptosis. *Free Radic. Biol. Med.* 51: 1492–1500.

58. Y.Z. Zhang, L. Wang, J.J. Zhang, et al., 2018. Vascular peroxide 1 promotes ox-LDL-induced programmed necrosis in endothelial cells through a mechanism involving beta-catenin signaling. *Atherosclerosis* 274: 128–138.

59. Y. Tang, Q. Xu, H. Peng, et al., 2015. The role of vascular peroxidase 1 in ox-LDL-induced vascular smooth muscle cell calcification. *Atherosclerosis* 243: 357–363.

60. H. Peng, K. Zhang, Z. Liu, et al., 2018. VPO1 modulates vascular smooth muscle cell phenotypic switch by activating extracellular signal-regulated kinase 1/2 (ERK 1/2) in abdominal aortic aneurysms. *J. Am. Heart Assoc.* 7: e010069.

61. Z. Liu, Q. Xu, Q. Yang, et al., 2019. Vascular peroxidase 1 is a novel regulator of cardiac fibrosis after myocardial infarction. *Redox Biol.* 22: 101151.

62. Y.S. Zhang, L. He, B. Liu, et al., 2012. A novel pathway of NADPH oxidase/vascular peroxidase 1 in mediating oxidative injury following ischemia-reperfusion. *Basic Res. Cardiol.* 107: 266.

63. B. You, Y. Liu, J. Chen, et al., 2018. Vascular peroxidase 1 mediates hypoxia-induced pulmonary artery smooth muscle cell proliferation, apoptosis resistance and migration. *Cardiovasc. Res.* 114: 188–199.

64. G. Sirokmany, H.A. Kovacs, E. Lazar, et al., 2018. Peroxidasin-mediated crosslinking of collagen IV is independent of NADPH oxidases. *Redox. Biol.* 16: 314–321.

65. S. Colon, H. Luan, Y. Liu, et al., 2019. Peroxidasin and eosinophil peroxidase, but not myeloperoxidase, contribute to renal fibrosis in the murine unilateral ureteral obstruction model. *Am. J. Physiol. Renal Physiol.* 316: F360–F371.

66. C. He, W. Song, T.A. Weston, et al., 2020. Peroxidasin-mediated bromine enrichment of basement membranes. *Proc. Natl. Acad: Sci. U.S.A.* 117: 15827–15836.

67. S. Colon, P. Page-McCaw, G. Bhave, 2017. Role of hypohalous acids in basement membrane homeostasis. *Antioxid. Redox Signal.* 27: 839–854.

68. B. Bathish, M. Paumann-Page, L.N. Paton, A.J. Kettle, C.C. Winterbourn, 2020. Peroxidasin mediates bromination of tyrosine residues in the extracellular matrix. *J. Biol. Chem.* 295: 12697–12705.

69. D.I. Pattison, M.J. Davies, 2004. Kinetic analysis of the reactions of hypobromous acid with protein components: implications for cellular damage and use of 3-bromotyrosine as a marker of oxidative stress. *Biochemistry* 43: 4799–4809.

70. C.D. Young, L.J. Zimmerman, D. Hoshino, et al., 2015. Activating PIK3CA mutations induce an epidermal growth factor receptor (EGFR)/extracellular signal-regulated kinase (ERK) paracrine signaling axis in basal-like breast cancer. *Mol. Cell Proteomics* 14: 1959–1976.

71. Y.Z. Zheng, L. Liang, 2018. High expression of PXDN is associated with poor prognosis and promotes proliferation, invasion as well as migration in ovarian cancer. *Ann. Diagn. Pathol.* 34: 161–165.

72. V. Castronovo, D. Waltregny, P. Kischel, et al., 2006. A chemical proteomics approach for the identification of accessible antigens expressed in human kidney cancer. *Mol. Cell Proteomics* 5: 2083–2091.

73. Y. Liu, E.B. Carson-Walter, A. Cooper, et al., 2010. Vascular gene expression patterns are conserved in primary and metastatic brain tumors. *J. Neurooncol.* 99: 13–24.

74. H. Medfai, A. Khalil, A. Rousseau, et al., 2019. Human peroxidasin 1 promotes angiogenesis through ERK1/2, Akt, and FAK pathways. *Cardiovasc. Res.* 115: 463–475.

75. I. Pastushenko, C. Blanpain, 2019. EMT transition states during tumor progression and metastasis. *Trends Cell Biol.* 29: 212–226.

76. A. Jayachandran, P. Prithviraj, P.H. Lo, et al., 2016. Identifying and targeting determinants of melanoma cellular invasion. *Oncotarget* 7: 41186–41202.

77. E. Briem, Z. Budkova, A.K. Sigurdardottir, et al., 2019. MiR-203a is differentially expressed during branching morphogenesis and EMT in breast progenitor cells and is a repressor of peroxidasin. *Mech. Dev.* 155: 34–47.

78. U. Santanam, N. Zanesi, A. Efanov, et al., 2010. Chronic lymphocytic leukemia modeled in mouse by targeted miR-29 expression. *Proc. Natl. Acad. Sci. U.S.A.* 107: 12210–12215.

79. L.H. Oliveira, J.L. Schiavinato, M.S. Fraguas, et al., 2015. Potential roles of microRNA-29a in the molecular pathophysiology of T-cell acute lymphoblastic leukemia. *Cancer Sci.* 106: 1264–1277.

80. J. Dougan, O. Hawsawi, L.J. Burton, et al., 2019. Proteomics-metabolomics combined approach identifies peroxidasin as a protector against metabolic and oxidative stress in prostate cancer. *Int. J. Mol. Sci.* 20: 3046.

81. P. Barnett, R.S. Arnold, R. Mezencev, et al., 2011. Snail-mediated regulation of reactive oxygen species in ARCaP human prostate cancer cells. *Biochem. Biophys. Res. Commun.* 404: 34–39.

82. M.J. Davies, C.L. Hawkins, D.I. Pattison, M.D. Rees, 2008. Mammalian heme peroxidases: from molecular mechanisms to health implications. *Antioxid. Redox Signal.* 10: 1199–1234.

83. M. Zamocky, S. Hofbauer, I. Schaffner, et al., 2015. Independent evolution of four heme peroxidase superfamilies. *Arch. Biochem. Biophys.* 574: 108–119.

84. D. Sarr, E. Toth, A. Gingerich, B. Rada, 2018. Antimicrobial actions of dual oxidases and lactoperoxidase. *J. Microbiol.* 56: 373–386.

85. L.S. Garver, Z. Xi, G. Dimopoulos, 2008. Immunoglobulin superfamily members play an important role in the mosquito immune system. *Dev. Comp. Immunol.* 32: 519–531.

86. M. Soudi, M. Paumann-Page, C. Delporte, et al., 2015. Multidomain human peroxidasin 1 is a highly glycosylated and stable homotrimeric high spin ferric peroxidase. *J. Biol. Chem.* 290: 10876–10890.

87. H. Li, Z. Cao, D.R. Moore, et al., 2012. Microbicidal activity of vascular peroxidase 1 in human plasma via generation of hypochlorous acid. *Infect. Immun.* 80: 2528–2537.

88. V. Pedchenko, O. Bondar, A.B. Fogo, et al., 2010. Molecular architecture of the Goodpasture autoantigen in anti-GBM nephritis. *N. Engl. J. Med.* 363: 343–354.

89. D.B. Borza, O. Bondar, S. Colon, et al., 2005. Goodpasture autoantibodies unmask cryptic epitopes by selectively dissociating autoantigen complexes lacking structural reinforcement: novel mechanisms for immune privilege and autoimmune pathogenesis. *J. Biol. Chem.* 280: 27147–27154.

90. R. Vanacore, V. Pedchenko, G. Bhave, B.G. Hudson, 2011. Sulphilimine cross-links in Goodpasture's disease. *Clin. Exp. Immunol.* 164 Suppl 1: 4–6.

91. J.L. Beal, S.B. Foster, M.T. Ashby, 2009. Hypochlorous acid reacts with the N-terminal methionines of proteins to give dehydromethionine, a potential biomarker for neutrophil-induced oxidative stress. *Biochemistry* 48: 11142–11148.

92. K. Tsuge, M. Kataoka, Y. Seto, 2000. Cyanide and thiocyanate levels in blood and saliva of healthy adult volunteers. *J. Health Sci.* 46: 343–350.

93. M. Donaghy, A.J. Rees, 1983. Cigarette smoking and lung haemorrhage in glomerulonephritis caused by autoantibodies to glomerular basement membrane. *Lancet* 2: 1390–1393.

94. G.J. Beirne, J.T. Brennan, 1972. Glomerulonephritis associated with hydrocarbon solvents: mediated by antiglomerular basement membrane antibody. *Arch. Environ. Health.* 25: 365–369.

95. G.J. Bombassei, A.A. Kaplan, 1992. The association between hydrocarbon exposure and anti-glomerular basement membrane antibody-mediated disease (Goodpasture's syndrome). *Am. J. Ind. Med.* 21: 141–153.

96. J.B. Levy, T. Hammad, A. Coulthart, T. Dougan, C.D. Pusey, 2004. Clinical features and outcome of patients with both ANCA and anti-GBM antibodies. *Kidney Int.* 66: 1535–1540.

97. S.W. Olson, C.B. Arbogast, T.P. Baker, et al., 2011. Asymptomatic autoantibodies associate with future anti-glomerular basement membrane disease. *J. Am. Soc. Nephrol.* 22: 1946–1952.

98. A.S. McCall, G. Bhave, V. Pedchenko, et al., 2018. Inhibitory anti-peroxidasin antibodies in pulmonary-renal syndromes. *J. Am. Soc. Nephrol.* 29: 2619–2625.

99. C.F. Cummings, V. Pedchenko, K.L. Brown, et al., 2016. Extracellular chloride signals collagen IV network assembly during basement membrane formation. *J. Cell Biol.* 213: 479–494.

PART FIVE

Prevention of Myeloperoxidase-Induced Damage

Structure, Function, and Mechanistic Insights into a Novel Family of Myeloperoxidase Inhibitory Proteins Expressed by Staphylococci

Molly Allison, Nitin Mishra, and Brian V. Geisbrecht
Kansas State University

CONTENTS

INTRODUCTION

Neutrophils are the earliest acting cellular components of the human innate immune system. Though they serve many roles in defense and repair, they are best known for their ability to engulf and kill invading microorganisms. Neutrophils rapidly sense and respond to pathogen-derived molecular patterns (e.g. formylated peptides), as well as danger or damage-associated molecular patterns (e.g. C5a) through a series of high-affinity receptors exposed on their plasma membrane. This allows neutrophils to be the first leukocytes to infiltrate sites of nascent infection or damaged tissues in the process of healing [1–4]. Activation of neutrophils results in remarkable morphological changes. It also triggers mobilization and secretion of their cytosolic granules [5]. Chief among these are the azurophilic granules, which contain critical components of the neutrophil antibacterial arsenal. Two of the most abundant components of azurophilic granules are the enzyme myeloperoxidase (MPO), which converts hydrogen peroxide (H_2O_2) into cytotoxic hypohalous acids (e.g. HOCl), and a series of chymotrypsin-like serine proteases, called neutrophil serine proteases (NSPs), which can directly attack the pathogen cell, its contents, or secreted products [6,7]. This concerted action of MPO and NSPs forms a foundation of neutrophil-mediated defense against invading bacteria.

Since they are immediately confronted by the host innate immune system, there is strong selective pressure for invading bacteria to evolve the molecular means to disrupt the host immune system or escape it altogether. Although studies on various pathogens have identified a diverse array of these so-called immune evasion strategies [8,9], the Gram-positive bacterium *Staphylococcus aureus* is particularly noteworthy for the sheer number of different proteins it produces to interfere with opsonization and phagocytosis [8–12]. Some studies have also shown that a population of *S. aureus* cells are resistant to killing within the phagosome [13]. Given the biochemical complexity of the phagosome and the extreme environment it presents [14–17], the fact that *S. aureus* can survive there at all implies that its physiological changes

DOI: 10.1201/9781003212287-23

must be multifaceted. It also suggests that the components of the staphylococcal innate immune evasion program that act within the phagosome must be somewhat protective. Indeed, the recent identification of a potent family of secreted NSP inhibitors that promote *S. aureus* virulence is consistent with this premise [15]. Nevertheless, this also raises questions of whether *S. aureus* targets other components of the neutrophil antibacterial arsenal that act primarily within the phagosome.

SPIN: A NOVEL MYELOPEROXIDASE INHIBITORY PROTEIN EXPRESSED BY *STAPHYLOCOCCUS AUREUS*

MPO serves a central role in the innate defense against pathogens [14–17]. It therefore represents an extremely attractive target for elaboration of an *S. aureus* innate immune evasion strategy. Since no MPO-inhibitory evasion protein had yet been identified, a secretome phage display library from *S. aureus* strain Newman was probed for proteins that bound to human neutrophil degranulate fluid [18,19], of which MPO is a predominant constituent. A single, highly enriched clone representing the gene NWMN_0402 was isolated following several rounds of enrichment [19]. NWMN_0402 encodes a pre-protein of 105 residues that contains a 32-residue signal peptide, leaving a predicted matured protein of 73 residues and a molecular mass of 8,380 Da. A recombinant form of NWMN_0402 protein bound specifically to immobilized human MPO in ELISA studies. Subsequent surface plasmon resonance experiments revealed an equilibrium dissociation constant of 10 ± 0.6 nM, with association and dissociation rate constants on the order of 10^5 $M^{-1}s^{-1}$ and $10^{-3}s^{-1}$, respectively [19]. Significantly, this same protein inhibited the peroxidase activity of MPO with an IC_{50} value of approximately 7 nM [19]. This value was in excellent agreement with the affinity measured by surface plasmon resonance (SPR), strongly suggesting that NWMN_0402 might act as a competitive inhibitor of MPO. Consequently, NWMN_0402 was renamed SPIN for S̲taphylococcal P̲eroxidase I̲nhibitor.

The SPIN protein has no obvious sequence homology to other characterized proteins [19]. This was a major impediment to developing hypotheses concerning its mechanism of MPO inhibition. To address this limitation, SPIN was crystallized bound to a recombinant form of human MPO (hereafter rhMPO) [19]. The SPIN/rhMPO structure was solved to 2.4 Å limiting resolution and refined to R_{work}/R_{free} values of 18.4% and 24.1%, respectively [19]. This structure revealed that SPIN was comprised of a peculiar β-hairpin at the SPIN N-terminus, followed by a compact α-helical bundle domain that is common among staphylococcal innate immune evasion proteins [19,20], including Efb-C [21], Ehp [22], and SCINs [23,24]. Since the approximately ten-residue β-hairpin lacked any intrinsically stabilizing features of its own, it was predicted to be disordered prior to binding MPO [19]. This turned out to be the case, as will be further described in a separate section of this text.

Examination of the SPIN/rhMPO structure revealed two distinct interfaces that contribute to complex formation [19] (Figure 18.1). The first interface involves the SPIN α-helical bundle domain and lies at the side of the MPO active site channel entrance. This interface buries 726 Å² of the inhibitor or approximately 45% of the 1,633 Å² of SPIN surface area buried in the complex. The second interface involves the SPIN β-hairpin, which lies entirely within the MPO active site channel. This interface buries 907 Å² or approximately 55% of the total SPIN surface area buried in the complex. For reasons that remain unclear, the heme occupancy of the rhMPO in this structure was negligible [19]; however, it was possible to infer the location of the heme prosthetic group using the structure of native human MPO as a guide [25]. This indicated that the invariant glycine residue found within the SPIN β-hairpin serves the role of a hinge [26]. Not only does this permit the β-hairpin to return toward the opening of the MPO active site channel, it also appears to allow for complete occlusion of access to the catalytic heme [19]. Indeed, visualization of the SPIN/rhMPO complex as a molecular surface led to the attractive model that SPIN acts as a molecular plug, thereby preventing solute exchange from the MPO catalytic center [19].

EXPRESSION AND FUNCTION OF SPIN IN STAPHYLOCOCCAL EVASION OF NEUTROPHIL DEFENSE

The *S. aureus* gene that encodes SPIN (hereafter denoted *spn*) is located on genomic island α that encodes staphylococcal superantigen-like (*ssl*) proteins and other evasion proteins, such as

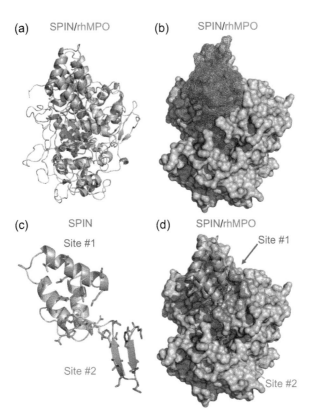

(a) SPIN/rhMPO (b) SPIN/rhMPO

(c) SPIN (d) SPIN/rhMPO

Site #1 Site #1

Site #2 Site #2

Figure 18.1 Structure of the staphylococcal peroxidase inhibitor, SPIN, bound to a recombinant form of human MPO. Ribbon representation of the final model for *S. aureus* SPIN (orange) bound to a recombinant form of human MPO (olive), as rendered from the PDB entry 5UZU [19]. The location of the heme prosthetic group (drawn as yellow sticks) was inferred from PDB entry 1CXP [25]. (b) Representation of the SPIN/rhMPO structure where SPIN is drawn as an orange space-filling mesh and rhMPO is an olive molecular surface. Note the complete occlusion of access to the catalytic heme by the N-terminal β-hairpin of SPIN. This feature is a key determinant of MPO inhibition by SPIN. (c) Representation of the *S. aureus* SPIN protein illustrating the nature of the two distinct rhMPO interfaces. Interface #1 (labeled "Site #1") is comprised of residues within the α-helical bundle domain and is colored light purple. Interface #2 (labeled "Site #2") is comprised of residues within the β-hairpin and is colored silver. The side chains of residues that form contacts with rhMPO in the structure are shown as ball-and-stick models. (d) Representation of the SPIN/rhMPO structure where the two distinct SPIN-binding surfaces on MPO are colored according to their participation in either Interface #1 or Interface #2.

hemolysin-α and leucocidin AB [11,19]. At the time of its initial discovery, a *spn*-like coding sequence was identified in the genome of 83 out of 84 strains in an *S. aureus* clinical isolate collection [19]. The SPIN protein produced by these various *S. aureus* strains is also approximately 92% identical across all clonal lineages. This high level of conservation suggested that SPIN likely serves an important role in host colonization and pathogenesis by *S. aureus*. Subsequent serological examination of 20 different healthy humans showed substantial levels of anti-SPIN antibodies. This demonstrated that the SPIN protein is produced at some level during asymptomatic colonization or active infection of the human host [19].

As with many other staphylococcal innate immune evasion proteins, the SPIN pre-protein contains a canonical export signal that directs its secretion into the extracellular environment [19]. Its target (i.e. solubilized rather than granular MPO), however, is localized within the phagosomal compartment. This suggested that expression of the *spn* gene might be upregulated in response to phagocytosis by neutrophils. qPCR studies using *S. aureus* strain USA300 cells showed an eight-fold increase in *spn* mRNA levels following phagocytosis when compared with free-living bacteria [19]. Analogous experiments using a USA300 strain lacking the SaeR/S gene system that regulates production of numerous immune evasion molecules showed no significant difference in *spn* expression level between phagocytosed and non-phagocytosed bacteria [19]. Examination of a USA300 reporter strain, where the gene encoding green fluorescent protein (*gfp*) was placed downstream of the *spn* promoter, revealed a time-dependent, statistically significant increase in the presence of GFP when phagocytosed bacteria were compared with their planktonically grown counterparts [19]. Together, these results demonstrated that production of SPIN is regulated in response to the environment and is enhanced after entering the neutrophil phagosome.

Under normal circumstances, MPO contributes to bacterial killing within the neutrophil phagosome by catalyzing production of highly cytotoxic HOCl from hydrogen peroxide (H_2O_2) [15,16]. However, the increase in SPIN production by *S. aureus* following phagocytosis and the ability of SPIN to inhibit MPO raised questions about the contribution of SPIN to bacterial survival following phagocytosis. Given the biochemical complexities of the phagosome, a combination of *in vitro* and *ex vivo* models was used to address this issue. Replicating the conditions that lead to efficient bacterial killing in purely *in vitro* models involves many challenges. As far as MPO function is concerned, perhaps the greatest of these is ensuring a steady-state level of H_2O_2 substrate that is normally provided by the NADPH oxidase system that assembles during phagosome maturation. In this regard, fungal glucose oxidase (GO) [27] was used in lieu of NADPH oxidase to supply sublethal levels of H_2O_2 substrate for MPO in an *in vitro* assay system designed to interrogate the protective effects of SPIN on *S. aureus* killing [19]. Whereas the addition of increasing levels of MPO to this assay system resulted in increasingly greater levels of killing for a laboratory strain of *S. aureus* (i.e. Newman) as well as a clinical MRSA isolate (i.e. USA300), both strains of *S. aureus* showed a significant decrease in killing when a fixed concentration of SPIN was included in the assay system [19]. Furthermore, both the Newman and USA300 strains also showed a significant increase in survival compared with controls when progressively higher concentrations of SPIN were added to assays containing a fixed concentration of MPO [19]. Together, these data provided proof of concept that SPIN could protect *S. aureus* from MPO-mediated killing within the neutrophil phagosome.

Although SPIN supported *S. aureus* survival in the reconstituted killing assay described above, its ability to affect a similar outcome in a more physiologically relevant scenario remained unclear. A normally favored approach for addressing such considerations would have been to compare wild-type versus *spn*-deleted strains of *S. aureus* in a laboratory animal infection model where neutrophils play a crucial role in the host response (e.g. the murine liver abscess model [28,29]). Yet as with several other staphylococcal innate immune evasion proteins including SCIN-class complement inhibitors [30–32] and leukocidins [33–35], SPIN displayed remarkable selectivity for human MPO as a target [19]. SPIN from *S. aureus* failed to bind or inhibit rodent, bovine, or equine MPO [19]. Consequently, further assessments of the physiological contributions of SPIN required use of isolated human neutrophils in *ex vivo* bacterial killing assays.

MPO is generally considered a major contributor in neutrophil-mediated defense against *S. aureus*, as killing of the organism by MPO-deficient neutrophils occurs at a slower rate and is markedly less effective than seen for normal leukocytes [14,16,17]. However, to provide additional insight into this phenomenon prior to more detailed studies, the extent to which *S. aureus* killing depends on MPO was also quantified using the membrane-permeable MPO inhibitor, AZM198 [36]. Whereas 82% of *S. aureus* cells were killed within 1 h following exposure to in-tact neutrophils and serum (to facilitate opsonophagocytosis), approximately 56% of the *S. aureus* cells were killed in an identical experiment using AZM198-treated neutrophils [19]; these results suggested that MPO contributes only roughly 26% of the *S. aureus* killing activity of the phagosome under these experimental conditions. However, they must be interpreted with caution for several reasons. For example, the relative imprecision of these measurements underscores the fact that this system is intrinsically variable. Similarly, the complex nature of the protocol, the numerous components involved, and their intricate dependence on one another suggest that this system is difficult to manipulate experimentally even under the most rigorous conditions. Finally, such experiments could not account for any confounding synergistic effects between various antimicrobial components of the phagosome that do not require MPO-derived oxidants to manifest themselves.

Given the limitations presented above and the small dynamic range of the killing assay, three different genetically modified strains of *S. aureus* were employed to assess the role of SPIN in promoting bacterial survival within neutrophils – a wild-type Newman strain overexpressing *spn* from a plasmid (i.e. WT PlukM-*spn*), a *spn*-deleted Newman strain overexpressing *spn* from a plasmid (i.e. Δ*spn* PlukM-*spn*), and a *spn*-deleted Newman strain overexpressing *gfp* from a plasmid (i.e. Δ*spn* PlukM-*gfp*) [19]. Enzyme inhibition studies showed that both *spn*-overexpressing strains produced approximately fivefold more SPIN than the parental Newman strain, while the *gfp*-overexpressing strain was devoid of MPO-inhibitory activity [19]. Congruent to this observation, both strains that overexpressed *spn* showed enhanced survival at 1 h following exposure to human neutrophils and serum when compared with the strain that lacked *spn* [19]. Furthermore, comparison of the two *spn*-deleted strains that expressed either plasmid-borne *spn* or *gfp* to one another revealed a roughly 10% increase in bacterial survival in the presence of SPIN that was statistically significant (P≤0.05) [19]. Although the magnitude of this effect appears mild at best and unimpressive at worst, it is impossible to ignore the fact that matured neutrophil phagosomes have been estimated to contain levels of MPO approaching 1 mM [37]. It therefore seems unlikely that this enormous amount of MPO could be completely inactivated by a single immune evasion protein acting as a simple competitive inhibitor, rather than one that could instead enzymatically inactivate its target via proteolysis, ADP ribosylation, glycosylation, etc. Nevertheless, these data clearly show that SPIN provides a modest but significant contribution to *S. aureus* survival within the neutrophil phagosome under the experimental conditions employed.

DEFINING THE STRUCTURE/FUNCTION RELATIONSHIPS OF THE SPIN PROTEIN

The initial biochemical studies on SPIN demonstrated that this novel protein acts as a nanomolar-affinity, competitive inhibitor of MPO. Thereafter, determination of a SPIN/rhMPO co-crystal structure provided a useful basis for further dissection of SPIN's structure/function relationships. In this regard, the lack of stabilizing structural features within the SPIN β-hairpin strongly suggested that this region might be disordered prior to binding MPO. If so, this would imply that the initial SPIN interaction with MPO must be driven by its α-helical bundle domain. To test these ideas, a combination of structural methods and deletion mutagenesis was used to great effect.

Since attempts to crystallize SPIN in the unbound state were unsuccessful, solution NMR spectroscopy was used an alternative structural approach [38,39] (Figure 18.2). The small size (i.e. 8,380 Da) and favorable solubility properties of SPIN provided high-quality multidimensional NMR spectra that facilitated assignment of the SPIN backbone and side-chain ^{1}H, ^{15}N, and ^{13}C resonances [39]. Aside from Phe^{48} and Leu^{49}, all other resonances were identifiable in the ^{1}H-^{15}N HSQC fingerprint spectrum of SPIN collected at 700 MHz (^{1}H). The TALOS-N platform was then used to calculate the secondary structure of SPIN based upon the longitudinal (R$_1$) and transverse (R$_2$) relaxation time constants for backbone resonances in the ^{1}H-^{15}N HSQC spectrum, since these values are sensitive to the backbone structural rigidity of a protein. Internally rigid structures are expected to have homogeneous relaxation time constants. While SPIN was characterized by a composite average R$_1$ value 2.49±0.58, the average R$_1$ of the N-terminal region was 2.90±0.78; oppositely, the composite average R$_2$ value for SPIN was 8.97±1.29 but was 7.64±1.33 for the N-terminal region. Similarly, the overall average R$_2$/R$_1$ was 3.72±0.73 but was 2.76±0.59 for the N-terminal region. Such localized deviation of these values when compared with the protein overall was indicative of backbone flexibility within the N-terminal region of SPIN. To further define the solution structure of SPIN, chemical shift index (CSI) values for Cα and Cβ SPIN resonances were calculated and compared with the BioMagResBank (BMRB) statistical database values for CSI. Residues in α-helical structures show a positive CSI for Cα and negative for Cβ, while residues in β-strands show a negative CSI for Cα and positive for Cβ; neutral CSI values are associated with residues in random coil-like structures [40]. Residues within the SPIN N-terminus exhibited significantly lower and less variable CSI values when compared with the protein as a whole [38]. This confirmed the absence of regular secondary structure within the SPIN N-terminal region in the unbound state.

Although the SPIN β-hairpin is responsible for a majority of the buried surface area in the SPIN/rhMPO complex [19], the NMR studies described above implied that the SPIN α-helical bundle predominates in terms of initial binding to MPO. To assess this experimentally, two SPIN mutants with altered N-terminal regions

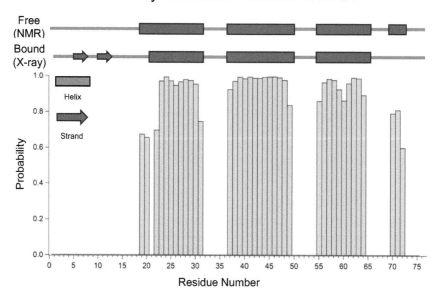

Figure 18.2 Comparison of secondary structural features of SPIN in the free and MPO-bound states. Nuclear magnetic resonance (NMR) spectroscopy was used to characterize the structure of S. aureus SPIN in the unbound state. Following spectral assignment using standard approaches [39], the chemical shift values of resonances were used to calculate the secondary structure via the TALOS platform [52]. The residue-dependent probabilities of various secondary structure elements are given on a scale from 0 to 1. Whereas the NMR data are consistent with the presence of three prominent α-helices also seen in the X-ray structure [19], the unusual β-hairpin found in the MPO-bound form of SPIN is not seen in the free state [38]. These data, along with supporting biochemical studies [38], indicate that the inhibitory N-terminal β-hairpin must form following initial binding of the SPIN α-helical bundle to MPO.

were developed [38]. The first mutant had its N-terminus completely removed and was comprised of SPIN residues Ala[46]-Lys[105] inclusive (hereafter SPIN[46–105]). The second mutant was used to determine how His[43], Asp[44], and Asp[45] impacted binding. Each of these residues was simultaneously replaced with Ala (hereafter SPIN[43–45→AAA]), as these residues are highly conserved among SPINs [26] and form polar interactions with MPO side chains in the SPIN/rhMPO crystal structure [19]. Surface plasmon resonance studies revealed that SPIN[46–105] and SPIN[43–45→AAA] had approximately 3.2-fold and 3.4-fold weakened affinities for native MPO, respectively [38], which arose from enhanced dissociation rates when compared with wild-type SPIN (Figure 18.3). A subsequent crystal structure of SPIN[46–105] bound to rhMPO determined at 2.3 Å limiting resolution and refined to R_{work}/R_{free} values of 17.9% and 22.9%, respectively, showed essentially no variance from SPIN/rhMPO [38], as the Cα positions from each model superimposed with an r.m.s.d. of 0.16 Å.

Together, these observations reinforced the concept that the N-terminus is not essential for SPIN binding to MPO.

Further comparison of these mutants to the wild-type protein provided additional insight into the structure/function relationships of SPIN. To begin, all three proteins were examined in a functional assay where MPO-catalyzed reduction of H_2O_2 was linked to oxidation of the chromogenic substrate o-dianisidine (Figure 18.4). Since wild-type SPIN, SPIN[46–105], and SPIN[43–45→AAA] all exhibited similar K_D values for MPO [38], MPO enzyme activity was measured in the presence of each SPIN protein at a single concentration sufficient to promote MPO binding (i.e. 74 nM). Although the wild-type protein inhibited MPO activity by over 90% under these conditions (P≤0.0001), neither mutant conferred any inhibition of MPO [38]. These same proteins were also examined in the in vitro GO-MPO killing model [19], as well as a phagocytosis-dependent assay that measures bleaching of GFP-expressing S. aureus cells [41]. Each of these assays is designed to mimic HOCl-dependent killing within

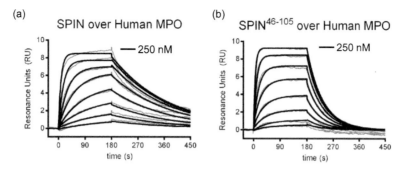

Figure 18.3 The N-terminal region of SPIN is dispensable for binding to human MPO. Surface plasmon resonance was used to assess the interaction of soluble SPIN proteins with immobilized forms of human MPO [38]. The reference-corrected sensorgrams (gray lines) obtained by injecting a twofold concentration series ranging from 1.95 to 250 nM were analyzed by fitting to a Langmuir binding model (black lines) to derive estimates for the association rate (k_{on}), dissociation rate (k_{off}), and equilibrium dissociation constants (K_D) for each interaction. (a) Wild-type SPIN over native human MPO; $k_{on} = 4.9 \pm 0.6 \times 10^5$ M^{-1}s^{-1}, $k_{off} = 5.1 \pm 0.2 \times 10^{-3}$ s^{-1}, and $K_D = 10.5 \pm 1.8$ nM. (b) SPIN$^{46-105}$ over native human MPO; $k_{on} = 5.2 \pm 1.3 \times 10^5$ M^{-1}s^{-1}, $k_{off} = 16.8 \pm 2.4 \times 10^{-3}$ s^{-1}, and $K_D = 32.5 \pm 3.7$ nM. Note that the roughly threefold increase in the dissociation rate for this protein is responsible for the commensurate decrease in its apparent affinity for human MPO.

the neutrophil phagosome. Again, only wild-type SPIN showed any ability to significantly inhibit MPO in either assay. Taken together, these data established that the N-terminus of SPIN is necessary, but not sufficient, for inhibiting MPO activity. In that regard it was somewhat surprising that the SPIN$^{43-45 \rightarrow AAA}$ mutant had lost its capacity to inhibit

MPO, since this protein bound MPO well and had an otherwise wild-type N-terminal region. This suggests that residues His^{43}, Asp^{44}, and Asp^{45} may be critical to guiding the nascently folding SPIN N-terminus into a productive inhibitory conformation, such as that seen in the SPIN/rhMPO co-crystal structure [19,38].

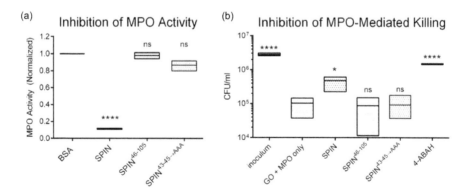

Figure 18.4 The N-terminal region of SPIN is necessary but not sufficient for inhibiting MPO. The influence of wild-type SPIN, SPIN$^{46-105}$, and SPIN$^{43-45 \rightarrow AAA}$ was compared with two different assays for MPO function [38]. Each experiment is represented as a box with the mean (center line) and range of the data (n = 3). (a) SPIN proteins were included at a fixed concentration of 74 nM in a chromogenic assay for MPO activity. This value lies far above the K_D of each protein for MPO, so that the activity of each SPIN-bound form of MPO was measured in this experiment [38]. Whereas wild-type SPIN significantly inhibited MPO activity when compared with control (BSA), neither SPIN$^{46-105}$ nor SPIN$^{43-45 \rightarrow AAA}$ had any significant effect on MPO activity. (b) SPIN proteins were also included in an assay where killing of *S. aureus* cells occurs via MPO-catalyzed generation of HOCl [19]. Only wild-type SPIN significantly inhibited MPO in this system, as judged by the nearly tenfold increase in survival of *S. aureus* cells when compared with GO-MPO alone. The small molecule, 4-aminobenzoic acid hydrazide (4-ABAH), was included as positive control for inhibition of MPO. Note that the SPIN$^{43-45 \rightarrow AAA}$ mutant behaved similarly to the SPIN$^{46-105}$ mutant in each assay. This demonstrated that simply having a full-length N-terminus is not enough to drive inhibition of MPO by SPIN.

IDENTIFICATION AND CHARACTERIZATION OF SPIN HOMOLOGS FROM OTHER STAPHYLOCOCCI

Whereas the *spn* gene was found to be highly conserved across human- and animal-derived *S. aureus* strains [19], the distribution of homologous *spn* genes throughout more distantly related species of staphylococci was unclear. To address this question, the SPIN protein sequence from *S. aureus* strain Newman was used to query the NCBI nonredundant protein database for any uncharacterized molecules with sequence identity great enough to suggest they might also function as MPO inhibitors. Eight proteins from various staphylococcal species pathogenic to humans, livestock, and/or domestic companion animals were identified from this search [26]. The putative secretion signal peptide cleavage site was determined for each protein using SignalP [42]. Thereafter, multiple sequence alignment of the matured sequences revealed that this cohort of uncharacterized proteins had amino acid identities with one another that ranged from a low of 29% to a high of 91% [26].

Phylogenetic analyses revealed multiple relationships among the sequences of these SPIN homologs [26] (Figure 18.5). For example, the SPIN proteins from *S. hyicus* and *S. agnetis* show approximately 85% identity with one another. This aligns with a previous report, which proposed an

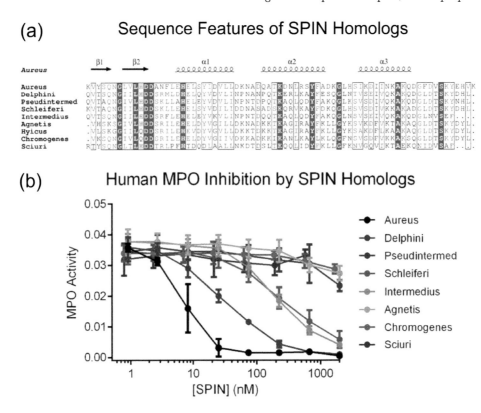

Figure 18.5 Sequence features of a panel of SPIN homologs and their inhibition of human MPO. (a) BLAST searching in the NCBI nonredundant protein database was used to identify uncharacterized proteins with homology to *S. aureus* SPIN [26]. The predicted matured forms of all proteins were aligned using Clustal Omega and are presented beneath the secondary structure elements of *S. aureus* SPIN in the MPO-bound form [19]. Invariant residues are shown as white letters inside blue fields, while residues found in a majority these sequences appear in magenta letters. Only 10 of the 73 residues comprising the matured form of *S. aureus* SPIN are invariant among these sequences. (b) Recombinant forms of various SPIN homologs were included in an assay for human MPO activity over a broad range of concentrations [26]. In addition to *S. aureus* SPIN, the homologs from *S. delphini*, *S. schleiferi*, and *S. intermedius* exhibited dose-dependent inhibition of human MPO. The remaining homologs failed to inhibit human MPO at the highest concentrations tested. This observation is in accordance with prior results, which suggest that the inhibitory activities of the SPIN protein are host restricted [19]. The y-axis represents the initial velocity of the chromogenic reaction.

evolutionary relationship between these two species [43]. Oppositely, SPIN from S. sciuri shows comparatively weaker conservation with other SPIN sequences at only 29%–39% identity. Again, this observation is in agreement with previous work, which suggested that S. sciuri represents a more distant evolutionary branch of these otherwise closely related bacteria [44,45]. Finally, the SPIN proteins from S. schleiferi and members of the Staphylococcus intermedius group (SIG), which includes S. intermedius, S. pseudintermedius, and S. delphini, share approximately 59% sequence identity with one another. These SPIN proteins are also noteworthy since they share the highest overall sequence identities with SPIN-aureus, ranging from 53% to 57%.

Despite their significant levels of sequence identity to S. aureus SPIN, it remained to be determined if any of these SPIN-like proteins could also bind MPO and inhibit its enzymatic activity. To that end, a synthetic coding sequence for the matured form of each SPIN homolog was produced and used to express and purify a recombinant form of the protein [26]. SPR was then used to examine the ability of each SPIN homolog to bind native human MPO that had been immobilized on the biosensor surface. Initial experiments revealed that several of these proteins exhibited dose-depending binding to native human MPO (as will be described below), but that SPINs from S. chromogenes, S. pseudintermedius, and S. sciuri failed to do so. These three proteins, along with SPIN from S. hyicus that was unstable and prone to degradation, were therefore excluded from further interaction analysis [26].

Full kinetic profiling of the interactions between immobilized human MPO and the SPINs from S. delphini, S. intermedius, S. schleiferi, and S. agnetis was carried out alongside S. aureus SPIN as a comparator. This allowed for determination of the association (k_a) and dissociation (k_d) rate constants, as well as the apparent equilibrium dissociation constant (K_D) for each interaction pair. While the K_D of 15.9 ± 2.1 nM for SPIN-aureus was in agreement with previous observations [19,38], the affinities of the other interactions were much more variable. Significantly, none of the homologs bound human MPO as strongly as did SPIN from S. aureus [26]. SPIN from S. agnetis displayed the next highest affinity with a K_D of 41.8 ± 1.1 nM, followed by the homologs from S. schleiferi, S. delphini, and S. intermedius at 230 ± 42.1, 310 ± 41.5, and 984 ± 274 nM, respectively. These values

corresponded to decreases in affinity for human MPO that ranged from 2.6- to 61.9-fold when compared with the S. aureus protein. Although the dissociation rate constants for the SPIN homologs were consistent as a group and ranged from $2.36 \pm 0.10 \times 10^{-3}$ to $3.34 \pm 0.17 \times 10^{-3}$ s^{-1}, the association rate constants were more variable. These values ranged from $20.10 \pm 2.22 \times 10^4$ M^{-1}s^{-1} for SPIN-aureus to $0.35 \pm 0.08 \times 10^{-4}$ M^{-1}s^{-1} for SPIN-intermedius. Consequently, the differences in affinity for human MPO among this cohort of SPIN homologs can be attributed primarily to variations in their respective association rate constants.

Previous studies on mutants of S. aureus SPIN showed that binding to MPO is necessary but not sufficient for inhibiting MPO enzymatic activity [38]. Select members from this panel of SPIN homologs were therefore examined in a colorimetric assay for MPO activity [26]. In line with previous observations [19,38], SPIN from S. aureus inhibited the peroxidase activity of human MPO with an IC$_{50}$ value very near its K_D for MPO (i.e. ~10 nM). Each of the homologs that failed to bind human MPO (i.e. SPIN-sciuri, SPIN-chromogenes, and SPIN-pseudintermedius) similarly failed to inhibit MPO activity. However, three SPIN variants, including those from S. delphini (IC$_{50}$ ~29.7 nM), S. intermedius (IC$_{50}$ ~222 nM), and S. schleiferi (IC$_{50}$ ~261 nM), inhibited the peroxidase activity of human MPO in a dose-dependent manner. Although the reason underlying the discrepancy between the observed equilibrium dissociation constant and half-inhibitory concentration for these SPIN homologs remains unclear, each of these proteins shows an ability to both bind and inhibit human MPO. The same cannot be said for the S. agnetis homolog, which did not inhibit human MPO even though it binds with a robust affinity (K_D ~41.8 nM). Indeed, the properties of SPIN from S. agnetis resembled the site-directed mutant, SPIN$^{43-45\rightarrow AAA}$, which also failed to inhibit MPO despite a near wild-type affinity [38]. Despite these differences in affinity for and potency against human MPO, a subset of these homologs clearly maintained the inhibitory activity first reported for the S. aureus SPIN protein. This strongly suggests that the ability to inhibit MPO activity is broadly distributed among this branch of staphylococci and not restricted to organisms such as S. aureus, which exhibit substantial preference for the human host.

STRUCTURE OF SPIN FROM *S. DELPHINI* BOUND TO RECOMBINANT HUMAN MPO PROVIDES A BASIS FOR COMPARATIVE STUDIES ON SPIN-CLASS MPO INHIBITORS

Considering the entire cohort of recently identified homologs, SPIN from *S. delphini* inhibited human MPO with an IC_{50} value second only to that of *S. aureus* SPIN. This suggested that further study of SPIN from *S. delphini* could not only define the conserved physical properties that manifest as inhibition of MPO but also help to identify features that lead to differences in structure/activity profiles among SPINs. To that end, SPIN from *S. delphini* was crystallized with rhMPO, and the

structure was solved at 2.4 Å limiting resolution and refined to R_{work}/R_{free} values of 18.5% and 21.8%, respectively [26] (Figure 18.6). Unlike the structure of *S. aureus* SPIN bound to rhMPO [19], the structure of this complex contained a covalently bound heme modeled at full occupancy within the rhMPO active site; this observation ruled out the possibility that binding of SPIN-class inhibitors to MPO might somehow promote loss of heme from the MPO active site and thereby inhibit MPO activity by displacing the essential heme cofactor. That difference aside, further comparison of the *S. delphini* SPIN/rhMPO complex with that of *S. aureus* SPIN/rhMPO revealed extensive similarities between the two structures.

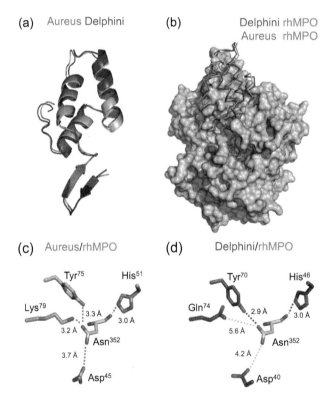

Figure 18.6 Structural characterization of SPIN from *S. delphini* bound to a recombinant form of human MPO. SPIN from *S. delphini* was crystallized bound to rhMPO and the structure was solved to 2.4 Å limiting resolution [26]. (a) Superposition of the SPIN proteins from *S. aureus* (orange) and *S. delphini* (purple), drawn as ribbon diagrams. The inhibitory N-terminal β-hairpin appears at the bottom of the image. (b) Superposition of the crystal structure of SPIN from *S. delphini* bound to rhMPO (PDB code 6BMT [26]) with that of *S. aureus* SPIN bound to rhMPO (PDB code 5UZU [19]). The SPIN proteins are drawn as Cα wires using the same coloring scheme as panel a. This illustrates the conserved positing of each SPIN inhibitor relative to rhMPO (olive surface). (c) *S. aureus* SPIN residues (carbon atoms colored orange) and the contacts formed with Asn³⁵² of rhMPO (carbon atoms colored olive). Likely polar interactions, along with their distances, are shown as orange dashed lines. (d) *S. delphini* SPIN residues (carbon atoms colored purple) and the contacts formed with Asn³⁵² of rhMPO. Likely polar interactions and distances are shown as purple dashed lines, while interactions that fail to form due to excessive distance are shown as gray dashed lines. These observations suggest that the decreased affinity of *S. delphini* SPIN for human MPO arises partly from local structural changes when compared with the *S. aureus* SPIN protein [26].

Not only did 539 of the corresponding Cα positions within each complex superimpose with an r.m.s.d. of 0.289 Å, 61 Cα positions from the two different SPIN molecules superimposed with an r.m.s.d. of 0.812 Å. In this regard, the only noteworthy regions of tertiary structural divergence between the S. delphini and S. aureus SPIN proteins were found in the extreme N- and C-termini of the respective polypeptides.

The SPIN protein from S. delphini shares 53% amino acid identity to its S. aureus counterpart but binds comparatively weakly to and is a less potent inhibitor of human MPO [26]. Consequently, the S. delphini SPIN/rhMPO complex was analyzed for any sequence-dependent differences in local structure features that could explain the partial impairment of its function [26]. The entire contact interface between S. delphini SPIN and rhMPO displayed a similar level of shape complementarity to the S. aureus SPIN complex, with s.c. coefficients of 0.715 and 0.704, respectively [46]. Restricting this analysis to the helical-bundle domains alone, however, revealed a far greater level of shape complementary for the S. aureus complex, with recalculated s.c. coefficients of 0.715 and 0.774, respectively. The difference in shape complementary between the two helical-bundle domains resulted in a lower overall buried surface area of 1,365 Å² for the S. delphini protein when compared with 1,633 Å² for S. aureus SPIN [19]. As shape complementarity and buried surface area provide reasonable benchmarks for the hydrophobic interactions that are a major determinant in driving binding affinities, the observations presented above suggest that the S. aureus SPIN protein is simply a better fit for human MPO than is S. delphini SPIN.

The sequence differences between the S. delphini and S. aureus SPIN proteins also changed the polar interactions they formed with rhMPO [26]. Whereas 14 residues from S. aureus SPIN formed one or more polar interactions with groups found on rhMPO, only 11 residues from S. delphini SPIN did the same. Further inspection showed that 7 of these 11 residues were conserved between these two SPINs and formed essentially identical interactions with rhMPO. Another conserved residue, Asp⁴⁵ in S. aureus and Asp⁴⁰ in S. delphini, was positioned too far in the structure of S. delphini SPIN bound to rhMPO to interact with the Asn³⁵² side chain derived from the enzyme (i.e. 3.7 Å versus 4.2 Å, respectively). Three other residues from S. delphini found at the interface with rhMPO (i.e. Gln²⁸, Thr³⁰, and Gln⁷⁴) constitute significant changes in side-chain properties with their corresponding positions in S. aureus SPIN (i.e. Lys³³, Tyr³⁵, and Lys⁷⁹), and thus fail to form equivalent polar interactions with rhMPO. Of these, only Gln⁷⁴ from S. delphini is part of the α-helical bundle domain that drives the initial interaction between SPIN and MPO [38]. Interestingly, the change from Lys⁷⁹ in S. aureus to Gln⁷⁴ in S. delphini prevents formation of a hydrogen bond with the Asn³⁵² side chain of rhMPO. This situation is reminiscent of the relationship between S. aureus Asp⁴⁵ and S. delphini Asp⁴⁰ described earlier in this paragraph, which also target the same Asn³⁵² sidechain or rhMPO [26]. Thus, the quantitative differences in function between the S. aureus and S. delphini SPIN proteins appear to arise from sequence-dependent changes in local structural features that influence both surface complementarity and the orientation of key functional groups at the inhibitor interface with human MPO.

CONCLUSION

Specific small-molecule inhibitors of MPO have been known for a decade and perhaps longer [36,47,48], yet the only proteinaceous inhibitor of MPO described prior to the identification of SPIN was plasma-resident ceruloplasmin [49–51]. The discovery of SPIN therefore provided the first evidence that inhibition of MPO activity by a pathogen-derived molecule could be advantageous in helping diminish a critical defense mechanism of the host [12,19]. While studies on SPIN as well as other staphylococcal innate immune evasion proteins that act within neutrophil phagosome have expanded understanding of the molecular basis of pathogenesis, SPIN also provides a unique tool for dissecting the structure/function relationships of a protein whose only known activity is inhibition of MPO in situ. Though much work remains to be done, comparative studies on S. aureus SPIN and its homologs have already identified conserved features that provide for high-affinity binding and inhibition of MPO. They have also provided a biologically relevant basis for defining quantitative structure/activity relationships of MPO inhibitors and a powerful means for defining the physical basis behind the host selectivity of virulence proteins. In many ways, the story of this novel MPO inhibitor is only beginning to be told, with many important insights certain to follow throughout the years ahead.

REFERENCES

1. P. Martin, 1997, Wound healing – Aiming for perfect skin regeneration, *Science* 276: 75–81.

2. A.J. Singer, R.A. Clark, 1999, Cutaneous wound healing, *N. Engl. J. Med.* 341: 738–746.

3. S. Frantz, K.A. Vincent, O. Feron, R.A. Kelly, 2005, Innate immunity and angiogenesis, *Circ. Res.* 96: 15–26.

4. B.L. Garcia, B.J. Summers, K.X. Ramyar, et al., 2013, A structurally dynamic N-terminal helix is a key functional determinant in staphylococcal complement inhibitor (SCIN) proteins, *J. Biol. Chem.* 288: 2870–2881.

5. B. Amulic, C. Cazalet, G.L. Hayes, K.D. Metzler, A. Zychlinsky, 2012, Neutrophil function: From mechanisms to disease, *Annu. Rev. Immunol.* 30: 459–489.

6. B. Korkmaz, M.S. Horwitz, D.E. Jenne, F. Gauthier, 2010, Neutrophil elastase, proteinase 3, and cathepsin G as therapeutic targets in human disease, *Pharmacol. Rev.* 62: 726–759.

7. C.T.N. Pham, 2006, Neutrophil Serine Proteases: Specific regulators of inflammation, *Nat. Rev. Immunol.* 6: 541–550.

8. J.D. Lambris, D. Ricklin, B.V. Geisbrecht, 2008, Complement evasion by human pathogens, *Nat. Rev. Microbiol.* 6: 132–142.

9. B.L. Garcia, S.A. Zwarthoff, S.H.M. Rooijakkers, B.V. Geisbrecht, 2016, Novel evasion mechanisms of the classical complement pathway, *J. Immunol.* 197: 2051–2060.

10. V. Thammavongsa, H.K. Kim, D. Missiakas, O. Schneewind, 2015, Staphylococcal manipulation of host immune responses, *Nat. Rev. Microbiol.* 13: 529–543.

11. A.N. Spaan, B.G.J. Surewaard, R. Nijland, J.A.G. van Strijp, 2013, Neutrophils versus *Staphylococcus aureus*: A biological tug of war, *Annu. Rev. Microbiol.* 67: 629–650.

12. N.W.M. de Jong, K.P.M. van Kessel, J.A.G. van Strijp, 2019, Immune evasion by *Staphylococcus aureus*, *Microbiol. Spectr.* 7: doi: 10.1128/microbiolspec.GPP3-0061-2019.

13. G.E. Thwaites, V. Gant, 2011, Are bloodstream leukocytes trojan horses for the metastasis of Staphylococcus aureus? *Pathogens* 9: 215–222.

14. S.J. Klebanoff, A.J. Kettle, H. Rosen, C.C. Winterbourn, W.M. Nauseef, 2013, Myeloperoxidase: A front-line defender against phagocytosed microorganisms, *J. Leukoc. Biol.* 93: 185–198.

15. W.M. Nauseef, 2007, How human neutrophils kills and degrade microbes: An integrated view, *Immunol. Rev.* 219: 88–102.

16. W.M. Nauseef, 2014, Myeloperoxidase in human neutrophil host defense, *Cell Microbiol.* 16: 1146–1155.

17. S.J. Klebanoff, C.B. Hamon, 1972, Role of myeloperoxidase-mediated antimicrobial systems in intact leukocytes, *J. Retic. Soc.* 12: 170–196.

18. C. Fevre, J. Bestebroer, M.M. Mebius, et al., 2014, *Staphylococcus aureus* proteins SSL6 and SEIX interact with neutrophil receptors as identified using secretome phage display, *Cell. Microbiol.* 16: 1646–1665.

19. N.W.M. de Jong, K.X. Ramyar, F.E. Guerra, et al., 2017, Immune evasion by a Staphylococal inhibitor of myeloperoxidase, *Proc. Natl. Acad. Sci. U.S.A.* 114: 9439–9444.

20. B.L. Garcia, K.X. Ramyar, D. Ricklin, J.D. Lambris, B.V. Geisbrecht, 2012, Advances in understanding the structure, function, and mechanism of the SCIN and Efb families of Staphylococcal immune evasion proteins, *Adv. Exp. Med. Biol.* 946: 113–133.

21. M. Hammel, G. Sfyroera, D. Ricklin, et al., 2007, A structural basis for complement inhibition by *Staphylococcus aureus*, *Nat. Immunol.* 8: 430–437.

22. M. Hammel, G. Sfyroera, S. Pyrpassopoulos, et al., 2007, Characterization of Ehp: A secreted complement inhibitory protein from *Staphylococcus aureus*, *J. Biol. Chem.* 202: 30051–30061.

23. S.H.M. Rooijakkers, F.J. Milder, B.W. Bardoel, et al., 2007, Staphylococcal complement inhibitor: Structure and active sites, *J. Immunol.* 179: 2989–2998.

24. B.L. Garcia, B.J. Summers, L. Zhuoer, et al., 2012, Diversity in the C3b contact residues and tertiary structures of the Staphylococcal Complement Inhibitor (SCIN) protein family, *J. Biol. Chem.* 287: 628–640.

25. T.J. Fiedler, C.A. Davey, R.E. Fenna, 2000, X-ray crystal structure and characterization of halide-binding sites of human myeloperoxidase at 1.8 A resolution, *J. Biol. Chem.* 275: 11964–11971.

26. N.T. Ploscariu, N.W.M. de Jong, K.P.M. van Kessel, J.A.G. van Strijp, B.V. Geisbrecht, 2018, Identification and structural characterization of a novel myeloperoxidase inhibitor from *Staphylococcus delphini*, *Arch. Biochem. Biophys.* 645: 1–11.

27. G.A. Denys, P. Grover, P. O'Hanley, J.T.J. Stephens, 2011, In vitro antibacterial activity of E-101 solution, a novel myeloperoxidase-mediated antimicrobial, against gram-positive and

gram-negative pathogens, J. Antimicrob. Chemother. 66: 335–342.

28. C. Li, F. Sun, H. Cho, et al., 2010, CcpA mediates proline auxotrophy and is required for Staphylococcus aureus pathogenesis, J. Bacteriol. 192: 3883–3892.

29. D.A.C. Stapels, K.X. Ramyar, M. Bischoff, et al., 2014, Staphylococcus aureus secretes a novel class of neutrophil-serine-protease inhibitors that promote bacterial infection, Proc. Natl. Acad. Sci. U.S.A. 111: 13187–13192.

30. S.H. Rooijakkers, M. Ruyken, A. Roos, et al., 2005, Immune evasion by a Staphylococcal complement inhibitor that acts on C3 convertases, Nat. Immunol. 6: 920–927.

31. I. Jongerius, J. Köhl, M.K. Pandey, et al., 2007, Staphylococcal complement evasion by various convertase-blocking molecules, J. Exp. Med. 204: 2461–2471.

32. N.W.M. de Jong, M. Vrieling, B.L. Garcia, et al., 2018, Identification of a Staphylococcal complement inhibitor with broad host specificity in equid Staphylococcus aureus strains, J. Biol. Chem. 293: 4468–4477.

33. A.N. Spaan, J.A.G. van Strijp, V.J. Torres, 2017, Leukocidins: Staphylococcal bi-component pore-forming toxins find their receptors, Nat. Rev. Microbiol. 15: 435–447.

34. A.N. Spaan, T. Henry, W.J.M. van Rooijen, et al., 2013, The Staphylococcal toxin paton-valentin leukocidin targets human C5a receptors, Cell Host Microbe 13: 584–594.

35. H. van de Velde, 1894, Etude sur le mécanisme de la virulence du staphylocoque pyogène, La Cellule 10: 403–460.

36. H. Bjornsdottir, A. Welin, E. Michaelsson, et al., 2015, Neutrophil NET formation is regulated from the inside by myeloperoxidase-processed reactive oxygen species, Free Radic. Biol. Med. 89: 1024–1035.

37. C.C. Winterbourn, M.B. Hampton, J.H. Livesey, A.J. Kettle, 2006, Modeling the reactions of superoxide and myeloperoxidase in the neutrophil phagosome, J. Biol. Chem. 281: 39860–39869.

38. N.W.M. de Jong, N.T. Ploscariu, K.X. Ramyar, et al., 2018, A structurally dynamic N-terminal region drives function of the Staphylococcal Peroxidase Inhibitor (SPIN), J. Biol. Chem. 293: 2260–2271.

39. N.T. Ploscariu, A.I. Herrera, S. Jayanthi, et al., 2017, Backbone and side-chain ^{1}H, ^{15}N, and ^{13}C resonance assignments of a novel Staphylococcal inhibitor of myeloperoxidase, Biomol. NMR Assign. 11: 285–288.

40. D.S. Wishart, B.D. Sykes, F.M. Richards, 1991, Relationship between nuclear magnetic resonance chemical shift and protein secondary structure, J. Mol. Biol. 222: 311–333.

41. J. Schwartz, K.G. Leidal, J.K. Femling, J.P. Weiss, W.M. Nauseef, 2009, Neutrophil bleaching of GFP-expressing Staphylococci: Probing the intraphagosomal fate of individual bacteria, J. Immunol. 183: 2632–2641.

42. H. Nielsen, 2017, Predicting secretory proteins with SignalP, in: D. Kihara (Ed.), Protein Function Prediction (Methods in Molecular Biology, vol. 1611), pp. 59–73. Springer.

43. S.K. Taponen, K. Supre, V. Piessens, et al., 2012, Staphylococcus agnetis sp. nov., a coagulase-variable species from bovine subclinical and mild clinical mastitis, Int. J. Syst. Evol. Microbiol. 62: 61–65.

44. W.E. Kloos, K.H. Schleifer, R.F. Smith, 1976, Characterization of Staphylococcus sciuri sp. nov. and its subspecies, Int. J. Syst. Bact. 26: 22–37.

45. S. Stepanovic, I. Dakic, D. Morrison, et al., 2005, Identification and characterization of clinical isolates of members of the Staphylococcus sciuri group, J. Clin. Microbiol. 43: 956–958.

46. M.C. Lawrence, P.M. Colman, 1993, Shape complementarity at protein/protein interfaces, J. Mol. Biol. 234: 946–950.

47. L.V. Forbes, T. Sjogren, F. Auchere, et al., 2013, Potent reversible inhibition of myeloperoxidase by aromatic hydroxamates, J. Biol. Chem. 288: 36636–36647.

48. A.K. Tiden, T. Sjogren, M. Svensson, et al., 2011, 2-Thioxanthines are mechanism-based inactivators of myeloperoxidase that block oxidative stress during inflammation, J. Biol. Chem. 286: 37578–37589.

49. A.L. Chapman, T.J. Mocatta, S. Shiva, et al., 2013, Ceruloplasmin is an endogenous inhibitor of myeloperoxidase, J. Biol. Chem. 288: 6465–6477.

50. M. Segelmark, B. Persson, T. Hellmark, J. Wieslander, 1997, Binding and inhibition of myeloperoxidase (MPO): A major function of ceruloplasmin? Clin. Exp. Immunol. 108: 167–174.

51. V.R. Samygina, A.V. Sokolov, G. Bourenkov, et al., 2013, Ceruloplasmin: Macromolecular assemblies with iron-containing acute phase proteins, PLoS One 8: e67145.

52. Y. Shen, A. Bax, 2013, Protein backbone and sidechain torsion angles predicted from NMR chemical shifts using artificial neural networks, J. Biomol. NMR 56: 227–241.

INDEX

thyroid peroxidase (TPO) 6, 8, 26
    biological functions of 54–55
    iodinated lipids 108
    substrate specificities of 56
tissue biogenesis 122
tissue fibrosis 295–297
triple-helical collagen IV protomers 46
triploblastic *Bilateralia* 47
type IV collagen 45, 46

unilateral ureteral obstruction (UUO) 296
uracil DNA glycosylase (UDG) 89

vascular cell adhesion molecule 1 (VCAM-1) 229
vertebrate clade, peroxidase domain 5
von Willebrand factor C domain (vWFC) 42

Weibel–Palade body mobilization 102
wire hang method 264
Wolff–Chaikoff effect 107

X-ray crystal structure 22

zebrafish 48
zymosan exposure 157

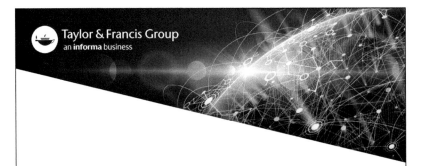